The Nursing Process in Orthopaedics

The Nursing Process in Orthopaedics

Delores C. Schoen, R.N., Ph.D.
Nursing Faculty
Parkland College
Champaign, Illinois

ACC APPLETON-CENTURY-CROFTS/Norwalk, Connecticut

0-8385-7043-7

Notice: The author(s) and publisher of this volume have taken care that the information and recommendations contained herein are accurate and compatible with the standards generally accepted at the time of publication.

86 87 88 89 90 / 10 9 8 7 6 5 4 3 2 1

Prentice-Hall of Australia, Pty. Ltd., Sydney
Prentice-Hall Canada, Inc.
Prentice-Hall Hispanoamericana, S.A., Mexico
Prentice-Hall of India Private Limited, New Delhi
Prentice-Hall International (UK) Limited, London
Prentice-Hall of Japan, Inc., Tokyo
Prentice-Hall of Southeast Asia (Pte.) Ltd., Singapore
Whitehall Books Ltd., Wellington, New Zealand
Editora Prentice-Hall do Brazil Ltda., Rio de Janeiro

Library of Congress Cataloging-in-Publication Data
Schoen, Delores Christina Harmon, 1938–
The nursing process in orthopaedics.

Includes index.
1. Orthopedic nursing. I. Title. [DNLM: 1. Nursing Process. 2. Orthopedics—nursing. WY 157.6 S356n]
RD753.S36 1986 617'.3 86-7991
ISBN 0-8385-7043-7

Design: Jean Sabato-Morley
Cover: M. Chandler Martylewski

PRINTED IN THE UNITED STATES OF AMERICA

CONTENTS

PREFACE

This book is designed to meet the needs of nurses by presenting care for the adult orthopaedic patient. It views the modern nurse as an autonomous member of the health team, and the patient as the subject, rather than the object of nursing care. The book is based on the nursing process model, which recognizes the new and expanded role of the nurse by focusing on assessment, nursing diagnosis, goal formulation, planning, intervention, evaluation, and reassessment. Chapter 1 introduces the reader to the nursing process and to the four major areas of orthopaedic nursing concern: (1) alleviating pain, (2) increasing mobility, (3) preventing complications, and (4) providing patient teaching. Together they are used throughout the book to organize the material in a way that I hope will be both meaningful and easy to understand.

Chapter 2 focuses on assessment, as it is the basis of all nursing care and has usually not been given the in-depth treatment it deserves. Chapters 3 and 4 examine trauma and pathology, the basic categories into which adult orthopaedic conditions fall. Chapters 5 through 11 examine orthopaedic conditions for each anatomical region of the body, and Chapter 12 concludes with a brief overview of the rapidly growing and changing field of orthopaedics. To provide technical details on the most important and widely used procedures, three appendices discuss traction, casts, and crutch and cane walking.

Four special features should be noted. First, this book is unique in its use of the nursing process approach in orthopaedics. Second, for quick reference, tables are provided that highlight the application of the nursing process to the care of the major traumatic and pathological conditions affecting each region of the body. Third, Chapters 5 through 11 are self-contained in that they present a review of the anatomy of that part of the body and of the most common traumatic and pathological conditions that are encountered. Fourth, Chapters 8 through 11 provide extensive discussions of the ankle and foot, the shoulder and upper arm, the elbow and lower arm, and the wrist and hand, areas that have largely been ignored by most orthopaedic nursing books.

This book can be used as a basic orthopaedic text. Because most undergraduate nursing programs only require a medical- surgical nursing text, it can serve as a supplementary text. At the graduate level, it can be a basic text for nurses specializing in orthopaedics. The book is also intended to be useful in continuing education programs for nurses, to staff nurses already working in orthopaedics, and to nurses orienting to orthopaedics.

ACKNOWLEDGMENTS

I would like to express my appreciation to all of my past students, faculty and clinical colleagues, and patients whose questions and suggestions have influenced the content of the book and motivated me to write it. I would also like to thank the reviewers whose comments helped to improve the book.

My greatest debt is to my husband, Robert Schoen, for his encouragement, support, and constructively critical reading of the manuscript. his help was invaluable.

1

INTRODUCTION

Modern medicine and health care delivery have greatly changed the role of the nurse. Staff nurses are becoming more autonomous in applying nursing theory and skills to assess patient needs and provide nursing care. To meet those new demands, nursing has adopted the nursing process model. That approach recognizes the new role of the nurse by incorporating the assessment of the patient, the formulation of a nursing diagnosis, the formulation of patient-centered goals, the planning of nursing care, the implementation of nursing interventions, the evaluation of the outcomes of care, and the reassessment of nursing care based on that evaluation.

This chapter presents a brief historical view of orthopaedics, a discussion of the major principles underlying orthopaedic nursing, and a definition and description of the seven steps in the nursing process. It concludes by identifying the four major areas of concern confronting orthopaedic nurses, which are alleviating pain, increasing patient mobility, preventing complications, and providing patient teaching.

THE FIELD OF ORTHOPAEDIC NURSING

Orthopaedics is derived from two Greek words, "orthos" meaning straight and "paidos" meaning child. It was introduced in 1741 by Nicholas Andre in a two-volume work entitled *Orthopaedia, or The Art of Correcting and Preventing Deformities in Children.* The first Orthopaedic Institute was founded in Switzerland in 1780.

For many years, orthopaedic practitioners were known as "strap-and-buckle" doctors, because of the appliances they used to straighten body and limbs. In Liverpool, Hugh Owen Thomas (1834–1891) became known for his ability to set broken bones and reduce dislocated joints. A number of appliances in use today, including the Thomas splint, bear his name. His nephew, Sir Robert Jones (1857–1933), was an orthopaedic surgeon who helped to establish orthopaedic surgery as a speciality. In the United States, orthopaedic surgery was pioneered by Dr. Virgil P. Gibney, Surgeon-in-Chief of the New York Hospital for the Ruptured and Crippled, and in 1887 the American Orthopaedic Association was founded as a professional society for orthopaedic surgeons (Larson & Gould, 1978, p.1).

Relatively little is known about the pioneers of orthopaedic nursing, but one name, Agnes Hunt (1862–1948), stands out. Known as the "Florence Nightingale" of orthopaedic nursing, she suffered an orthopaedic deformity in childhood, but went on to open the "Baschurch Home" in Oswestry, England in 1900. From modest beginnings, the home grew into a large orthopaedic hospital with a school for training orthopaedic nurses.

The first professional association of orthopaedic nurses in the United States, the Orthopedic Nurses' Association (ONA), was not established until 1972. The ONA later dissolved and was succeeded in 1980 by the National Association of Orthopaedic Nurses (NAON). NAON seeks to meet the professional needs of orthopaedic nurses by promoting high standards of practice, encouraging continuing education, and furthering research in orthopaedic nursing.

Standards of Orthopaedic Nursing Practice have been established by the Orthopedic Nurses' Association and the American Nurses' Association Division on Medical–Surgical Practice (ONA & ANA, 1975). Orthopaedic nursing practice was defined as the nursing care of individuals with known and/or predicted neuromusculoskeletal alterations. Orthopaedic nursing takes into account related physiological, social, and behavioral problems resulting from or affecting the individual's response and adjustment to the neuromusculoskeletal alterations. The scope of orthopaedic nursing encompasses those activities that assist individuals to modify their life-styles and environments so that they can attain the optimum neuromusculoskeletal function compatiable with their life goals. Modern orthopaedic nursing has moved well beyond dealing with broken or malformed bones. It has grown rapidly as technological innovations have expanded the field of orthopaedics, and today is one of the most demanding and challenging fields of nursing practice.

THE MAJOR PRINCIPLES UNDERLYING ORTHOPAEDIC NURSING CARE

Four important principles that underly orthopaedic nursing care are (1) standards of practice, (2) the philosophy of rehabilitation, (3) health teaching, and (4) the interrelations between the musculoskeletal system and the rest of the body.

Standards of Practice

Standards of Practice are objective criteria, established by the profession, by which the quality of nursing practice can be measured. Since 1973, the American Nurses' Association (ANA) Congress for Nursing Practice and the several Divisions on Practice (Medical–Surgical, Gerontological, Maternal–Child, Psychiatric–Mental Health, and Community Health) have published materials setting forth the baselines of acceptable practice, the rationales for the establishment of those standards, and the specific critieria by which practice in any setting can be evaluated to determine whether the Standards are being met. In 1975, the Orthopedic Nurses' Association in collaboration with the ANA Division on Medical–Surgical Nursing Practice developed the Standards of Orthopedic Nursing Practice.

The Standards emphasize the nursing process as the means by which nursing care should be delivered. Although the setting in which care is provided and the observable outcomes of care are considered, the focus of the Standards is on evaluating the implementation of the nursing process. The Standards (ONA & ANA, 1975, p. 3) state that to implement the nursing process effectively, orthopaedic nurses should (1) base nursing practice on principles and theories of biophysical and behavioral sciences; (2) continuously update knowledge and skills, applying new knowledge generated by research, changes in health care delivery systems, and changes in social profiles; (3) determine the range of practice by considering the patient's needs, the nurse's competence, the setting for care, and the resources available; and (4) insure patient and family participation in health promotion, maintenance, and restoration. The Standards explicitly recognize that ongoing revisions of their contents will be necessary to reflect changes in the scope of practice and the extent of knowledge. Soon to be released are Standards that have been revised by the National Association of Orthopaedic Nurses (NAON) and ANA.

Philosophy of Rehabilitation

In the words of the National Council on Rehabilitation (Stryker, 1972, p. 11), rehabilitation is the "restoration of the individual to the fullest physical, mental, social, vocational, and economic capacity of which he is capable." Broadly speaking, rehabilitation seeks to prevent further disability, to maintain the patient's remaining abilities, and to restore lost functions. It is a dynamic process that begins with the onset of a disabling injury or disease and continues throughout its presence.

A disabling injury or disease may be one of the three major types: temporary, permanent, and progressive (Sakalys, 1971, p. 272). A temporary disability is typically one of short duration, with rapid improvement and ultimate removal of all etiological factors, for example, recovery from a simple fracture. In a permanent disability, the individual never fully regains premorbid levels of function, as in the case of an amputation following trauma. A progressive disability is a nontemporary affliction that produces a fast or slow, but continuing and irreversible loss of function. As is the case in rheumatoid arthritis, there may be periods of both exacerbation and remission.

No matter which type of disabling injury or disease, the patient will go through a period of adjustment and even grieving. The psychological stages the patient goes through in adapting to a disability are closely related to those described in the literature on death and dying. Five stages are usually identified: psychological shock, denial, depression, anxiety, and acceptance. The stages are mixed, there may be progression and regression, and the length in any stage may vary from days to months and even years. Only by carefully observing the patient's behavior can the nurse determine the stage the patient is in and help the patient through to final acceptance.

A number of factors can affect the impact of a disability and how a person will respond and move through the five stages of adjustment. Significant personal characteristics include (1) age and sex, (2) marital/family status, (3) occupation, (4) educational level, and (5) personality before the disability. Significant characteristics of the disability include (1) suddenness of onset, (2) severity and prognosis, and (3) degree of physical dependency. Important environmental factors include (1) the degree of family and community support available and (2) the financial resources available (Stryker, 1972, pp. 15–18). The role of the patient's family and significant others is often crucial. They, like the nurse, should adopt the philosophy that "It is never how high one rises that determines one's merit, but rather how far one has come, considering his difficulties" (Brunner & Suddarth, 1980, p. 179).

Health Teaching

Teaching is a special kind of communication that produces learning. Teaching should take into account the perceptions, feelings, and specific needs of the learner, and should respond to feedback. Learning is the development of new behavior patterns as a result of acquiring new knowledge, skills, or attitudes. Learning is active, not passive, and requires the full participation of the learner. It is through the teaching–learning process that the nurse assists patients in acquiring behaviors necessary to their ability to meet their own health needs. Although adults are certainly not a homogeneous group, there are four basic principles of adult learning that are broadly applicable (Kidd, 1973). These are (1) adult learners see themselves as responsible, self-directing, capable individuals who will resent being treated like children; (2) adults have accumulated a great many experiences on which to base new learning, but some of those experiences may interfere with new learning; (3) adults are interested in learning what is relevant to them "here and now"; and (4) teachers of adult learners should relate to them as individuals with individual needs.

Health teaching is an integral part of health care and it is the responsibility of all nurses, individually and collectively, to provide relevant, effective, and consistent health education to the patient, and to the patient's family or significant others. Health teaching requires a well-developed plan that includes (1) an assessment of the patient's needs and readiness for health education, (2) a diagnosis of why and in what areas the patient is deficient in knowledge, (3) a formulation of the short- and long-term educational goals, (4) planning to properly present the material to the patient, (5) intervention in carrying out the presentation, (6) an evaluation of the effectiveness of the presentation by such means as written or verbal responses or a return demonstration, and (7) a reassessment to renew the effort if the goals are not met. In other words, the nursing process, which will be discussed in detail in the next section, is central to health teaching as it is to all other aspects of nursing care.

Interrelations Between the Musculoskeletal System and the Rest of the Body

The musculoskeletal system is composed of bones, muscle, cartilage, joints, ligaments, tendons, fascia, and bursa, organized into a complex system that protects the body, gives it shape and structural framework, and provides its ability to move. The muscle mass accounts for approximately half of normal body weight, and the body structures and connective tissue add an additional 25 percent. Thus, the musculoskeletal system collectively constitutes the largest organ system in the body.

There are 206 bones in the human body. They can be divided into four categories: long bones (i.e., the humerus), short bones (i.e., the tarsals), flat bones (i.e., the sternum), and irregular bones (i.e., the vertebrae). More than 99 percent of total body calcium and a substantial portion of body phosphorous are present in bones, which serve as the main storage place for these minerals. Bone also works as a chemical buffer to prevent rapid changes in hydrogen ion concentrations in body fluids. After birth, the red bone marrow is the only tissue capable of red blood cell formation, and the yellow bone marrow produces some white blood cells. Muscles serve as a repository for glycogen, the body's stored energy.

Bones as living tissue have the characteristics of all living material, including respiration, nutrition, excretion, reproduction, and response to stimulation. Respiration for bone cells is the taking in of oxygen and the giving off of carbon dioxide. Nutrition in the form of protein, fat, carbohydrates, water, mineral salts, and vitamins must reach bone cells in a steady supply in order that growth, replacement of worn cells, and other activities can occur. Excretion of by-products of metabolism, such as excess water, carbon dioxide, lactic acid, and urea, occurs continuously. Reproduction in the adult skeleton is the steady process of cell division and production of new bone cells to replace worn out cells. The skeletal system responds to stimulation or stress by improving its strength and by repairing itself when broken or damaged.

Because the musculoskeletal system serves to support the other systems of the body, a disabling injury or illness to the musculoskeletal system can greatly affect other systems of the body. In particular, immobility has serious and far reaching consequences. With regard to the cardiovascular system, it can lead to orthostatic hypotension, increased workload on the heart, and thrombus formation. The respiratory system may be affected by decreased respiratory movement, decreased movement of secretions, and disturbed oxygen–carbon dioxide balance. The gastrointestinal system may encounter dysfunctions in ingestion, digestion, and elimination, which can result in a stress ulcer, a paralytic ileus, or constipation. In the urinary system, there may be difficulty in urine formation, urinary tract stones, and difficulty in micturation. The psychosocial effects can also be severe, as boredom, loss of morale, loss of independence, and negative self-image take their toll (Olson et al., 1967).

THE NURSING PROCESS

The nursing process is a problem-solving approach, a systematic method for organizing nursing care. Although several variations of the nursing process have been used, this book follows the version used in the American Nurses' Association Standards of Nursing Practice (ANA, 1973). Accordingly, the nursing process involves the steps of assessment, nursing diagnosis, goal formulation, planning, intervention, evaluation, and reassessment. Each step is a necessary one, and the order in which those steps are taken is important. Even in crisis situations, when nurses will rarely consciously articulate each step in the nursing process, professional standards require that the nursing process underly the actions taken.

Assessment

The assessment step of the nursing process involves the collection of information relevant to the patient's health status. The necessary data are obtained in several ways. The most direct is by interviewing, observing, and examining the patient. Other methods include available records, including the results of diagnostic tests, and information provided by family, significant others, and other health care providers. The data are usually classified into two categories: subjective and objective. Subjective data cannot be observed or measured, and can only be obtained directly or indirectly from the patient. For example, only patients can say whether they are in pain, nauseous, or dizzy. On the other hand, objective data are observable and measurable by others. When an individual who has had a total hip replacement complains of severe pain in the hip following a turn to the unaffected side, subjective information is being given. The nurse cannot measure or observe the pain, but the nurse can objectively observe and measure whether the affected leg is shorter, internally rotated, or adducted.

The nursing history is the part of the assessment that assembles information about the patient's past and present health status. The nursing history, as distinct from the medical history, focuses on the meaning of illness and health care to the patient, instead of on the pathology (Murray et al., 1980, p. 20). The nursing history frequently includes information on the patients' (1) previous experience with illness and hospitalization, (2) understanding of their health problems and treatments, (3) educational level and ability to learn, (4) ability to communicate, (5) occupation, (6) usual behavioral patterns (e.g., diet, exercise routines, religious observances, hours of sleep, personal hygiene practices, recreational activities), (7) ability to deal with stress, and (8) significant others who might provide support (Bower, 1972).

At first, one might think that conducting a lengthy assessment, which includes a nursing history, is too time consuming and impractical. On the contrary, the nurse–patient relationship is begun during the assessment, which should convey the nurse's interest and concern, and the effort helps to establish a sense of mutual trust. During the first contact with the patient, family, or significant other, the initial or "first-level" assessment may focus on determining the perceived health threat, the patient's adjustment to the threat, and the information needed for immediate nursing actions. In some instances, depending on the health status of the patient, this assessment is very brief. The ongoing or "second-level" assessment is the assessment that continues throughout the time the nurse is in contact with the patient. The patient needs time to build a relationship of trust with the nurse before a complete nursing history can be taken, and changes in the patient's condition must be continually observed. Assessment, no matter how thorough, is never complete because the patient and the patient's environment are constantly changing. Thus nursing assessment is a continual process of collection and reassessment.

Nursing Diagnosis

Once the data have been collected in the assessment step, they need to be analyzed and interpreted so that explicit statements about the patient's health can be made. A diagnosis is "a careful examination and analysis of the facts in an attempt to understand or explain something" (Webster's Dictionary, 1978, p. 388). Accordingly, nursing diagnosis involves the identification of existing or potential threats to the patient's health.

Although nurses have been making judgments about existing or potential health problems for many years, it is important to distinguish between nursing diagnoses and medical diagnoses. A key distinction, as pointed out by Murchison and Nichols (1970, p. 97), is that different courses of action are open to each professional after the decision from the observation is made. Some nurses have a more restricted view of a nursing diagnosis. Gordon (1976, p. 1299) reserves the term for problems "which nurses by virtue of their education and experience are capable and licensed to treat." In this text the broader view of the term is seen as more appropriate, although in most instances the text's focus on nursing care limits its coverage to the narrower sense.

The nurse should state the nursing diagnosis in a sufficiently precise way so that goals can be established, nursing interventions planned, and the underlying problem identified. For example, a nursing diagnosis of "skin breakdown" is not specific enough. A more complete nursing diagnosis, which specifically states what, where, and why, would be "sacral decubitus related to immobility."

Goal Formulation

After assessment and diagnosis, various nursing actions need to be considered to develop a plan of care for promoting, maintaining, and restoring the patient's health. Based on the collected and analyzed data, the goal formulation phase establishes patient-centered goals, which describe the observable outcomes that the nurse, in consultation with the patient and the patient's significant others, considers desirable and attainable outcomes. Both immediate or short-term goals and long-term goals are usually identified. Short-term goals can be accomplished in a short span of time, whereas long-term goals state the ultimate desired result of nursing intervention.

Planning

After goals have been formulated, they must be placed in priority order, based on the severity of existing or potential threats to the patient's health. With the goals established and the priorities set, specific ways to meet those objectives are set forth, identifying (1) what is to be done, (2) how it is to be done, (3) when it is to be done, (4) where it is to be done, and (5) who is to do it. Thus the planning step prescribes the nursing actions necessary to achieve the formulated goals.

Intervention

Nursing intervention is the action step of the nursing process, when the nurse implements the plans of the preceding step. Interventions include all therapeutic actions taken by the nurse on behalf of the patient; including nursing procedures; measures for patient comfort; teaching, counseling, and purposeful socializing; and coordinating or collaborating with other health team members. Whenever possible, the patient and the patient's significant others should be encouraged to take an active part in the intervention, and the rationale for the measure should be explained. Every nursing intervention must be properly authorized. In areas where independent nursing action is permitted, nurses can act on the basis of their own professional abilities. In other areas, the nurse must work in conjunction with the physician, or on the basis of standing medical orders.

Evaluation

The evaluation compares the post intervention health status of the patient with the observable outcomes specified in the goals. The patient, the patient's family, and significant members of the health team should contribute to the evaluation, and they should be kept informed of the progress toward goal achievement.

Reassessment

Reassessment serves to reorient and renew the nursing process when the evaluation indicates that the patient is not making satisfactory progress toward goal attainment or new data on the health status of the patient becomes available.

The nursing process is thus a continuing and dynamic one, which typically is repeated in its entirety many times in the course of caring for a patient.

MAJOR AREAS OF NURSING CONCERN

The four major areas of concern confronting orthopaedic nurses are alleviating the patient's pain, increasing patient mobility, preventing complications, and providing patient teaching. The orthopaedic patient may have soft tissue, muscle, nerve, or bone pain due to trauma, surgery, or a disease process. The type and degree of pain vary greatly, and a wide variety of nursing measures must be utilized.

Orthopaedic patients frequently have greatly decreased mobility, whether it be in their ability to walk and bear weight, move their arms to care for themselves, or have the spinal flexibility to work and earn a living. The role of the nurse is to help the patient regain mobility through positioning, turning, exercising, ambulating, and dealing with the activities of daily living.

Preventing complications includes averting problems due to surgery, trauma, disease, or immobility. Those potential problems involve not only the musculoskeletal system, but all other systems of the body.

Patient teaching strives to increase the patient's knowledge of the disease or injury, the methods of care, and the rehabilitation process to help reduce the patient's anxiety and enable the patient to become an active participant in the recovery efforts. The teaching plan includes the patient, family, and significant others and focuses on care in the hospital setting, at-home care, and ways to prevent the occurrence of future injuries.

REFERENCES

American Nurses' Association Congress for Nursing Practice. *Standards of nursing practice.* Kansas City, Mo.: American Nurses' Association, 1973.

Bower, F. *The process of planning nursing care; A theoretical model.* St. Louis: C. V. Mosby, 1972.

Brunner, L. S., & Suddarth, D. S. *Medical–surgical nursing* (4th ed.). Philadelphia: Lippincott, 1980.

Gordon, M. Nursing diagnoses and the diagnostic process. *American Journal of Nursing,* 1976, *76* (8), 1298–1300.

Kidd, J. R. *How adults learn.* New York: Association Press, 1973.

Larson, C. B., & Gould, M. *Orthopedic nursing* (9th ed.). St. Louis: C. V. Mosby, 1978.

Murchison, I., & Nichols, T. *Legal foundations of nursing practice.* New York: Macmillan, 1970.

Murray, R., Huelskoette, M. M., & O'Driscoll, D. *The nursing process in later maturity.* Englewood Cliffs, N.J.: Prentice-Hall, 1980.

Olson, E. V. (Ed.). The hazards of immobility. *American Journal of Nursing,* 1967, *67* (4), 779–797.

Orthopedic Nurses' Association and American Nurses' Association Division on Medical–

Surgical Nursing Practice. *Standards of orthopedic nursing practice.* Kansas City, Mo.: American Nurses' Association. 1975.

Sakalys, J. A. Stages of adaptation to illness and disability: A psychosocial view. In M. Duffy et al. (Eds.), *Current concepts in clinical nursing.* St. Louis: C. V. Mosby, 1971.

Stryker, R. P. *Rehabilitative aspects of acute and chronic nursing care.* Philadelphia: Saunders, 1972.

Webster's new world dictionary of the American language (2nd college ed.). Cleveland, Ohio: William Collins, World Publishing, 1978.

BIBLIOGRAPHY

Atkinson, L. D., & Murray, M. E. *Understanding the nursing process.* New York: Macmillan, 1980.

Carpenito, L. J. *Nursing diagnosis: Application to clinical practice.* Philadelphia: Lippincott, 1983.

Christopherson, V., Coulter, P., & Wolamin, M. *Rehabilitation nursing: Perspectives and applications.* New York: McGraw-Hill, 1974.

Coken, M. M. *Interactions for patients.* New York: Appleton-Century-Crofts, 1979.

Dossey, B., & Guzzetta, C. E. Nursing diagnosis. *Nursing 81,* 1981, *11* (6), 34–38.

Fadden, T. C., & Seiser, G. K. Nursing diagnosis: A matter of form. *American Journal of Nursing,* 1984, *84* (4), 470–472.

Francis, G. M., & Munjas, B. *Promoting psychological comfort* (3rd ed.). Dubuque, Iowa: Wm. C. Brown, 1979.

Gordon, M., Sweeney, M. A., & McKeehan, K. Nursing diagnosis: Looking at its use in the area. *American Journal of Nursing,* 1980, *80* (4), 672–676.

Gordon, M. *Nursing diagnosis: Process and application.* New York: McGraw-Hill, 1982.

Harris, R. B. A strong vote for nursing process. *American Journal of Nursing,* 1979, *79* (10), 1999.

Hirschberg, G. G., Lewis, L., & Vaughan, P. *Rehabilitation: A manual for the care of the disabled and elderly* (2nd ed.). Philadelphia: Lippincott, 1976.

Jones-Walton, P. Orthopaedic health promotion: Injury and disability prevention. *Orthopaedic Nursing,* 1984, *3* (6), 35–42.

Lunney, M. Nursing diagnosis: Refining the system. *American Journal of Nursing,* 1982, *82* (3), 456–459.

McCormick, R-M. D., & Gilson-Parkevich, T. (Eds.). *Patient and family education: Tools, techniques, and theory.* New York: Wiley, 1979.

Moss, R. H. *Coping with physical illness.* New York: Plenum, 1977.

Murray, R. B., & Zentor, J. P. *Nursing concepts for health promotion* (2nd ed.). Englewood Cliffs, N.J.: Prentice-Hall, 1979.

Neuman, M. A. Nursing diagnosis: Looking at the whole. *American Journal of Nursing,* 1984, *84* (12) 1496–1499.

O'Sullivan, S. B., Cullen, K. E., & Schmitz, T. J. *Physical rehabilitation: Evaluation and treatment procedures.* Philadelphia: F. A. Davis, 1981.

Pohl, M. L. *The teaching function of the nursing practitioner.* Dubuque, Iowa: Wm. C. Brown, 1981.

Price, M. R. Nursing diagnosis: Making a concept come alive. *American Journal of Nursing,* 1980, *80* (4), 668–671.

Shoemaker, J. How nursing diagnosis helps focus your care. *RN,* 1979, *42* (8) 56–61.

Shontz, F. C. *The psychological aspects of physical illness and disability.* New York: Macmillan, 1975.

Smitherman, C. *Nursing actions for health promotion.* Philadelphia: F. A. Davis, 1981.

Stevens, C. B. *Special needs of long-term patients.* Philadelphia: Lippincott, 1974.

Stryker, R. P. *Rehabilitative aspects of acute and chronic nursing care.* Philadelphia: Saunders, 1972.

Tucker, S. M., Breeding, M. A., Canobbio, M. M., et al., *Patient care standards* (3rd ed.). St. Louis: C. V. Mosby, 1984.

Walsh, A. *The expanded role of the rehabilitation nurse.* Thorofare, N. J.: Charles B. Slack, 1980.

Werner-Beland, J. A. *Grief responses to long-term illness and disability: Manifestations and nursing interventions.* Reston, Va.: Reston, 1980.

Yura, H. & Walsh, M. B. *Human needs 2 and the nursing process.* Norwalk, Conn.: Appleton-Century-Crofts, 1982.

Yura, H. & Walsh, M. B. *The nursing process: Assessing, planning, implementing, evaluating* (4th ed.). Norwalk, Conn.: Appleton-Century-Crofts, 1983.

2

MUSCULOSKELETAL ASSESSMENT

Assessment is the first step in the nursing process, and thus influences all phases of nursing practice. Even before the nursing process was articulated, nurses were expected to assess patients, but the recognition of assessment as a nursing skill and a nursing responsibility was not stressed or even widely accepted.

The muscoloskeletal system is very complex and is usually evaluated in conjunction with other systems. This chapter concentrates on the musculoskeletal system alone. In discussing musculoskeletal assessment, history taking is simply defined, diagnostic procedures are discussed briefly, and the emphasis is placed on the physical examination of the patient.

An assessment of the musculoskeletal system is directed toward both function and structure, primarily by inspection, palpation, determination of active range of motion, and the assessment of muscle strength against resistance. Here the focus is on the healthy, "normal" patient and the identification of abnormalities. Specific assessments for pathological and traumatic conditions are disucussed in depth in later chapters.

HEALTH HISTORY

The health history serves as the foundation for the physical and laboratory assessment by directing the examiner toward the areas that should be examined. In the health history, patients are asked to give information on their past and present health status and their present concerns.

In a musculoskeletal assessment, there are four specific areas that must be examined in detail: (1) onset of symptoms, (2) pain, (3) deformity, and (4) paralysis. Important points to know about the onset of symptoms are: (1) when the symptoms started, (2) how they started, (3) what they were, (4) whether the onset was gradual or sudden, and whether anything specific was associated with the onset of the symptoms, (5) how the symptoms have progressed, (6) what has increased or decreased symptoms, and (7) what specific treatments have been used and whether they have been effective in the immediate and long term.

Pain, the most common symptom in orthopaedics, must be evaluated closely. Have the patient point to the specific location of the pain. Use the patient's own words (e.g., sharp, dull, stabbing, or aching) to describe the character of the pain. Determine what effect the pain has on the patient's life-style and ability to perform activities of daily living. Determine if the pain radiates, and if so to what location. Find out what precipitates or relieves the pain, the frequency of occurrence, how long the pain lasts, and if there are any associated symptoms.

In obtaining information about a deformity, it is essential to know when the changes were first noted and whether there was any pain, swelling, or stiffness associated with onset. Determine if there is family history of those or similar symptoms.

In collecting data about paralysis, it is important to note the time of onset, extent of involvement, progression or regression, and presence or absence of sensory disturbances.

Besides the above four areas of concern, the present and past medication history is important. Be clear about what has been prescribed, what the patient is actually taking, and why past medications were discontinued. For an in-depth discussion of history taking, see the references on assessment at the end of this chapter.

PHYSICAL EXAMINATION

Examination Techniques

Inspection and palpation are the principal techniques used to examine the musculoskeletal system. Inspect and palpate each body part; then test its range of motion and muscle strength. Examine each muscle and joint bilaterally, comparing the two sides of the patient's body. Remember that both sides of the body must be in the same position before a comparison can be made.

Inspection of the musculoskeletal system includes visual scanning of the two sides of the body for symmetry, contour, and size. Look for gross deformities, areas of swelling or inflammation, skin changes such as ecchymosis or other discolorations, and muscle atrophy. The patient's posture and body alignment should be viewed from both front and back. Note the structural relationship of the feet to the legs, the hips to the pelvis, the hands to the arms, the arms to the shoulders, and the shoulders to the upper trunk. Inspect the shape of the spine and its structural opposition to the shoulder girdle, thorax, and pelvis. When a deformity is present, another body part may shift to compensate for the imbalance, e.g., the pelvis may tilt when one leg is shorter than the other. The nurse should look for such compensatory changes.

Palpation is utilized to detect pain, tenderness, swelling, localized temperature changes, marked changes in shape, and muscle tone. Pain and tenderness in a bone may indicate a tumor, inflammation, or the aftermath of trauma. An angulated bone, one that is out of its original alignment, may be the result of abnormal bone development, injury, or an old fracture that healed in improper alignment. While palpating a muscle, the examiner should be alert to fasciculations, involuntary contractions, or twitchings of groups of muscle fibers. Ask patients about any sensation that they feel while their muscles and tendons are being palpated. Their descriptions of pain or tenderness on palpation should be recorded.

Measuring Range of Motion

After inspecting and palpating each body part with the patient at rest, test the active and passive range of motion of the joints. During passive range-of-motion testing, evaluate the patient's muscle tone by feeling the movements of the muscles with your hands. This adds to the information obtained during the earlier palpation of the muscles at rest.

To measure the patient's range of motion, use a goniometer (Fig. 2–1). Place the center, or zero point, on the joint to be measured, and the axis (the fixed part of the goniometer) along the 0 degree line. Use the movable arm to measure degrees of movement. For example, in measuring degrees of flexion at the elbow, place the zero point on the lateral epicondyle of the humerus, align the axis with the shaft of the humerus, and use the movable arm to measure the number of degrees the forearm departs from the fully extended position.

Muscle Strength

Knowledge of muscle strength and tone is helpful in diagnosing musculoskeletal conditions and gives information about the amount of assistance a patient may need when ambulating or doing activities of daily living. Muscle strength is assessed throughout the full range of motion for each muscle or group of muscles. Muscle strength is tested by asking the patient to resist movement or to move against restrictions applied by the examiner. Strength is

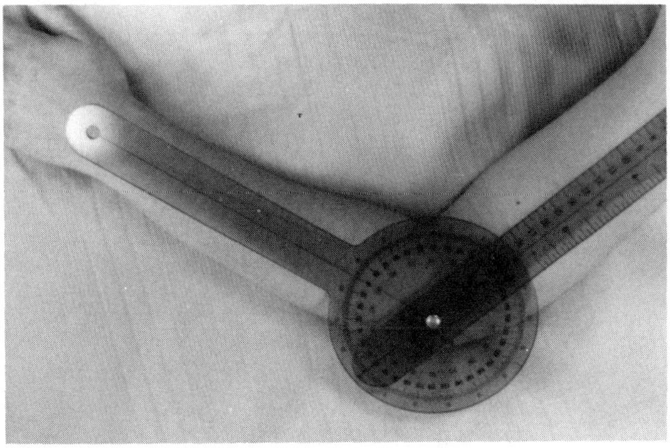

Figure 2–1. Goniometer used to measure joint motion.

graded according to the examiner's judgment by observing for muscular contraction and feeling the patient's muscle strength exerted. Grading is usually based on a scale of 0 to 5 (Table 2–1). Disability is considered to exist if muscle strength is less than grade 3, and external support may be required to make the involved part functional. It is expected that muscle strength will be greater in the dominant arm and leg (e.g., the right arm and leg for right-handed persons).

Measuring Muscle Mass

The difference between the firm, hypertrophic muscle of the athlete and the limp, atrophic muscle of the paralytic is obvious both on inspection and by palpation. Only in the very obese patient is muscle mass difficult to assess. Although muscle size is largely a function of the use or disuse of muscle fibers, a change in the size of a muscle may be indicative of disease. Malnutrition tends to reduce muscle size as well as weaken the strength of muscle contraction. Lack of neural input due to lesions of the spinal cord may also lead to a reduction in muscle size.

Measurements taken of extremities at their maximum circumference may provide a basis for comparison when swelling or atrophy are suspected. In making such a comparison, the measurements are taken with the extremities placed in the same position and with the muscles in the same state of tension. Measurements should be made at several corresponding points above and below the patella or the olecranon process. For example, authorities routinely measure 5 cm below and 5 cm and 10 cm above, or 10 cm below and 10 cm and 20 cm above the midpatella. Differences in symmetry or extremity size of less than 1 cm are not significant.

TABLE 2–1. CRITERIA FOR GRADING MUSCLE STRENGTH

Grade	Lovett Scale	Muscular Reaction	Notation in Charting
0	0 (zero)	No evidence of contractility felt or seen	0/5
1	T (trace)	Only slight contractility; no joint motion	1/5
2	P (poor)	Complete range of motion with gravity eliminated	2/5
3	F (fair)	Complete range of motion against gravity	3/5
4	G (good)	Complete range of motion against gravity and some resistance	4/5
5	N (normal)	Complete range of motion against gravity and full resistance	5/5

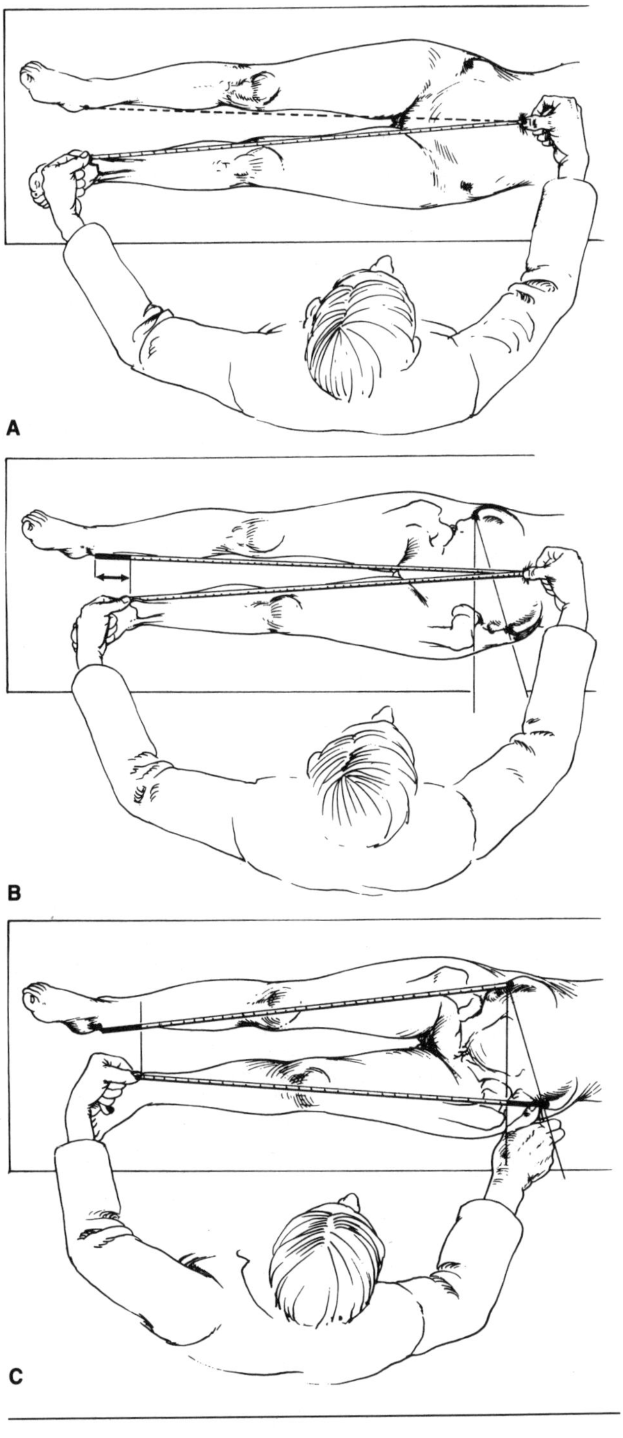

A

B

C

Figure 2–2. A. Measure from a nonfixed point to a fixed point to determine an apparent leg length discrepancy. **B.** An apparent leg length discrepancy associated with pelvic obliquity. **C.** True leg length measurements are equal despite the apparent leg length discrepancy. *(Figures 2–2 through 2–4, and 2–7 through 2–17 are reproduced from Hoppenfeld, S., 1976, with permission.)*

Measuring Extremity Length

Measurements of patient extremity lengths are best made with the patient lying relaxed on an examining table with pelvis level, hips and knees fully extended, and both hips equally adducted. The length of the lower extremity is the distance from the lower edge of the anterosuperior iliac spine to the tibial malleolus (Fig. 2–2). The length of the upper extremity is the distance from the tip of the acromion process to the tip of the middle finger, with the shoulder adducted and the other joints in neutral position. (Table 2–2).

Testing Reflexes

In the musculoskeletal system there are five major reflexes to evaluate. They are the biceps, triceps, brachioradialis, patellar, and Achilles reflexes (Figs. 2–3 and 2–4). The *biceps reflex* tests the C5–6 spinal nerve response. The patient's arm is flexed at the elbow and held by the examiner. The examiner then places his or her thumb horizontally over the biceps tendon. A blow on the examiner's thumb is delivered with a percussion hammer. There will be slight flexion of the elbow, and the examiner will be able to feel the bicep's contraction through the thumb. Spinal nerve responses can be graded using the scale in Table 2–3.

The *brachioradialis reflex* also tests the C5–6 spinal nerve response. The patient's forearm can rest on either the examiner's forearm or the patient's leg. A percussion hammer strikes the radius 2 to 5 cm (1 to 2 inches) above the wrist. The patient is observed for flexion and supination of the forearm, and the fingers of the patient's hand may also extend slightly.

The *triceps reflex* tests the C7–8 spinal nerve response. The patient's arm is flexed at the elbow. The examiner palpates the triceps tendon about 2 to 5 cm (1 or 2 inches) above the elbow, and then delivers a blow with a percussion hammer directly to the tendon. The patient is observed for a contraction of the triceps tendon and a slight extension of the elbow.

The *patellar knee jerk reflex* tests the L2–4 spinal nerve response. The patient should be sitting up with the legs dangling over the side of a bed or table. If the patient is unable to sit up, the examiner should slide the arm under the

TABLE 2–2. MEASURING EXTREMITY LENGTH

Extremity	Points of Measurement
Arm	
Arm length	Tip of acromion process to tip of middle finger
Upper arm length	Tip of acromion process to tip of olecranon process
Forearm length	Tip of olecranon process to styloid process of ulna
Leg	
Leg length	Lower edge of anterosuperior iliac spine to tibial malleolus
Thigh length	Lower edge of anterosuperior iliac spine to medial aspect of the knee
Lower leg length	Medial aspect of knee to tibial malleolus

(Adapted from Malasanos, L. et al. Health assessment. *St. Louis: C.V. Mosby, 1977, p. 312.)*

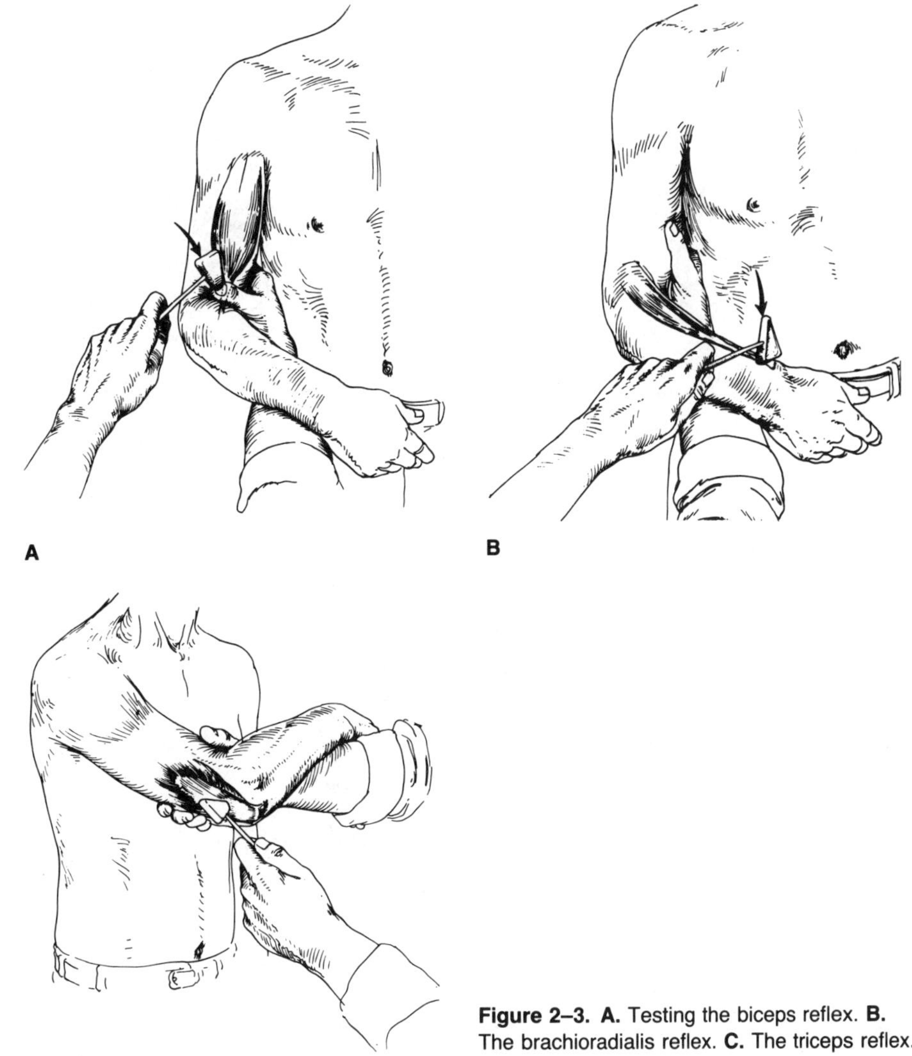

A B C

Figure 2–3. A. Testing the biceps reflex. **B.** The brachioradialis reflex. **C.** The triceps reflex.

patient's knee and lift the patient's leg to flex the knee. The patellar tendon is then tapped with a percussion hammer. The tendon is usually found directly below the patella itself. If no response is obtained, the patient's legs may not be relaxed enough. In that case, ask the patient to interlock the fingers and pull. That allows the patient to relax the legs so that the reflex can be obtained.

The *Achilles tendon reflex* tests the S1–2 spinal nerve response. That reflex should be checked after the patellar reflex so that the patient can remain in the same position. With the patient's foot dorsiflexed, the examiner strikes the

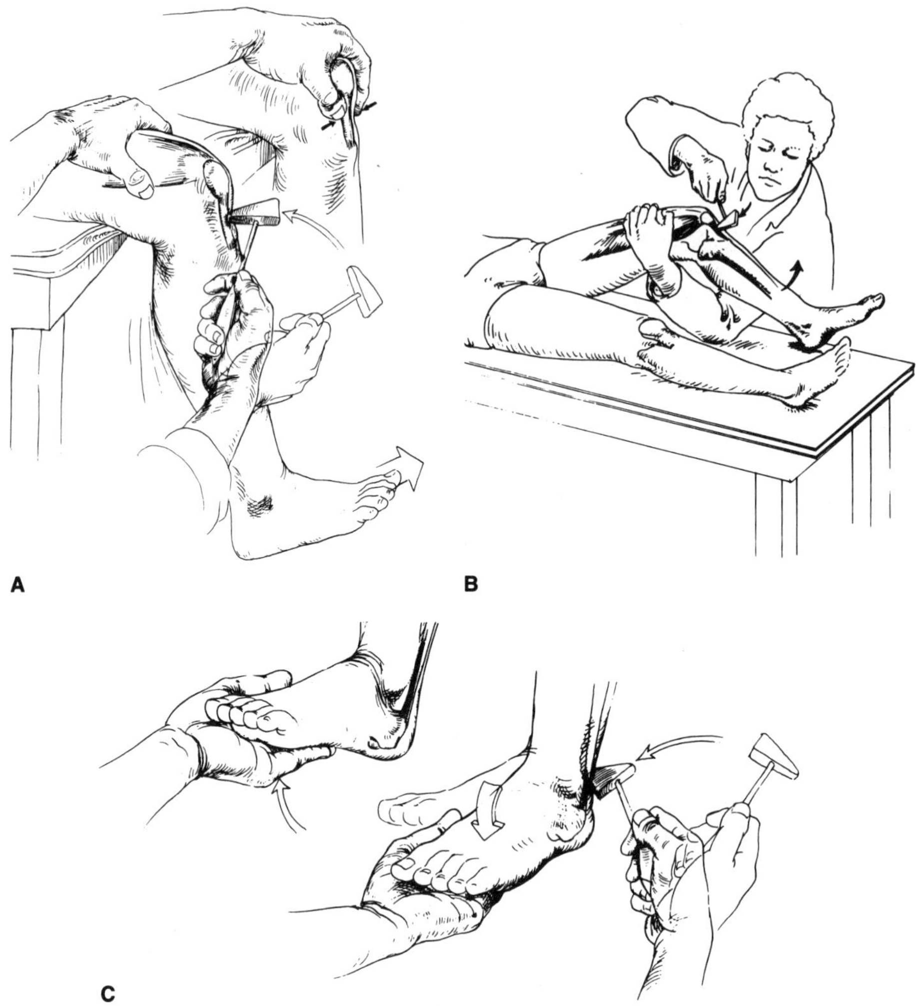

Figure 2–4. A. The patellar reflex. **B.** Position to elicit the patellar reflex on a bed patient. **C.** Testing the Achilles tendon reflex.

Achilles tendon with a percussion hammer just above the heel. The examiner should see and feel the foot plantar flex. If the patient is unable to sit up, the examiner can take the foot and place it on the patient's other shin, which will dorsiflex the foot.

Neurovascular Assessment

In doing a neurological assessment of the upper extremities, it is important to check the five major nerves, i.e., the circumflex, the musculocutaneous, the median, the ulnar, and the radial. The *circumflex nerve* supplies sensation to the

TABLE 2–3. A SCALE FOR REFLEX RESPONSES

Rating	Description
U	No reflex response
+1	Below normal
+2	Average
+3	Stronger than average
+4	Very intense response (may resemble clonus)

(Adapted from Malasanos L. et al. Health assessment. *St. Louis: C.V. Mosby, 1977, p. 410.)*

skin over the deltoid and is the motor nerve to the deltoid muscle. Check the sensory portion of the nerve by determining the patient's sensation over the deltoid area. Have the patient do an abduction of the arm at the shoulder to test the motor function of the circumflex nerve. The *musculocutaneous nerve* supplies motor function to the biceps and the brachioradialis muscles. To check the sensory portion, determine the patient's sensation at the radial side of the forearm. The patient's ability to flex the arm at the elbow is the test for motor function. The *median nerve* innervates most of the flexor muscles of the forearm, particularly the muscles of the thenar eminence. To determine the sensory portion of the median nerve, check the sensation of the entire palmar surface of the thumb, index, and long fingers. To check motor function, have the patient oppose the thumb to the little finger. The *ulnar nerve* supplies motor function to the flexor muscles of the ulnar side of the arm and to the intrinsic muscles of the hand, particularly the interossei and the lumbricals of the third and fourth fingers. For sensory function, check the patient's sensation along the palmar surface of the little finger. To determine motor function, have the patient abduct and adduct all of the fingers. The *radial nerve* has a small sensory distribution and an extensive motor function. Virtually all of the extensor muscles of the arm from the triceps down are supplied by the radial nerve. To assess the sensory portion, determine sensation in the area over the web space between the patient's thumb and index finger. For an assessment of the motor function of the radial nerve, have the patient extend the wrist and fingers.

In doing a neurological assessment of the lower extremities, it is important to check the three major nerves: the femoral, the obturator, and the sciatic. Each *sciatic nerve,* with its two major divisions the *posterior tibial* and the *common peroneal,* supplies motor and sensory function to much of the entire leg. The sciatic nerve supplies the hamstring muscles in the thigh and the division of those muscles below the knee. The *tibial nerve* supplies the gastrocnemius muscle, the soleus muscle, and the flexors of the toes, and it provides sensation along the dorsum of the foot. Check the motor function of the tibial nerve by having the patient plantarflex the ankle and flex the toes. To assess the sensory portion, prick the medial and lateral surfaces of the sole of the foot. The *common peroneal nerve* innervates the peroneal and anterior tibial muscles of the leg and provides sensation along the lateral aspect of the leg below the knee and to the sole of the foot. To determine the motor function of the peroneal nerve have the patient dorsiflex the ankle and extend the toes. Assess the sensory portion by pricking the lateral surface of the great toe and the medial surface of the second toe.

If the major trunk of the sciatic nerve is injured, the site of the injury is usually in the buttock or thigh. The patient will have an anesthetic foot and be unable to move that foot and toes. If the nerve is injured high in the thigh, loss of hamstring function and weakness of knee flexion may also occur. Injury to the tibial branch usually occurs at the posterior calf or the popliteal space and produces anesthesia over the lateral aspect of the calf and the foot. The patient has a loss of sensation over the heel and sole of the foot, and cannot plantarflex the ankle. Eversion and dorsiflexion of the foot at the ankle are also lost.

The *femoral nerve* supplies motor function of the quadriceps femoris and sensation along the medial side of the foot and leg, extending as low as the medial malleolus. The femoral nerve is usually injured at the inguinal ligament in the anterior aspect of the thigh. Loss of femoral nerve function produces anesthesia along the medial aspect of the foot and an inability to extend the knee.

The *obturator nerve* supplies the adductor muscles of the thigh, with a small sensory distribution along the medial side of the thigh. The obturator nerve is rarely injured, as it lies deep in the pelvis. However, injury to the obturator nerve should be kept in mind when penetrating wounds of the perineum occur. Injury to that nerve can result in an inability to adduct the thigh.

To assess the vascular function of the extremities, check the patient's pulse, color, and temperature. The first steps in assessing circulatory status are to note if there is any swelling of the hands and fingers, or the feet and toes, abnormal color (i.e., pallor or cyanosis), or abnormal temperature (i.e., coldness or increased warmth). Determine circulation to the fingers and toes by checking capillary refill (or blanching). Pinch the end of a finger or toe and then let go. The patient's nail bed should first turn white and then return to pink in less than 3 seconds. Take the patient's pulse, and note if there is any weakness or disappearance of the pulse. Compare the neurovascular status of one side of the body with the other.

There are three major pulses in the upper extremity: the radial, the ulnar, and the brachial (Fig. 2–5). The radial artery extends down the radial side of the forearm to the wrist. The *radial pulse* is the most commonly palpated and is located on the flexor surface of the wrist laterally (to describe the strength of a pulse, see Table 2–4). The ulnar artery extends down the ulnar side of the forearm to the wrist. It then divides into two branches, which anastomose with branches of the radial artery to form the arterial arches of the hand. The *ulnar pulse* is located on the flexor surface of the wrist medially. It is usually palpated only when arterial insufficiency is suspected. The *brachial pulse* is palpated in the groove between the biceps and triceps muscles. It too is usually palpated only when arterial insufficiency is suspected. Just below the elbow, the brachial artery branches into the radial and ulnar arteries.

There are four major pulses in the lower extremity: the femoral, the pop-

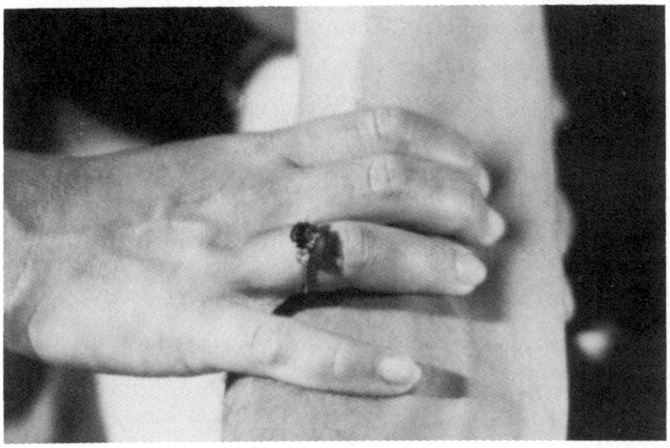

A

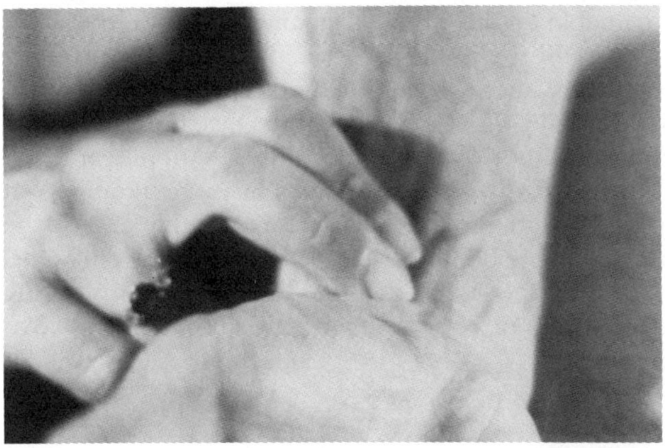

B

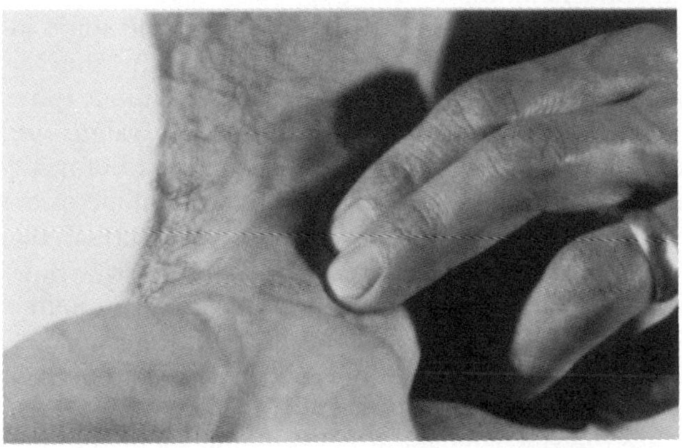

C

Figure 2–5. A. The brachial pulse. **B.** The radial pulse. **C.** The ulnar pulse. *(From Block, G.J., et al., 1986, p. 236, with permission.)*

TABLE 2–4. PULSE STRENGTH

Rating	Description of Pulse
0	No pulse
1	Pulse is thready, weak, and difficult to palpate; it may fade in and out and is easily obliterated with pressure
2	Pulse is difficult to palpate and may be obliterated with pressure, so light palpation is necessary; once located, it is moderately strong
3	Pulse is easily palpable, does not fade in and out, and is not readily obliterated by pressure; considered to be a normal pulse
4	Pulse is strong and bounding, easily palpated, and not obliterated with pressure; it may reflect a pathological condition such as aortic regurgitation

(From Block, G.J., et al., 1986, pp. 227–228, with permission.)

liteal, the posterior tibial, and the dorsalis pedis (Fig. 2–6). The *femoral artery* arises at the level of the inguinal ligament and extends downward through the thigh. The *femoral pulse* is palpable at the inguinal ligament midway between the anterior–superior iliac spine and the pubic tubercle. The popliteal artery is a continuation of the femoral artery and is located behind the knee. To palpate the *popliteal pulse,* the patient should be asked to slightly flex the knee. The examiner then presses the fingers of both hands deeply into the popliteal fossa. This pulse is often difficult to locate. The posterior tibial artery extends down the posterior aspect of the leg around the medial malleolus to the side of the foot. The *posterior tibial pulse* is palpable behind and below the medial malleolus. The *dorsalis pedis pulse* is felt in the groove between the first two tendons on the medial side of the dorsum of the foot. It is congenitally absent in approximately 10 percent of the population.

Abnormal Findings

A variety of deformities and abnormalities occur in the musculoskeletal system, and are described by a number of standard terms. Deviations in the spine include (1) *kyphosis,* an increased convex curve ("hunchback") in the thoracic spine, (2) *lordosis,* an increased concave curve ("swayback") in the lumbar spine, and (3) *scoliosis,* a lateral curve of the spinal column. The terms valgus and varus describe deviations of the joints of the extremities. *Valgus* is a deformity in which the distal portion of a joint is angulated away from the midline of the body, e.g., *genus valgus* describes "knock-knees," *talipes valgus* describes feet turned outward, and *cubitus valgus* is when the forearm deviates laterally (at a "carrying angle"). *Varus* is a deformity in which the distal portion of a joint is angled toward the midline of the body, e.g., *genus varus* describes "bowlegs," *talipes varus* describes feet turned inward ("pigeon toes"), and *cubitus varus* is when the forearm deviates medially (the "gunstock deformity"). The terms eversion and inversion are used to describe abnormal positionings of the foot. *Eversion* is a "turning out" position where the foot is rotated along its longitudinal axis so that increased weight is borne on the medial side. *Inversion* is a

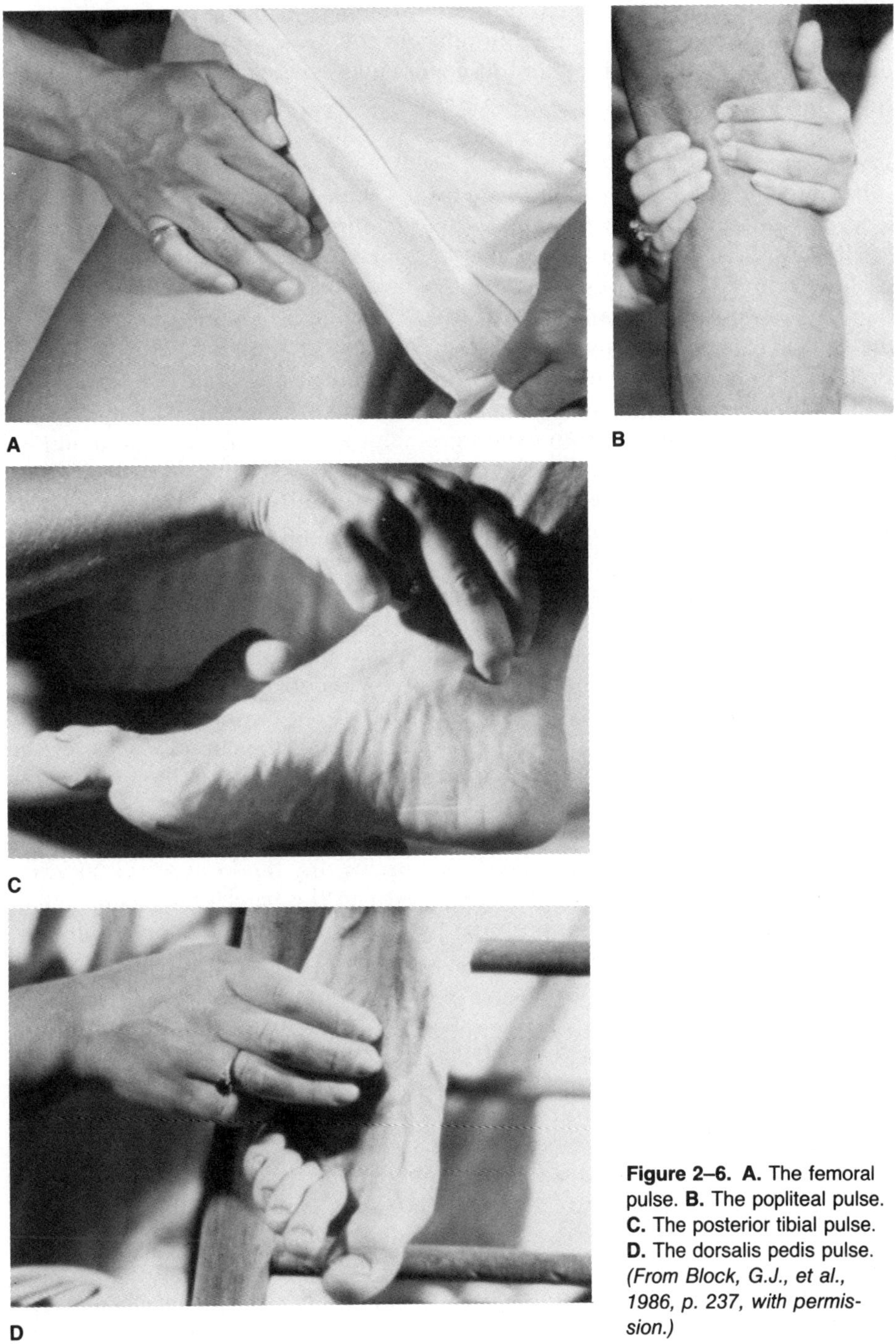

Figure 2–6. A. The femoral pulse. **B.** The popliteal pulse. **C.** The posterior tibial pulse. **D.** The dorsalis pedis pulse. *(From Block, G.J., et al., 1986, p. 237, with permission.)*

"turning in" position where the foot is rotated along its longitudinal axis so that increased weight is borne on the lateral side.

The most common abnormal findings in the musculoskeletal system relate to swelling and inflammation, and to pain. Their assessment is discussed in the following two sections.

Swelling and Inflammation

Inflammation results from injury to tissues, and swelling occurs as exudate from an inflammation that forms to defend the tissues from further injury. Swelling within the musculoskeletal system may be local or diffuse. Localized swelling is most often present as a lump or a small, specific mass under the skin, e.g., a swollen olecranon bursa, where swelling is confined to the area of the bursa. Diffuse swelling is more widespread. As a general rule, localized swelling is contained within a joint capsule or bursa and does not extravasate into nearby tissues, whereas diffuse swelling is more widespread and may involve the entire region. Inflammation of a joint typically produces pain and an increase in temperature and erythema (redness). A joint appears swollen when there is a thickened synovial membrane, an increase in synovial fluid, blood or purulent material within the joint capsule, or swelling in the surrounding soft tissue.

It is important to know whether a joint is enlarged from soft tissue swelling or from an increase in fluid within the joint. This is especially true for the knee, because many knee injuries involve swelling that may be due to either swollen tissue or to fluid in the joint. To check for increased fluid, the examiner can "milk" the medial aspect of the knee by two or three upward strokes with the ball of the hand. The knee is then tapped just behind the lateral margin of the patella. A bulge on the median side indicates fluid returning to the hollow area medial to the patella (Bates, 1979, p. 291). Another method of checking for fluid in the knee joint is ballottement for a "floating patella." Firmly grasp the thigh just above the knee with one hand, forcing any fluid out of the superior portion of the joint space into the space between the patella and femur. With the fingers of the other hand, push the patella sharply back against the femur. A palpable tap indicates fluid within the knee joint (Hoppenfeld, 1976, p. 195).

Pain

The critical features of pain are (1) type, (2) location, (3) severity, (4) duration, and (5) precipitating factors (Meinhart & McCaffery, 1983, p. 174ff).

Type. Have the patient describe in his or her own words just what the pain is like. Pain may be described as "being stabbed with an ice pick" or with such words as "heavy," "crushing," "sharp," "burning," and "throbbing." Deep as opposed to superficial pain is a diffuse aching sensation such as that produced by squeezing the Achilles tendon, and is often described by expressions like "being in a vise," or "having an iron band round my chest." You may have to ask the patient for more details if you receive an answer such as "like a headache," because there are many types of headaches.

Location. Try to ascertain where the patient's pain is perceived. The patient may need help in locating the exact point of the pain, in part because of different degrees of sensitivity in different areas of the body. On the finger tip, two pinpoints can be distinguished from one another when they are only 3 mm apart, but on the back, the minimum distance for distinguishing two pinpricks may be 50 mm. Often the patient will add nonverbal descriptions such as pointing with a finger tip or spreading an outstretched hand over an area. The location of the pain should include whether it is superficial or deep, and whether or not it radiates to another anatomical site (e.g., pain radiating from the lower back down the posterior thigh is associated with the sciatic nerve).

Severity. In some diseases pain is characteristically severe, whereas in others it is mild or may vary in severity. Individuals vary so much in their tolerance to pain that a mere statement of severity is insufficient, and thus severity is generally best described by having the patient tell how the pain affects normal activities. In evaluating severity, it must be remembered that the intensity of pain depends greatly upon the patient's state of mind. Mental depression, anxiety, and introspection tend to aggravate pain.

Duration. The assessment of pain should include its duration and frequency. Estimates of time made without actual measurements are often very inaccurate, but even such estimates may be helpful. In some instances, pain occurs at regular intervals. It is sound practice to ask if the pain recurs at any special times, e.g., at night or upon wakening. Arthritis pain, for example, is generally more severe after activity, whereas bone pain occurs more often at night.

Precipitating Factors. Many factors are associated with the onset and relief of pain. The patient's accounts should be carefully assessed for reliability. For example, if bending is alleged to bring on pain, is bending always painful, is it always the same type of pain, and so on. Ask questions that can be answered by "yes" or "no." Remember that patients may believe their condition has improved from treatment or activities that have had no real effect.

Phantom Limb Pain

Phantom limb sensations include tingling, itching, and sweating in the amputated limb. They occur in almost all patients who have had a body part amputated either surgically or traumatically, and in those who have had an interruption or denervation of sensory pathways in the spinal cord or brain. Phantom limb pain occurs much less frequently, with estimates varying from 2 percent (Sternback, 1968) to 35 percent (Melzack, 1973), depending on the criteria used. Phantom limb pain is most common immediately following the amputation, but occasionally the "limb" gradually becomes more painful over time. Seiden (1981, p. 54) reported that 5 to 10 percent of patients experience permanent phantom limb pain. A patient may have stump pain (postoperative discomfort at the surgical site) in addition to the phantom limb pain, but the two are not necessarily related.

The quality and characteristics of phantom limb pain vary. The pain may be described as severe, burning, crushing, cramping, a sensation that the limb is edematous, or a sensation that the limb is in a distorted position that the patient is unable to change. Craig (1978, p. 86) reports four features associated with phantom limb pain. First, it is more likely to occur if the patient had pain in the limb prior to amputation. Second, if pain was present prior to amputation, the phantom limb pain will be qualitatively similar to the preamputation pain. Third, individuals experiencing traumatic injuries, especially those who do not regain consciousness prior to their amputation, rarely experience phantom limb pain. Fourth, the individual may experience the limb as being in the same position it was in immediately prior to the amputation.

Phantom limb pain may be triggered by many things, including touching the amputated stump, the occurrence of another illness, fatigue, atmospheric changes, and emotional stress. Phantom limb pain that does not resolve with time may be evoked by many stimuli, including touching healthy areas of the body.

The pathophysiology of phantom limb pain is not fully known. Transecting the spinal cord, sympathectomy, and other surgical procedures to interrupt the sensory pathways may not completely eliminate phantom limb pain.

Physical Assessment

When doing a complete musculoskeletal assessment, organize the examination so that it progresses smoothly, with minimal position changes for the patient. A good way is to begin with the patient sitting so you can examine the neck, shoulders, and upper extremities. Then examine the back, ilium, and gait with the patient both standing and walking. Finally, have the patient lie supine while you examine the hips, knees, ankles, and feet. For clarity of presentation, a slightly modified order is followed in subsequent sections.

Gait and Posture

Observe how the patient sits, stands, and walks. The assessment of the patient's gait should begin when the patient walks into the room, because the patient is then less apt to be conscious that his or her gait is being assessed. Gait varies from person to person, but normally there is a certain rhythm to a person's walk. Observe the patient walk several steps away and then turn and walk back. Observe the patient's posture, the swing of the arms, the stride length and rhythm, and any associated movements (Fig. 2–7). A distance of 2 to 4 inches should separate the patient's heels as they pass during walking, and the stride length should be about 15 inches, depending on the patient's height and body structure (Fig. 2–8). The patient's arms should swing freely at the side, the body should be well balanced, and posture should be erect. When the patient turns, the face and head should turn before the rest of the body.

Thoracic and Lumbar Spine

With the patients's back and buttocks exposed, inspect the curvature of the spinal column from both posterior and lateral views. Note any prominence of

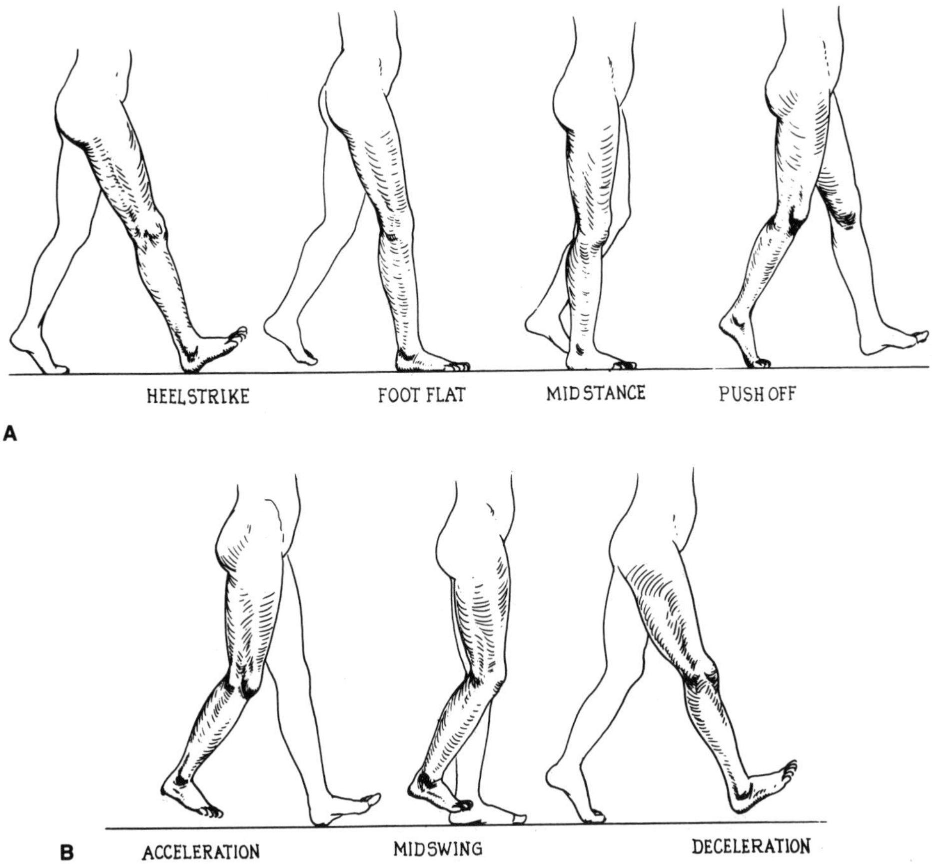

Figure 2–7. The phases of gait. **A.** Stance phase: *(1)* heel strike, *(2)* foot flat, *(3)* midstance, and *(4)* push-off. **B.** Swing phase: *(1)* acceleration, *(2)* midswing, *(3)* deceleration.

the scapulae and whether the shoulders are level. Palpate the spinous processes and paravertebral muscles, noting any tenderness or swelling. Use the flat of your hand to detect muscle hardening from spasm. Have the patient perform active range of motion of the trunk (Fig. 2–9).

ASSESSING RANGE OF MOTION IN THE THORACIC AND LUMBAR SPINE

Spinal Movements and Normal Range of Motion	*Instructions to Patient*	*Procedure for Testing Muscle Strength*
Flexion: 70–90 degrees	"Bend over and touch your toes without flexing your knees"	With one hand stabilizing the patient's pelvis, apply resistance with the other hand to the center of the patient's chest

(continued)

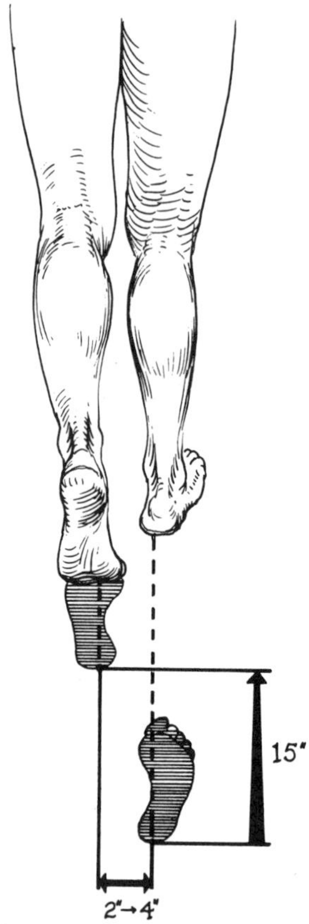

Figure 2–8. The width of a normal base measures from 2 to 4 inches. Normal step length is approximately 15 inches.

ASSESSING RANGE OF MOTION IN THE THORACIC AND LUMBAR SPINE—*(Continued)*

Spinal Movements and Normal Range of Motion	*Instructions to Patient*	*Procedure for Testing Muscle Strength*
Extension: 30 degrees when standing; 20 degrees when prone	"Bend your head and shoulders back as far as you can"	With the pelvis stabilized, apply resistance between the patient's scapulae
Lateral: 35 degrees	"Bend your trunk as far to the side as possible"	With the pelvis stabilized, apply resistance to the deltoid area
Rotation: 30–45 degrees	"Twist your shoulders as far to the right as possible and then as far to the left as possible"	With the pelvis stabilized, apply resistance to the shoulders

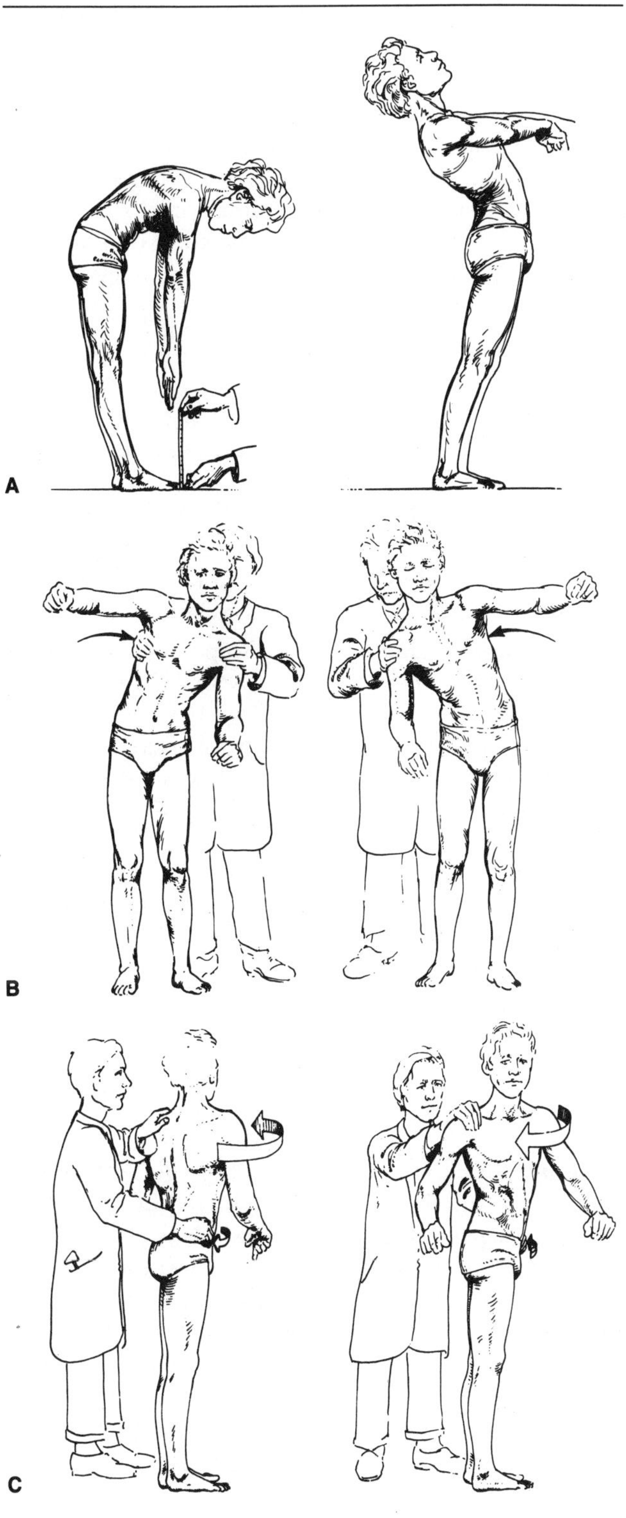

Figure 2–9. A. *Left.* Range of flexion in the lumbar spine. *Right.* Range of extension in the lumbar spine. **B.** Range of lateral bending in the lumbar spine should be equal on both sides. **C.** Range of rotation in the lumbar spine.

Cervical Spine

Inspect the front, back, and sides of the neck for size and for symmetry in the patient's neck muscles. Compare the neck muscles, particularly the sternocleidomastoid and trapezius. Note any abnormalities, such as deviations in the bone structure or muscle masses. Palpate along the spinous processes of the cervical spine and along the supraclavicular fossa for any nodules or points of tenderness and swelling. Have the patient perform active range of motion of the cervical spine (Fig. 2–10).

ASSESSING RANGE OF MOTION IN THE CERVICAL SPINE

Spinal Movements and Normal Range of Motion	*Instructions to Patient*	*Procedure for Testing Muscle Strength*
Flexion: 45 degrees	"Bend your head down to touch your chest"	Apply resistance to the forehead
Extension: 55 degrees	"Lift your head and bend it back as far as you can"	Apply resistance to the occipital prominence
Lateral bend: 40–45 degrees	"Bend your head so that your ear touches your shoulder. Do not bring your shoulder up to meet your ear"	Apply resistance to the temporal bone
Rotation: 70 degrees	"Turn your head as far as you can to the right and then turn it as far as you can to the left"	Apply resistance to the temple

Shoulder

Inspect and compare the patient's shoulders and shoulder girdle anteriorly, noting bony or muscular asymmetry, swelling, masses, deformities, muscular atrophy, discolorations, and scars. Inspect and compare the clavicles for symmetrical alignment. Inspect the scapulae and related muscles posteriorly. Inspect the deltoid muscles for atrophy, for prominence of the greater tuberosity of the humerus, and for the presence of hollows in the muscle (which could indicate displacement of the humerus). Observe the rhythm of the patient's shoulder movements. Normal motion has a smooth, even flow with no jerky or irregular movements. Palpate the shoulder to determine bony landmarks, and note any tenderness, bogginess, or crepitation around the joint. Have the patient perform active range of motion of the shoulder (Fig. 2–11).

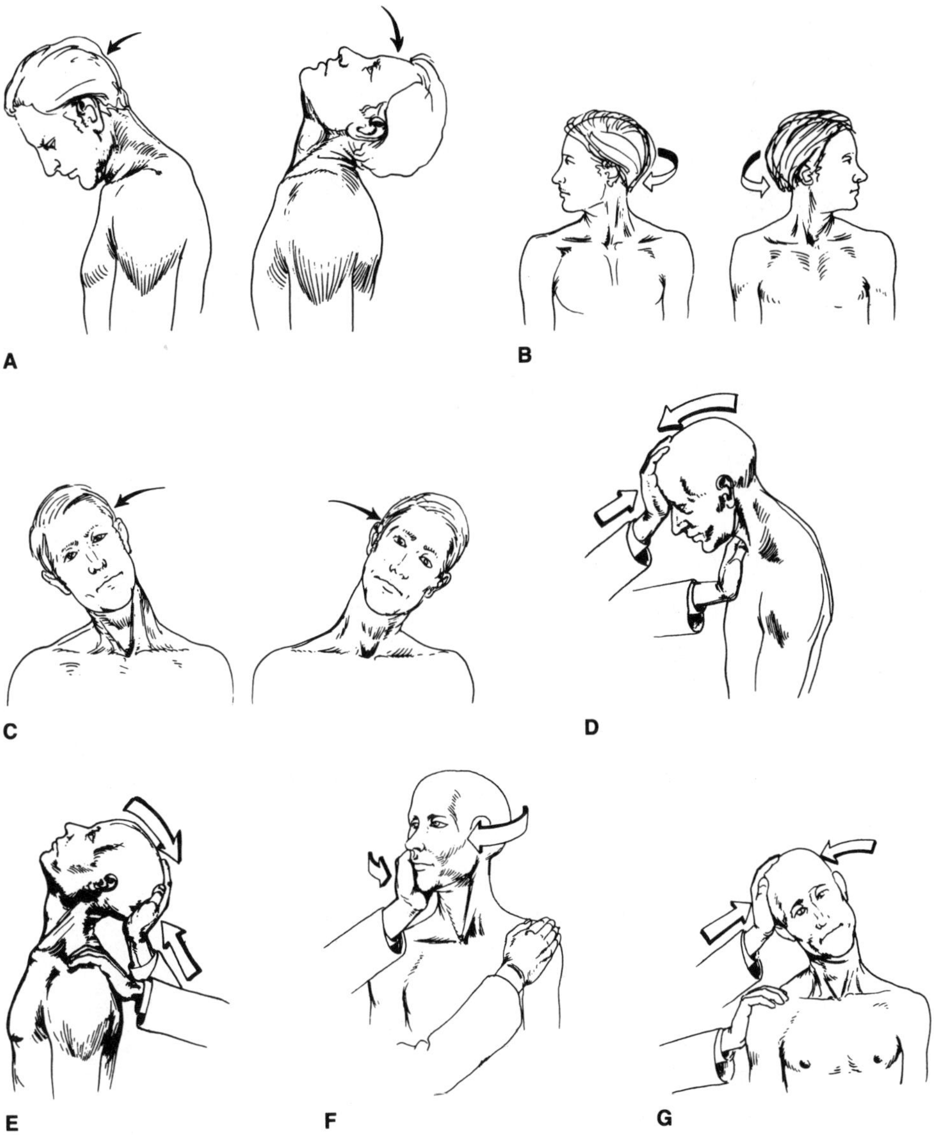

Figure 2–10. A. *Left.* Normal range of neck flexion. *Right.* Normal range of neck extension. **B.** Normal range of neck rotation. **C.** Normal range of lateral bending. **D.** Hand positions for neck flexion muscle test. **E.** Hand positions for neck extension muscle test. **F.** Hand positions for testing the sternocleidomastoid muscles for lateral rotation. **G.** Muscle test for lateral bending of the neck.

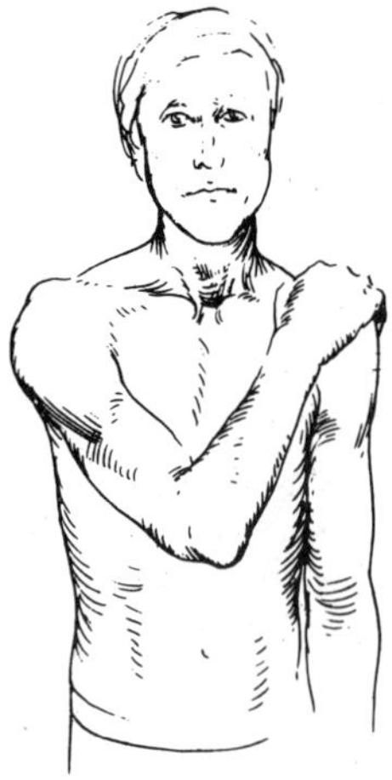

A

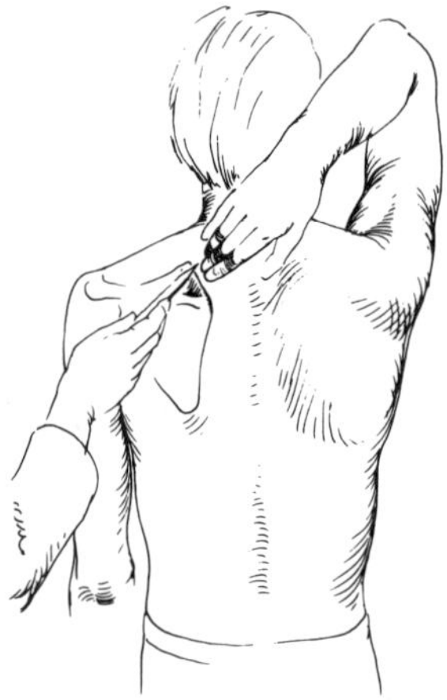

B

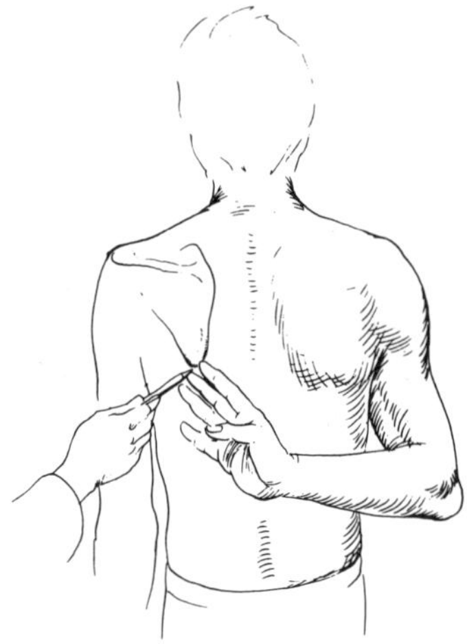

C

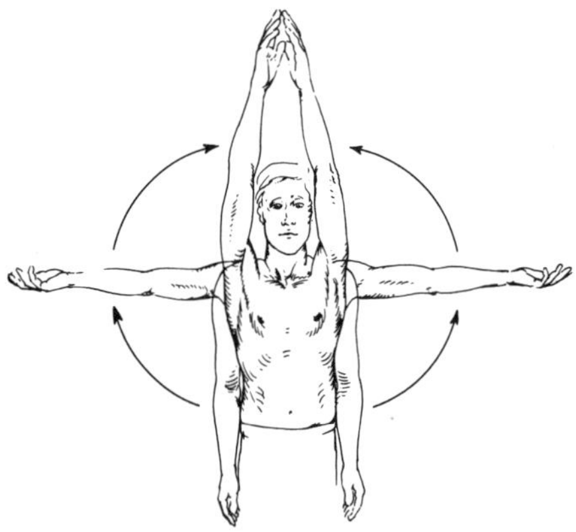

D

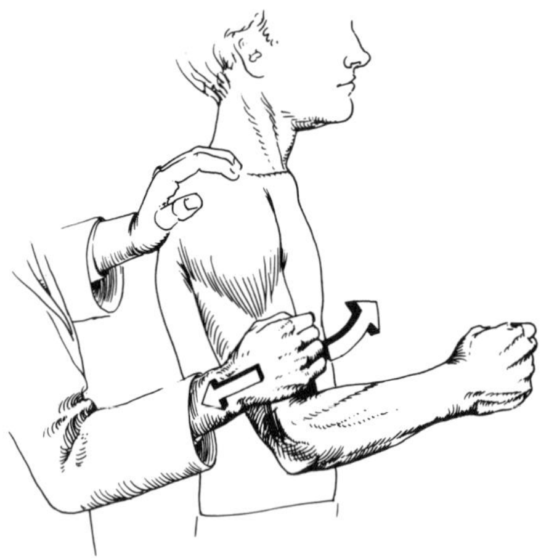

E

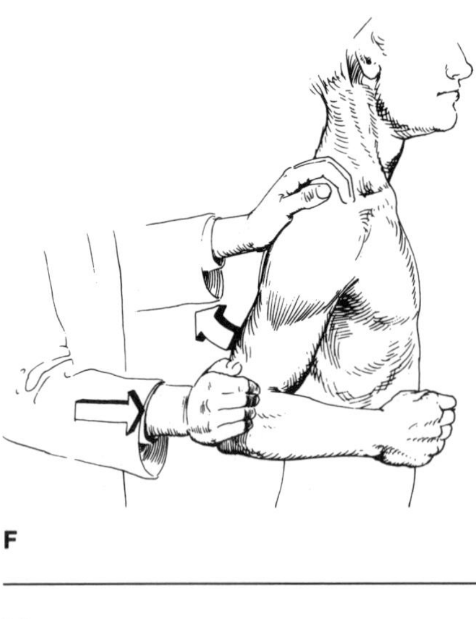

F

Figure 2–11. A. Test for internal rotation and adduction. **B.** The Apley scratch test: external rotation and abduction. **C.** Internal rotation and adduction. **D.** Test for shoulder flexion. **E.** Test for shoulder extension. **F.** Range of motion. *(continued)*

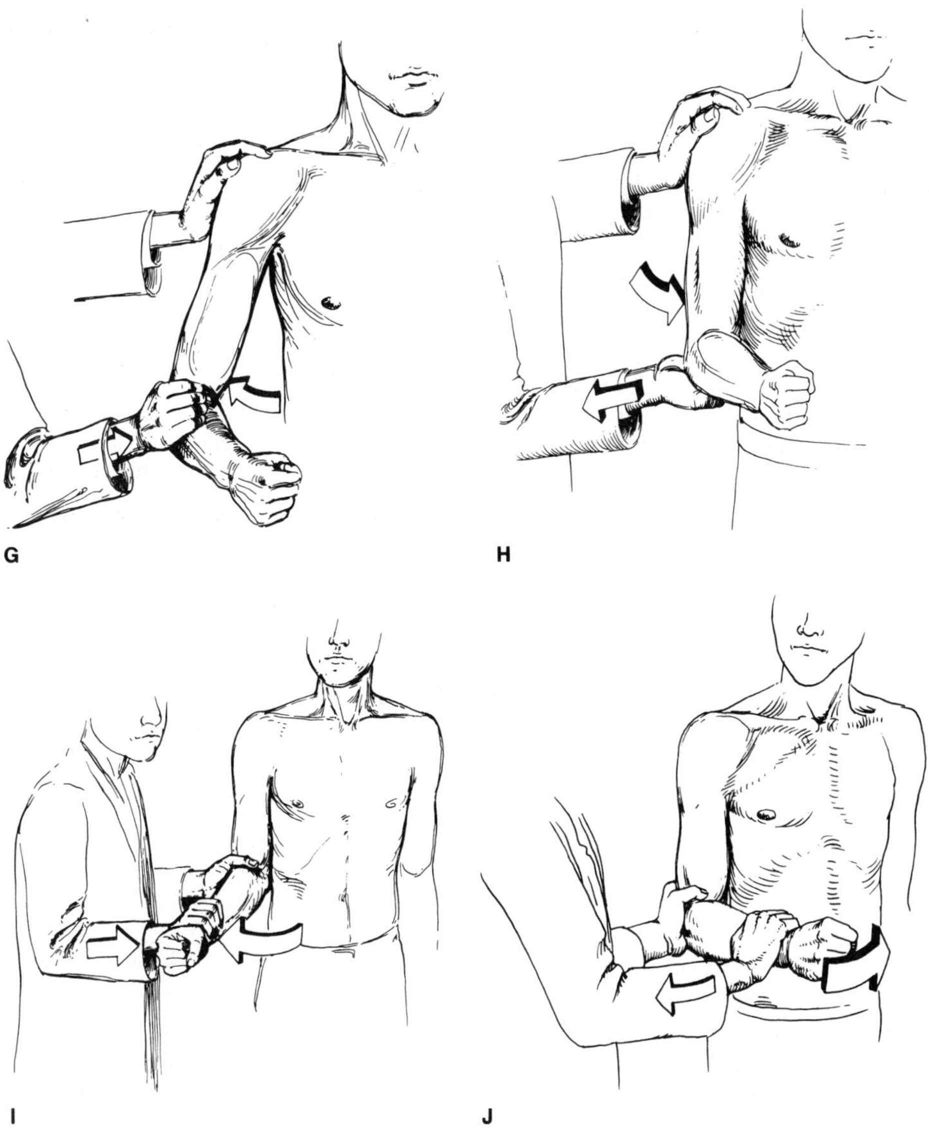

Figure 2–11. G. Test for shoulder adduction. **H.** Test for shoulder adduction. **I.** Test for external rotation of the shoulder. **J.** Test for internal rotation of the shoulder.

ASSESSING RANGE OF MOTION IN THE SHOULDER

Shoulder Movements and Normal Range of Motion	*Instructions to Patient*	*Procedure for Testing Muscle Strength*
Forward flexion: 180 degrees	"Move your arms forward and up"	Apply resistance to the anterior aspect of the arm proximal to the elbow
Backward extension: 50–60 degrees	"Move your arms downward and back"; "Clasp your arms behind your back"	Apply resistance to the posterior aspect of the arm proximal to the elbow
Abduction: 120 degrees	"Lift your arm straight out from your side, away from your body"	Apply resistance to the lateral aspect of the arm proximal to the elbow
Horizonal adduction: 45 degrees	"Bring your straight arm over your chest"	Apply resistance to the medial side of the arm proximal to the elbow
Horizonal abduction: 180 degrees	"Keeping your straight arm at shoulder height, move it backward as far as you can"	Apply resistance to the posterior surface of the arm proximal to the elbow
Internal rotation	"Rotate your shoulder inward and swing your arm backward with your palm upward, pointing your fingers toward the ceiling"	Apply resistance to the volar surface of the wrist
External rotation	"Rotate your shoulder outward with your palm down and bring your arm up"	Apply resistance to the dorsum of the wrist

Elbow and Forearm

Flex the patient's elbow to 90 degrees, noting any redness, swelling, nodules, or deformities. Compare the two elbows, noting any differences between the elbow joint angles and the muscular structures of the forearm and upper arm. Palpate the elbow in positions of flexion and extension, checking for subcutaneous nodules, bogginess, crepitation, and tenderness or enlargement of the supracondylar lymph nodes. (Lymph nodes are located above the epicondyles and are not palpable unless there is an infection below the elbow.) Palpate the muscle bodies for tenderness or muscle spasm. Have the patient perform active range of motion of the elbow (Fig. 2–12).

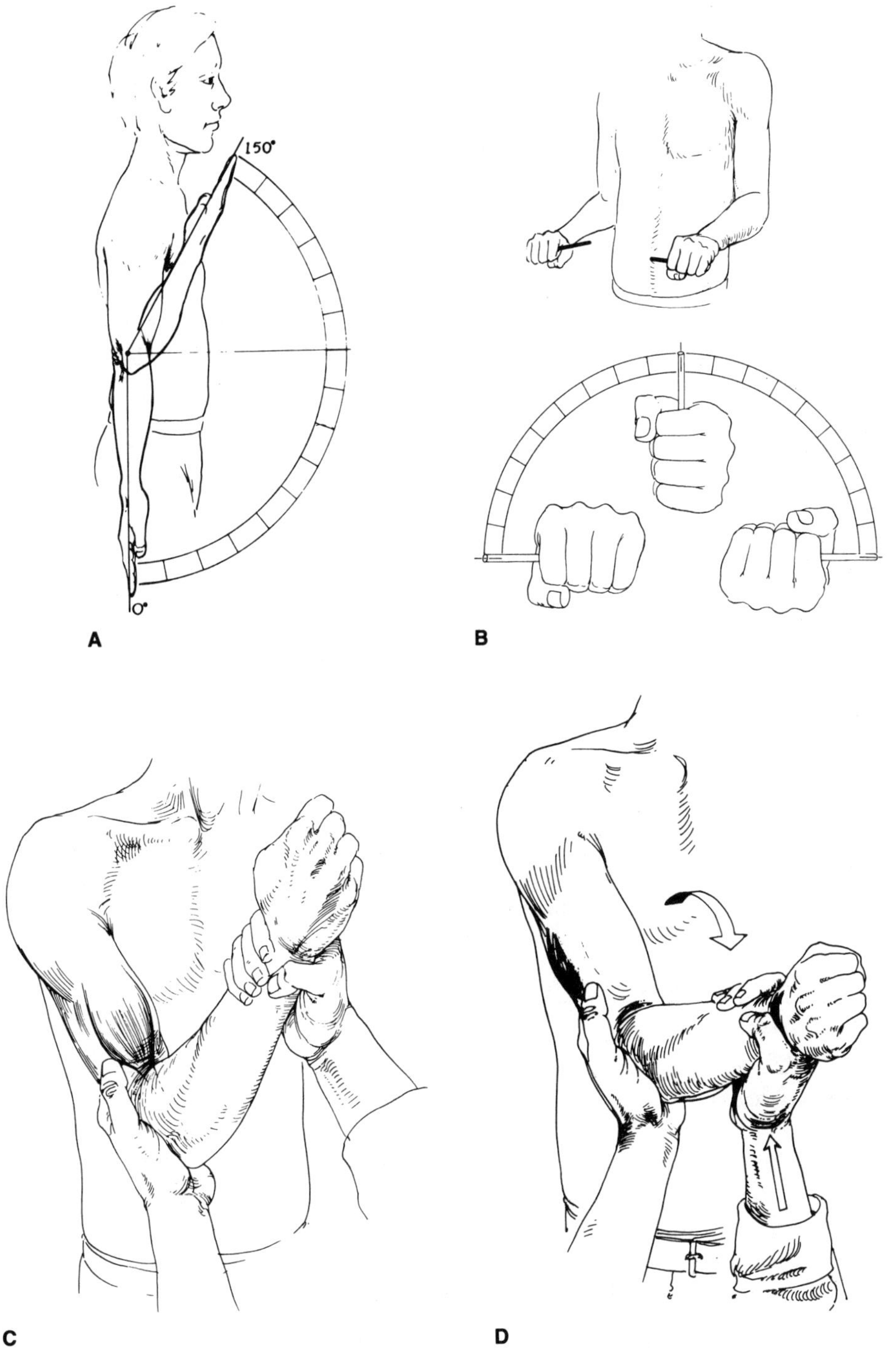

Figure 2–12. A. The elbow range of motion in flexion and extension. **B.** The elbow range of motion in supination and pronation. **C.** Muscle test for flexion. **D.** Muscle test for extension.

ASSESSING RANGE OF MOTION IN THE ELBOW

Elbow and Forearm Movements and Normal Range of Motion	*Instructions to Patient*	*Procedure for Testing Muscle Strength*
Elbow		
Flexion: 150 degrees	"Move your right (left) hand to your right (left) shoulder"	Apply resistance to the lower arm
Extension: 0 degrees	"Straighten out your right (left) arm"	Apply resistance to the dorsal surface of the arm
Forearm		
Pronation: 90 degrees	"Rotate your right (left) hand inward so that your palm is downward"	Apply resistance at the base of the thumb on the volar surface
Supination: 90 degrees	"Rotate your right (left) hand outward so that the palm is upward."	Apply resistance over the dorsal surface of the hand
Hyperextension: 0–15 degrees	Motion not present in all individuals	

Wrist

Inspect each wrist for shape, deformity, swelling, lumps, or redness, and then compare their contour and bony prominences. Palpate both wrists, checking for bogginess, crepitation, tenderness, and enlargement. Have the patient perform active range of motion of the wrist (Fig. 2–13).

ASSESSING RANGE OF MOTION IN THE WRIST

Wrist Movements and Normal Range of Motion	*Instructions to Patient*	*Procedure for Testing Muscle Strength*
Flexion: 80 degrees	"Bend your right (left) hand down toward you"	Apply resistance to the volar surface of the hand
Extension: 70 degrees	"Bend your right (left) hand back on itself"	Apply resistance to the dorsum of the hand
Lateral (ulnar) deviation: 30–50 degrees (Ulnar deviation is usually measured with the wrist in pronation. When measured in supination, ulnar deviation is increased)	"Rotate your hand laterally outward from your body (toward the ulna)"	Apply resistance to the ulnar surface of the hand

(continued)

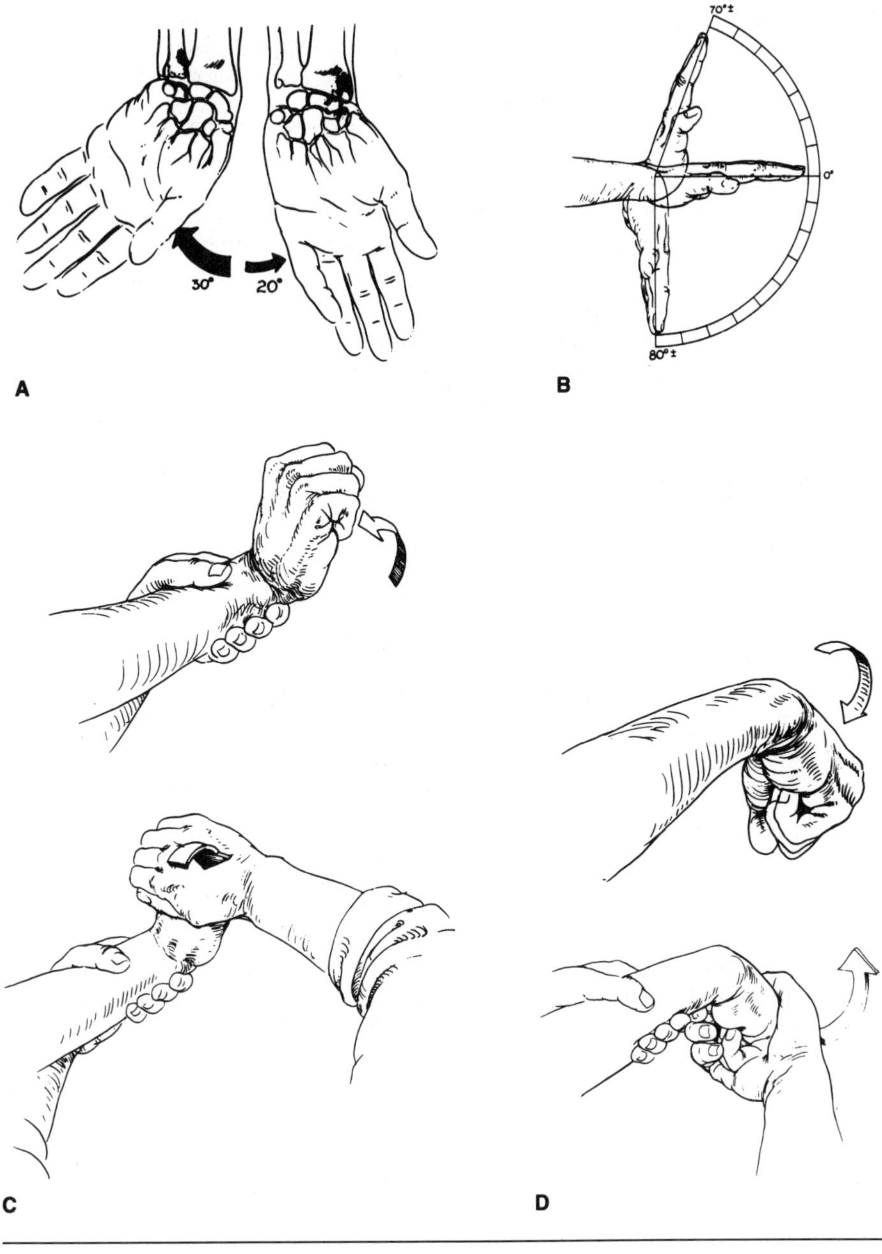

Figure 2–13. **A.** Ulmar and radial deviation of the wrist. **B.** Wrist flexion and extension range of motion. **C.** Muscle test for wrist extension. **D.** Muscle test for wrist flexion.

ASSESSING RANGE OF MOTION IN THE WRIST—*(Continued)*

Wrist Movements and Normal Range of Motion	*Instructions to Patient*	*Procedure for Testing Muscle Strength*
Lateral (radial) deviation: 20 degrees	"Rotate your hand laterally inward toward your body (toward the radius)"	Apply resistance to the radial surface of the hand

Hand and Fingers

Inspect and compare the hands in terms of their bony and muscular structures, noting any swelling, redness, nodules, and deformities, such as extra fingers (polydactyly), missing fingers, partially amputated fingers, or webbing between fingers (syndactyly). Inspect the thenar and hypothenar eminences for atrophy, which deepens the palmar depression. Palpate the hand and fingers for bony landmarks, noting any tenderness, bogginess, or nodules. Have the patient perform active range of motion of the hand and fingers (Fig. 2–14).

ASSESSING RANGE OF MOTION IN THE HAND AND FINGERS

Hand and Finger Movements and Normal Range of Motion	*Instructions to Patient*	*Procedure for Testing Muscle Strength*
Thumb		
Metacarpophalangeal joint		
Flexion: 50 degrees	"Bend your thumb to touch your palm"	Apply resistance to the volar surface of the thumb
Extension: 0 degrees	"Straighten out your thumb as if thumbing a ride"	Apply resistance to the dorsal surface of the thumb
Abduction: 70 degrees	"With your palm up, raise your thumb to the ceiling"	Apply resistance to the lateral surface of the thumb
Adduction: 0 degrees	"Bring your thumb against the index finger"	Apply resistance to the medial surface of the thumb
Opposition—touching each fingertip with the tip of the thumb	"Touch the top of the right (left) thumb to the tip and then to the base of the little, ring, middle, and index fingers"	Apply resistance to the volar surfaces of the thumb and fingers
Interphalangeal joint		
Flexion: 90 degrees Extension: 20 degrees		
Hand		
Metacarpophalangeal joint		
Flexion: 90 degrees	"Bend your fingers at the first joint"	Apply resistance to the volar surface of the proximal and distal phalanges

(continued)

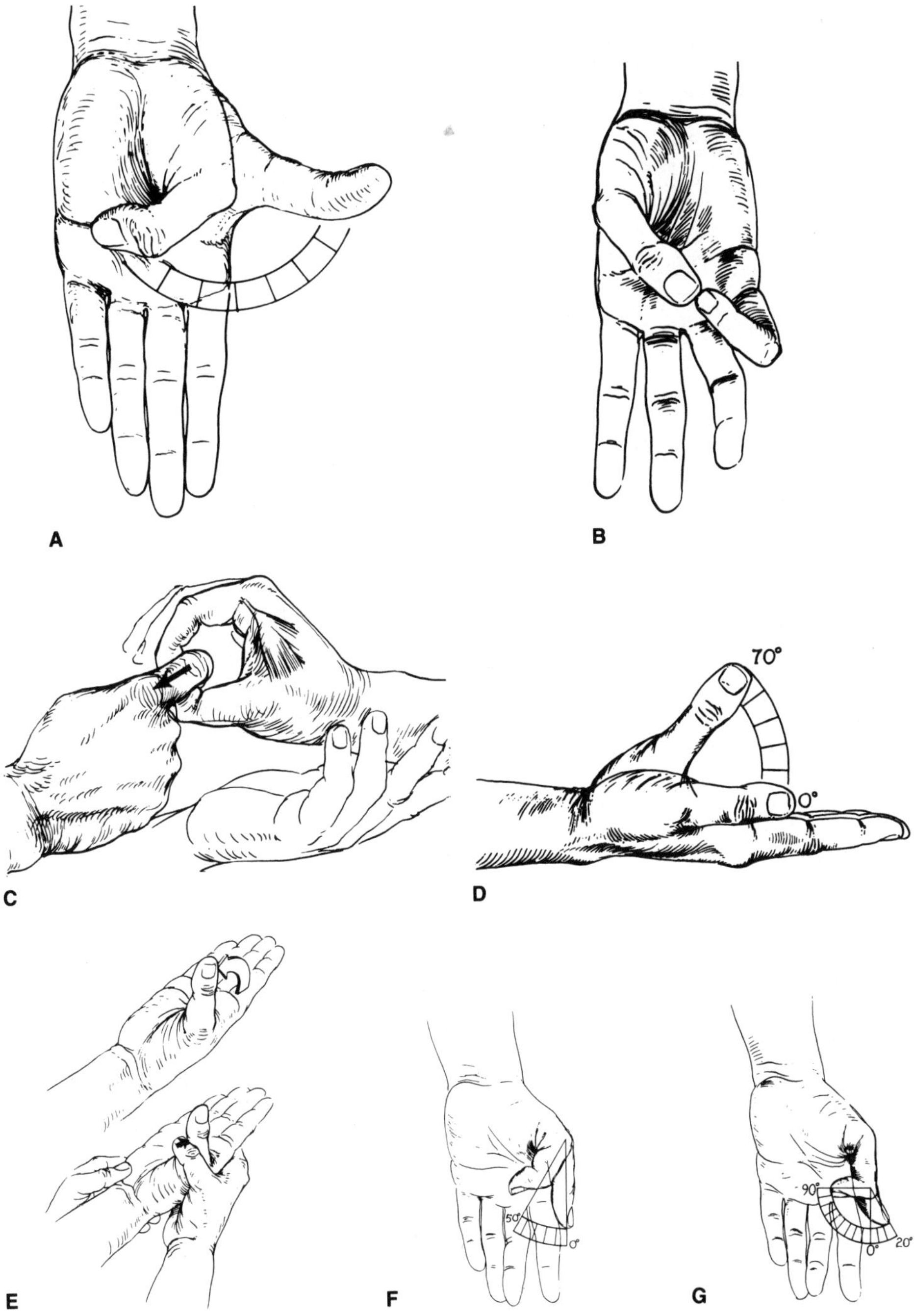

Figure 2–14. A. Thumb flexion and extension. **B.** Opposition of the thumb and fingertips. **C.** Muscle test for the pinch mechanism. **D.** Palmar abduction–adduction of the thumb. **E.** A muscle test for thumb abduction. **F.** Thumb flexion and extension, metacarpophalangeal joint. **G.** Thumb flexion and estension, interphalangeal joint. *(continued)*

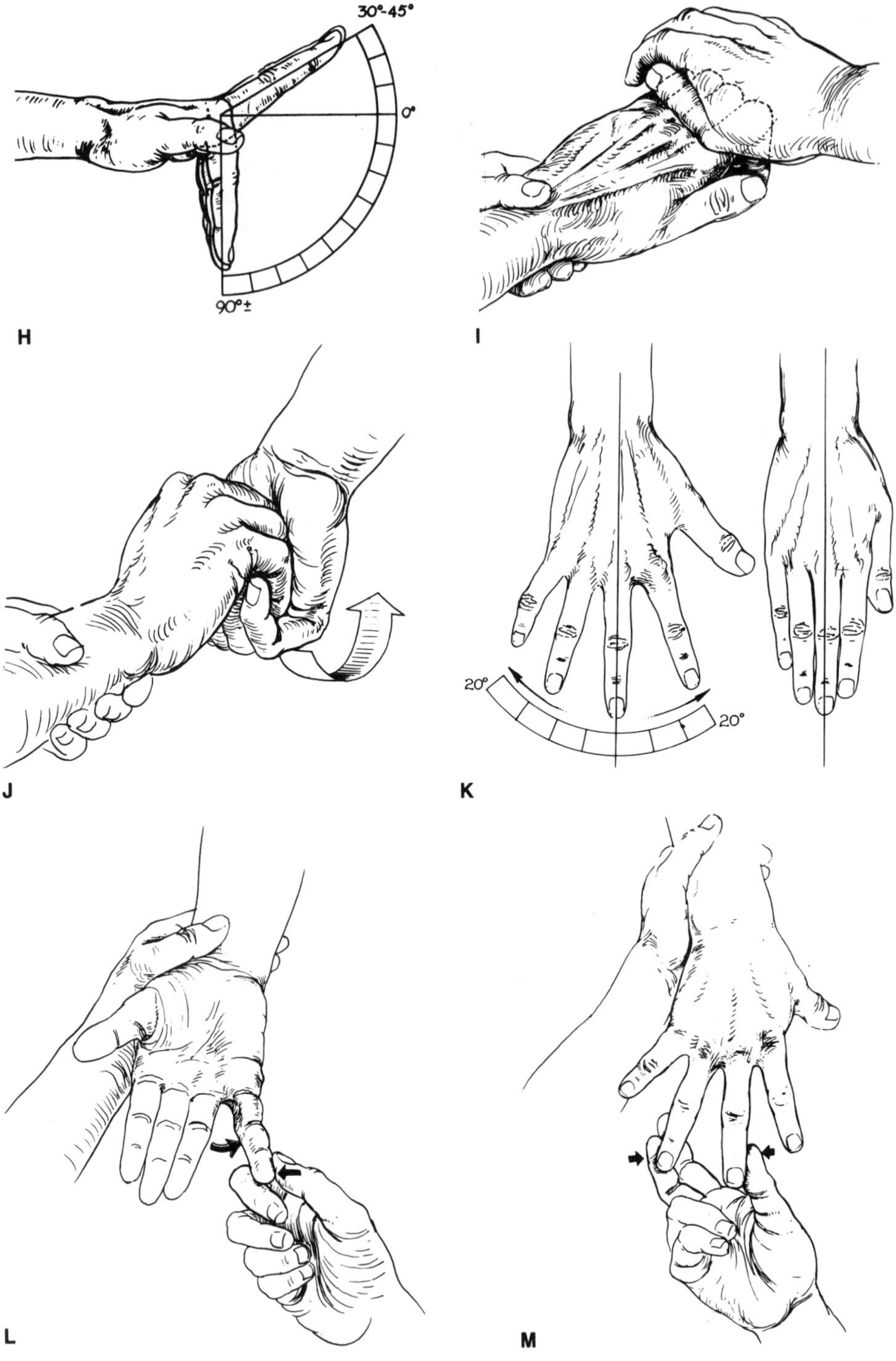

Figure 2–14. H. Metacarpophalangeal joint range of motion, flexion–extension. **I.** Muscle test for finger extension. **J.** Muscle test for finger flexion. **K.** Finger abduction and adduction. **L.** Muscle test for finger abduction. **M.** Muscle test for finger abduction. *(continued)*

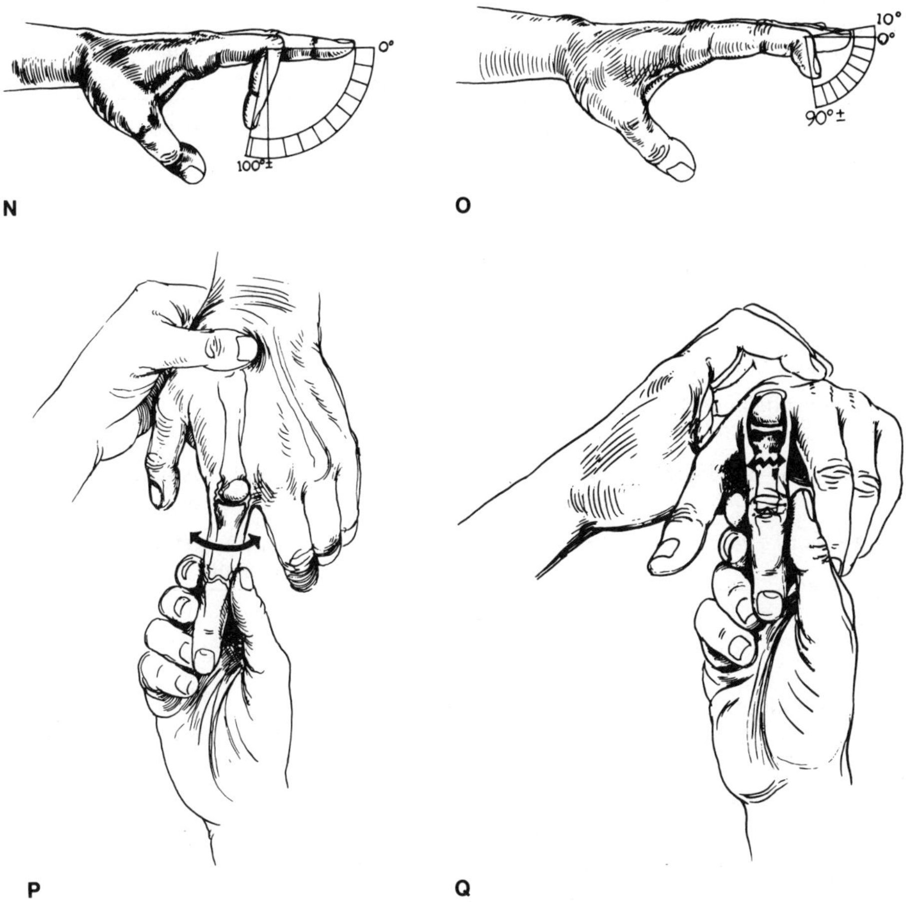

Figure 2–14. N. Proximal interphalangeal joint range of motion, flexion–extension. **O.** Distal interphalangeal joint range of motion, flexion–extension. **P.** The metacarpophalangeal joints can be moved laterally a few degrees when extended. **Q.** There is no motion in the metacarpophalangeal joints when they are flexed.

ASSESSING RANGE OF MOTION IN THE HAND AND FINGERS—*(Continued)*

Hand and Finger Movements and Normal Range of Hand Motion	*Instructions to Patient*	*Procedure for Testing Muscle Strength*
Extension: 30–45 degrees	"Straighten out your fingers"	Apply resistance to the dorsal surface of the proximal and distal phalanges
Abduction: 20 degrees between fingers	"Spread your fingers as far apart as possible"	Apply resistance against the medial and lateral surfaces of the fingers being tested

ASSESSING RANGE OF MOTION IN THE HAND AND FINGERS—*(Continued)*

Hand and Finger Movements and Normal Range of Hand Motion	*Instructions to Patient*	*Procedure for Testing Muscle Strength*
Adduction: fingers should touch	"Put your fingers together"	Apply resistance by attempting to pull the fingers apart
Proximal interphalangeal joint		
Flexion: 100–120 degrees	"Bend your fingers at the middle joint"	Apply resistance to the volar surface of the middle phalanx
Extension: 0 degrees		
Distal interphalangeal joint		
Flexion: 80–90 degrees	"Bend your distal finger joint"	Apply resistance to the volar surface of the fingertip
Extension: 20 degrees	"Straighten your finger as much as possible"	Apply resistance to the fingernails

Hip and Pelvis

Observe the patient's ability to move, sit, get onto the examination table, and lie supine. Note if the movements are smooth or if the patient has any difficulty performing them. Look for any bruising, abrasions, or swelling. With the patient's legs aligned symmetrically, check for equal leg length (if they appear unequal, measure; see p. 17–18). With the patient lying supine, palpate the iliac crests, the anterior spines of the pelvis, and the symphysis. With the patient lying prone, palpate the ischial tuberosities and feel along the spine for tenderness, swelling, or nodules. Have the patient perform active range of motion of the hip and pelvis (Fig. 2–15).

ASSESSING RANGE OF MOTION IN THE HIP AND PELVIS

Hip and Pelvis Movements and Normal Range of Motion	*Instructions to Patient*	*Procedure for Testing Muscle Strength*
Flexion: 110–120 degrees	"Draw your knees up to your chest" (while sitting or supine)	Apply resistance to the anterior surface of the leg proximal to the knee

(continued)

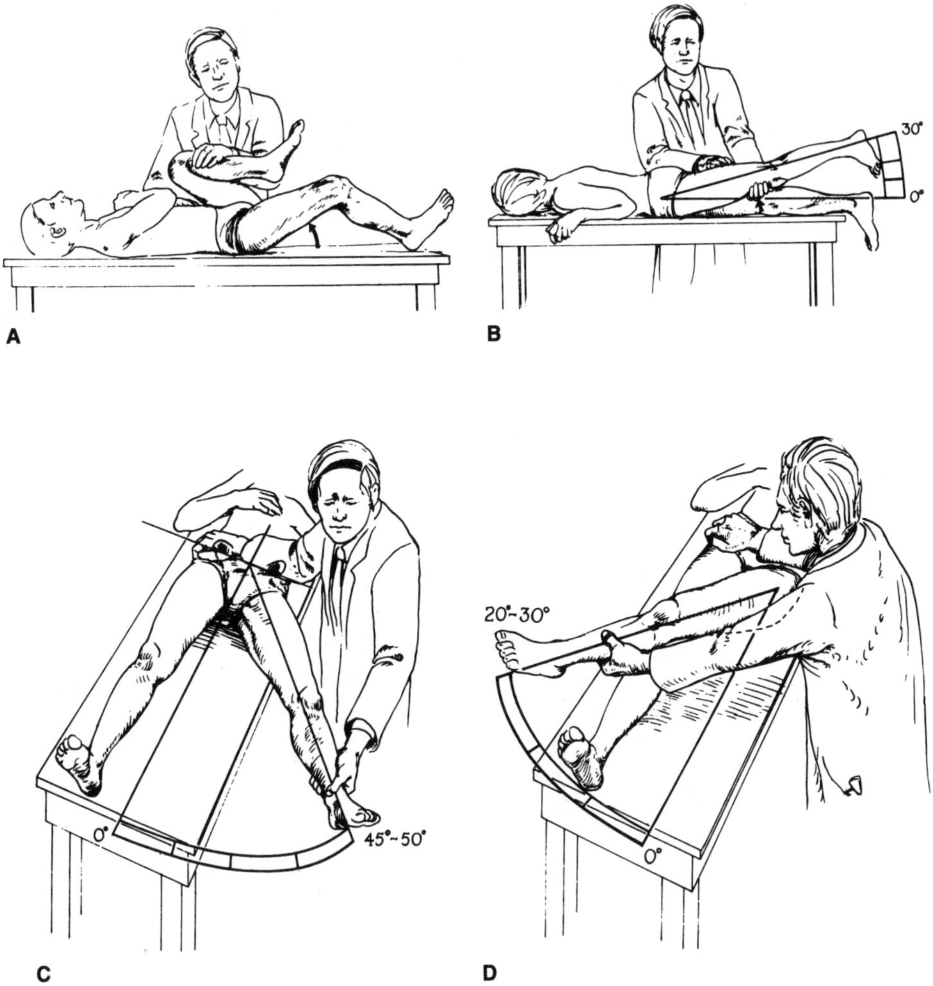

Figure 2–15. A. The normal limit for hip flexion is approximately 135 degrees. **B.** Test for hip extension. **C.** Normal limits for hip abduction are 45 to 50 degrees. **D.** Normal limits for hip adduction are 20 to 30 degrees. *(continued)*

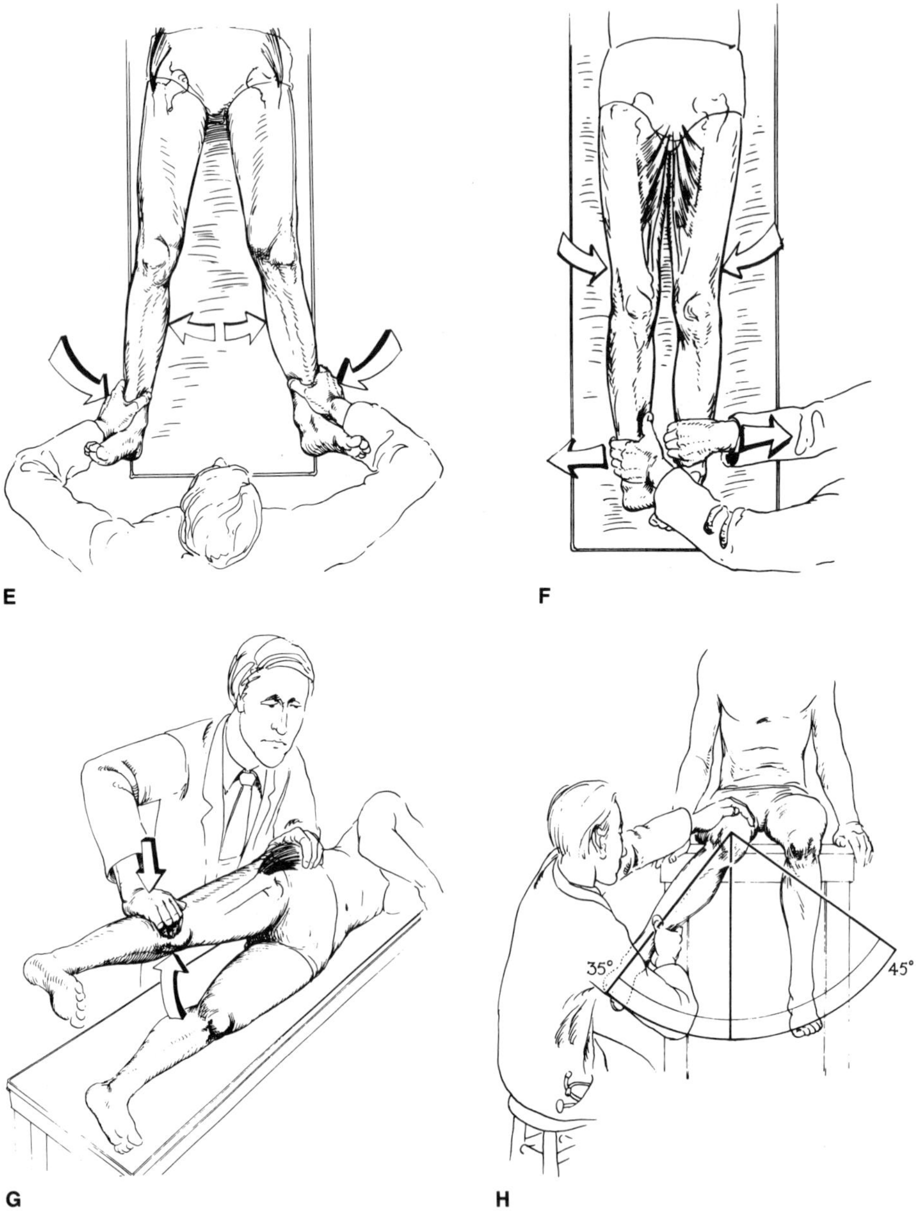

Figure 2–15. E. Alternate muscle test for abduction (gluteus medius). **F.** Test for adductor muscle strength. **G.** Muscle test for abduction. **H.** Test for internal and external femoral rotation on the flexed position.

ASSESSING RANGE OF MOTION IN THE HIP AND PELVIS—*(Continued)*

Hip and Pelvis Movements and Normal Range of Motion	*Instructions to Patient*	*Procedure for Testing Muscle Strength*
Extension: 30 degrees or less	"Lift your leg toward the ceiling" (while lying prone)	Apply resistance to the posterior surface of the leg proximal to the knee
Abduction: 45–50 degrees	"Move your upper leg toward the ceiling" (while lying on a side)	Apply resistance to the lateral surface of the upper leg
Adduction: 20–30 degrees	"Try to bring your legs together"	Apply resistance to the medial surfaces of the upper legs
Internal rotation: 45 degrees (with knee extended)	"Pivot your hip inward by turning your foot away from your body" (while sitting)	Apply resistance against the lateral surface of the ankle and foot
External rotation: 35 degrees (with knee extended)	"Rotate your hip outward by turning your foot toward your body" (while sitting)	Apply resistance to the medial ankle and foot

Knee

Inspect the patient's knee while the patient is supine, observing the contour and alignment. Note any deformities (such as knock-knees or bowlegs), redness, swelling, or nodules. Observe the quadriceps muscles for contour, symmetry, and atrophy, and look for the normal hollows around the patella. If muscle atrophy is present, measure the circumference of the leg (see p. 16); it is normal for the dominant leg to be up to 1 cm (0.4 inches) larger. Palpate each knee by placing your thumb and forefinger over the suprapatellar pouch on both sides of the quadriceps. Check for any bogginess or tenderness in the synovial membrane. Observe the muscle structures around the knee, and note any bony enlargements or points of tenderness in the joint, muscles, and tendons. Compare the two knees. Palpate the quadriceps muscles, starting at the uppermost aspect of each thigh and moving lengthwise in a circular motion to cover the anterior, posterior, medial, and lateral aspects. The thigh muscles should be firm and continuous from origin to insertion. Palpate the popliteal space to check for swelling or cysts. Have the patient perform active range of motion of the knee (Fig. 2–16).

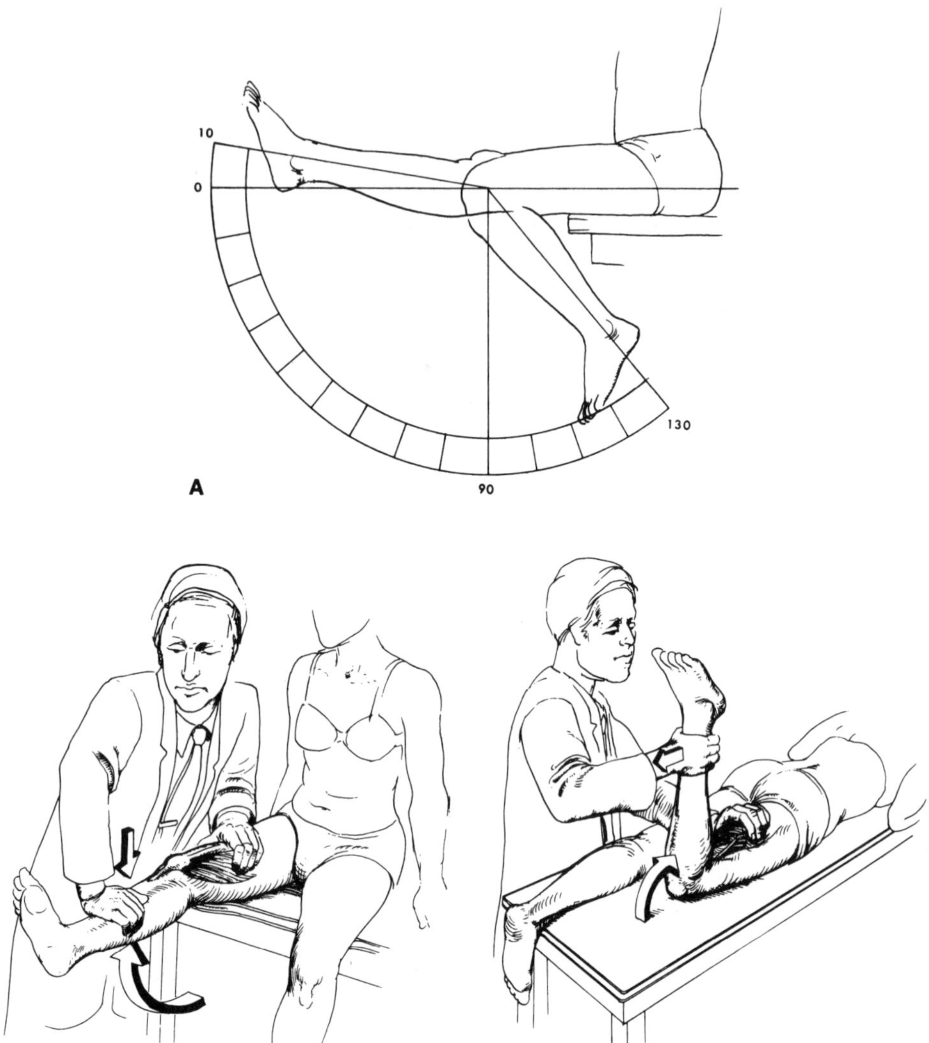

Figure 2–16. A. The range of knee motion in flexion and extension. **B.** Quadriceps muscle test. **C.** Hamstring muscle test.

ASSESSING RANGE OF MOTION IN THE KNEE

Knee Movements and Normal Range of Motion	*Instructions to Patient*	*Procedure for Testing Muscle Strength*
Flexion: 130 degrees	"Bend your right (left) leg. Try to touch your heel to the back of your leg" (while prone or sitting)	Apply resistance to the posterior ankle
Extension: 10 degrees	"Straighten out your right (left) leg as far as you can"	Apply resistance to the anterior ankle
Internal rotation: 10 degrees	"Turn your foot inward toward the midline"	Apply resistance against the medial side of the foot
External rotation: 10 degrees	"Turn your foot outward from the midline"	Apply resistance against the lateral side of the foot

Ankle and Foot

Inspect the patient's ankles and feet for swelling, tenderness, redness, nodules, and other deformities. Check the arch of each foot, look for any toe deformities, and note any skin changes. Check the position of the ankles, noting whether the medial malleolus angles in or out abnormally. Note any edema, calluses, bunions, corns, ingrown toenails, plantar warts, trophic ulcers, hair loss, or unusual pigmentation. Palpate the bony and muscular structures of the patient's ankles and feet and check for any areas of tenderness. Ask the patient to perform active range of motion of the ankle, foot, and toes. Several of the motions may need to be done passively, or at least with assistance (Fig. 2–17).

ASSESSING RANGE OF MOTION IN THE ANKLE AND FOOT

Ankle and Foot Movements and Normal Range of Motion	*Instructions to Patient*	*Procedure for Testing Muscle Strength*
Ankle		
Flexion (dorsiflexion): 20 degrees	"Bend your toes toward your knees"	Apply resistance to the dorsal aspect of the foot
Extension (plantarflexion): 45–50 degrees	"Point your toes away from you (downward) as far as you can"	Apply resistance to the ball of the foot
Inversion: 5 degrees (passive)	"Point your toes and rotate them inward along the long axis of your foot"	Apply resistance against the medial aspect of the first metatarsal
Eversion: 5 degrees (passive)	"Point your toes and rotate them outward along the long axis of your foot"	Apply resistance against the lateral aspect of the fifth metatarsal

(continued)

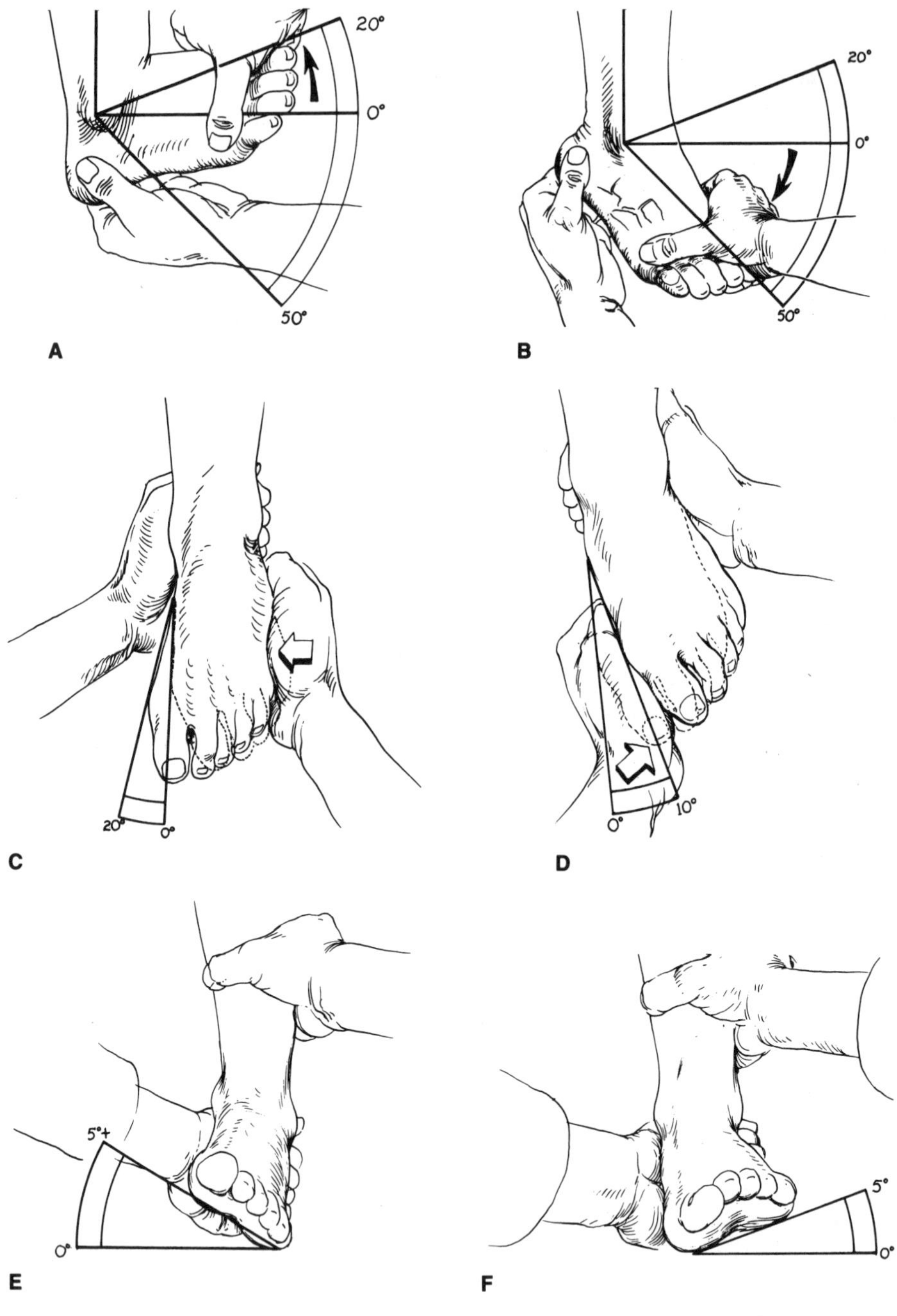

Figure 2–17. A. Range of ankle dorsiflexion. **B.** Range of ankle plantar flexion. **C.** Forefoot adduction test. **D.** Forefoot abduction test. **E.** Foot inversion test. **F.** Foot eversion test. *(continued)*

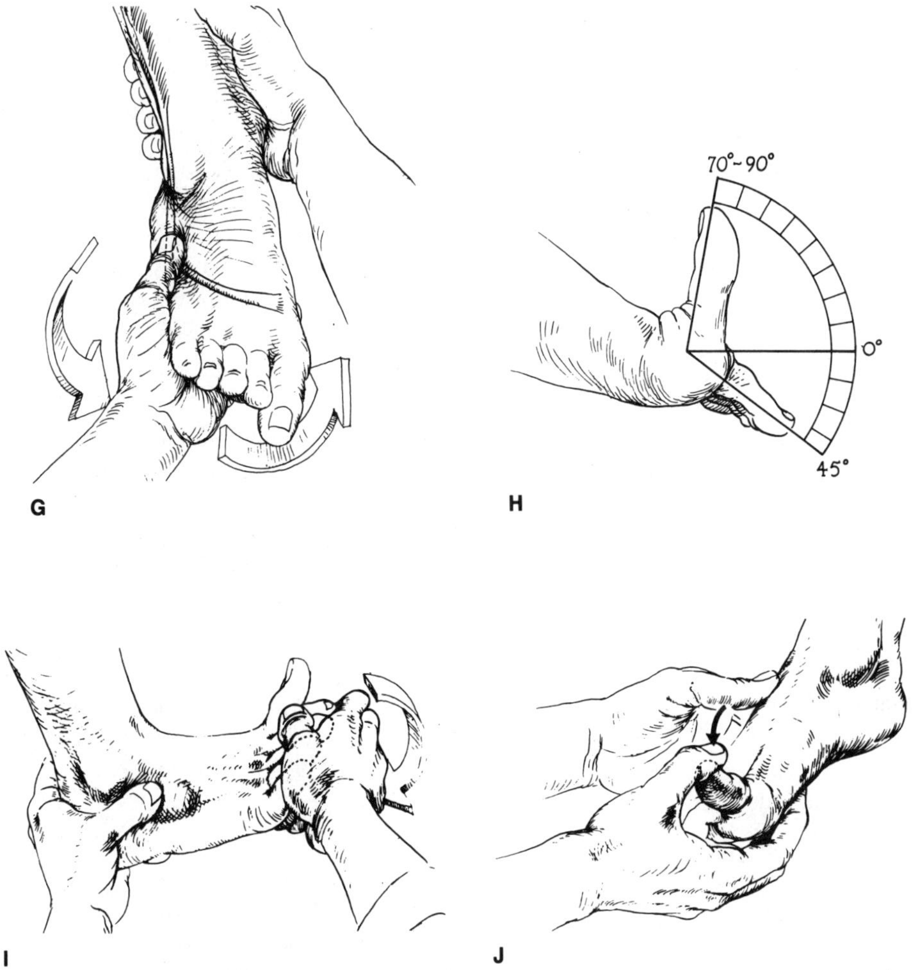

Figure 2–17. G. The peronei muscle test. **H.** The normal flexion–extension range of the first metatarsophalangeal joint. **I.** Testing the strength of the digitorum longus muscle. **J.** The extensor hallucis longus muscle test.

ASSESSING RANGE OF MOTION IN THE ANKLE AND FOOT—*(Continued)*

Ankle and Foot Movements and Normal Range of Motion	*Instructions to Patient*	*Procedure for Testing Muscle Strength*
Abduction: 10 degrees (passive)	"Point your toes; then move them outward"	Apply resistance against the fifth metatarsal
Adduction: 20 degrees (passive)	"Point your toes; then move them inward"	Apply resistance against the first metatarsal
Great toe Metatarsophalangeal joint		
Flexion: 45 degrees	"Bend your big toe downward"	Apply resistance to the plantar side of the great toe
Extension: 70–90 degrees	"Bend your big toe upward"	Apply resistance to the dorsum of the great toe
Toes Metatarsophalangeal joints		
Flexion: 40 degrees	"Bend all your toes downward"	Apply resistance to the plantar surface of the proximal phalanges
Extension: 40 degrees	"Straighten out your toes and point them upward"	Apply resistance to the dorsum of the proximal phalanges
Interphalangeal proximal joints		
Flexion: 35 degrees	"Bend your toes downward"	Apply resistance to the plantar surface of the medial phalanges
Extension: 0 degrees		
Interphalangeal distal joints		
Flexion: 60 degrees	"Bend your toes downward"	Apply resistance to the plantar surface of the distal phalanges
Extension: 30 degrees	"Point your toes upward"	Resistance is applied to the dorsum of the distal phalanges
Abduction: degrees vary	"Try to spread your toes apart"	

DIAGNOSTIC PROCEDURES

A third source of information on the patient is gained from diagnostic procedures. The major diagnostic techniques are (1) joint aspirations, (2) biopsies, (3) arthroscopies, (4) roentgenographic examinations, (5) electromyographies, and (6) laboratory studies.

Joint Aspiration

Joint aspiration is performed to obtain samples of synovial fluid from within the joint cavity. The procedure is performed by introducing a needle into the joint cavity and withdrawing fluid. It aids in determining the presence of aseptic inflammatory processes, such as rheumatoid arthritis, and septic processes, such as bacterial arthritis.

The synovial fluid samples are cultured and examined microscopically and chemically. Synovial fluid is normally straw-colored and clear. Its viscosity resembles that of motor oil. In the presence of inflammation, it becomes turbid and more watery; the number of white blood cells, the protein content, and the number of polymorphonuclear cells are increased; and the glucose content is decreased.

A local anesthetic is usually administered before the procedure. After the procedure, the joint is often dressed and an elastic bandage applied for 8 to 24 hours. If infection is present in the joint and there is drainage from the joint following aspiration, precautions should be taken with the wound dressings to prevent the possible spread of infection.

Biopsy

A biopsy is the removal of tissue for purposes of microscopic examination to confirm a diagnosis, to follow the course of a disease, or to determine the effectiveness of treatment. Specimens may be obtained by means of a special needle or punch, a surgical incision, or the aspiration of fluid. Needle or punch biopsies may be done at the patient's bedside, in a physician's office, an outpatient clinic, or in surgery. When a needle biopsy is done on an internal lesion, however, there is no certainty that the area sampled contains cells from the lesion. Therefore, an open incision, where the lesion is visualized, may be the method of choice. The incisional biopsy is an operative procedure under general or local anesthesia.

Muscle Biopsy

A muscle biopsy is performed to aid in the diagnosis of myopathic disorders. In most instances the muscle to be biopsied has previously been examined by gross muscle testing and electromyography (EMG). Histochemical staining of biopsied muscle tissue may reveal features of lower motor neuron disease (such as atrophy of groups of fibers innervated by single motor units), degeneration, inflammatory reactions, or involvement of specific fibers that indicate myopathic disease.

A muscle biopsy is an operative procedure usually performed under a local or general anesthetic. Following the procedure, the patient will experience minor to moderate discomfort, depending on the location of the muscle biopsied. The discomfort may be in the form of stiffness or pain at or around the operative site. If the muscle biopsied is in the lower extremity (i.e., one of the gluteals or quadriceps), the patient is usually encouraged to resume ambulation within 4 hours to avoid stiffness.

Synovial Biopsy

A synovial biopsy is helpful in differentiating various forms of arthritis. The specimen of synovium is examined histologically for evidence of inflammation, and a sample of the synovial fluid obtained at the same time is sent for culture and other studies. The biopsy may be performed as a closed biopsy with a special synovial biopsy needle (such as the Parker–Pearson) or as an open biopsy done in surgery. When a closed biopsy is performed, the patient is given a local anesthetic. Afterwards, a small compression dressing with an elastic bandage is usually applied around the joint, and the patient is asked to rest the joint for 24 hours to prevent hemorrhage or effusion.

Other Biopsies

In the musculoskeletal system, biopsies also involve bone, skin, the buccal mucosa, and the temporal artery. A bone biopsy may be accomplished by an open or needle biopsy to diagnose or follow a bone disease or lesion. A punch biopsy may be taken of the skin to diagnose connective tissue disorders. The buccal mucosa may be biopsied to help diagnose Sjögren's syndrome, and the temporal artery may be biopsied to diagnose temporal arteritis.

Arthroscopy

Arthroscopy, a procedure performed in surgery, is the examination of a joint through a special fiberoptic endoscope called an arthroscope. The instrument has lenses and a light source that permits visualization, photography, and surgical procedures within the joint. After the administration of a local anesthetic and the application of a tourniquet (to reduce the blood flow), the endoscope is inserted into the joint cavity through a small incision. Normal saline is instilled to provide a viewing medium, enabling the physician to see the structure and contents of the joint. In the past, the usefulness of the procedure was limited mainly to the knee, but it is now being used for other joints, especially the shoulder. The procedure permits biopsy or removal of a torn meniscus, removal of loose bodies, and in some instances biopsy of a synovium or cartilage.

Once the procedure is completed, a compression dressing with an ace bandage is applied. Following a knee arthroscopy, the patient may be allowed weight bearing, but must avoid excessive use of the joint for 24 to 48 hours, depending upon the procedure done. Because an arthroscopy is frequently done on an outpatient basis, make sure the patient knows the signs of infection and who to contact if a problem should arise.

Roentgenographic Examinations

Roentgenograms of Bones and Joints

Roentgenographic (x-ray) examination provides data important to the identification and treatment of fractures and the identification and observation of a number of pathological conditions, including rheumatoid arthritis, spondylitis, avascular necrosis, and tumors. Joint changes, such as erosion of joint margins, joint space narrowing, bone spurs, loose bodies, and dislocations can also be detected. Injuries to soft tissues, such as tendons and ligaments, do not show on roentgenograms, but soft tissue swelling can be observed.

No special preparation is required for roentgenograms of bones and joints. Some orthopaedic patients have significant mobility restrictions, however, and may be unable to lie on a hard x-ray table for any length of time. In particular, persons with arthritis, who frequently experience joint stiffness and pain, may require extensive roentgenographic examinations. Careful planning should be given in scheduling their roentgenograms, and several sessions with one or two days of rest in between may be required for patients with severe joint involvement. Analgesics before, and analgesics or local heat applications afterwards, may be necessary for relief of joint pain. When a fracture is suspected, the patient should be carefully moved to and from the table to prevent further injury. Having the suspected extremity splinted is very helpful.

Arthrogram

An arthrogram is a roentgenographic and fluoroscopic examination of a joint (usually the knee but occasionally the shoulder). Following the injection of air (pneumoarthrography), a radiopaque contrast medium is injected into the joint space, which permits the imaging of components within the joint that are not normally seen on bone and joint roentgenograms. This imaging helps to detect injuries of the meniscus, cartilage, and ligaments of the knee, and structures of the joint capsule, rotator cuff, and subacromial bursa of the shoulder.

An arthrogram of the knee is accomplished by first cleansing the skin around the puncture site and then anesthetizing the area. A needle is inserted into the joint space between the patella and the femoral condyle, and synovial fluid is aspirated. The needle is not withdrawn, and a fluoroscopic examination is done to verify correct needle placement. Dye is then injected into the joint space. After the needle is removed, the puncture site is cleansed and sealed with collodion. The patient is asked to walk a few steps or to move the knee through the normal range of motion to distribute the dye throughout the joint space. A series of films is then taken, with the knee in various positions, before the contrast medium can be absorbed by the joint tissue. Once the film series is completed, a dressing with an elastic bandage is applied to the knee. Postcare involves keeping the knee joint at rest for at least 12 hours and the dressing in place for several days. The patient may experience some swelling, discomfort, or crepitus in the joint, but the symptoms usually disappear after a day or two. Ice applied to the knee helps reduce swelling, and analgesics help reduce pain.

Myelogram

Myelogram is the roentgenographic and fluoroscopic examination of the spinal cord and subarachnoid space following the injection of a contrast medium. A myelogram is helpful in the identification of lesions in the intradural and extradural compartments of the spinal canal and in the diagnosis of abnormalities such as a herniated disc or tumor.

The myelogram involves a cisternal or lumbar spinal puncture, the removal of cerebrospinal fluid for analysis, and the injection of a radiopaque contrast medium into the subarachnoid space. The flow of the radiopaque dye through the subarachnoid space is observed using fluoroscopy. Lesions in the spinal cord or the subarachnoid space usually produce a complete or incomplete blockage in the spinal canal. The exact configuration of the defect causing the blockage is helpful in determining whether the lesion is intramedullary or extramedullary. Turning the patient in various positions helps to secure a more complete visualization. After the fluoroscopic examination and roentgenograms are completed, the dye is removed as it can cause serious irritation to the meninges.

Radioisotope Scan

A radioisotope scan permits an imaging of the skeleton by a scanning camera following the intravenous injection of a radioactive tracer compound. The tracer of choice is usually Tc-99m–sodium pertechnetate, which concentrates at sites of abnormal bone metabolism, such as sites of abnormal osteoblastic activity. In malignancies, osteoblastic activity is accelerated, and those sites appear as "hot spots" 3 to 6 months before roentgenography can reveal any lesion. A bone scan is primarily indicated in patients with symptoms of metastatic bone disease, but it is helpful for bone trauma patients, patients with bone grafts, and patients with known degenerative disorders that require monitoring for signs of progression. Bone scans can also help detect an infection after a total hip arthroplasty.

To reduce anxiety and make the procedure more comfortable, describe it to the patient, family, and significant others. The patient is required to drink several glasses of water or tea in the one- to three-hour period after the injection of the tracer and before the scan to facilitate excretion of tracer that is not absorbed by bone tissue. Advise the patient not to drink large amounts of fluid before the injection. The scan itself takes about an hour and is painless. Postcare involves checking the injection site for redness or swelling. If a hematoma develops, discomfort may be eased by warm soaks.

Computerized Axial Tomography

Computerized axial tomography (CAT scan) provides cross-sectional views of the body by passing a narrow roentgenographic beam from a computerized scanner through the body at different angles. CAT scanning may be done with or without an injected radioiodine contrast agent, which highlights blood vessels and allows greater visual discrimination. The CAT scan is a series of x-ray photographs, translated by a computer and displayed on an oscilloscope, representing the cross-sectional images of various layers (or slices) of the body. The technique can reconstruct cross-sectional, horizontal, and sagittal plane images.

CAT scans are at least a hundred times more sensitive than ordinary roentgenograms, and can discriminate even slight variations in tissue densities to help diagnose a disease at an earlier stage in the disease process. For example, a lumbar CAT scan presents sharper images than a myelogram, and provides cross-sectional displays that are not possible with myelograms.

The CAT scan can be done on an outpatient or inpatient basis. For a scan without a contrast medium, there is no physical preparation of the patient, but educating the patient about the procedure is essential. The patient lies on a hydraulically adjustable couch, which is moved into a doughnutlike scanner opening. When the patient is positioned, the scanner revolves around the body. The patient usually lies supine during the scan. During the scan, the patient will hear clicking noises that are normal scanner sounds. The procedure is painless but the patient may become uncomfortable as the scan takes 10 to 45 minutes. If the patient is very restless, the physician may order a sedative as movements during the scan cause a streaking of the image.

Electromyography

Electromyography measures electrical activity across muscle membranes by means of needle electrodes. The procedure yields information on the condition of nerve impulses to muscles, as well as the response of those muscles to the nerve impulses. No electrical activity is present in normal muscles at rest, but electrical activity can be detected during volitional movements. During the procedure, electrical activity is recorded with the muscle at rest, during voluntary movement, and during electrical stimulation. The electrical activity can be heard over a loudspeaker, viewed on an oscilloscope, or printed on a graph called an electromyogram (EMG). In primary myopathic and neuropathic disorders, there are specific patterns of electrical activity, and in neurogenic atrophy there may be fibrillations in resting muscles. An EMG is thus particularly helpful in the diagnosis of lower motor neuron disease, primary muscle disease, and diseases involving defects in the transmission of electrical impulses across neuromuscular junctions, such as myasthenia gravis. However, electromyography cannot be used to differentiate specific disease entities in either the myopathic or neuropathic categories.

There is no special preparation for the procedure. The patient should be informed, however, that small needles will be inserted into the skin and muscles which may cause some discomfort, though there is no danger of an electrical shock.

Blood Tests

Tests on the patient's blood provide information useful in diagnosing and following the course of many disease processes. Even though routine blood tests, such as white blood counts and hematocrits, are used in orthopaedic practice, only tests that are commonly used for musculoskeletal conditions are presented in Table 2–5.

TABLE 2–5. DIAGNOSTIC TESTS USED FOR MUSCULOSKELETAL CONDITIONS

Laboratory Test	Normal Values	Indications for Abnormal Values
Blood		
Alkaline phosphatase	1.5 to 4.0 Bodansky units/dl 4 to 13.5 King–Armstrong units/dl	Increased in osteoblastic bone tumors (osteogenic sarcoma and metastatic carcinoma), inflammatory conditions, rickets, osteomalacia, hyperparathyroidism, and during fracture healing
Acid phosphatase	0.5 to 2.0 Bodansky units/dl 1 to 5 King–Armstrong units/dl	Increased in Paget's disease and carcinoma of the bone
Calcium (Ca)	7 to 12 mg/dl 4.5 to 5.5 mEq/L	Increased in metastatic bone cancer, acute osteoporosis, multiple myeloma, prolonged immobilization, and during fracture healing Decreased in hypoparathyroidism, osteomalacia, and rickets
Creatine phosphokinase (CPK)	15 to 57 units/L in women 23 to 99 units/L in men 0 to 12 Sigma units/cc	Increased in necrosis or atrophy of skeletal muscles, traumatic muscle injury, strenuous exercise, and progressive muscular dystrophy
Lactic dehydrogenase (LDH)	80 to 120 Wacker units 48 to 115 IU/L 150 to 450 Wroblewskin units	Increased in muscular dystrophy, damage to skeletal muscles (0–14 days postinjury), after a pulmonary embolism, and during skeletal muscle malignancy
Phosphorus (P)	3.0 to 4.5 mg/dl 1.8 to 2.6 mEq/L	Increased in fracture healing, osteoporosis, and hypoparathyroidism
Serum glutamic oxaloacetic transaminase (SGOT)	8 to 20 units/L 5 to 40 Karmen units	Increased in skeletal muscle damage and muscular dystrophy
Serum glutamic pyruvic transaminase (SGPT)	5 to 40 Karmen units	Increased in skeletal muscle damage
Uric acid	2.3 to 6.0 mg/dl in women 4.3 to 8.0 mg/dl in men	Increased in gout, multiple myeloma, arthritis, and hyperparathyroidism Decreased in acromegaly
Creatine	0–40 mg/24 hours in men 0–100 mg/24 hours in women	Increased in active rheumatoid arthritis and skeletal muscle damage

(continued)

TABLE 2–5. *(Continued)*

Laboratory Test	Normal Values	Indications for Abnormal Values
C-Reactive protein	Negative	Positive in any acute inflammatory change or necrosis, widespread metastasis, and rheumatoid arthritis
Antinuclear antibodies (ANA)	Negative	Positive in rheumatoid arthritis
Human lymphocyte antigen B27 (HLA-B27)	Negative	Positive in ankylosing spondylitis and rheumatoid arthritis
Lupus erythematosis cell preparation (LE prep)	Negative	Positive in rheumatoid arthritis
Serum rheumatoid factor (RF)	Negative	Positive (titers in the 1:100 to 1:160 range) in rheumatoid arthritis and some chronic inflammatory diseases
Urine		
Calcium	1^+ to 2^+ 275 mg/24 hours in men 250 mg/24 hours in women	Increased in hyperparathyroidism, osteolytic bone disease, and osteoporosis Decreased in hypoparathyroidism and osteomalacia

(Sources: Bryne, J. C. et al., 1981; Donahoo, C. A., & Dimon, J. H. 1977, p. 14; Mourad, L., 1980, pp. 430–439.)

REFERENCES

Bates, B. *A guide to physical examination.* Philadelphia: Lippincott, 1979.

Block, G. J., & Nolan, J. W. *Health assessment for professional nursing: A developmental approach.* Norwalk, Conn.: Appleton-Century-Crofts, 1986.

Bryne, J. C., Saxton, D. F., Pelikan, P. K., & Nugent, P. M. *Laboratory tests: Implications for nurses and allied health professionals.* Menlo Park, Calif: Addison-Wesley, 1981.

Craig, K. D. Social modelling influences on pain. In R. A. Sternbeck (Ed.), *The psychology of pain.* New York: Raven, 1978.

Donahoo, C. A., & Dimon, J. H. *Orthopedic nursing.* Boston: Little, Brown, 1977.

Hoppenfeld, S. *Physical examination of the spine and extremities.* New York: Appleton-Century-Crofts, 1976.

Malasanos, L., Barkaukas, V., Mass, M., & Stoltenberg-Allen, K. *Health assessment.* St. Louis: C. V. Mosby, 1977.

Meinhart, N. T., & McCaffery, M. *Pain: A nursing approach to assessment and analysis.* Norwalk, Conn.: Appleton-Century-Crofts, 1983.

Melzack, R. *The puzzle of pain.* New York: Basic Harper Torchbooks, 1973.

Mourad, L. *Nursing care of adults with orthopedic conditions.* New York: Wiley, 1980.

Seiden, M. R. *Practical management of chronic neuralgic problems.* New York: Appleton-Century-Crofts, 1981.

Sternback, R. A. *Pain: A psychophysiological analysis.* New York: Academic Press, 1968.

BIBLIOGRAPHY

Byerman, K. Flawed perceptions about pain. *American Journal of Nursing,* 1982, *82*(2), 302–304.

Corbett, J. V. *Diagnostic procedures in nursing practice.* Norwalk, Conn.: Appleton-Century-Crofts, 1983.

De Gowin, E. L., & De Gowin, R. L. *Bedside diagnostic examination* (3rd ed.). New York: Macmillan, 1976.

Deutsch, S. D., & Gandsman, E. J. The use of bone scanning for the diagnosis and management of musculoskeletal trauma. *Surgical Clinics of North America,* 1983, *63*(3), 567–586.

Dossey, B. Perfecting your skills for systematic patient assessment. *Nursing 79,* 1979, *9* (2), 42–45.

Dunn, B. H. Musculoskeletal assessment: Gait assessment. *Orthopedic Nursing,* 1982, *1* (1), 33–37.

Dunn, B. H. Musculoskeletal assessment: Components of musculoskeletal examination. *Orthopedic Nursing,* 1982, *1* (6), 33–37.

Farrell, J. Orthopedic pain: What does it mean? *American Journal of Nursing,* 1984, *84* (4), 466–469.

Gillies, D. A., & Alyn, I. B. *Patient assessment and management by the nurse practitioner.* Philadelphia: Saunders, 1976.

Haughey, C. W. What to say—And do—When your patient asks about CT scans. *Nursing 81,* 1981, *11* (12), 72–76.

Hubbard, L. F. Computed tomography in orthopedics. *Surgical Clinics of North America,* 1983, *63* (3), 587–598.

Jacox, A. Assessing pain. *American Journal of Nursing,* 1979, *79* (5), 895–901.

Laughlin, R. M., & Clancy, G. J. Musculoskeletal assessment: Neurovascular examination of the injured extremity. *Orthopedic Nursing,* 1982, *1* (1), 43–48.

Lowe, E. B., Jr. Diagnostic and operative arthroscopy. *Surgical Clinics of North America,* 1983 *63* (3), 599–606.

Macleod, J. *Clinical examination.* New York: Churchill Livingstone, 1976.

McCaffery, M. Relieving pain and noninvasive techniques. *Nursing 80,* 1980, *10* (12), 54–58.

McCaffery, M. When your patient's still in pain, don't just do something—Sit there. *Nursing 81,* 1981, *11* (6); 58–61.

McCaffery, M. Would you administer placebos for pain? *Nursing 82,* 1982, *12* (2), 80–85.

McGuire, L. A short simple tool for assessing your patient's pain. *Nursing 81,* 1981, *11* (3), 48–49.

Meissner, J. E. McGill–Melzack pain questionnaire. *Nursing 80,* 1980, *10* (1), 50–52.

Moore, D. E., & Blacker, H. M. For chronic pain? *American Journal of Nursing,* 1983, *83* (8), 1175–1177.

Nurses Reference Library. *Diagnostics.* Springhouse, Pa.: Nursing 81 Books, Intermed Communications, 1981.

Nurses Reference Library. *Procedures.* Springhouse, Pa.: Nursing 83 Books, Intermed Communications, 1983.

Nursing 81 Books. *Nursing photobook: Assessing your patients.* Springhouse, Pa.: Nursing 81 Books, Intermed Communications, 1981.

Nursing 83 Books. *Nursing photobook: Carrying out special procedures.* Springhouse, Pa.: Nursing 83 Books, Intermed Communications, 1983.

Sauvé, M. J., & Percherer, A. *Concepts and skills in physical assessment.* Philadelphia: Saunders, 1977.

Sherman, J. L., & Fields, S. K. *Guide to patient evaluation.* Flushing, N.Y.: Medical Examination, 1974.

Storlie, F. Pointers for assessing pain. *Nursing 78,* 1978, *8* (5), 37–39.

Taylor, A. G., West, B. A., Simon, B., et al. How effective is TENS for acute pain? *American Journal of Nursing,* 1983, *83* (8), 1171–1174.

Thompson, J. M., & Bowers, A. C. *Clinical manual of health assessment.* St. Louis: C. V. Mosby, 1980.

Vanderbeck, K. A. Getting the facts: A guide to orthopedic assessment. *Orthopaedic Nursing,* 1984, *3* (5), 31–34.

3

MUSCULOSKELETAL TRAUMA

Chapter 3 discusses the effects of trauma on the musculoskeletal system. It examines soft tissue trauma, including contusions, strains, sprains, and dislocations, and fractures, including first-aid measures, methods of repair, complications from fractures, and complications from imposed immobility. In-depth discussions of specific injuries, methods of treatment, and associated nursing care are provided in later chapters.

Musculoskeletal injuries are relatively common occurrences. Many injuries occur at home from lifting heavy objects, slipping in the bathtub or on a wet or waxed floor, tripping over rugs or pets, falling off chairs or ladders, and falling down stairs. Other injuries occur in motor vehicle accidents, during recreational activities, and on the job. Musculoskeletal injuries can even occur during "normal" activities, as when violent coughing fractures a rib. Factors that increase the possibility of musculoskeletal injuries are age, because older persons have more fragile bones, and pathological conditions that weaken the musculoskeletal system.

SOFT TISSUE TRAUMA

Contusions

A contusion is a soft tissue injury or bruise produced by a blunt force such as a blow, kick, or fall. There is always some hemorrhage into the injured part due to the rupture of small blood vessels. That hemorrhage (ecchymosis) produces skin discolorations ("black and blue" marks), which gradually turn purplish, then yellow, and finally disappear as absorption becomes complete. When the hemorrhage is sufficient to cause an appreciable collection of blood, a hematoma forms with local symptoms of pain, swelling, and discoloration.

Treatment of a contusion consists of elevating the affected part and applying moist or dry cold for the first 8 to 10 hours to produce vasoconstriction and a consequent decrease in hemorrhage and edema. Cold applications should be kept in place for 20 to 30 minutes at a time. After the first 24 hours, heat is usually applied for 20 minutes at a time to promote absorption and repair. Because heat can cause swelling and increase tissue fluid, hot compresses may be followed by cold applications to minimize those effects. Pressure in the form of an elastic bandage can also help reduce the hemorrhage and swelling.

Strains

A strain is an injury to the musculotendinous structures surrounding a joint, produced by an excessive force or stretching, which causes hemorrhage into the tissues. Strains may be classified as first-degree strains (mild strains or slightly pulled muscles), second-degree strains (moderate strains or moderately pulled muscles), and third-degree strains (severely pulled muscles).

A first-degree strain causes a low-grade inflammation and some disruption of muscle–tendon tissue, but little hemorrhage. The patient has local pain in the area, which is aggravated by movement or muscle tension. Other symptoms include swelling, ecchymosis, local tenderness, and a minor loss of function and strength in the affected joint. Complications, which can occur following a mild strain, are recurrence of the strain, tendinitis, and periostitis at the tendinous attachment site.

A second-degree strain involves the tearing of musculotendinous fibers without a complete disruption of the muscle or the tendon. The patient has local pain, which is aggravated by movement or muscle tension, moderate muscle spasm, swelling, ecchymosis, local tenderness, and impaired muscle function. Complications are the same as those for a first-degree strain.

Patients with a third-degree strain have a ruptured muscle or tendon with the separation of muscle from muscle, muscle from tendon, or tendon from bone. There is severe pain and disability, severe spasm, swelling, ecchymosis, hematoma, tenderness, loss of muscle function, and usually a palpable defect in the joint. Roentgenograms are usually necessary as they can demonstrate soft tissue swelling and an avulsion fracture at the tendinous attachment.

Treatment of strains focuses on decreasing the swelling and immobilizing the joint with the disrupted tissues approximated. It usually consists of elevating and resting the affected part, with cold compresses applied for 15 to 20 minutes four times a day. The vasoconstricting effect of the cold retards the extravasation of blood and lymph and reduces pain. Sometimes additional support is provided by temporary splinting or an elastic bandage. In third-degree strains, surgery may be required occasionally to suture the muscle and surrounding fascia. The joint is then immobilized until healing occurs.

Sprains

A sprain is an injury to the ligamentous structures surrounding a joint, caused by a wrench or a twist. Blood vessels are ruptured, resulting in rapid swelling due to the extravasation of blood within the tissues. Movement of the joint becomes painful. The function of a ligament is to maintain stability while permitting mobility, and a torn ligament causes the joint to lose functional stability.

Sprains are classified as first-degree (or mild) sprains, second-degree (or moderate) sprains, and third-degree (or severe) sprains. A mild sprain consists of a minor tearing of ligamentous fibers causing mild, focused tenderness, no abnormal motion, little or no swelling, minimal hemorrhage, and minimal functional loss. The principal complication is the recurrence of a mild sprain.

A moderate sprain, the partial tearing of a ligament, involves focused tenderness, moderate loss of function, slight to moderate abnormal motion, swelling, and localized hemorrhage. Complications following a moderate sprain are a tendency toward recurrent sprains, persistent instability, and traumatic arthritis.

A severe sprain, the complete tearing of a ligament, involves a loss of function, marked abnormal motion, possible deformity, tenderness, swelling, and hemorrhage. Stress roentgenograms, done when pain is adequately relieved, demonstrate a loss of joint stability. Complications following a severe sprain are the same as those following a moderate sprain.

The immediate treatment of sprains includes rest and elevation of the affected part and the use of intermittent cold compresses to retard the extravasation of blood vessels and lymph and to reduce pain. After 24 hours, mild heat may be applied at 15- to 30-minute intervals four times a day to promote absorption. For mild or moderate sprains, additional support is usually provided by a temporary splint or an elastic bandage. If the sprain is severe, surgical repair or cast immobilization is necessary to restore joint stability. Ligaments are relatively avascular, so healing is slow. The larger ligaments must be protected until there is maturation of the scar, usually 8 to 16 weeks. (For further information on sprains of specific joints, see later chapters.)

Dislocations

A dislocation is when the articular surfaces of the bones forming a joint are out of anatomical position. Dislocations may be congenital (such as a congenital dislocated hip), pathological (i.e., due to a disease of the articular or periarticular structures), or traumatic (i.e., from an external force). Signs of a dislocation are pain, changes in the contour of the joint, changes in the length of an extremity, loss of mobility, and changes in the axis of the dislocated bones.

Treatment involves the reduction of the dislocation (i.e., the return of the joint to anatomical alignment), which is usually done under anesthesia. The joint is then immobilized by bandages, splints, or a cast to keep it in a stable position until healing takes place.

FRACTURES

A fracture is a break in the continuity of a bone. Most fractures occur as the result of *trauma.* When sufficient force is applied to a bone it breaks, dissipating the original force through nearby soft tissue, and usually embedding small fragments of bone in adjacent muscles, blood vessels, and nerves.

A *pathological* fracture may occur in normal activity or following minimal injury when the bone is weakened by a disease process. A *fatigue* or *stress* fracture occurs in normal bone that has been subjected to repeated stresses, such as those arising from long and strenuous activities.

Fractures are classified according to the nature of the injury and the type of bone discontinuity. A *closed* (or simple) fracture is one in which the skin over the injury site remains intact, with no connnection between the bone and the skin surface. An *open* (or compound) fracture is one in which the skin over the injury site is broken. An open wound is caused either by the fracture fragments piercing the skin or by an outside force penetrating through the skin. An open fracture has a high risk of contamination that may lead to infection.

Fractures may be either complete or incomplete. In an *incomplete* fracture, only a portion of the bone is broken. A fracture is *complete* when there is a separation of the bone into two or more major parts. The part of the bone nearest the body is termed the proximal fragment, and the one most distant from the body is called the distal fragment. The proximal fragment is also called the uncontrollable fragment because its location and muscle attachments prevent it from being moved or manipulated during reduction of the fracture. The distal fragment is referred to as the controllable fragment because usually it can be moved and manipulated to bring it into alignment with the proximal fragment. Fractures in long bones are usually designated as being in the proximal, middle, or distal thirds of the bone. When the two major fragments remain in good alignment, the fracture is referred to as a fracture without displacement, whereas if they are separated, it is a fracture with displacement.

Fractures may be classified into 12 major types. *A greenstick* fracture involves only part of the thickness of a bone. It typically occurs in young children with soft bones. An *oblique* fracture has a fracture line at an oblique angle to the bone shaft. A *transverse* fracture involves a break perpendicular to a bone's long axis. In a *spiral* fracture, the fracture lines encircle the bone, spiraling or coiling toward the torso. A *comminuted* fracture involves multiple bone fragments, usually several small pieces between two large ones. A *linear* or *longitudinal* fracture is a fracture along the long axis of a bone. An *impacted* (or telescoped) fracture occurs when the fracture fragments are forcibly pushed against and into one another. An *avulsion* fracture is when a fragment of bone connected to a ligament breaks off from the rest of the bone. A *compression* fracture is when a bone, most commonly a vertebra, is deformed by compression. A *depression* fracture occurs when bone fragments are forced below their normal level. It most commonly occurs in the skull. An *articular* fracture is a fracture involving an articulating surface of a bone. A *segmental* fracture is a fracture of a small feature of a bone, typically a styloid process.

The signs and symptoms of fractures vary according to the type of fracture, the location of the fracture, the function of the involved bone, and the amount of related soft tissue damage. Fractures may occur without displacement, with little swelling, and with pain occurring only when direct pressure is applied. In most cases, however, the following signs and symptoms can be observed: (1) pain or tenderness at the site of the injury, (2) loss of function from pain, muscle spasm, or bone instability, (3) deformity, such as a change in the alignment or contour of a bone or the appearance of soft tissue swelling, (4) abnormal motility, particularly noticeable in long bones, (5) crepitus, a grating sensation that can be felt or heard, which is caused by bone fragments rubbing against each other, (6) ecchymosis, and (7) roentgenographic evidence of a fracture.

First-Aid Measures

The immediate management of a fracture may determine the patient's outcome and make the difference between complete recovery and disability or even death. Incorrectly moving an accident victim from one position to another may make a closed fracture an open one, puncture a lung, or sever the spinal cord or a major blood vessel. Look for fractures and dislocations in the extremities, check neurovascular status by palpating pulses distal to the injury (Chap. 2), and look for the classic signs of arterial insufficiency, a decreased or absent pulse, pallor, paresthesia, pain, and paralysis. In examining for fractures, handle the limb gently and as little as possible. Keep in mind that the victim may have multiple fractures accompanied by head, chest, and other injuries.

Before a patient can be moved, the extent of the injuries must be assessed, and all fractures immobilized by splints or backboards. Evaluate the patient for respiratory difficulties, take measures to control hemorrhage, and treat for shock. A conscious victim may be able to describe specific areas of pain. Pain over a bone or a joint should be treated as a fracture until proven otherwise, even if the victim can move the extremity. Inspect all fracture sites, relieve pain, improve circulation, minimize further tissue injury, and prevent a closed fracture from becoming an open one. Splints can be improvised using a variety of materials, including pillows, pieces of board, rolled-up newspapers, rifle barrels, golf clubs, and tennis rackets. If an open fracture is present, the wound should be covered by a clean cloth or dressing. Investigate any complaints of pain or pressure, and then transport the patient carefully and gently.

The following paragraphs discuss how trained personnel can move a victim with fractures of the spine, pelvis, hip, arm, and leg.

Fractures of the Spine

Any questionable injury to the neck or back, even in the absence of signs of paralysis, should be treated as a fracture of the spine. Check for paralysis by pinching or pricking the victim's toes and fingers with a pin or sharp object (see neurovascular assessment, Chap. 2). If the victim is lying flat, the vertebrae are examined by sliding a hand under the back without turning the victim. Observe for complications of spinal fractures, such as spinal cord damage, neurogenic shock, and interference with respiration.

If a cervical fracture is suspected, gentle traction may be applied to the neck and maintained until the neck can be supported by a cervical collar. A collar may be improvised by newspaper rolled up into a triangular bandage. The neck should not be flexed, twisted, or hyperextended. If no respiratory difficulties are present, the neck can be splinted in the position in which the victim was found. (Some authorities say, however, that the only first-aid reason to move a victim with an injured cervical spine is to improve an inadequate airway.) To support the cervical spine during a move, place your hands on each side of the victim's head, cupping the victim's ears in your hands. The thumb should be in the temporal region, the index finger just below the zygoma, the third finger along the zygoma, and the fourth finger beneath the mandible. Keep the head in line with the victim's body. Slide the supine victim onto a flat, rigid surface, moving the entire body as a unit. Avoid twisting, turning, or pulling the spine. Watch for inadequate respiratory exchange due to paralysis of chest muscles or neurogenic shock. Once the victim is on a backboard, the victim's head can be additionally supported by placing sand bags, rolled towels, or rolled blankets on each side. A cravat can be placed through or around the backboard and over the forehead. In that way the victim's head, neck, and backboard will move as a unit.

If a lumbar fracture is suspected, the victim should be carefully placed on a flat, rigid surface such as a long backboard. Avoid flexion, extension, or rotation of the spine. The victim should be transported on a backboard as discussed in moving a victim with a cervical fracture.

Pelvic Fractures

An accident victim with a suspected pelvic fracture first must be turned carefully onto the back. Place padding between the victim's legs, splint them together to prevent unnecessary motion, and then turn the victim's body as a single unit. The supine victim should be placed on a firm, flat surface or stretcher. Immobilize the pelvis by binding a folded blanket around it.

Hip Fractures

A victim with a possible fractured hip must be splinted from the axilla to the ankle on the affected side. A board works very well, but if one is not available, bind the victim's legs together. If a half-ring traction is available, the half-ring is slipped around the leg and placed at the groin and gluteal fold, and traction can be applied by means of a clove hitch around the victim's foot and ankle. The victim can then be transported on a stretcher or firm surface.

Leg Fractures

The leg of a victim with a femoral shift or knee fracture can be immobilized using a Thomas ring splint. The ring engages the ischial tuberosity for countertraction, and traction is applied to the end of the splint with an ankle hitch. If no ring splint is available, use boards or other devices to immobilize the victim's leg from the pelvis to the ankle.

A Jones compression splint can also be used for acute knee trauma and for ankle injuries. Alternatively, ankle injuries may be immobilized by tying the victim's lower legs, ankles, and feet together. If possible, transport the victim on a stretcher. The victim should not be allowed to bear weight on the affected leg.

Arm Fractures

For most fractures of the arm, place the victim's elbow at a right angle and apply a sling. The arm and sling should then be bound to the victim's body with a circular bandage or binder. Do not compromise the circulation in the antecubital area with the bandage; check the radial pulse. Fractures of the clavicle may later be immobilized by a figure-of-eight clavicular strap, and shoulder dislocations, humeral fractures, and certain elbow fractures may later be immobilized by a Velpeau bandage. If the victim's injured elbow is in extension, bandage the extremity to the body in the position in which it is found. Always check the radial pulse in an elbow injury.

Fractures below the elbow can be immobilized with a newspaper splint or with a commercial or inflatable air splint. The victim's arm is then placed in a sling with the elbow at a right angle. The air splint is closed over the extremity by its zipper and inflated by blowing air into the mouth tube. Skin maceration will occur if air splints are used for any extended period.

Methods of Fracture Repair

Objectives in the care and treatment of patients with a fracture include (1) reduction of the fracture, (2) maintenance of the fragments in the correct position while healing takes place, (3) prevention of excessive loss of joint mobility and muscle tone, (4) prevention of complications, and (5) maintenance of good general health so that when the fracture heals the patient is restored to the preinjury level of health.

Reduction is the term used to designate the return of the bone fragments to their normal anatomical position. That may be accomplished by closed manipulation, traction, or open reduction. Closed manipulation is effected by the physician exerting a pulling force on the distal fragment while applying counteraction to the proximal fragment until the bone fragments engage or fall into their normal alignment. Pressure may also be applied over the site of the fracture to correct angulation or lateral displacement of a fragment. The fracture is then immobilized in a splint or cast. Closed manipulation is used to reduce closed fractures.

Traction, as a method of reduction, is accomplished by placing a continuous pull on the affected part for a period of hours, days, or even weeks to overcome muscle spasms and reduce the fracture (Appendix A). Skeletal traction is usually involved, and it may be a definitive method of treatment or a temporary method pending internal fixation. Skeletal traction is especially useful for fractures of the femur and severely displaced, unstable fractures of the humerus.

Open reduction is a method in which the fracture site is surgically opened and the fracture fragments replaced into correct anatomical position. The fractured bone is immobilized by the use of nails, rods, plates, screws, or pins, which hold the fragments together. Among the devices most commonly used for internal fixation are intramedullary nails and compression plates. Intramedullary nails are generally used in fractures of the middle two-thirds of the femur, the humerus, and occasionally the tibia and the radius. They have the advantage of providing good fixation without damaging the periosteum, which is a major source of callus for the healing bone. Compression plates applied to the bone cortex provide rigid fixation, and with proper techniques substantial compression can be applied to the fracture site, which may speed healing. They are most suitable for fractures of the radius and the ulna and, less often, the humerus, the tibia, and the femur. Intra-articular fractures, for example, malleolar fractures of the ankle, are best fixed by screws. Certain hip fractures may require prosthetic replacement of the femoral head or, occasionally, a total joint replacement.

Methods of Immobilization

The purpose of immobilization is to hold the reduced bone fragments in contact with each other until healing takes place. Any activity that involves the movement of the bone fragments must be restricted. Usually immobilization includes the joints immediately proximal to and distal to the fracture site. Bandages, adhesive tape, splints, casts, skeletal traction, internal fixation, and external fixation are the most common methods of immobilization.

External fixation devices are used to hold fracture fragments in alignment when there is extensive soft tissue damage, in large open fractures where inspection of soft tissues is essential, where vascular repair has been carried out in an open wound, and in burns with underlying fractures. Pins are surgically inserted through the skin and through the bone above and below the fracture. The pins are then clamped to the external framework that maintains the fracture fragments in correct alignment. In the upper extremity, the olecranon, the ulna, the distal third of the radius, and the second and third metacarpals are the usual sites for the insertion of pins. In the lower extremity, the supracondylar areas of the femur, the region of the tibial tubercle, the supramalleolar area of the tibia, and the os calcis are usually selected. For example, in a comminuted fracture of the tibia with a large soft tissue wound requiring debridement, fixation is secured by the insertion of two or more pins through the tibia in the area of the tibial tubercle, which are then connected with external fixation bars. Fixation is then secure, the patient may be turned readily, and the wounds inspected and dressed while alignment of the comminuted fracture is maintained.

Fracture Healing

Fracture healing is a continuous process that begins immediately after a fracture. The injury causes a hemorrhage into the fracture site from ruptured vessels within the bone, torn periosteum, and surrounding soft tissues. Within 24 hours, a hematoma is formed that fills the fracture site and the surrounding area. The coagulated blood of the hematoma gives rise to a loose fibrin mesh that seals off the fracture site and, at the same time, serves as a framework for the ingrowth of fibroblasts and capillary buds. During the first 24 to 48 hours following injury, the progressive disintegration of red blood cells provides a continuing inflammatory stimulus that results in significant edema, vascular congestion, and an infiltration of leukocytes, chiefly neutrophils. Two days after the injury, large numbers of macrophages begin the phagocytosis of the tissue and red cell debris. At the same time, fibroblasts and chondroblasts from the surrounding connective tissue, the periosteum, and the medullary cavity invade the margins of the clot and begin to form a soft tissue callus in and about the fracture site (Robbins, 1974, p. 1440).

After the first few days, newly formed cartilage and bone matrix are evident in the fibrovascular response. By the end of the first week, well-developed new bone and cartilage are dispersed throughout the soft tissue callus. During the following days, these bone spicules become sufficiently numerous and aggregated to create a large, fusiform, temporary bony union of the fracture fragments known as the provisional callus or procallus. By that time, the inflammatory reaction has mostly subsided and the repair is well underway.

The provisional callus is considerably wider than the normal diameter of the bone, and extends up over the fractured ends to create a spindle-shaped, splint-like support. In uncomplicated fractures, the provisional callus reaches its maximal size about 14 to 21 days after injury, but continues to increase in strength from the precipitation of bone salts. At the same time the procallus is remolded by osteoblastic and osteoclastic activity, which reacts to the muscle and weight-bearing stresses imposed upon the bone. If the fracture has been well aligned and weight-bearing stresses gradually restored, virtually perfect reconstruction of the bone is accomplished. However, the repair may be impeded or prevented by many complications.

Complications of Fractures

The immediate complications following a fracture are (1) shock, which may be fatal in the first few hours after injury, (2) fat embolism, (3) pulmonary embolism, (4) compartmental syndrome, (5) neurological complications, and (6) infection. Late fracture complications, such a malunion, delayed union, nonunion, avascular necrosis, and chronic osteomyelitis, are primarily matters of orthopaedic reconstruction. Prevention of those complications, however, is best accomplished by avoiding errors in the early care of the injured patient.

Shock

Hypovolemic or traumatic shock, resulting from hemorrhage (both external and internal) and loss of extracellular fluid into damaged tissues, may occur in fractures of the extremities, thorax, pelvis, and spine. Because bone is very vascular, large quantities of blood may be lost as a result of bone trauma, especially in femoral and pelvic fractures. Treatment of shock consists of replacing depleted blood volume, relieving pain, providing adequate splinting of the fracture, and protecting the patient from further injury.

Fat Embolism

Fat emboli occur when fat in the blood becomes entrapped in the lung capillaries. There may also be occlusions of small vessels that supply the brain, kidneys, and other organs. The fat may originate at the fracture site and gain access to the venous circulation through ruptured marrow veins, or may be formed by an alteration of lipid stability in the blood caused by the stress of trauma. Occlusion of a large number of small vessels in the lungs causes pulmonary pressure to rise, possibly even resulting in acute right-sided heart failure. Edema and hemorrhage in the alveoli impair oxygen transport, leading to hypoxia.

Fat emboli are more likely to occur following comminuted fractures of long bones (especially the femur and the tibia) and the pelvis. The onset usually occurs 12 to 48 hours after injury or surgery. An early symptom of fat emboli is abnormal behavior, varying from mild agitation and confusion to delirium and coma, caused by the hypoxia. When personality changes occur following trauma or surgery, blood gas studies should be done to help confirm a diagnosis of fat emboli. Other symptoms are an increase in respiratory rate, sudden severe pericardial chest pain, dyspnea, pallor, exhaustion, and even collapse. With systemic embolization, petechiae can usually be detected in the buccal membranes and conjunctival sacs, on the hard palate, on the fundus of the eye, and over the chest, neck, shoulders, and anterior axillary folds. Free fat may also be found in the urine when fat emboli affect the kidneys.

There is no specific treatment for systemic fat emboli. The primary objective of care is to support the respiratory system, which is usually accomplished by placing the patient in high Fowler's position and administering oxygen at high concentrations. Oxygen lowers the surface tension of the fat globules and reduces local anoxia. In some instances controlled volume ventilation with positive end-expiratory pressure (PEEP) may be used to assist in decreasing pulmonary edema. Steroids may be administered to reduce lung inflammation and help control cerebral edema. Intravenous fluids may be given for their emulsifying effect. Low molecular weight dextran may be given to improve pulmonary and capillary flow. Blood transfusions may be necessary to relieve shock and maintain an adequate hemoglobin level. Patients are kept as quiet as possible and subjected to no unnecessary movement. Some experts feel that immobilization and careful handling of patients with bone injuries are important in preventing the occurrence of fat emboli.

Pulmonary Embolism

Pulmonary embolism is a complication that frequently occurs following fractures of the pelvis, hip, and femur, particularly where prolonged immobilization is required. Following a fracture, pulmonary emboli may occur as early as 2 to 3 days or as late as several weeks after injury.

Pulmonary embolism refers to the obstruction of one or more pulmonary arteries by a thrombus (or thrombi), which originates somewhere in the venous system or the right side of the heart, becomes dislodged, and is carried to the lung. An infarction of lung tissue occurs due to the interruption of the lung's blood supply. The majority of thrombi originate in the deep veins of the legs, but other sources include the pelvic veins and the right atrium of the heart. A statis, or slowing of the blood flow because of damage to the blood vessel wall (particularly the endothelial lining), and changes in the blood coagulation mechanism, are conditions that can lead to the development of a thrombus.

The symptoms of pulmonary embolism depend on the size of the thrombus and the location of the occlusion. A massive embolism at the bifurcation of the pulmonary artery usually produces pronounced dyspnea, sudden substernal pain, rapid and weak pulse, shock, syncope, and even sudden death. If one or more branches of the right or left pulmonary arteries are obstructed, the patient usually experiences dyspnea, mild substernal pain, anxiety, weakness, and tachycardia from the pulmonary infarction. The patient may also have a fever, cough, and hemoptysis. When the terminal pulmonary arteries are occluded, a pleuritic type of pain, a cough, and hemoptysis develop. Multiple small emboli can lodge in the terminal pulmonary arterioles and produce multiple small infarctions, giving a clinical picture similar to bronchopneumonia. In some instances, however, the condition presents very few symptoms.

The best treatment is prevention. Every effort should be directed toward preventing venous stasis by keeping the patient well hydrated, doing active and passive exercises, and beginning ambulation as early as possible. Patients may wear elastic stockings to increase blood flow to the deep leg veins. Anticoagulation therapy (e.g., heparin, warfarin, low-molecular dextran, and aspirin) may also be used.

Compartmental Syndrome

A compartmental syndrome is a condition in which high pressure within a closed fascial space (or muscle compartment) reduces capillary blood perfusion below the level necessary for tissue viability. Compartmental syndromes develop in skeletal muscles enclosed by relatively noncompliant, osseofascial boundaries. A build-up of pressure within the muscle compartment is not easily dissipated, because of the inelasticity of the fascia. If pressure remains high for several hours, normal muscle and nerve function is jeopardized, myoneural necrosis results, and permanent loss of function and limb contracture may occur. A prompt diagnosis of the condition and decompression of the compartment are essential to reinstate capillary perfusion and prevent irreversible sequelae. It is essential that the nurse look for the signs and symptoms of increased compartmental pressure (see pp. 387–388). Decompression can be accomplished by a fasciotomy, which allows the muscles to swell out of their tight fascial enclosure. The four compartments of the lower leg are most frequently involved, but compartmental syndromes can occur in the forearm, hand, arm, shoulder, thigh, and buttocks (Mubarak & Hargens, 1983; Schoen, 1977).

Neurological Complications

A variety of neurological complications may occur, especially in long bone fractures. In general, satisfactory reduction of the fracture relieves the stress placed on nerves, because most nerve injuries following fractures are due to stress rather than laceration. Fractures of the humerus, particularly displaced fractures of the distal third, can compress the radial nerve. When the nerve loss is complete and recovery has not occurred within a few weeks following fracture reduction, exploratory surgery may be necessary to try to relieve the symptoms. Lesions of the sciatic nerve, especially of the perineal branch, are associated with fracture dislocations of the hip in which a fracture fragment from the posterior acetabulum is driven into the sciatic nerve. Such fragments need to be surgically removed. Damage to the perineal branch of the sciatic nerve can also occur in fractures of the tibia and fibula, particularly proximal fractures of the fibula. The primary role of the nurse is to be alert to possible neurological abnormalities. For a discussion on how to assess neurological function, see Chapter 2.

Infections

An infection at a fracture site can cause poor fracture healing, nonunion, or malunion. Any fracture can become infected, but open fractures are particularly susceptible to infection. If an infection involves an internal fixation or prosthesis, the device may need to be removed, leaving a disability rather than a functional bone. Infections of the bone are extremely difficult to eradicate, so prevention must be the goal.

A patient with an open fracture is taken to the operating room where the wound is cleansed, debrided, and irrigated. Devitalized bone fragments are removed, the fracture reduced, and internal or external fixation used to stabilize the fracture. At the time of surgery, cultures are taken for sensitivity studies. Heavily contaminated wounds may be left open and later closed by suturing or by autogenous skin or flap grafts.

The most common infections are osteomyelitis, tetanus, and gas gangrene. For more information on osteomyelitis, see pp. 101–103. Tetanus is caused by the bacillus *Clostridium tetani,* which is found in soil, especially where horses and cattle are present. The organism usually enters the body through penetrating or crush wounds. The symptoms usually occur 4 to 21 days after contamination, with an average of 10 days. Chemotherapy usually consists of tetanus immune globulin (TIG) and penicillin G (or an alternative antibiotic). Prophylactic treatment is the debridment of the wound and the administration of toxoid booster injection for patients previously immunized or separate tetanus toxoid and TIG injections for nonimmunized patients.

Gas gangrene is a severe infection caused by several species of gram-positive clostridia that may complicate trauma, open fractures, contusions, and lacerated wounds by producing exotoxins that destroy tissue. The organisms are anaerobic and spore-forming and are found normally in soil and in the human intestinal tract. They grow primarily in deep wounds where the oxygen supply is reduced, a situation enhanced by the presence of foreign bodies or necrotic tissue. Those anaerobic bacilli are highly resistant to heat, cold, sunlight, drying, and many chemical agents. Because they normally inhabit the intestinal tract, they are likely to be the infecting organisms in thigh wounds and following amputations, especially when the patient is incontinent of feces.

Gas gangrene may be prevented if all devitalized and infected tissue is thoroughly debrided to render the wound unsuitable for the growth of *Clostridium.* Penicillin may be administered intravenously as a preventive measure. If gas gangrene develops, hyperbaric oxygen, i.e., oxygen administered under greater than atmospheric pressure in specially designed chambers, may be used. That increases the dissolved oxygen in the arterial system by increasing the partial pressure of oxygen breathed by the patient, and reduces toxin formation and microbial reproduction.

Malunion

Malunion is when union occurs with the fragments in a deformed or angulated position, and is usually the result of inadequate reduction and immobilization. If malunion is severe, it may become necessary to manually or surgically manipulate the fracture site, realign the fragments, immobilize the fracture site, and allow the bone to recalcify.

Delayed Union

Delayed union (or delayed healing) is used to describe a fracture that is slow to heal but does demonstrate some calcification. Some reasons for delayed union are infection, inadequate immobilization or reduction that allows movement at the fracture site, inadequate blood supply, or metabolic disturbances that affect the protein and the vitamins available for bone healing. Treatment consists of discovering the cause and correcting the underlying problem.

Nonunion

Nonunion is when the fracture fragments do not calcify together. Nonunion may occur if: (1) the space between the fracture fragments is too large for either callus or bone cells to bridge, (2) muscles or fascia are between the fracture fragments, (3) the callus is broken or torn by excessive activity, (4) an infection develops, (5) there is inadequate blood supply to the fracture site, and (6) there is marked dietary deficiency. Occasionally, nonunion occurs with no apparent reason.

Treatment for nonunion includes surgical intervention to debride and revise the fracture ends and implant a bone graft. In recent years, electrical stimulation has proven very effective in treating nonunion. One method is noninvasive, and employs an electrode placed over the patient's skin or cast. Patients use the device 10 to 12 hours a day at home, usually while they sleep. The treatment may continue for 3 to 8 months.

Avascular Necrosis

Avascular necrosis may occur from infection or when bone loses its blood supply. It may be idiopathic or follow a fracture or dislocation. An interruption of blood supply may be an unpreventable complication that occurs at the time of injury. Healing can occur in the presence of avascular necrosis when dead bone is reabsorbed and replaced by new bone, but the patient usually develops a painful arthritis later.

Avascular necrosis is particularly common following fractures of the head and neck of the femur. The blood supply to the head and neck may be disrupted by an injury to blood vessels, and bone death can result. To permit weightbearing, the head of the femur is removed and replaced by a prosthesis.

Complications of Immobility

Respiratory Complications

Recumbency, drugs used for pain relief that depress respiration, a decrease in the body's need for oxygen, and the resistance of the bed against the chest wall are some of the factors that can lead to respiratory complications. Limited movement of the chest wall, collection of secretions, creation of dead spaces in the lung, and collapse of alveoli can lead to stasis pneumonia, pneumothorax, and oxygen–carbon dioxide imbalance. Patients recovering from hip surgery may have added respiratory manifestations due to circulatory problems such as pulmonary embolism (see pp. 72–73) or fat embolism (see p. 72).

The best method of treatment is prevention and quick observation of abnormalities. The procedures of turning, coughing, and doing deep breathing exercises are essential to facilitate respiratory hygiene. Elevating the head of the bed assists the patient in coughing and doing deep breathing exercises. When the patient turns to the side, give a vigorous back rub to stimulate circulation, including some clapping and vibration to loosen secretions if the patient's condition allows. Keeping the patient well hydrated assists in bringing up secretions. Other techniques to help inflate the lungs and promote gas exchange are incentive respiratory devices (e.g., spirometers) and intermittent positive pressure breathing (IPPB) (Table 3–1).

Circulatory Complications

Circulatory Overload. Intravenous fluids ordered postoperatively are a method to administer antibiotics and to keep the patient hydrated until oral fluid intake is adequate. The general rate of flow is usually 80 to 100 cc per hour. It may be advisable (based on the assessment of the patient), to run the intravenous fluids more slowly to prevent circulatory overload and strain on the heart, which may have a limited cardiac reserve. That is especially true in some elderly patients. Encourage oral fluids, in small portions, as soon as possible to reduce the need for IV fluids after the initial 24 to 48 hours (Table 3–2).

Orthostatic Hypotension. Orthostatic hypotension or postural hypotension occurs when the patient is on prolonged bedrest and the muscles and blood vessels in the lower extremities lose their tone. After such a period of recumbency, the veins in the lower extremities will accept a large volume of blood when the patient stands. That large amount of blood deprives the other parts of the body, especially the brain, of an adequate blood supply, and can cause the patient to become dizzy or possibly faint. In an effort to keep or develop good muscle tone and therefore more efficient vascular return, have the patient do

TABLE 3–1. NURSING PROCESS FOR POTENTIAL ALTERATION IN RESPIRATORY FUNCTION

Assessment	Nursing Diagnosis	Goal Formulation	Planning and Intervention	Evaluation and Reassessment
Auscultate the chest for clearness of lungs and for any cardiac abnormalities. Check respirations for depth, rate, and rhythm. Assess the patient's ability to cough and deep breathe. Assess fluid intake and output. Determine the use of accessory muscles of respiration (in the chest, abdomen, and neck). Note any nasal flaring. Check for any sputum. Assess for signs of confusion.	Potential alterations in respiratory function: ineffective airway clearance related to trauma or immobility postsurgery.	Short-term goal: no problems with respiratory function due to immobility. Long-term goal: free of respiratory problems.	Explain rationale for preventing respiratory complications. Teach coughing and deep breathing. Teach the use of assistive breathing devices. Encourage the patient to turn and move in bed. Facilitate early ambulation. Increase fluid intake as indicated. Provide for the proper level of environmental humidity. Encourage good oral hygiene. Teach breathing exercises. Elevate the head of the bed. Give back rubs with clapping and vibration.	Determine that the patient is well hydrated and has no signs of confusion. Observe respirations for rhythm, rate, and no shortness of breath. Auscultate the chest for clear breath sounds. Determine that the patient gives a deep cough and has no secretions. The patient should have no nasals flaring and should not make excessive use of accessory muscles. The patient should have good color and normal temperature.

TABLE 3–2. NURSING PROCESS FOR POTENTIAL ALTERATIONS IN FLUID VOLUME: EXCESSIVE FLUID

Assessment	Nursing Diagnosis	Goal Formulation	Planning and Intervention	Evaluation and Reassessment
Assess for shortness of breath, pulmonary congestion, abnormal breath sounds, and changes in respiratory pattern. Note any jugular venous distention. Check for any increased pulse volume or increase in blood pressure. Check whether fluid intake is greater than output. Note any change in mental status. Note any restlessness or anxiety. Assess for fatigue. Check for taut, shiny skin.	Potential alteration in fluid volume: excessive fluid related to parental fluid intake.	Short-term goal: have fluid volume maintained within normal limits. Long-term goal: free of any circulatory complication.	Give fluids with caution. If fluids are restricted, set up a 24-hour schedule for fluid intake. Monitor vital signs, weight, and urine output. Observe for signs of congestive heart failure. Place in semi-Fowler's position. Allow patient frequent rest periods. Administer skin and mouth care. Restrict sodium intake. Take safety precautions for periods of confusion.	Vital signs should be within normal limits. There should be no signs of congestive heart failure, and fluid output should be within normal range compared to intake. Patient should be well hydrated with good skin turgor. There should be no sign of confusion or injury.

active flexion of all muscle groups, particularly in the lower extremities (e.g., quadriceps setting, ankle dorsiflexion, and plantar flexion). Other procedures to help reduce the effect are to have the patient sit on the side of the bed for a few minutes before ambulating, or use a tilt table. Exercises in turning and lifting with the aid of the trapeze increase general circulation and should be encouraged (Table 3–3).

Venous Stasis. When a patient is immobile, venous return is slowed, partly because of the decreased muscular activity in the lower extremities which would normally assist the return of blood from the legs back to the heart. When the walls of the vessels lose their tone, there may be stasis of some of the heavier components in the blood leading to inflammation of the veins and the formation of clots (thrombi). Thrombophlebitis, intravascular clotting in an inflamed vein, can easily occur in patients postoperatively. Thrombophlebitis and the formation of thrombi can lead to pulmonary emboli (see pp. 72–73).

Measures used to help prevent venous stasis are leg movement, leg exercises, and assisting the patient in changing positions. Elastic stockings are usually worn. They support the venous circulation and help to prevent dependent edema. The stockings must go from the toe to the groin and be the correct size, tight enough to assist with venous return but not so tight as to be constricting to the skin, nerves, and vascular system. The stockings should be removed for ½ to 1 hour mornings and evenings, and the legs, especially the heels, checked for any redness. The patient needs at least two pairs of stockings so they can be changed and cleansed. Another measure employed is the use of antiocoagulation therapy (e.g., heparin, warfarin, low-molecular dextran, and aspirin). With this treatment, the nurse should observe for signs of bleeding, especially around the site of the incision. That area should also be checked for edema, hardness, and increased temperature which could indicate a hematoma. Keep the patient well hydrated, as patients with dehydration will have more problems with venous stasis (Table 3–3).

Gastrointestinal Complications

Paralytic Ileus. Paralytic ileus is an infrequent complication of immobility following surgery or trauma. It involves an absent or diminished peristalsis of the bowel due to the traumatic disturbance of the autonomic nervous system. However, there is no physical obstruction or interruption of blood supply to the intestines. Prophylactically, intravenous fluids and minimal oral fluids are utilized until peristalsis is established after surgery. Abdominal setting exercises and bed exercises increase circulation and muscle tone. Abdominal exercises are done from the supine position. With hands on the abdomen, the neck and shoulders are raised far enough to tighten the stomach muscles. Depending on the patient's age and general musculature, the exercise can be made more vigorous by lifting the head and shoulders even further. If no actual flexion of the spine is desired, the exercise can be done by only lifting the head and neck off the pillow, just enough to tighten the stomach and abdominal muscles. An

TABLE 3–3. NURSING PROCESS FOR POTENTIAL ALTERATION IN FLUID VOLUME: DEFICIT OF FLUID

Assessment	Nursing Diagnosis	Goal Formulation	Planning and Intervention	Evaluation and Reassessment
Assess vital signs. Observe the patient's color and temperature. Check skin turgor and mucous membrane texture. Assess fluid intake and output. Check specific gravity of urine. Assess muscle tone and strength.	Potential alteration in fluid volume: deficit related to decreased intake and lack of muscle tone.	Short-term goal: fluid volume maintained within normal limits. Long-term goal: free of any circulatory complications.	Maintain hydration. Offer fluids the patient likes. Set up a 24-hour schedule for fluid intake. Explain the need for fluid intake. Teach muscle setting exercises. Turn and reposition frequently. Do passive and encourage active range-of-motion exercises. Facilitate early ambulation. Teach use of elastic stockings. Administer anticoagulant drugs.	The patient should not have any dryness of skin, poor skin turgor, or dryness of mucous membranes. The patient should not have a furrowed tongue. The patient should not have any decrease in lacrimal secretions or saliva. Determine the patient's muscle tone and strength in ability to move and reposition self. Observe for side effects of drug therapy.

TABLE 3–4. NURSING PROCESS FOR POTENTIAL ALTERATION IN BOWEL ELIMINATION: INEFFECTIVE BOWEL FUNCTION

Assessment	Nursing Diagnosis	Goal Formulation	Planning and Intervention	Evaluation and Reassessment
Auscultate for bowel sounds. Check for expulsion of flatus. Assess for abdominal softness. Assess for abdominal distention by measuring the abdominal girth. Check fluid intake and output. Assess for nausea or anorexia. Assess for pain.	Potential alteration in bowel elimination: ineffective bowel function related to immobility secondary to surgery or trauma.	Short-term goal: normal peristalsis and the ability to expel waste products. Long-term goal: free of any problems with bowel elimination.	Restrict oral intake if there are no bowel sounds. Teach abdominal exercises. Explain rationale for exercises. Teach exercises for movement and early ambulation, and encourage the patient to turn and move in bed. Teach active range-of-motion exercises. Maintain fluid and electrolyte balance. For use of rectal tube and the use of a heating pad on the abdomen, seek medical consultation.	Determine bowel sounds and the patient's ability to pass flatus. Determine that the patient's abdomen is soft with no increase in abdominal girth. The patient should have no nausea or vomiting.

TABLE 3–5. NURSING PROCESS FOR POTENTIAL ALTERATION IN BOWEL ELIMINATION: CONSTIPATION

Assessment	Nursing Diagnosis	Goal Formulation	Planning and Intervention	Evaluation and Reassessment
Assess for hard formed stool. Check frequency and consistency of stools. Determine normal elimination routine. Assess for bowel sounds. Note any straining while defecating. Check for any complaints of pressure in the rectum or pain on defecation. By manual examination, palpate for possible impaction.	Potential alteration in bowel elimination: constipation related to immobility secondary to surgery or trauma.	Short-term goal: bowel elimination on a regular basis without pain or discomfort. Long-term goal: have bowel elimination return to pre-morbid pattern.	Set up specific time for elimination. Provide for comfort and privacy. Assist patient in achieving a suitable position on the bedpan or commode. Provide stimulus to defecate (e.g., coffee, hot lemonade or prune juice early in the morning). Discuss the need for a well-balanced diet high in fiber content (e.g., whole grains, nuts, raw and coarse vegetables, and fresh fruits with skins).	Evaluate bowel sounds and the form and consistency of stools. Determine that elimination occurs without straining, pain, or discomfort. The patient should have a regular bowel elimination routine. Evaluate the amount of fluid intake and type and amount of food intake. Determine how often and how long the patient exercises.

Note pain medications and stool softeners utilized. Determine food and fluid intake.	Explain the need for 2 liters or more of fluid per day. Explain the role of exercise in assisting with bowel elimination. Teach abdominal exercises and active range-of-motion exercises. Encourage early ambulation and movements in bed. If the above measures are ineffective, a mild laxative or stool softener may be needed temporarily. Explain the effect of pain medication on elimination. Explain the rationale for stool softeners and laxatives.

exercise that puts even less strain on the body involves tightening the abdominal muscles for a count of three and then relaxing for a count of three. If a paralytic ileus should occur, the gastrointestinal tract is rested by allowing nothing by mouth and using intravenous fluids to prevent dehydration. A heating pad on the abdomen may be used to increase circulation in the area. A rectal tube may be used to help reduce distention, and a nasogastric tube may be necessary. The complication is usually resolved within 72 hours (Table 3–4).

Constipation. Constipation is a potential problem for most surgical and immobile patients because of their decreased mobility and drug therapy (e.g., sedatives and pain medications). Elderly patients are at increased risk because the aging process slows bowel function. The usual preventive measures are increased fluid intake, a diet with increased roughage and fiber and less carbohydrates, exercises in bed, and ambulation. Stool softeners are usually ordered, but laxatives and enemas are almost invariably indicated (Table 3–5).

Genitourinary Complications

Lower urinary tract infection is one of the most common problems of the aged, and immobile patients are potential candidates. Both men and women are susceptible. Older men usually have an enlarged prostate and an atonic decompensated bladder. Women may have interstitial cystitis and a contracted bladder. Older women may also have stress incontinency due to a prolapsed uterus, or, when on prolonged bedrest, may have urine collect in the vagina.

To help prevent infection, and give an acid-ash diet, encourage fluids, based as much as possible on preferences, to keep the urine acidic and to facilitate voiding. Assist with bedpan use on a schedule (even during the night) to prevent bladder distention and problems with overflow continence. Getting the patient out of bed to use a bedside commode or the bathroom facilitates a more complete emptying of the bladder. Every effort must be made to avoid having to use a cathether. If that is not possible, include a program for cleansing around the catheter and the meatus. The meatus area provides a good medium for bacterial invasion and subsequent infection (Table 3–6).

Musculoskeletal Complications

A contracture, the inability to passively stretch a muscle, is a serious and permanent deformity that can easily develop in an inactive patient. The beginning stages of a contracture have been known to develop within 36 hours after injury. Keeping the patient in correct alignment, encouraging independent movement as much as possible, and doing exercises help to prevent contractures. Both active and passive exercises of all joints must be encouraged. There should be frequent changes of position with appropriate joint support and correct alignment. The feet should be supported with a footboard, flexion pillow, or some other support device, and there should be no pillow under the knees. Make sure the position of the hip, with the head of the bed elevated, differs from the position the hip is in when the patient is lying on a side. All contractures can be prevented (Table 3–7).

TABLE 3–6. NURSING PROCESS FOR POTENTIAL ALTERATION IN URINARY ELIMINATION

Assessment	Nursing Diagnosis	Goal Formulation	Planning and Intervention	Evaluation and Reassessment
Assess for bladder distention. Note the frequency, amount, color, and odor of urine. Assess whether urination is accompanied by any pain. Assess fluid intake and output.	Potential alternation in urinary elimination: infection due to urinary stasis related to immobility secondary to surgery or trauma.	Short-term goal: ability to void without pain or discomfort. Long-term goal: free of any urinary complication.	Provide for privacy during elimination. Offer bedpan on a 24-hour schedule. Assist patient into a comfortable position for voiding. Maintain fluid and electrolyte balance. Explain the rationale for drinking liquids that alter the acidity of the urine (e.g., cranberry juice). Teach perineal care.	The patient should not have bladder distention or urinary incontinence after voiding. The patient should take in adequate fluids. The patient should void 200–300 ml every 4–6 hours. Determine if there is any pain or discomfort on voiding.

TABLE 3–7. NURSING PROCESS FOR POTENTIAL ALTERATION IN MOBILITY: CONTRACTURES

Assessment	Nursing Diagnosis	Goal Formulation	Planning and Intervention	Evaluation and Reassessment
Assess range of motion of all joints. Assess the patient's ability to move and change position independently. Assess the patient's general muscular development and strength. Assess how frequently the patient changes position. Assess the patient's ability to perform activities of daily living.	Potential alteration in mobility: contracture related to immobility secondary to surgery or trauma.	Short-term goal: ability to move freely in bed without restriction. Long-term goal: free of any mobility complications that could impede joint function.	Teach patient correct positioning and how to change position. Make sure joints actually change position (flexion and extension) when the patient changes position. Teach patient how to do active range-of-motion exercises. Do passive range-of-motion exercises when indicated. Demonstrate muscle setting exercises.	Evaluate the patient's range of motion in all joints. Determine how much of the 24-hour day the patient has different joints in extension. Evaluate how well the patient is able to perform the exercise program. Determine how well the patient is able to perform activities of daily living.

TABLE 3–8. NURSING PROCESS FOR POTENTIAL IMPAIRMENT OF SKIN INTEGRITY: PRESSURE AREAS

Assessment	Nursing Diagnosis	Goal Formulation	Planning and Intervention	Evaluation and Reassessment
Assess for any reddened areas over bony prominences. Note any complaints of pain or discomfort at the heel, sacrum, elbow, trochanter, scapula, ears, and occiput. Assess for nutritional intake. Assess skin for dryness, edema, thinness, or obesity. Assess for hydration.	Potential impairment of skin integrity: pressure areas related to immobility secondary to surgery or trauma.	Short-term goal: free of pain or discomfort from pressue due to immobility. Long-term goal: free of any skin problems due to immobility.	Encourage range-of-motion exercises to increase blood flow. Utilize a turning schedule that relieves pressure on vulnerable areas. Massage vulnerable areas during each position change. Turn or shift weight every 30 minutes to 2 hours. Limit Fowler's position to reduce pressure on the sacrum. Use foam blocks or pillows to provide a bridging effect to support the body above and below high-risk areas so they do not touch bed surface. Reduce the pressure on skin surfaces by using alternating pressure mattresses, sheepskins, eggcrates, and foam protectors.	Determine that no reddened areas exist. The patient should have a well-balanced diet with adequate fluid intake. Determine that the turn/repositioning schedule is utilized 24 hours a day. Evaluate how often the patient exercises. Determine that the skin is dry but well hydrated.

Integumentary Complications

Immobility, especially in older patients, can rapidly lead to pressure areas and skin breakdown. The skin over bony prominences is especially susceptible. It is essential that preventive measures be taken before pressure areas develop. Put a circulating mattress, sheepskin, egg crate mattress, or other similar material on the bed before the patient returns from surgery. Schedule turns so the patient's position is changed every 2 to 3 hours. Discourage the patient from sitting all day with the head of the bed elevated, as this increases pressure on the coccyx. (Sitting on the side of the bed with feet on the floor or being in a chair does not have the same effect on the coccyx.) Encourage fluids and a well-balanced diet. Fluids keep the skin hydrated and the balanced diet keeps the patient's tissues in a healthy state and thus less susceptible to breakdown from pressure (Table 3–8).

REFERENCES

Mubarak, S. J., & Hargens, A. R. Acute compartment syndromes. *Surgical Clinics of North America,* 1983, *63* (3), 539–566.

Robbins, S. L. *Pathologic basis of disease.* Philadelphia: Saunders, 1974.

Schoen, D. C. Compartmental syndrome. *Orthopedic Nurses Association Journal,* 1977, *4* (8), 208–210.

BIBLIOGRAPHY

Aaron R. K., & Ciombar, D. Venous thrombaembolism in the orthopedic patient. *Surgical Clinics of North America,* 1983, *63* (3), 529–539.

Anderson, W. A. D., & Kissane, J. M. *Pathology* (7th ed.). St. Louis: C. V. Mosby, 1977.

Barry, J. *Emergency nursing.* New York: McGraw-Hill, 1979.

Bailey, M. Emergency! First aid for fractures. *Nursing 1982,* 1982, *12* (11), 72–81.

Brooker, A. New techniques in fracture management. *Surgical Clinics of North America,* 1983, *63* (3), 607–628.

Cameron, G. Pressure sores: What to do when prevention fails. *Nursing 79,* 1979, *9* (1), 42–47.

Clissold, G. *The body's response to trauma: Fractures.* New York: Springer, 1973.

Compere, E. L. *Orthopaedic surgery—A handbook of operative surgery.* Chicago: Year Book Medical, 1974.

Crossland, S., & Deyerle, W. M. Compartmental syndrome. *Nursing 80,* 1980, *10* (11), 51–54.

Dimon, J. H., & Donahoe, C. Trauma. *Orthopedic Nurses Association Journal,* 1979, *6* (3), 100–113.

Duncan, C. Initial care of the trauma patient. *Orthopedic Nurses Association Journal,* 1979, *6* (11), 450–452.

Edmonson, A. S., & Crenshaw, A. M. (Eds.). *Campbell's operative orthopaedics,* (6th ed.). St. Louis: C. V. Mosby, 1980.

Epps, C. A. *Complications in orthopedic surgery.* Philadelphia: Lippincott, 1978.

Evarts, C. McC. Thromboembolic disease. *Current Practice in Orthopaedic Surgery,* 1977, 7, 246.

Folcik, C., & Dumos, K. Identifying a standard for pin care using the quality assurance approach. *Orthopaedic Nursing,* 1984, *3* (3), 17–24.

Fulkerson, J. P., & Phillips, S. B. Complications of closed suction-irrigation: A case report. *Orthopedics,* 1979, *2* (2), 128–129.

Gartland, J. J. *Fundamentals of orthopaedics* (3rd ed.). Philadelphia: Saunders, 1979.

Ghista D. N., & Roof, R. *Orthopaedic mechanics, procedures and devices.* San Francisco: Academic Press, 1978.

Gilroy, A., & Caldwell, E. Initial assessment of the multiply injured patient. *Nursing Clinics of North America,* 1978, *13* (4), 117–190.

Iverson, L. D., & Clawson, D. K. *Manual of acute orthopaedic therapeutics.* Boston: Little, Brown, 1977.

Johnston, C. (Ed.). *Advances in external fixation.* Chicago: Year Book Medical, 1980.

Kerr, A. *Orthopedic nursing procedures, part 1: Initial and emergency care* (3rd ed.). New York: Springer, 1980.

Kryschyshen, P. L., & Fischer, D. A. External fixation for complication fractures. *American Journal of Nursing,* 1980, *80* (2), 256–259.

Larson, C. B., & Gould, M. *Orthopedic nursing* (9th ed.). St. Louis: C. V. Mosby, 1978.

Love-Mignogna, S. Taping and splinting: Seven common problems—And how to avoid them. *Nursing 80,* 1980, *10* (4), 88–92.

Lupin, A. E. Head off compartment syndrome before its too late. *RN,* 1980, *43* (12), 38–41.

Mackey, C., & Hopefl, A. W. Keeping infections down when risks go up. *Nursing 80,* 1980, *10* (6), 69–73.

Matsen, F. A., Winquist, R. A., & Krugmire, R. B., Jr. Diagnosis and management of compartmental syndrome. *Journal of Bone and Joint Surgery,* 1980, *62A* (2), 286–291.

Mock, M. S. Sprains and strains: Orthopedics in the emergency room. *Orthopedic Nurses Association Journal,* 1979, *6* (8), 318–319.

Miller, M. E. Cycle trauma. *Nursing 80,* 1980, *10* (7), 26–31.

Mubarak, S. J., Owen, C. A., Hargens, A. R., et al. Acute compartmental syndromes: Diagnosis and treatment with the aid of the wick catheter. *Journal of Bone and Joint Surgery,* 1978, *60A* (8), 1091–1095.

Price, S. A., & McCarty, W. L. *Pathophysiology, Clinical concepts of disease processes.* New York: McGraw-Hill, 1978.

Reilly, M. M. Let's set the record straight: Preparing the discharge summary and the patient's instruction sheet. *Nursing 79,* 1979; *9* (1), 56–61.

Richter-Davies, L., Barnett, K., & Reid, D. Emergency management of lower extremity fractures. *Assessment and fracture management of the lower extremities.* Pitman, N. J.: Anthony J. Jannetti, 1984.

Roaf, R., & Hodkinson, L. J. *Textbook of orthopaedic nursing* (2nd ed.). Oxford: Blackwell Scientific, 1975.

Ross, N. Whose contracture? *Nursing 78,* 1978, *8* (6) 20.

Schneider, F. R. *Orthopaedics in emergency care.* St. Louis: C. V. Mosby, 1980.

Shires, G. T. *Care of the trauma patient* (2nd ed.). New York: McGraw-Hill, 1979.

Sproles, K. J. Nursing care of skeletal pins: A closer look. *Orthopaedic Nursing,* 1985, *4* (1), 11–19.

Turek, S. L. *Orthopaedics, principles and their applications* (3rd ed.). Philadelphia: Lippincott, 1977.

4

MUSCULOSKELETAL PATHOLOGY

Chapter 4 presents a brief overview of the major pathological conditions affecting the musculoskeletal system; including arthritis; infections due to tuberculosis, osteomyelitis, and other causes; neoplasms; and other orthopaedic abnormalities such as osteoporosis, osteomalacia, and Paget's disease. In contrast to the later anatomical chapters, Chapter 4 gives a more generalized view of the condition and how it affects the entire body. General symptomatology, diagnostic tests, treatment methods, and complications are discussed.

ARTHRITIS

Rheumatoid Arthritis

Rheumatoid arthritis (RA) is a chronic systemic inflammatory disease characterized most prominently by recurrent inflammations involving the synovia or linings of joints, and leading to destructive changes in the joints. RA is the most virulent form of arthritis and afflicts more than 7 million people in the United States alone. It occurs more frequently in women, with a women to men ratio of 4:1. Although RA can occur at any age and has been diagnosed in children only a few months old, the primary ages of onset are 20 to 40.

In spite of intensive research, the etiology of RA is still unknown. Three hypotheses being considered are: (1) a virus or other microorganism (e.g., mycoplasma), (2) a metabolic aberration, and (3) an immunological response. There is also a possiblity that there is a genetic base for a predisposition to RA, because it tends to occur in families.

RA commonly involves the peripheral joints, but it is a systemic disease, attacking connective tissues throughout the body. Degenerative lesions may occur in collagen in the lungs, heart, muscles, blood vessels, pleura, and tendons. Vasculitis may occur in the eyes, nervous system, and skin, producing ischemia and thrombosis. In most patients, the disease follows an intermittent course, with periods of remission and exacerbation. Some patients experience a relatively brief period of illness, lasting only a few days or months, and then have their symptoms subside for several months or even years. Periods of remission, which allow normal activity, tend to appear more frequently in the early course of the disease. Occasionally permanent spontaneous remissions occur. According to Engleman et al. (1969), 10 years after onset, 15 percent of persons with arthritis are likely to be bedridden, 35 percent may be ambulatory but are unable to earn a living, and 50 percent may be employable and capable of self-care. In general, the disease becomes more severe with the development of nodules, vasculitis, and high titers of rheumatoid factors. RA usually requires lifelong treatment and, in some instances, surgery.

RA usually develops insidiously, but onset often coincides with disturbances that deplete the patient's physical and emotional reserves (e.g., worry, exposure, overwork, divorce, and acute illness). Initially RA produces nonspecific symptoms, such as malaise, early afternoon fatigue, vasomotor disturbances, anorexia, weight loss, persistent low-grade fever, enlarged lymph nodes, enlarged spleen, mental depression, vague articular symptoms, and subcutaneous nodules. Then more specific localized articular symptoms develop, such as joint deformities and ocular manifestations. Atrophy of the muscles and the skin around the involved joint ensue. The patient develops flexion contractures from spasms of the flexor muscles around the inflamed joints and atrophy of the antagonistic extensor muscles. Typically, RA initially involves the proximal interphalangeal (PIP), metacarpophalangeal (MCP), and metatarsophalangeal (MTP) joints of the hands and feet. Those symptoms usually occur bilaterally and symmetrically, and may extend to the wrists, knees, elbows, and ankles. The pain produced by RA is variable in intensity and tends to be most persistent upon use of the involved joints. Stiffness is often the most constant symptom, especially upon rising in the morning. The fingers may assume a spindle shape from marked edema and congestion in the joints. The joints become tender and painful, at first only when the patient moves them, but eventually even at rest. The involved joints often feel hot to the patient, a sign of active disease. Ultimately, joint function is diminished.

If unarrested, the disease process within the joint passes through four main stages (1) synovitis, (2) pannus formation, (3) fibrous ankylosis, and (4) bony ankylosis. In the stage of synovitis the involved joint develops a proliferative type of inflammation that is initially localized in the joint capsule, primarily in the synovial membrane. Edema and congestion then thicken the synovial tissue. In the second stage, pannus formation, a layer of granulation develops in the inflamed synovial tissue. The pannus extends over the surface of the articular cartilage into the interior of the joint, and adheres tightly to the underlying cartilage of the joint. The rough, granular pannus erodes and destroys the cartilage of the joint by invasion, lysis, and decreased nutrition. Additional destruction occurs as granulation develops in subchrondral bone. In the third stage, fibrous ankylosis, there is subluxation and distortion of the affected joint as the granulation spreads throughout the joint. The fibrous tissue of the joint is toughened and scarred by the continuing inflammation. The result is a joint with decreased motion due to subluxation and the inhibiting effects of the fibrous tissue. In the fourth state, bony ankylosis (union) develops as the fibrous tissue becomes calcified and changes into osseous tissue.

Deformities are inevitable if the disease process is allowed to progress. In the hand, the PIP joints can develop flexion or hyperextension deformities. The MCP joints can swell dorsally, and volar subluxation and stretching of tendons can pull the fingers to the ulnar side ("ulnar drift"). The fingers may develop "swan's neck" or "boutonniere" deformity. The hands may appear shortened and the wrists boggy. Carpal tunnel syndrome may develop from synovial pressure on the median nerve, causing tingling paresthesias in the fingers.

A less common complication is degeneration of the odontoid process, a part of the second cervical vertebra. In rare instances, cord compression occurs, particularly in patients with longstanding, deforming RA. Upper motor neuron weakness and a positive Babinski sign occur infrequently. RA can also cause temporomandibular disease, which impairs chewing and causes earaches.

The most common extra-articular symptom is the gradual appearance of rheumatoid subcutaneous nodules. The nodules, which may be present for weeks or months, most commonly develop over bony prominences, especially near the elbows. Vasculitis can lead to skin lesions, leg ulcers, and multiple complications. Peripheral neuropathy may produce numbness, tingling, weakness, and loss of sensation in the feet and hands. Stiff, weak, or painful muscles are common. Other extra-articular effects include pericarditis, pulmonary nodules or fibrosis, pleuritis, scleritis, and behavioral changes (e.g., depression and anxiety). General body reactions to treatment can include renal calculi, cushingoid features from steroids, and gastrointestinal bleeding from salicylates.

Diagnosis

Besides the typical features of RA observed on physical examination, laboratory findings and diagnostic tests are necessary to confirm the diagnosis. Serum protein electrophoresis frequently shows elevated serum globulin. Rheumatoid factors (RF), large antibody-like protein molecules, are found in 75 to 80 percent of the patients, as indicated by a titer of 1:160 or higher. The erythrocyte sedimentation rate (ESR) is elevated in 85 to 90 percent of the patients with RA. C-Reactive Protein and ESR are both elevated during acute and chronic phases. A complete blood count (CBC) usually shows a moderate anemia and a slight leukocytosis. A hypochromic, normocystic anemia is common. Usually the white blood cell (WBC) count is slightly elevated or normal, though leukopenia may be present (e.g., with splenomegaly). When synovial (joint) fluid is aspirated, abnormalities are found. Roentgenograms show soft tissue swelling early in the course of the disease. As the disease progresses, roentgenograms can reveal osteoporosis around the involved joint, erosion of the cartilage at the periphery of the joint surface, joint space narrowing due to erosion of cartilage, and bony cysts from the invasion of granulation tissue. After several years, degenerative changes from secondary osteoporosis become apparent.

Treatment

As RA is a chronic and potentially crippling disease, it is difficult for a patient to accept. When the diagnosis is presented to the patient, attempts should be made to realistically discuss how the illness will affect the patient's life. Given the variable nature of the disease process, precise forecasts cannot be made, but it should be emphasized that many persons with RA continue to lead active, productive lives and that with early, intensive treatment only slight modifications in life-style may be necessary. Arthritis does not need to be a "hopeless" disease. If treatment is delayed or avoided, however, it typically worsens, and patients who cannot or will not accept their limitatons and modify their lives accordingly tend to do more poorly than those who are able to adapt.

Treatment goals are the preservation of function, the reduction of pain and inflammation, and the prevention or correction of deformities. Initially the treatment of RA is usually conservative, employing salicylates, rest, and physical therapy. An important aspect of that treatment is a successful patient education program that teaches the patient about illness and the best methods for dealing with it. Patients with RA should be alerted to the pitfalls of "quack" cures, and be informed of local assistance efforts, such as those of the Arthritis Foundation, which may be of help.

Salicylates. Salicylates (aspirin) are the most effective drug used in the treatment of RA. They have analgesic and anti-inflammatory properties, in addition to being relatively safe and inexpensive. Aspirin is available in plain, enteric-coated, or buffered tablets, and as a suppository. Aspirin should be taken with food because of its irritating effects on the stomach.

With the advancement of the disease, additional medications may be used. They include nonsteroidal, anti-inflammatory agents (such as indomethacin, fenoprofen, and ibuprofen), antimalarial drugs (chloroquine and hydroxychloroquine), gold salts, penicillamine, adrenocorticosteroids (prednisone), cytoxic agents (cyclophosphamide), and immunosuppressives (azathioprine).

Rest. Rest for a patient with RA should include complete physical and emotional rest, not just rest of the involved joints. The amount of systemic rest needed depends on the stage of the disease and the number of joints involved. With mild RA, 2 to 4 hours of rest daily (in addition to the normal 8 to 10 hours of rest at night) is usually adequate. That amount of rest may be reduced as the patient's condition improves. For rest to be effective, the bed needs to be firm and the patient should lie in correct body alignment to prevent flexion or extension deformities. Sandbags, splints, footboards, pillows, and other supportive devices may be used to maintain correct body alignment.

Physical Therapy. Physical therapy helps to (1) prevent and correct deformities, (2) control pain, and (3) strengthen weakened muscles and improve function. Physical therapy helps to prevent or correct deformities by teaching positioning and an active exercise program and sometimes, by splinting and casting. Pain control is accomplished by teaching the patient methods of regulating activities so as to minimize pain. Strengthening of weakened muscles is accomplished by isometric exercises. Joint function can be improved by identifying patient needs and teaching patients more effective methods of daily living. A variety of self-help appliances are also available to help the patient maintain a high level of independence.

Other treatment modalities are hot and cold applications. Heat has an analgesic effect and helps to relax muscles. Heat may also relieve joint stiffness and swelling. After heat applications, exercises can usually be performed more effectively. Various forms of heat therapy, which can be used, are moist heat (whirlpools, jacuzzis, hot tubs, showers, hot packs, and hot towels), dry heat (electric heating pads, hot water bottles, and infrared heat lamps), diathermy, ultrasound, and paraffin baths. Cold applications (e.g., crushed ice packs) induce a local anesthesia. They are effective during acute episodes.

Advanced stages of the disease may require surgical repair, often including arthroplasties of major joints. Other useful surgical procedures include metatarsal head and distal ulnar resection arthroplasties; insertion of a Silastic prosthesis between MCP and PIP joints to free and stabilize them; arthrodesis (joint fusion), usually in the wrists, feet, or spine; synovectomy (removal of a destructive, proliferating synovium), usually in the wrists, knees, and fingers to delay the course of the disease; osteotomy (cutting or excising bone) to realign joint surfaces and redistribute stresses; and tendon transfers to prevent deformities or relieve contractures.

Osteoarthritis

Osteoarthritis (also known as osteoarthrosis, degenerative arthritis, and hypertrophic arthritis) is an idiopathic, slowly progressive noninflammatory disease of diarthrodial (synovial-lined) joints, characterized by deterioration and erosion of articular cartilage and the formation of new bone, or spurs, at the articular margins. It generally occurs late in life and is the most common of all forms of arthritis, estimated to afflict well over 40 million Americans. Only a small fraction of that number, however, are significantly incapacitated. Osteoarthritis is almost as inevitable a concomitant of aging as gray hair.

Aging is the single most important factor in the development of osteoarthritis, and virtually all persons over the age of 50 have at least a trace of it. However, some older persons have little evidence of the disease, whereas other, relatively young, persons may become incapacitated. The precise nature of the aging influences are uncertain, but it has generally been attributed to cumulative stress and mechanical trauma. It is twice as prevalent in the obese, and mainly affects the weight-bearing joints. In men, a single weight-bearing joint is usually involved, but in obese men the disease often assumes the generalized pattern more typical of women. Osteoarthritis tends to appear earlier and to be more severe in patients with diabetes, ochronosis, and acromegaly, and there are some indications of a familial tendency.

Pathology

Osteoarthritis may involve one joint or many joints. The hips and knees are particularly susceptible. The spine is a common site, especially in the midcervical, midthoracic, and midlumbar areas, which are the regions of greatest movement in the spine. Osteoarthritis of the first metatarsophalangeal (MTP) joint of the foot and the distal interphalangeal joints of the hand is common. In the hand, osteoarthritis leads to Heberden nodes in the distal joints and Bouchard's nodes in the proximal joints.

Principally, osteoarthritis involves degeneration of cartilage rather than inflammation of the synovia. The first changes are fissuring and irregularity of the articular cartilaginous surfaces, followed by microfractures and the separation of small fragments of cartilage. After the destruction of the articular cartilage, the underlying bone is exposed. That subarticular bone is thickened by compression and new bone formation. The marrow spaces become filled with fibrous tissue and small pieces of cartilage. Some cartilage fragments become ossified and project above the surface of the articular cartilage, usually at the margins, producing the characteristic bony spurs of osteoarthritis. Those spurs are responsible for the "lipping" found in the vertebral body when the spine is affected. The calcific spurs may break off to form free intra-articular foreign bodies known as "joint mice." The capsule and ligaments of the joints often undergo calcification that further limits mobility (Robbins, 1974, pp. 1470–1471).

The patient with osteoarthritis usually does not appear ill and is commonly obese. Symptoms usually do not appear before age 40, unless the involved joints have been subjected to trauma. Commonly the onset is gradual. An aching pain is the most common symptom. Other symptoms are limitation of motion, contractures, and muscle spasms. Pain occurs with use and is more pronounced after exercise. Pain at rest may be caused by muscle spasms, and night pain and morning stiffness may also occur. A flexion contracture of the hip and a loss of ability to extend the knee are the most common disabling symptoms. The severity of the symptoms and the degree of degenerative joint changes are often not correlated. Therefore, a patient with minor degenerative changes may be quite uncomfortable, whereas a patient with advanced changes may have few or no symptoms. Affected joints may appear normal but be locally tender. Creaking, grating, and crepitus are often detectable in osteoarthritic joints. Occasionally, bony enlargement is evident. Limitation of motion is common, but ankylosis does not occur.

Treatment

Osteoarthritis progresses slowly. Even though there is no "cure" for the disorder, effective joint function can usually be maintained. Treatments include the reduction of stress on the joints, medications, physical therapy, orthopaedic appliances, and orthopaedic surgical procedures that may completely relieve the discomforts of osteoarthritis for some patients.

Reduction of Stress. Reducing the stress on affected joints can be accomplished in a number of ways. First, weight reduction in obese patients greatly relieves the strain on affected weight-bearing joints. The involved joint should be rested to reduce compression and shear stress and to allow any synovial inflammation to subside. During an acute inflammatory episode, the patient may be placed on bedrest with the involved joint positioned to relax the capsule and ligamentous structures, thereby minimizing compression of the articular surfaces. In rare instances, traction may be used to separate the joint surfaces and stretch the contracted capsule until the inflammation subsides.

Vertical loads on weight-bearing joints in the legs may be reduced by using assistive devices. A cane can be used in the hand of the uninvolved side to reduce stress. With advanced disease or bilateral joint involvement, the patient may require two canes, crutches, or a walker. The patient will need instruction on the proper gait (Appendix C).

Medications. There are a number of medications that help to relieve the pain of osteoarthritis. Acetylsalicylic acid (aspirin) is the most effective. Indomethacin (Indocin) or phenylbutazone (Butazolidin) may be used if salicylates fail. Muscle spasms may be relieved with diazepam (Valium), methocarbamol (Robaxin), or other such antispasmodics. Systemic corticosteroid therapy is not usually given for osteoarthritis, but intra-articular injections (e.g., of hydrocortisone acetate) may be helpful in treating inflamed large joints.

Physical Therapy. Physical therapy is of major importance in the management of osteoarthritis to help relax muscles and relieve aching and stiffness. Physical therapy usually consists of moist heat followed by massage and range-of-motion exercises, both passive and active. Forcible attempts to regain lost range of motion should be avoided, as excessive motion will put too much pressure on the joint surfaces. Isometric rather than isotonic exercises are usually preferred to build muscle power while minimizing joint stress.

Orthopaedic Appliances. A number of orthopaedic appliances may be used to eliminate faulty posture and maintain joint function. Supportive shoes can improve posture. A removable plaster or plastic splint can rest a joint while permitting daily physical therapy. An ordinary elastic bandage applied about an affected joint restricts motion while permitting some use. A simple plastic or fabric corset may provide sufficient support to the lower back, though a brace is a more effective form of immobilization. A long ischial-weight-bearing caliper brace may be used to reduce stress on the joint of the leg, and a leather cuff about the knee can provide additional support.

Orthopaedic Surgical Procedures. Surgical measures are aimed at the relief of pain, improving and maintaining joint movement, correcting deformity and malalignment, reducing vertical loads and shear stresses, removing intra-articular causes of erosion of articular surfaces, or creating a new joint with artificial implants. Arthrodesis is the only certain way of relieving pain and providing joint stability, and should be considered when other forms of surgery are not feasible or have failed. Special surgical considerations are applicable to each joint, and are described in later chapters.

Gout (Gouty Arthritis)

Gout is a hereditary condition of abnormal purine metabolism, which produces urate deposits in articular, periarticular, and subcutaneous tissues that cause painfully arthritic joints. It is characterized by recurring acute attacks, intervals of freedom from pain, and, in the later stages, by crippling, deforming arthritis, nephritis, urinary calculi, and cardiovascular lesions. Gout can affect any joint but tends to involve those in the feet and the legs. Primary gout occurs predominately in men over 40 years of age. It rarely occurs in women, and when it does the women are usually postmenopausal. Secondary gout occurs in the elderly. Even though gout can lead to chronic disability or incapacitation, prognosis is good with treatment.

Gout develops in four stages: asymptomatic, acute, intercritical, and chronic, In asymptomatic gout, serum urate levels rise but produce no symptoms. The first acute attack of gout occurs suddenly and peaks quickly. Although it generally involves only one or two joints, it is extremely painful. Affected joints appear hot, tender, inflamed, and dusky-red or cyanotic. The MTP joint of the great toe usually becomes inflamed first, but the disease frequently affects the instep, ankle, heel, knee, and wrist. The patient may develop a low-grade fever. Mild acute episodes often subside quickly, but tend to recur at irregular intervals. Severe episodes may persist for days or weeks. As the disease progresses, it may cause hypertension, nephrolithiasis, and severe back pain.

Intercritical periods are the symptom-free intervals between gout attacks. Most patients have a second attack within 6 months to 2 years, but in some the attack is delayed for 5 to 10 years. Subsequent attacks are more common in those who are untreated, and tend to be longer and more severe than initial attacks. Such attacks are also polyarticular, invariably affecting joints in the feet and legs, and are sometimes accompanied by fever. Some attacks are migratory, sequentially affecting various joints and the Achilles tendon, and are associated with either subdeltoid or olecranon bursitis (Turek, 1977 pp. 194–200).

Eventually, chronic polyarticular gout develops. That final, unremitting stage of the disease is marked by persistent painful polyarthritis, with large, subcutaneous, tophaceous (uric acid) deposits in cartilage, synovial membranes, tendons, and soft tissue. The classic site is the helix of the ear (above the earlobe), but urate deposits also form in fingers, hands, knees, feet, ulnar sides of the forearms, Achilles tendons, and, rarely, in internal organs such as the kidneys. The skin over the tophus may ulcerate and release a chalky, white exudate or pus. Chronic inflammation and tophaceous deposits cause joint degeneration, with eventual deformity and disability. Kidney involvement, with associated tubular damage, leads to chronic renal dysfunction. Hyptertension and albuminuria occur in some patients; urolithiasis is common.

Diagnosis

The main factors in making a diagnosis of gout are family history, repeated attacks with intervals of freedom from pain, renal disturbances such as urate calculus, and hyperuricemia. Urate deposits in or near affected joints, bursae, the helixes of the ears, distal finger joints, Achilles tendons, or elsewhere strongly suggest chronic gout. Aspiration of synovial fluid (arthrocentesis) or of tophaceous material reveals needle-like intracellular crystals of sodium urate. Serum uric acid is above normal; urinary uric acid values are usually higher in secondary gout than in primary gout.

Roentgenograms show clearly defined "punched out" areas of bone lysis. Similar erosions occur in other diseases (including rheumatoid arthritis [RA], degenerative joint disease, and tuberculosis), but only gout manifests outward displacement of the overhanging margin from the bone contour. A positive test for the rheumatoid factor distinguishes RA from gout.

Treatment

The objectives of gout management are to relieve acute discomfort and prevent the development of chronic gouty arthritis, renal calculi, and renal damage. The treatment of gout falls into two categories: acute and long-term management.

During an acute attack, treatment is directed toward relieving pain and inflammation by means of anti-inflammatory drugs. The patient is placed on bedrest and the affected extremity immobilized in a soft pillow splint. An ice pack effectively reduces pain. A bed cradle over the foot of the bed helps to relieve pressure from the bed linen on the affected leg. Occasionally hot packs may be used. Medications such as colchicine (an analgesic and diuretic), ACTH, phenylbutazone, indomethacin, oxyphenbutazone, most steroidal anti-inflammatory agents, ibuprofen, naproxen, and fenoprofen are used to reduce inflammation. Narcotics or analgesics may be used for severe pain until anti-inflammatory therapy becomes effective. The patient should eat a diet high in carbohydrates and fluids and avoid alcohol. The patient may be allowed to rest in a chair, with the affected extremity protected and elevated. Weight bearing is to be avoided until the attack subsides.

Long-term management is to lower serum uric acid levels to the normal range. The therapy involves either inhibiting production of uric acid or increasing the excretion of uric acid. Drugs that result in increased excretion of uric acid are probenecid (Benemid) and sulfinpyrazone (Anturane). The effectiveness of both drugs can be reduced if the patient receives aspirin or other salicylates. Allopurinal (Zyloprim) is a xanthineoxidase inhibitor that reduces the production of uric acid.

INFECTIONS

Extrapulmonary Tuberculosis

Tuberculosis in areas other than the lungs is called extrapulmonary tuberculosis. In the past, tuberculosis was the most common chronic joint disease, and this is still the case in many countries. Tuberculosis of bones and joints is always secondary to a focus of tuberculosis elsewhere in the patient's body. For further discussions on tuberculosis, see the references at the end of the chapter.

The onset of tuberculosis is usually insidious. The patient has loss of weight and general malaise followed by the gradual development of pain, muscle spasms, restricted movement, and deformity in the affected joint. The classic joint symptom is night pain. There is marked wasting of the muscles adjacent to the joint, substantial limitation of joint movement, and ultimately the development of a fixed deformity. To prevent the deformity, it is essential that the diagnosis be made and treatment started at an early stage in the disease process. When tuberculosis of a joint is found on clinical and roentgenographic examination, diagnostic studies must be done to determine the primary focus of the disease. A direct biopsy of the synovial membrane may be done to confirm a diagnosis of joint tuberculosis.

Treatment

The treatment of bone and joint tuberculosis involves (1) rest (2) drug therapy (3) disease control and (4) nutrition. In the early stages, apart from diagnostic measures, surgical procedures are rare, but if there is a chronic thickening of the synovial membrane, it is usually excised. If there is extensive destruction of bone and joint cartilage, an arthrodesis of the joint may be done or, if the joint has assumed a position of fixed deformity, a corrective osteotomy may be necessary. For more details on the treatment and nursing care of tuberculosis of different parts of the skeletal system, see the following chapters.

Rest. In general, the patient is placed on bedrest, particularly during the acute stages of the infection. When it is demonstrated that antituberculin drugs are effective and the patient's condition is improving, limited activity is allowed. The involved joint is placed at rest, usually in a splint, until roentgenographic and clinical examination shows that the infection is subsiding and movement can be permitted. If the progress of the infection is arrested in time and proper immobilization is maintained, the prognosis for restoration of joint function is good.

Drug Therapy. Isoniazid, ethambutol, rifampin, and streptomycin are often referred to as the first line drugs against tuberculosis. However, other effective drugs are viomycin, capreomycin, kanamycin, ethionamide, pyrazinamide, para-aminosalicylic acid, and cycloserine. Currently there is no medication that can be given in amounts large enough to completely destroy all the tubercle bacilli in the body. However, persons receiving antituberculosis drug therapy rapidly become noninfectious. Drug therapy for patients with active tuberculosis requires uninterrupted, intensive, prolonged administration. It may require 2 to 3 years, or even longer if the lesions respond slowly.

Disease Control. Tuberculosis can spread through pus produced by bone and joint lesions. Dressings, exudate from sinuses or abscesses, and the debris obtained from the site at the time of surgery must be treated with the same care as any infected dressing. For the protection of the staff, other patients, and the patient's relatives and friends, all patients with tuberculous joints are investigated for a possible pulmonary lesion.

Irradiation of the upper room air with ultraviolet light is the most effective method of decontaminating the immediate environment. This procedure can rapidly make room air noninfectious. Good ventilation is important, but is usually much slower than ultraviolet light in reducing the concentration of airborne organisms.

Nutrition. Patients with tuberculosis may have had a loss of appetite for some months before the pathology was diagnosed; alternatively, they may have come from an environment where there was insufficient food. Good nutrition is a part of the treatment regime and requires a diet high in protein, especially meat, fish, and dairy products. Patients with poor appetites should be encouraged to eat frequent small meals. The patient's fluid intake should be higher than normal because of the drug therapy, to facilitate discarding toxins from the infection, and to prevent stasis and crystal deposits in the tubules of the kidney, which can lead to stone formation.

Complications of Tuberculosis of the Skeletal System

A common complication is the formation of a cold abscess, a painless collection of pus and debris. An abscess may occur at the site of the lesion or appear some distance away (e.g., in spinal tuberculosis, an abscess may form in the psoas sheath and appear in the groin). Another complication is the formation of a sinus. If an abscess is not surgically aspirated, the phagocytes of the blood create their own channel to the surface of the body. A third complication is Pott's paraplegia, when tuberculosis of the vertebral column results in the formation of an abscess that impinges upon the spinal cord (see pp. 167–168). A fourth complication is an amyloid disease, the presence of a chronic tubercular lesion that results in deposits of wax-like materials in the visceral organs of the body. That is associated with vitamin and protein deficiency, and is rarely seen today in developed countries. Amyloid disease primarily affects the kidneys, liver, intestines, and (rarely) the peripheral nerves.

Osteomyelitis

Osteomyelitis is an infection of bone, bone marrow, and surrounding soft tissue caused by pyogenic (pus-producing) bacteria. The infection may reach the bone directly (e.g., through an open fracture), through the bloodstream, or from infections in adjacent soft tissues. It can cause bone destruction, mobility limitations, and severe pain, and can be an acute or chronic condition.

Osteomyelitis is most often caused by *Staphyloccocus aureus,* with hemolytic *Streptococcus* the second most common cause. Other organisms that can cause osteomyelitis are *Salmonella, Neisseria gonorrhea, Hemophilus influenzae, Proteus,* and *Pseudomonas.* When the bacteria enter the bone, they multiply and destroy bone cells. In response, the body's macrophages enter to kill the bacteria. The collection of debris and resulting edema causes a rise in pressure within the rigid bone, and if the pressure reaches arterial pressure, blood and antibiotics cannot enter. Eventually, the infection extends from the marrow cavity through the cortex of the bone. Pressure elevates the periosteum, destroying its blood vessels and causing bone necrosis. The dead bone tissue (sequestrum) cannot easily be liquified and discharged as pus, nor can the necrotic cavity collapse and heal as is the case with soft tissue. The body's response is to attempt to heal the infected bone by laying down new bone cells over the sequestrum, forming a new covering called the involucrum. Even though healing appears to take place, the involucrum interferes with normal phagocytosis, acts as a barrier to antibiotics, and thus preserves a chronically infected sequestrum that can produce recurring abscesses throughout the life of the individual. The course of chronic osteomyelitis is characterized by asymptomatic remissions and exacerbations when pain and inflammation reoccur as the body tries to rid itself of sequestra. Sinus tracts may form between the sequestra and the skin or may lead into an adjacent joint, draining the purulent abscess into that joint.

Clinical Manifestations

Local symptoms of acute osteomyelitis are a sudden onset of severe pain in the affected bone, tenderness over the bone, heat, redness, swelling, painful movement, and involuntary restriction of movement. Muscle spasms may occur and cause the patient to hold the extremity in flexion and resist attempts to touch the painful area. General symptoms that often occur with acute severe bone infection are chills, high fever, headache, nausea, diaphoresis, rapid pulse, marked leukocytosis, an elevated ESR, and a positive blood culture. Evidence of bone infection may not appear on roentgenograms for at least 2 weeks.

In the chronic phase, an exacerbation is characterized by low-grade fever, pain, and persistent drainage from a sinus. A sinogram (a roentgenogram with dye) may be used to reveal the location of the sinus and the site of the primary infection.

Treatment

Early diagnosis is extremely important to prevent chronic osteomyelitis. With early treatment, the chances of effectively controlling acute osteomyelitis are quite good. Once osteomyelitis is suspected, antibiotics (usually a penicillinase-resistant penicillin) are given immediately. After blood cultures are obtained and the causative organism is identified, antibiotics specific to that organism are begun and continued for several weeks. It is important that the specific antibiotic reach the bone before bone necrosis occurs. If treatment is delayed, bone necrosis may develop and prevent the antibiotic from effectively combating the infection. With the patient on bedrest, the infected bone should be immobilized using a cast or traction until evidence of acute infection disappears.

In acute infectious osteomyelitis, if the response to antibiotics is slow and an abscess develops, an incision and drainage (I and D) may be done. If the patient has internal fixation devices for fracture repair, they may be removed at the time of the I and D. After an I and D, antibiotics may be instilled into the bone cavity daily. Catheters may also be placed in the wound for continuous drip instillation of an antibiotic solution or for irrigation of the wound. A closed irrigation and drainage system with low pressure suction is frequently used.

If chronic osteomyelitis develops, the wound usually needs to be exposed and all infected dead bone and cartilage carefully removed so permanent healing can take place. This operation, called a sequestrectomy, consists of the removal of the sequestrum and the overlying involucrum. The procedure is followed by continuous wound irrigation with an antibiotic solution. The joints above and below the affected part may be immobilized with a splint to decrease pain and muscle spasm until the wound heals. Hot packs may also be utilized to reduce swelling.

NEOPLASMS

Tumors involving the skeleton are by no means rare and are frequently malignant. Bone neoplasms may occur as primary benign or malignant lesions or as secondary (i.e., metastatic) lesions. The most common benign tumors include osteomas, chrondromas, giant-cell tumors (the most common), cysts, and osteoid osteomas. Benign tumors are usually well circumscribed, grow slowly, and seldom spread. Primary malignant bone tumors include osteogenic sarcoma (the most common), Ewing's sarcoma, multiple myeloma, reticulum cell sarcoma, and angiosarcoma. Multiple myeloma is considered by some authorities to be a disorder of the blood-forming organs (i.e., the bone marrow) rather than a primary bone tumor. In adults, the most common bone tumors are metastatic, with the primary lesion frequently in the breast, lung, prostate, kidney, ovary, or thyroid. Among tumors, carcinomas tend to metastasize to bone more frequently than sarcomas.

Certain bone tumors tend to occur at specific ages. For example, osteogenic sarcomas generally appear below age 25; giant-cell tumors usually occur between the ages of 21 and 35; and multiple myelomas occur more frequently between the ages of 50 and 70.

Symptoms

In general, bone tumors interfere with mobility and comfort. The major symptoms are a local swelling or mass, pain, restricted motion, aching, and fractures due to the weakening of the bone. In tumors of the lower extremity, the patient may walk with a limp due to pain. The bone pain may range from mild to severe and is frequently described as persistent pain. Pain usually occurs before the tumor is detectable on roentgenography.

Diagnosis

The diagnostic measures for detecting bone tumors are based on personal history, signs and symptoms, roentgenography, and bone biopsies with frozen sections. Once a malignant tumor is suspected, roentgenography such as radioisotope scanning or computed axial tomographic scan is done to look for additional lesions. The precise identification of the tumor type is extremely important in determining treatment.

Treatment

Bone tumors are usually treated by either chemotherapy, irradiation, or surgery. Sometimes a combination of treatments is required. Surgical procedures may range from small resections to radical amputations.

Benign Giant-Cell Tumor

A giant-cell tumor is an osteophytic tumor that occurs in young adults after the epiphyseal plate has ossified and longitudinal bone growth is completed, i.e., usually between ages 15 to 35. It occurs most frequently at the end of the long bones, especially the distal femur, proximal tibia, and distal radius. The cause is unknown.

The manifestations of the tumor are chronic, constant pain in the region of the joint. Pain becomes progressively more severe at night and with increased activity. Usually there is swelling and the overlying skin is stretched. In contrast to osteogenic sarcoma, the skin displays no dilated vessels. Pressure over the swelling produces audible and palpable crackling as the bone cortex is ruptured. The patient does not have limitation of motion or pathological fractures until the tumor has expanded and distorted the end of the affected bone.

Diagnosis. Diagnosis is based on the patient's personal history, signs and symptoms, and roentgenograms. Positive roentgenograms show a circumscribed osteolytic growth.

Treatment. The goal is to try and conserve the extremity when possible. The surgical procedure is usually to remove the tumor by curettage and then cauterize the cavity walls or fill the cavity with bone grafts. When the tumor is extensive, a resection of the bone is done and the remaining shaft may be arthrodesed to other bones at the joint. An intramedullary pin is sometimes utilized in the arthrodesis. Newer methods are cryotherapy after tumor excision, or cryotherapy and filling the cavity with methyl methacrylate bone cement (Connelly, 1981). Depending upon the extent of the tumor and its recurrence, amputation may be indicated.

Osteogenic Sarcoma

Osteogenic sarcoma (osteosarcoma) is a highly malignant bone tumor. It is the most common primary malignant bone tumor and usually occurs in patients between 10 and 25 years of age. It has been known to occur later in life secondary to Paget's disease, and in some instances following osteomyelitis or previous bone irradiation.

Osteosarcoma is manifested by pain, swelling, limitation of motion, and weight loss. There is intermittent pain, usually noted at night. The bony mass may be palpable and tender, with venous dilation leading to increased skin temperature over the mass. The patient may complain of fatigue.

The tumor is visible on roentgenograms, and bone scans can be used to demonstrate increased tumor growth. In 50 percent of patients, there is an elevation in the serum alkaline phosphatase. The primary lesion may involve any bone. The most common sites, however, are the distal femur, the proximal tibia, and the proximal humerus.

The goal of treatment is to destroy or remove the malignant tissue. The most effective method usually requires a combination of treatments. The surgical removal of the tumor may involve local bone resection, resection and implantation of metallic prostheses or allografts as bone replacements, or amputation. Chemotherapy and radiation may also be utilized.

Nursing should focus on interventions to assist the patient with the emotional reactions, especially with regard to the diagnosis and treatment that may result in a change in body image and self-concept.

OTHER PATHOLOGICAL PROCESSES

Osteoporosis

Osteoporosis occurs when the rate of bone resorption exceeds the rate of bone formation, causing a reduced bone mass. With rare exceptions, it is a systemic disorder that affects the patient's entire skeleton. It can occur locally when part of the body is immobilized by a fracture or paralysis. Systemic osteoporosis appears to be most marked in the spine, pelvis, and skull. The bone changes are characterized by a thinning of the cortical bone, resorption of cancellous bone, enlargement of the medullary cavity, and an overall loss of bone mass (Robbins, 1974, p. 1442). Bones become porous, brittle, and subject to fractures from minimal trauma. Compression fractures of the vertebrae are most common, but the ribs, wrist, and hip are also frequently fractured.

Osteoporosis has been classified as either primary or secondary. In primary osteoporosis there is no clearly identifiable cause, though poor diet, estrogen deficiency, and lack of exercise may be involved. Senile osteoporosis is the most common type of primary osteoporosis. Many of the patients are postmenopausal women, and women outnumber men by a ratio of 4:1. They usually seek medical attention because of back pain related to minor trauma. No satisfactory method of treatment is presently available. The most common method of treatment is to improve the patient's protein, calcium and vitamin D intake. Exercise, estrogen replacement, and high fluoride intake have also been used effectively.

Secondary osteoporosis has an identifiable cause. The list of those causes is long, but the three major ones are nutritional deficiencies, abnormal endocrine function, and disuse. Various abnormal nutritional states are known to cause osteoporosis, including vitamin C deficiency (scurvy), mild malabsorption syndrome (lactose intolerance), acid diets, and calcium-deficient diets. High-protein diets used for weight reduction may also increase bone resorption because the increased acidity resulting from a nitrogen imbalance is buffered by calcium from the bones.

Endocrine osteoporosis is caused by abnormal functioning of an endocrine gland. Persons with hyperthyroidism, hyperparathyroidism, Cushing's syndrome, acromegaly, and hypogonadism, are likely to have endocrine osteoporosis. Some medications, such as corticosteroids, cause an osteoporotic reaction similar to endocrine osteoporosis. Disuse osteoporosis, caused by bedrest and inactivity, is well-known, and elderly people who become less active are subject to it. Lack of sufficient stresses and strains appears to be the main factor, as stressing bones by exercise is known to strengthen them and increase bone mass.

Osteoporosis may be present for a long time before it is detected. Lukert (1982) states that 50 percent of women over age 65 have asymptomatic osteoporosis. The symptoms of osteoporosis may occur suddenly or insidiously. The patient usually has initial symptoms that include weakness, pain, unsteady gait, stiffness, and poor appetite (Richards, 1982). Back pain, usually in the lower thoracic or lumbar region, is the most common complaint. Other painful areas are the hips, pelvis, and legs. Physical changes in the spine cause a loss of height and a rounded back (kyphosis). Laboratory studies are usually within normal limits. Only after 30 percent of the bone has been lost is the loss visible on roentgenograms.

Medical treatment is prescribed according to the cause of the secondary osteoporosis. However, it usually includes a well-balanced diet, exercise, frequent rest periods, avoidance of severe fatigue, calcium, and vitamin C and D supplements. Estrogen is sometimes used, but is controversial because of the risk of endometrial carcinoma (Lukert, 1982). Sodium fluoride, in combination with calcium and vitamins, stimulates osteoblastic activity, increases bone strength, and decreases fracture risks (Lukert, 1982).

Osteomalacia

Osteomalacia, now a rare condition, literally means "softness of bone." It is the adult counterpart of childhood rickets and is characterized by inadequate mineralization of newly formed bone. The difference between rickets and osteomalacia is that in adults the mechanisms of bone growth are not involved and only bone turnover mechanisms are affected, so that the bones become softer and more fragile than normal. Fractures are common, but bending and stress deformities also develop because the bones have decreased rigidity (Robbins, 1974, p. 1443).

It is overly simplistic to say that osteomalacia is merely the result of a dietary deficiency of vitamin D. There are other possible mechanisms leading to inadequate mineralization of bone. They can be divided into three categories. First, there may be insufficient intake of vitamin D, which is the most common cause. Second, there are patients with hypophosphatemia, principally familial hypophosphatemia (vitamin D-resistant rickets), but also including Fanconi's syndrome and renal tubular acidosis. Third, there are patients with defective nucleation of preformed bone matrix, such as hypophosphatasia and fluoride and strontium intoxication. All three categories produce skeletal changes that cannot readily be distinguished from one another (Robbins, 1974, p. 1443).

In all cases, osteomalacia is characterized by a prolongation of the time interval between osteoid synthesis and mineralization. Instead of the normal 6 to 10 days, the time lag for mineralization may be as long as 2 to 3 months. Moreover, some areas completely fail to mineralize, leaving osteoid residuals.

Osteomalacia develops insidiously. It may be identified by reduced serum calcium and phosphorus levels, reduced urine calcium, bone deformities, bone pain and tenderness, and roentgenographic changes. A biopsy of the bone may help establish the diagnosis. The bones most commonly involved are the spine, pelvis, and lower extremities. Usually there is a history of bone or spinal pain from crush fractures.

Treatment of osteomalacia may involve large amounts of vitamin D and dietary measures to insure adequate intake of calcium and phosphorus, e.g., diets high in eggs, milk, fish, and vegetables. Calcium salts and phosphate supplements may also be given.

Paget's Disease

Paget's disease of the bone (osteitis deformans) is an acquired disorder of unknown etiology characterized by hyperactive bone destruction (osteoclastic activity) and formation (osteoblastic activity), with replacement of normal bone by expanded, soft, poorly mineralized, "honeycombed" osteoid tissue. Although the affected bones are increased in size, they are usually light, soft, and porous, and almost have the consistency of dry bread. The bone disease occurs in two patterns, monostotic and polyostotic, The tibia is the most common site in the monostotic pattern, and the pelvis and sacrum are typically the first bones involved in the polyostotic form. The entire skeleton is rarely involved (Robbins, 1974, p. 1445). Paget's disease rarely occurs in patients under the age of 40 and is more common in men than in women by a ratio of about 2:1.

When multiple bones are involved, Paget's disease usually produces readily identifiable characteristic deformities. The bone becomes shorter, broader, and weaker than normal bone and is more easily fractured. When the vertebral column is involved, grotesque dwarf-like distortions result. In the generalized form of the disease, the patient becomes shorter and, because the skull expands, may require a larger hat.

If only one or two bones are involved, the disease is commonly asymptomatic and is only discovered accidentally on roentgenographic examination. The onset of the disease is insidious. The initial complaint may be pain in the involved bone. The pain may be a dull ache, neurological discomfort, or a sharp stabbing sensation, and may be intermittent or constant. When pain is felt over the tibia, the bone may be found to be enlarged and bowed. The overlying skin is often warm to the touch, but the bone is not tender. Skull lesions may cause headaches, facial pain, and enlargement of the skull. Backache is a common accompaniment of spinal involvement.

Over time, the enlarged head contrasts with the relatively small face. One or both legs or thighs become bowed anterolaterally, as the enlarged tibiae increase the circumference of the legs. The femurs bend and the femoral necks may yield under pressure. The width of the chest is narrowed, and a kyphosis develops from compression of the vertebral bodies. The bones affected, in decreasing order of frequency, are the pelvis, skull, femur, spine, tibia, humerus, scapula and, only occasionally, other bones including the mandible.

Treatment. The treatment consists of drug therapy. Calcitonin (subcutaneously or intramuscularly) and etidronate are used to retard bone resorption and reduce serum alkaline phosphate and urinary hydroxyproline secretions. Although calcitonin involves long-term therapy, there is usually noticeable improvement after the first few weeks of treatment. Etidronate produces improvement after 1 to 3 months. Mithramycin, a cytotoxic antibiotic, is used to decrease calcium, urinary hydroxyproline, and serum alkaline phosphate. Mithramycin produces remission of symptoms within 2 weeks and biochemical improvement in 1 to 2 months. However, mithramycin may destroy platelets or compromise renal function. Drugs that usually help to control the pain are aspirin, indomethacin, and ibuprofen.

Patients may need surgery to reduce or prevent pathological fractures, correct secondary deformities, and relieve neurological impairment. Drug therapy may precede surgery to reduce the risk of excessive bleeding from hypervascular bones. Other treatments are symptomatic and supportive, and vary according to the symptoms.

Complications. The most common complication of Paget's disease is a fracture, especially of weight-bearing long bones, which usually occurs in the vascular soft (osteoblastic) stage of the disease process. Those fractures are usually found over the apex of the convexity of the bowed shaft. The fractures heal rapidly, although with a minimum of callus. When fractures occur in dense bone during the osteoclastic stage, union is delayed.

In at least 5 percent of patients with Paget's disease, the involved bone will undergo malignant degeneration (Turek, 1977, p. 653). The tumors are either osteogenic sarcoma, fibrosarcoma, or round-cell sarcoma. The development of a tumor is usually preceded by an increase in pain and a rapid increase in the size of a bone.

REFERENCES

Connelly, J. F. (Ed.). *De Palma's the management of fractures and dislocations: An atlas* (3rd ed.). Philadelphia: Saunders, 1981.

Engleman, E. P., Giansiricusa, J. E., & Chatton, M. J. Arthritis and allied rheumatoid disorders. In N. Brainerd, S. Margin, & M. J. Chatton (Eds.), *Current diagnosis and treatment.* Los Altos, Calif.: Lange Medical, 1969.

Lukert, B. P. Osteoporosis—A review and update. *Archives of Physical Medicine and Rehabilitation,* 1982, *63,* 480–487.

Richards, M. Osteoporosis. *Geriatric Nursing,* 1982, *3* (2), 98–102.

Robbins, S. L. *Pathologic basis of disease.* Philadelphia: Saunders, 1974.

Turek, S. L. *Orthopaedics, principles and their application* (3rd ed.). Philadelphia: Lippincott, 1977.

BIBLIOGRAPHY

Albright, J. A., & Brand, R. A. (Eds.). *The scientific basis of orthopaedics.* New York: Appleton-Century-Crofts, 1979.

Althoff, D. G. Diagnostic overview: Psoriatic arthritis. *Orthopaedic Nursing,* 1983, *2* (5), 50.

Anderson, W. A. D., & Kissane, J. M. *Pathology* (7th ed.). St. Louis: C. V. Mosby, 1977.

Arthritis Health Profession Section of the Arthritis Foundation. *Self-Help Manual for Patients with Arthritis.* Atlanta, Ga.: Arthritis Foundation, 1980.

Barnard, C. *Christiaan Barnard's program for living with arthritis, A Fireside Book.* New York: Simon & Schuster, 1984.

Barry, H. C. Orthopedic aspects of Paget's diseases of bone. *Arthritis and Rheumatism,* 1980, *23* (10),1128–1130.

Beary, J. F. Gout: Diagnosis and therapy. *Orthopedic Nurses' Association Journal,* 1979, *6* (8), 313–317.

Bik, P. An orthopedic case study: A patient with an osteoid osteoma. *Orthopedic Nurses' Association Journal,* 1978, *5* (5), 149–151.

Borzotta, A. P., Riddick, L., Sadlock, W., & Chun, B. Sudden death from massive tumor embolization of chondrosarcoma. *Journal of Bone and Joint Surgery,* 1978, *60A* (4), 561–563.

Brassell, M. P. Teaching patients to cope with polymyalgia rheumatica. *Nursing 78,* 1978, *8* (5), 22–28.

Brown-Skeers, V. How the nurse practitioner manages the rheumatoid arthritis patient. *Nursing 79,* 1979, *9* (6), 26–35.

Cave, L. Lowering the uncertainties of arthritis with a nurse-led support group. *Orthopaedic Nursing,* 1984, *3* (5), 39–42.

Clayton, M. L., & Kagan A., II, The rheumatoid knee. *Current Practice in Orthopaedic Surgery,* 1977, 7, 179–196.

Dalinka, M. K., Aronchick, J. M., & Hoddad, J. G. Paget's disease. *Orthopedic Clinics of North America,* 1983, *14* (1), 3–19.

DeGowon, E. L., & DeGowin, R. L. *Bedside diagnostic examination* (3rd ed.). New York: Macmillan, 1976.

Dickinson, G., & Gorman, T. K. The assessment (Adult arthritis). *American Journal of Nursing,* 1983, *83* (2), 262–265.

Drupp, M. A., & Chatton, M. J. (Eds.). *Current medical diagnosis and treatment 1982.* Los Altos, Calif.: Lange Medical, 1982.

Ebong, W. W. Acute osteomyelitis three years after a closed fracture in an adult with sickle-cell anemia. *Journal of Bone and Joint Surgery,* 1980, *62A* (7), 1196–1198.

Edmondson, A. S., & Crenshaw, A. H. (Eds.). *Campbell's operative orthopaedics* (6th ed.). St. Louis: C. V. Mosby, 1980.

Fries, J. F. *Arthritis, a comprehensive guide.* Menlo Park, Calif.: Addison-Wesley, 1982.

Frost, H. M. The evolution of osteoporosis therapy. *Orthopedic Clinics of North America,* 1981, *12* (3), 603–610.

Frost, H. M. Coherence treatment of osteoporosis. *Orthopedic Clinics of North America,* 1981, *12* (3), 649–669.

Frost, H. M. The evolution of pathophysiologic knowledge of osteoporosis. *Orthopedic Clinics of North America,* 1981, *12* (3), 477–478.

Gartland, J. J. *Fundamentals of orthopaedics* (3rd ed.). Philadelphia: Saunders, 1979.

Graham, B. A., & Gleit, C. J. Osteoporosis: A major health problem in postmenopausal women. *Orthopaedic Nursing,* 1984, *3* (6), 19–26.

Gruchacz, I. Case study: Reticulum cell sarcoma. *Orthopedic Nurses' Association Journal,* 1978, *5* (5), 165.

Johnston, C. C., Altman, R. D., Canfield, R. E., et al.: Review of fracture experience during treatment of Paget's disease of bone with etidronate disodium (ENDP). *Clinical Orthopedics and Related Research,* 1983, 186–194.

Kirns, L. L., & Simon, M. A. Surgical theory, staging, definitions and treatment of musculaskeletal sarcomas. *Surgical Clinics of North America,* 1983, *63* (3), 671–696.

Kim, E. E., Deland, F. A., & Maruyamo, Y. Decreased uptake in bone scans ("cold lesions") in matastatic carcinoma. *Journal of Bone and Joint Surgery,* 1978, *60A* (6), 844–846.

KleereKaper, M., Tolia, K., & Parfitt, A. M. Nutritional, endocrine and demographic aspects of osteoporosis. *Orthopedic Clinics of North America,* 1981, *12* (3), 547–558.

Koerner, M. E., & Dickinson, G. C. A look at some of its forms. *American Journal of Nursing,* 1983, *83* (2), 254.

Lane, J. M., & Vigorita, V. J. Current concepts review: Osteoporosis. *Journal of Bone and Joint Surgery,* 1983, *65A* (2), 274–278.

Lee, C. K., et al. Pathological fracture in chronic osteomyelitis. *Orthopedics,* 1979, *2* (1), 56–59.

Louther, S. A. Nursing case study: Osteoclastoma—giant-cell tumor. *Orthopedic Nurses' Association Journal,* 1978, *5* (2), 45–48.

Mankin, H. J., Cantley, K. P., Lippiello, L., et al. The biology of human chondrosarcoma: Part 1. *Journal of Bone and Joint Surgery,* 1980, *62A* (2), 160–176.

Mankin, H. J., Cantley, K. P., Schiller, A. L., & Lippiello, L. The biology of human chondrosarcoma: Part 2. *Journal of Bone and Joint Surgery,* 1980, *62A* (2), 176–188.

Mooney, N. G. Coping with chronic pain in rheumatoid arthritis: Patient behavior and nursing intervention. *Orthopedic Nursing,* 1982, *1* (3), 21–25.

Nowotny, M. L. If your patient's joints hurt, the reason may be osteoarthritis. *Nursing 80,* 1980, *10* (9), 39–42.

Peimer, C. A., Schiller, A. L., Mankin, H. J., & Smith, R. J. Multicentric giant-cell tumor of bone. *Journal of Bone and Joint Surgery,* 1980, *62A* (4), 652–656.

Porter S. F., Dapper, M. J., & Foran, C. Hand splints. *American Journal of Nursing,* 1983, *83* (2), 276–278.

Price, S. A., & McCarty, W. L. *Pathophysiology, clinical, concepts of disease process.* New York: McGraw-Hill, 1978.

Ricker, R. R. Continuous treatment of osteoporosis: Current status. *Orthopedic Clinics of North America,* 1981, *12* (3), 611–626.

Roof, R., & Hodkinson, L. J. *Textbook of orthopaedic nursing* (2nd Ed.). Oxford: Blackwell Scientific, 1975.

Ross, D. G. Paget's disease. *Orthopaedic Nursing,* 1984, *3* (3), 41–44.

Simpson, C. F. Heat, cold, or both? *American Journal of Nursing,* 1983, *83* (2), 270–272.

Simpson, C. & Dickinson, G. Exercise. *American Journal of Nursing,* 1983, *83* (2), 272–275.

Smith, E. L. Exercise for the prevention of osteoporosis: A review. *Physician and Sports Medicine,* 1983, *10,* 72–83.

Spruck, M. Gold therapy for rheumatoid arthritis. *American Journal of Nursing,* 1979, *79* (7), 1246–1249.

Strand, C. V., & Clark, S. R. Drugs and remedies. *American Journal of Nursing,* 1983, *83* (2), 266–269.

Swinson, D. R., & Swinburn, W. R. *Rheumatology.* New York: Wiley, 1980.

Tucker, R. E., Winter, W. G., & Wilson, H. D. Osteomyelitis associated with *Chromobacterium violaceum* sepsis. *Journal of Bone and Joint Surgery,* 1979, *61A* (6), 949–951.

Turek, S. L. *Orthopaedics, principles and their applications* (3rd ed.). Philadelphia: Lippincott, 1977.

Wallach, S. Treatment of Paget's disease. *Advances in Internal Medicine,* 1982, *27,* 1–43.

Warpus, J. M. Tuberculosis of bone joints. *Orthopedic Nurses' Association Journal,* 1978, *5* (3), 77–81.

Wu, K. K., & Guise, E. R. Ewing's sarcoma: A clinicial analysis of forty-six cases treated at Henry Ford Hospital. *Orthopedics,* 1979, *2* (3), 237–241.

Wu, K. K., & Guise, E. R. Extraosseous osteogenic sarcoma: A clinical analysis of ten cases. *Orthopedics,* 1980, *3,* 115–121.

Wu, K. K., Collon, D. J., & Guise, E. R. Extra-osseous chondrosarcoma. *Journal of Bone and Joint Surgery,* 1980, *62A* (2), 189–194.

5

THE SPINAL COLUMN, THORAX, AND PELVIS

Chapter 5 discusses the nursing care of patients with traumatic and pathological conditions of the spine, the thorax, and the pelvis. The spinal column is divided into three separate sections, the cervical, the thoracic, and the lumbar, and the chapter starts with a brief review of anatomy to help the nurse understand the rationale underlying nursing care. The emphasis is on orthopaedics, and there will be no discussion of paraplegia or quadriplegia.

ANATOMY

BONES

Spinal Column

The spine or vertebral column is a strong, flexible column that supports the head, provides a base for the ribs, and encloses the spinal cord. The 26 bones that comprise the adult spinal column are called the vertebrae, and are divided into five regions. The cervical region has 7 vertebrae, the thoracic 12, the lumbar 5, the sacral 1, and the coccygeal 1 (Fig. 5–1). A lateral view of the vertebral column shows four curves, alternately convex and concave ventrally.

The vertebrae differ from one another in size and shape, but in general show a uniform structure. A vertebra is composed of (1) a weight-bearing portion, the body, (2) a part that protects the spinal cord, the neural foramen, (3) three projections on which muscles pull, the spinous process, and the right and left transverse process, and (4) four projections, the two superior and two inferior articular processes, which restrict vertebral movements (Fig. 5–2).

The body of the vertebra is the central mass of bone that forms its anterior part. The arch is composed of two bony pedicles, which extend backward from

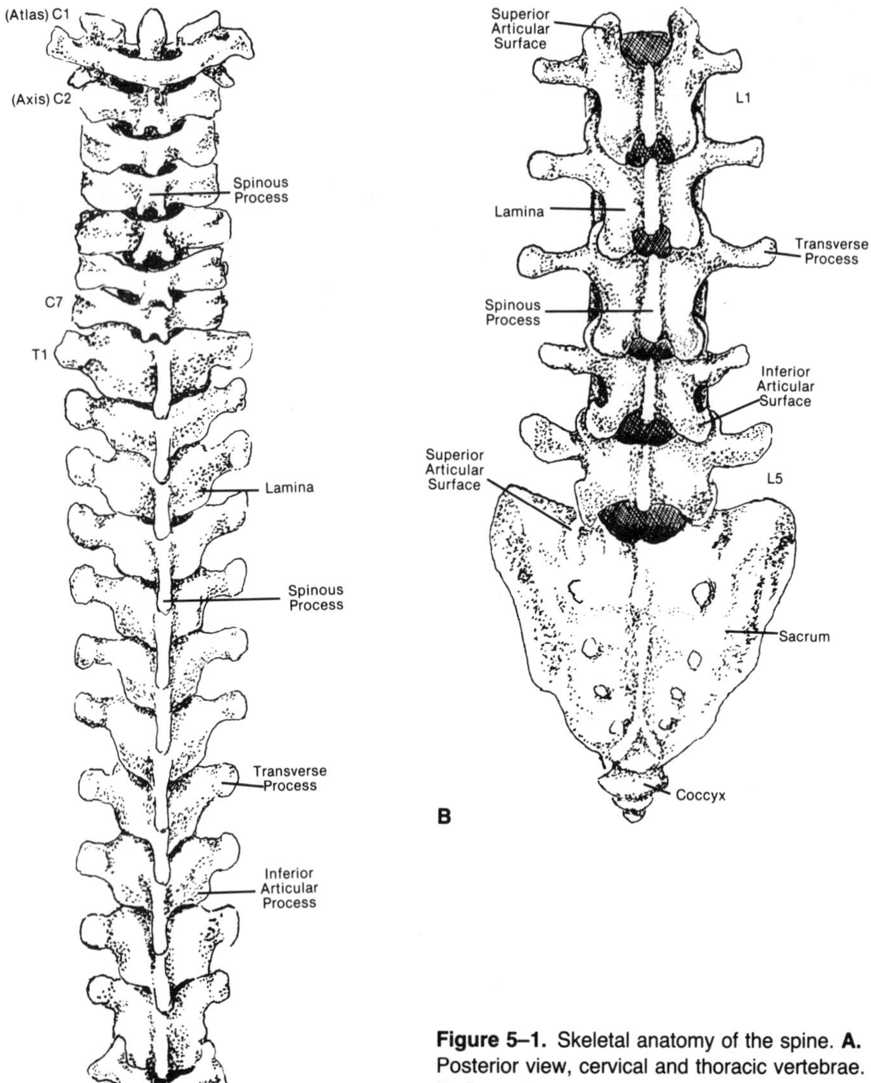

Figure 5–1. Skeletal anatomy of the spine. **A.** Posterior view, cervical and thoracic vertebrae. **B.** Posterior view, lumbar vertebrae and sacrum. *(From Brantley, P., & Analla, M., 1980, p. 50. Courtesy of Howmedica.)*

the body, and two bony laminae, which complete the arch. The body and the neural arch enclose the spinal foramen, through which the spinal cord passes. The spinous process extends backward from the point of union of the two laminae. The transverse processes project laterally from each side at the junction of a lamina and a pedicle. The articular processes arise near the junction of a pedicle and a lamina. The superior articular processes project upward, and the inferior project downward, with the inferior articular processes of the vertebra above fitting into the superior articular processes of the vertebra below. These are true joints, as their contact allows movement but prevents forward displacement of one vertebra with respect to another.

The vertebrae of the cervical region have foramina (openings) in the transverse processes (Fig. 5–3). In the first six vertebrae, those foramina transmit the vertebral arteries. The spinous processes of the cervical vertebrae are short, with the third, fourth, and fifth vertebrae having bifurcated spinous processes. The seventh cervical vertebra has an unusually long spinous process, which can be felt as a prominence at the back of the neck. In general, the bodies of the cervical vertebrae are small, and the vertebral foramina large and somewhat triangular. The first cervical vertebra, called the atlas, has no body but is composed of an anterior and a posterior arch and two lateral masses. The second cervical vertebrae, the axis, has a process (the odontoid process) on the upper surface of its body that forms a pivot on which the atlas rotates. The thoracic vertebrae have facets for articulation with the ribs. All of the processes in the thoracic region (Fig. 5–4) are larger and heavier than those in the cervical region, and the spinous processes are directed downward at a sharper angle. The vertebral foramen of the thoracic vertebrae are nearly circular. The lumbar vertebrae have bodies that are larger and heavier than other vertebrae (Fig. 5–5). The adult sacrum is composed of five fused preadult sacral vertebrae (Fig. 5–1). It is triangular in shape and fits like a wedge between the two halves of the pelvis. The coccyx is the terminal bone in the vertebral column. It is composed of four or five nodular pieces representing bodies of the preadult coccygeal vertebrae. The coccyx is triangular in shape, with its base attached to the sacrum (Fig. 5–1).

Thorax

The thorax is a bony, cartilaginous cage whose walls are formed at the back by the thoracic vertebrae, at the sides by the ribs, and in front by the costal cartilages and the sternum. The 24 ribs, 12 on a side, are long, flat bones that both curve and twist. The first seven pairs, which are attached directly to the sternum by costal cartilages, are called "true" ribs. The next five pairs are called "false" ribs. The eighth, ninth, and tenth ribs are attached to the sternum through the costal cartilages of the rib immediately above. The eleventh and twelfth ribs are unattached and have been termed "floating" ribs. The sternum or breast bone is composed of the manubrium or handle, the body or blade, and the xiphoid process.

Pelvis

Pelvis is a Latin word meaning basin, and the pelvis can be seen as a basin formed by the right and left innominate bones, the sacrum, and the coccyx. The innominate bones, which constitute the pelvic girdle, are built for stability and are firmly united to the vertebral column. The pelvic girdle serves to link

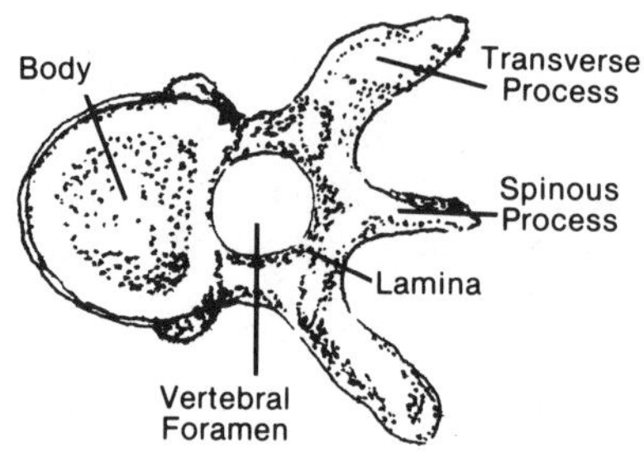

Figure 5–2. Superior view of thoracic vertebra. *(From Brantley, P., & Analla, M., 1980, p. 50. Courtesy of Howmedica.)*

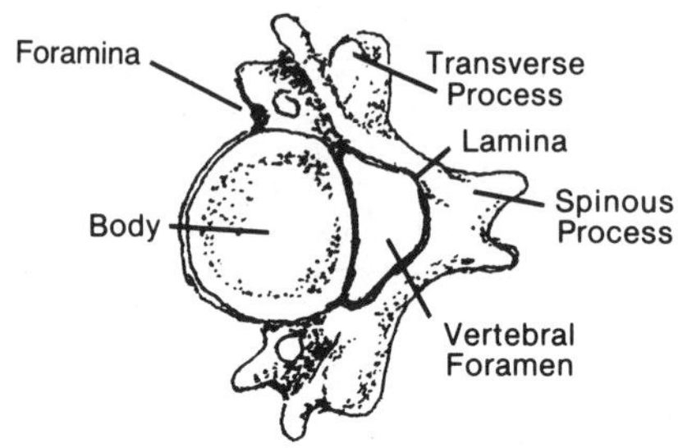

Figure 5–3. Superior view of cervical vertebra. *(From Brantley P., & Analla, M., 1980, p. 50. Courtesy of Howmedica.)*

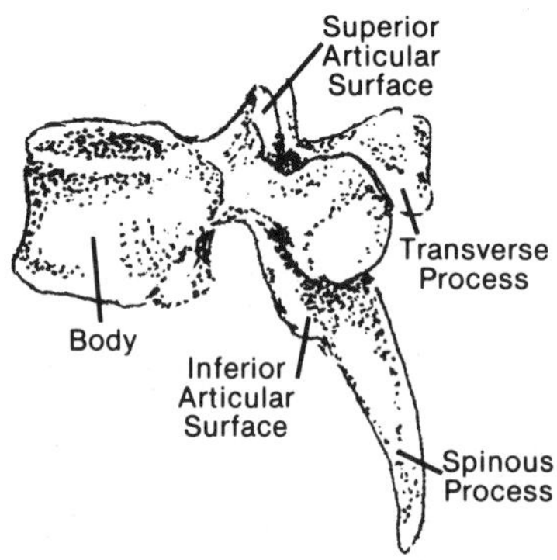

Figure 5–4. Lateral view of thoracic vertebra. *(From Brantley, P., & Analla, M., 1980, p. 50. Courtesy of Howmedica.)*

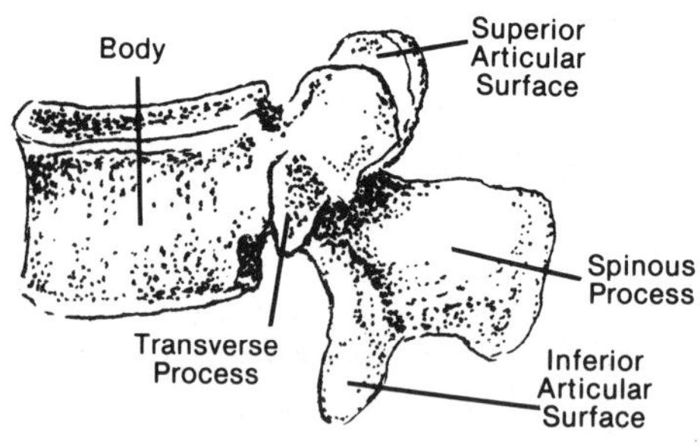

Figure 5–5. Lateral view of lumbar vertebra. *(From Brantley, P., & Analla, M., 1980, p. 50. Courtesy of Howmedica.)*

the legs to the spinal column. Each innominate bone is a large irregular bone. In children the innominate bone is composed of three separate bones (the ilium, the pubis, and the ischium), all of which come together at the acetabulum.

The *ilium,* the upper portion of the innominate bone, has a broad and expanded prominence, the iliac crest. A projection of the anterior tip of the crest forms the anterior superior spine of the ilium. The anterior inferior spine is immediately below. There are the posterior superior and the posterior inferior iliac spines on the posterior crest. Beneath the posterior inferior iliac spine is the greater sciatic notch.

The *pubic* bone comprises the anterior part of the innominate bone and forms a joint at the body's midline known as the symphysis pubis. The pubic bone is composed of a body and two arms, or rami. The body of the pubic bone comprises about one-fifth of the acetabulum. The upper, superior ramus is a rough ridge, the pubic crest. The inferior ramus passes downward and outward to meet the ischium. The pubic arch is formed by the inferior rami of both pubic bones, which converge at the symphysis.

The *ischium* forms the lower and back part of the innominate bone. It consists of a body and a ramus. The body of the ischium comprises a little over two-fifths of the acetabulum. The lower portion of the ischium is a large, rough process, the ischial tuberosity, which supports the body in a sitting position. The sharp projection above the tuberosity is the spine of the ischium. The ramus of the ischium passes upward to join the inferior ramus of the pubis. The ischium and the pubis combine to form a large aperture, the obturator foramen.

JOINTS OF VERTEBRAL COLUMN AND THORAX

The vertebrae from the second cervical to the first sacral articulate with one another by a series of cartilaginous joints between the vertebral bodies and through a series of synovial joints between the vertebral arches. The vertebral bodies are united by an anterior and a posterior longitudinal ligament, and by intervertebral discs of fibrocartilage known as symphyses. The anterior longitudinal ligament is a strong band that extends along the anterior surfaces of the vertebral bodies. The posterior longitudinal ligament is inside the vertebral canal on the posterior surfaces of the bodies of the vertebrae, and extends from the axis to the sacrum.

Intervertebral Discs

An intervertebral disc is interposed between the adjacent surfaces of vertebral bodies from the axis to the sacrum. The shape of the disc corresponds to that of the adjacent vertebral bodies, and its thickness varies from anterior to posterior and by region of the column. The fronts of the discs are thicker than the backs in the cervical and lumbar regions, and thus contribute to the anterior convexities of those levels. In the thoracic area, each disc is nearly uniform in thickness. The discs are thinnest in the thoracic region and thickest in the lumbar region.

For the most part, discs are avascular in adults and are supported by diffusion through the spongy bone of the adjacent surfaces of the vertebrae. Each disc consists of an outer laminated portion, the annulus fibrosus and an inner core, the nucleus pulposus. In teenagers, the intervertebral discs are so strong that when stress is applied to the vertebral column the bones ordinarily give way before the discs. After age 20, however, trauma may produce degenerative changes in the discs, leading to necrosis or sequestration of the nucleus pulposus, and to softening and weakening of the annulus fibrosus. After such trauma, a comparatively minor strain may cause either an internal derangement of the disc with an eccentric displacement or bulging of the nucleus pulposus, or the nucleus pulposus may actually burst through the annulus fibrosus, usually in a posterolateral direction. In the former case, the unequal tension within the vertebral joint is responsible for muscle spasm and acute low back pain. In the latter case, the projecting nucleus pulposus may press upon and irritate the adjacent spinal nerve roots, causing referred pain, such as sciatica. Derangements of that kind may occur at any level, but are most common in the lower lumbar region, especially at the lumbosacral joint, and at the level of the fifth to seventh cervical vertebrae. Motor effects, with loss of power and reflexes, may also ensue.

Vertebral Arches

The joints between the articular processes of the vertebrae are of two kinds, synovial and plain. Each joint has a thin, loose articular capsule, attached just outside the margins of the articular facets of the adjacent articulating processes. They are longer and looser in the cervical region than in the thoracic and lumbar regions.

The laminae of adjacent vertebrae are connected by broad thin ligaments, the *ligamenta flava.* They permit separation of the laminae in flexion and help to control movement. The ligamenta flava also assist in restoring the vertebral column to the erect position after flexion and in protecting the vertebral discs from injury. The transverse processes are connected by the *intertransverse ligaments.*

In the cervical region, the intertransverse ligaments consist of a few irregular, scattered fibers and are largely replaced by intertransverse muscles; in the thoracic region, they are rounded cords intimately connected with the deep muscles of the back; in the lumbar region they are thin and membranous. The spinous processes are connected by the *ligamentum nuchae* from the occiput to the seventh cervical vertebra. From the seventh cervical vertebra to the sacrum, they are connected by the *supraspinal ligaments.* Adjacent spinous processes are connected by *interspinal ligaments* that extend from the root to the apex of each process, and meet the ligamenta flava in front and the supraspinal ligaments behind. The ligamentum nuchae is a fibroelastic membrane (or intermuscular septum) that, in the neck, is homologous to the supraspinous and interspinous ligaments of other levels. It extends from the external occipital crest to the spinous process of the seventh cervical vertebra. The ligamentum nuchae plays an important role in holding the head erect.

Movements of the Vertebral Column

The range of movement possible between any two adjoining vertebrae is restricted by the limited flexibility in the intervertebral disc between the vertebral bodies. Although movement between adjoining vertebrae is small, the sum of the movements gives a relatively wide range of motion to the vertebral column as a whole.

Flexion (forward bending), extension (backward bending), lateral flexion (bending to one side), circumduction (turning), and rotation (twisting) are all possible movements of the vertebral column. In flexion, the anterior longitudinal ligament is relaxed and the anterior parts of the intervertebral discs are compressed. At the limit of flexion, the posterior longitudinal ligament, the ligamenta flava, and the intraspinous and supraspinous ligaments are stretched, and the posterior fibers of the intervertebral discs are decompressed. In extension, the opposite takes place. Extension is limited by the tension of the anterior longitudinal ligaments, and by the approximation of the spinous processes. In lateral flexion, the sides of the intervertebral discs are compressed, with the extent of motion being limited only by the tension of antagonist muscles and surrounding ligaments. Circumduction is merely a succession of the preceding movements. Rotation is produced by the twisting of the vertebrae relative to each other with torsional deformation of the intervening intervertebral discs.

Muscles Producing Vertebral Movements

The spinal column may be moved by muscles attached to it or by muscles attached to other bones that act on it. Flexion involves the longus cervicis, scaleni, sternocleidomastoid, and rectus abdominis of both sides. In extension, the erector spinae and the splenius and semispinalis capitis of both sides are involved. During lateral flexion, the longissimus and iliocostocervicalis components of the erector spinae and the oblique muscles of the side flexed are involved. In rotation, the rotarores, multifidus, and splenius cervicis are involved.

SPINAL NERVES

There are 31 pairs of spinal nerves; of which 8 pairs are cervical, 12 pairs are thoracic, 5 pairs are lumbar, 5 pairs are sacral, and 1 pair is coccygeal. The first pair of cervical nerves arises from the medulla oblongata and leaves the spinal canal between the occipital bone and the atlas. The other spinal nerves arise from the spinal cord, and each leaves the spinal canal through the intervertebral foramen behind the vertebra whose number it bears, e.g., the sixth thoracic nerve emerges through the foramen between the sixth and seventh thoracic vertebrae. The coccygeal nerve passes from the lower extremity of the spinal canal.

Nerve plexuses are formed in the cervical, brachial, lumbar, and sacral segments. The cervical plexus is formed by the anterior branches of the first four cervical nerves. There is communication from the cervical plexus to the hypoglossal, vagus, and accessory nerves of the head and neck. The brachial plexus is formed by the union of the anterior branch of the last four cervical and the first thoracic nerves. Important nerves formed from the plexus are the median, ulnar, and radial nerves that supply the upper extremity. The lumbar plexus is formed by a few fibers from the twelfth thoracic and the anterior primary divisions of the first four lumbar nerves. The largest peripheral nerves formed are the femoral and obturator nerves. The sacral plexus is formed by a few fibers from the fourth lumbar nerve and the first three sacral nerves. The largest peripheral nerve is the sciatic, which supplies the muscles of the lower extremity. Other major nerves from the sacral plexus are the medial and posterior popliteal and tibial nerves, and the lateral popliteal and anterior tibial nerves.

CERVICAL SPINAL COLUMN

The cervical spine is completely encircled by intricate layers of muscles that function to control its movement and stabilize it. In the upright position the cervical spine assumes a lordotic or convex inward curve known as the "relaxed" position. Any deviation from that position brings the muscles into play. The range of movement of the cervical spine is limited only by the length of the elongating muscles or by structural changes in a diseased spine.

Pain in and from the neck region can originate from many different tissue sites by many different mechanisms. Frequently the pain is not felt at its origin, e.g., pain originating in deep somatic structures is vague and diffuse in its distribution, and may be referred to as a distal site.

Pain is particularly likely at the periosteal site of muscular attachment, because neck muscles do not terminate in tendons but attach to the bone by myofascial tissue that blends into the periosteum. Sustained muscle contraction, which can occur with emotional tension or from maintaining an awkward posture for prolonged periods, produces sustained traction at the site of insertion and thus can cause pain and tissue tenderness. An acute muscle contraction or ligamentous stretch, which can occur in an accident or quick movement of the head, can have the same result. A common site of such tenderness is at the base of the skull where the muscles attach to the occiput at the site of emergence and passage of the superior occipital nerve. When irritated, the nerve will contract the muscles and transmit and refer pain across the top and side of the scalp to the frontal area. The so-called cervical tension state and tension headaches occur in the neck and the head as a direct result of a sustained muscular contraction of the cervical spine.

Pain and tenderness can also occur within the belly of a muscle as a result of contraction, either acute or sustained. Acute contraction of all the neck muscles resulting from trauma can cause excessive intramuscular pressure with or without muscle tear, with the end result of the increased internal pressure being an inflammation known as "myositis." Sustained muscular contraction in a static neck results in tension myositis.

Trauma

CERVICAL SPRAIN

Cervical sprain may be defined as a stretching disruption of the soft tissues that support the cervical spine. The degree of injury may vary from a slight separation of a few fibers to an actual interruption of the gross ligament structure. Injuries that stretch the ligaments also involve other structures (e.g., disc, articular cartilage, and bone), damage to which must be assessed in every case. The most common ways of injurying the cervical vertebrae are by hyperflexion and hyperextension of the neck.

In a *hyperflexion* injury, the most superficial stabilizing ligamentous structure on the posterior aspect, the ligamentum nuchae, bears the brunt of the stretching force. It may be stretched or torn, but usually heals rapidly. At times, however, it becomes elongated and permits excessive mobility of the cervical vertebrae at the affected level. An extreme forcible flexion injury, such as that sustained in a diving accident, usually tears the ligamentum nuchae at the lower cervical level (i.e., the C5–6, C6–7, or C7–T1) and can also involve the interspinous ligament. In such an extreme hyperflexion injury, the nuchal ligament may be torn from the tips of the spinous processes or avulsed.

The tear may extend deeply enough to involve the capsular structures about the interspinal articulations and the annulus, thus permitting vertebrae to displace forward. Nerve roots may be compressed by the swollen, injured capsular structures or by a protruding disc, and peripheral nerve symptoms may develop. The degree of soft tissue disruption is in direct proportion to the intensity of the force and fragility of the tissues. With advancing age, especially in the presence of degenerative disease, the tissues become inelastic and are easily torn. The disc substance may be damaged without actually being extruded externally, and then undergoes degeneration. Disc protrusion in the cervical region due to hyperflexion is rare, but when it does occur it almost always is a result of a severe acute flexion force, not a "whiplash" type of injury.

In a *hyperextension* injury, when the head is thrust backward, the vertebrae are forced into an extremely lordotic position, the superior articulating processes displace inferiorly to an extreme degree, and the capsular ligaments are stretched. The anterior longitudinal ligament, which is very strong except when softened by disease, is rarely disrupted. The apex of the lordotic curve, from C3 to C6 receives the maximum amount of stress and is therefore the site of the patient's symptoms. A considerable amount of hyperextension force is usually necessary to produce posterior subluxation of one vertebra upon another. When it does happen, however, fractures of the posterior articulations, or lamina and disc damage, often occur.

The most common mechanism producing a cervical sprain is the acceleration or deceleration force in a car collision. In the usual rear-end collision the occupants of the front car sit with their cervical muscles relaxed and, as the trunk of their bodies is suddenly thrust forward, the inertia of the head acutely hyperextends the neck, which then recoils forward. The reverse type of injury in a head-on collision causes a hyperflexion–extension movement. The ordinary "whiplash" phenomenon, in which no direct trauma to the head is sustained, generally results in a mild sprain in which muscle and ligament structures remain intact. The injury may be compounded by the presence of degenerative disease of the cervical spine. When the direction of the force is from the side, or when a frontal or rear force occurs while the head is turned to one side, the spine is less flexible and the force is expended upon the articulations where the small bone elements may be fractured. Displacement of vertebrae rarely occurs in rear-end car acceleration injuries.

Mild Sprain

A mild sprain, the most common type of cervical injury, involves mainly the muscles, and the symptoms usually last only a few days to a few weeks. The immediate discomfort is minimal at first but gradually intensifies in the hours after the injury. Motion in the neck becomes limited and painful, and the affected muscles are tender and painful when stretched. When these muscles are relaxed by heat and positioning, the discomfort is usually reduced.

Moderate Sprain

A moderate sprain involves the ligaments as well as the muscles, with symptoms that persist well beyond the usual time required for recovery from a mild sprain. The initial short period of acute pain is usually followed by an interval of aching pain that is intensified by movements that exert tension on the affected ligaments. Over the hours following the injury, the pain usually becomes more severe, and protective muscle spasms become intense and persistent even while the patient is recumbent. The patient usually complains of generalized pain about the neck and referred pain to some distant point such as the occiput, the scapula, the upper extremity, or even the upper anterior chest area where it may be confused with pain of cardiopulmonary origin. Only absolute immobilization and strong sedation are usually effective in reducing the pain. During the initial acute phase, there are frequently vague complaints such as blurred vision, diplopia, vertigo, nausea, and headache. Those symptoms rapidly subside, although the headache may persist for a few weeks.

Within a few days after the injury, the severe pain and muscle spasms lessen, and a point of tenderness can be identified. In the case of a forcible flexion injury, the tenderness is usually situated over an interspinous interval. In a hyperextension injury there is usually tenderness over the posterolateral articulations, generally at or above the midcervical level. The patient usually complains of inability to maintain the head upright when bending forward, difficulty in positioning the head on a pillow, and painful tension in the sprained ligaments. Within 3 to 6 weeks recovery of the ligaments is usually complete.

Severe Sprain

A severe sprain is one in which complete interruption of the ligaments takes place and is a result of a severe hyperflexion or hyperextension injury. The intensity of the trauma and the fragility of the tissues involved lead to a tearing of soft tissues and a displacement of the cervical vertebrae. Initially the patient's symptoms are like those of a patient with a moderate sprain, but additional symptoms demonstrate the severity of the injury. Headache is typically occipital although it may radiate forward. Vague symptoms, such as vertigo, nausea, tinnitus, and blurred vision, quickly subside, but the headache may continue indefinitely. Pain, paresthesia, and weakness in one or both upper extremities may develop at the time of injury or gradually over the first few hours. Those symptoms are often transitory, and usually subside before medical attention can be obtained. Persistence of those symptoms is serious, as they may indicate associated neurological damage.

After the acute episode has subsided, the patient may continue to complain of annoying and unrelenting discomfort, either about the neck or in the scapula, the occipiut, or the space between the neck and the shoulders. A persistent sensation of weakness in the neck and an inability to hold the head upright demonstrate ligamentous inadequacy. Characteristically, patients hold their head in their hands for support. Straightening the neck upward from the forward flexed position is extremely uncomfortable, and may cause protective muscle spasms that restrict such movement. After a few weeks, the site of the ligamentous damage becomes evident as a well-localized point of tenderness. In a hyperextension injury the points of tenderness are usually located over the posterolateral articulations at or just above the midcervical level. As the ligaments heal over a number of weeks, symptoms gradually subside, and full cervical motion gradually returns. Failure of healing of the ligament is rare but can lead to persistent pain and disability.

Treatment

The follow-up care for patients with cervical sprains varies depending on the severity of the sprain. A mild muscular sprain usually requires little or no treatment. An acceleration or deceleration injury, in the absence of severe direct trauma to the head and when the cervical spine is free of previous pathology, usually causes nothing more than ligamentous stretching. Care consists of a short period of bedrest with firm support for the cervical spine, such as a rolled-up towel placed behind the neck. For moderate and severe sprains, a hot pack several times daily and analgesics usually help reduce pain from muscle spasms. Cervical traction is contraindicated in most instances, because traction stretches the damaged ligaments. However, light cervical traction and sandbags placed about the head can prevent unguarded motion. After a few days, a cervical collar may be applied, and the patient is then allowed to be ambulatory. If pain is provoked by bending the neck forward, the collar should be higher in front to hold the neck in a slight degree of extension (Fig. 5–6). If extension is painful, the collar should be reversed. The collar is worn for several weeks or until all movement can be performed painlessly. Physical therapy modalities, such as infrared, diathermy, and ultrasound, may also be used, but some physicians doubt their efficacy. Massage and manipulation are contraindicated as they may tear the ligaments that are already softened by hemorrhage and edema. Restriction of cervical motion is continued until the ligaments are reconstituted and fixation is secured, which generally requires 4 to 6 weeks in cases of complete ligamentous separation.

When there is a chance that extensive ligamentous disruption has occurred, extreme caution should be taken to prevent displacement. The patient's neck should be supported continuously for 6 weeks in a brace or cast that includes the head. If instability persists after a period of immobilization, surgical stabilization may be necessary.

CERVICAL DISLOCATIONS AND FRACTURES

Trauma to the cervical spine may produce a variety of injuries varying from dislocations without fractures to massive fractures without dislocations. Fre-

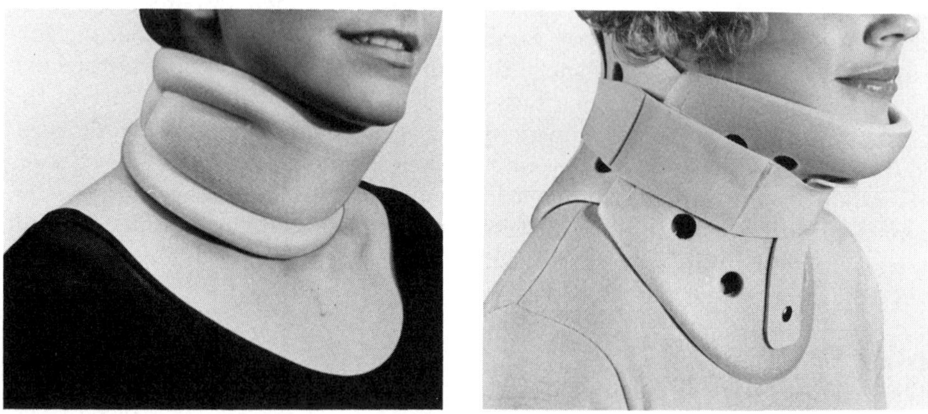

A B

Figure 5–6. A. Cervical collar with neck in hyperextension or reversed for flexion. **B.** Philadelphia cervical collar. *(Courtesy of Zimmer, Inc.)*

quently both a fracture and a dislocation are sustained. Dislocations vary from mild spontaneously reduced subluxations to complete dislocations of the articular facets. Fractures associated with dislocations vary from small chip fractures of the distal border of a vertebra to complete separation of the pedicles, fractures of the articular processes, or marked compression fractures of the vertebral body. Milder injuries, such as crush or compression fractures of vertebral bodies or subluxations of the articular facets, usually respond satisfactorily to traction followed by immobilization in a cast or brace. More severe injuries may require surgery (Edmondson & Crenshaw, 1980, p. 1955).

Fracture of the C1 Vertebra

A fracture of the C1 vertebra (Jefferson's fracture) occurs when a vertical compression force impacts downward on the articular facets of the skull, pushing the lateral masses outward and disrupting the ring of the atlas. Normally the articular processes of the atlas (C1 vertebra) face upward, inward, and slightly backward. The injury often results from a diving accident.

The patient's complaints may vary from minimal to severe pain, usually accompanied by gross limitation of movement. Tenderness is usually present posteriorly over the atlas. There is pain on extension of the neck, but rotation may be relatively pain free. There is a potential for injury to the suboccipital nerve, which crosses the posterior ring of the atlas to each lateral mass, and to the greater occipital nerve, which emerges just below the posterior ring of the atlas and supplies the skin over the occiput. If the fracture causes damage to the spinal cord, however, immediate death usually occurs (Iversen & Clawson, 1977, pp. 109–110).

Initial treatment is to place the patient in 5 to 8 pounds of traction while continuing to assess the extent of the injury. The patient is then usually immobilized in a Minerva or halo cast (see pp. 133–135) until healing of the fracture occurs, usually about 3 months.

Fracture of the Odontoid Process

The C1 vertebra and the odontoid process of the C2 vertebra are a single functional unit. When the cruciate ligaments on the posterior aspect of the odontoid process remain intact following a flexion or extension injury to the upper neck, the result can be a fracture of the base of the odontoid process. The skull, the C1 vertebra, and the odontoid process can then move independently of the rest of the cervical spine.

The patient may have only minimal pain, but in most instances there is severe pain behind the ears and stiffness of the neck. Patients often complain of a feeling of instability at the base of the skull, and hold or turn the head with the hands on top of the skull. There is usually no weakness or numbness of the extremities, but there is usually tenderness in the suboccipital region.

With an anteriorly displaced C1 vertebra, a fracture of the odontoid process may be reduced by allowing the patient's head to go into extension with the patient in a supine position. The reduction may be facilitated by sedating the patient and then inserting a pillow under the patient's shoulders to promote extension of the head and neck. Light traction using a head halter may then be applied. The use of traction beyond the first few days is contraindicated, as it may produce distraction (excessive separation of the vertebrae) and does not immobilize the fracture.

Once reduction is accomplished, the head and the neck are immobilized and held in position by a Minerva or halo cast. The cast is applied as soon as possible so that the patient can sit up and get out of bed. Immobilization is continued until the fracture is healed, usually about 3 months. Progressive mobilization of the neck is then initiated, and a soft collar is used until muscle strength has returned. If flexion and extension roentgenography do not demonstrate union 4 months after surgery, a posterior C1–2 fusion is usually done.

Fracture of the C2 Vertebra (Hangman's Fracture)

The classic hangman's fracture injury is a bilateral fracture that passes through the posterior part of the lateral masses and pedicles of the axis (C2 vertebra) and into the intervertebral notch. The body of the axis is then subluxated or dislocated in relation to the body of the C3 vertebra. The skull and the C1 vertebra move as a unit with the body of the C2 vertebra, whereas the posterior elements of the C2 vertebra move with the posterior elements of C3. Although hanging causes this injury by distraction and extension, other mechanisms that produce the same fracture occur in automobile accidents when persons catch their chin on the steering wheel or dashboard (causing flexion) or strike their forehead on the sun visor (causing extension) (Iversen & Clawson, 1977, pp. 111–112). If the spinal cord is involved, most persons do not survive the initial trauma. Those who do, may only complain of local pain, stiffness, and tenderness over the C2 spinous process. The injury is occasionally accompanied by other injuries in the lower part of the cervical spine.

Reduction of the fracture is usually accomplished with the neck in a neutral position. A Minerva or halo cast immobilization is applied and continued for 3 months. Traction can produce distraction and subsequent nonunion or ligamentous instability. Patients may require intubation or tracheostomy because of initial severe retropharyngeal swelling.

☐ NURSING PROCESS (Table 5–1)

Assessment

The initial nursing assessment of a typical patient following a fracture of a cervical vertebra and the application of a halo apparatus should focus on the patient's neurological well-being. The patient's neurological status is usually assessed every 15 minutes for the first hour after application, then every hour for the next 8 hours, and then every 4 hours for the next 2 days. (See Chapter 2 for neurovascular assessment of upper and lower extremities.) If there are no complications, the neurological checks can

TABLE 5–1. NURSING PROCESS FOR FRACTURE OF A CERVICAL VERTEBRA AND THE APPLICATION OF A HALO APPARATUS

Assessment	Nursing Diagnosis	Goal Formulation	Planning and Intervention	Evaluation and Reassessment
1. Assess the location, duration, and severity of pain. Observe for verbal and nonverbal cues of pain. Note any complaints of an unusual pulling sensation on the head or scalp. Check for any loosening of pins or screws. Assess for any pain on chewing or speaking.	1. Alteration in comfort: pain in the head and neck related to bone and soft tissue trauma.	1. Short-term goal: a decrease in the level of pain through immobilization. Long-term goal: free of any pain.	1. Alleviate Pain Keep the patient's body in correct alignment. Keep the halo apparatus correctly positioned. Discuss the rationale for the use of the halo apparatus. Teach relaxation techniques. Administer prescribed pain medications as indicated. Notify physician of any undue discomfort along sensory-motor pathways of the face or scalp.	1. The patient should have only minimal discomfort when the halo apparatus has proper pin placement and properly immobilizes the head and neck.
2. Check the patient's position in bed. Check that the halo apparatus is correctly positioned. Assess the patient's ability to do exercises. Assess the patient's ability to get out of bed and ambulate safely.	2. Impaired physical mobility: a decrease in neck function related to bone and soft tissue trauma.	2. Short-term goal: an increase in mobility through cervical immobilization. Long-term goal: regain full neck motion with no residual effects.	2. Increase Mobility *Position* Keep the patient supine (when in bed). Place pillows under the knees. *Exercises* Encourage active range-of-motion (AROM) exercises for the lower extremities for the first few days after application of the halo, do passive range-of-motion exercises to upper extremities twice a day (later AROM exercises can be done). Encourage exercising on a stationary bicycle twice a day for 15 to 20 minutes.	2. The patient should be comfortable in the supine position. Pillows under the knees should help reduce stress on the back.

(continued)

TABLE 5–1. *(Continued)*

Assessment	Nursing Diagnosis	Goal Formulation	Planning and Intervention	Evaluation and Reassessment
			Ambulation Teach the patient to turn the body instead of the head. Assist the patient in learning how to get out of bed. Assist the patient in learning how to balance and stabilize self while walking. Assist the patient in learning how to get in and out of a chair and to go up and down stairs.	The patient should be able to retain range of motion in the joints and to prevent a decrease in muscle tone and strength.
3. Assess for pain. Check vital signs. Assess for signs of infection (tenderness, heat, redness, swelling). Check for any drainage.	3. Potential for injury: infection related to soft tissue and bone trauma.	3. Short- and long-term goals: free of any signs of infection.	3. Prevent Complications *Integumentary* Do pin site care every shift. Wash the patient's hair on a regular basis. Administer antibiotics as prescribed. Culture any drainage and notify the physician.	3. The patient should remain free of any signs of infection.
Check pins and screws for loosening. Check the apparatus for any friction or wearing at sites of contact. Assess for any complaints of an unusual pulling sensation in the hair or scalp.	Potential for injury: instability of cervical vertebra related to loosening of apparatus.	Short- and long-term goal: have the halo apparatus remain intact without any signs of loosening.	*Loosening of Screws* Prevent jarring of the apparatus. Avoid getting clothing caught in the apparatus. Avoid any roughness while washing the patient's hair. Notify physician of any loosening. Keep a wrench at patient's bedside.	There should not be any loosening of screws; any loosened screws should be tightened.

Observe for periods of decreased concentration, fatigue, increased complaints or withdrawal from staff and others. Assess patient's verbalization and cooperation with the plan of care.	Potential for anxiety and depression related to adjustment to treatment method and rehabilitation.	Short- and long-term goals: a decrease in anxiety and depression.	*Psychological* Encourage patients to talk and listen to them express their feelings. Educate the patient about the halo apparatus. Teach the patient how to live with the apparatus in place. Encourage the patient and family or significant other to ask questions. Introduce the patient to others who are wearing or who have worn a halo. Encourage the patient to participate in planning daily activities.	The patient should verbalize an understanding of the treatment method. The patient should be able to express feelings of concern about the treatment method and rehabilitation process.
Assess range of motion in all extremities. Assess muscle strength. Assess ability to do exercises.	Potential for injury: decreased muscle tone related to lack of use.	Short- and long-term goals: free of any decrease in muscle tone or strength.	*Musculoskeletal* Encourage active range-of-motion exercises. Assist with passive range-of-motion exercises. Develop a program of exercises for home care.	The patient should not have any decrease in muscle tone or strength due to inactivity.
Check vital signs, level of consciousness, orientation, speech quality, hand grip strength, ability to raise the arms above the head, for numbness or tingling in upper extremities, for difficulties with jaw movements, extraocular movements and pupil reaction, peripheral vision, and for visual difficulties.	Potential for injury: neurological deficit related to application of halo apparatus.	Short- and long-term goals: free of neurological deficits.	*Neurological* Report any abnormal neurological sign. Do cranial nerve checks every 15 minutes for the 2 hours after application of the halo, every 30 minutes for the next 4 hours, every 2 hours for the next 18 hours, and then at the beginning of every shift.	The patient should have no neurological deficit.

(continued)

TABLE 5–1. ***(Continued)***

Assessment	Nursing Diagnosis	Goal Formulation	Planning and Intervention	Evaluation and Reassessment
Assess breathing rate, depth, and rhythm. Auscultate the chest for lung clearance. Assess for any shortness of breath or chest pain.	Potential impaired gas exchange related to immobility.	Short- and long-term goals: free of respiratory complications.	*Respiratory* Teach deep breathing but do not have patient cough. Utilize incentive spirometry. Change patient's position every 2 hours while awake and every 4 hours during the night. Encourage early ambulation. Keep patient well hydrated.	The patient should be able to obtain good gas exchange by deep breathing. The patient should not cough as coughing jars the apparatus which causes discomfort and loosening of the screws.
Auscultate for bowel sounds. Check for expulsion of flatus. Check for any nausea or vomiting. Assess abdomen for any distention. Measure abdominal girth.	Potential alteration in bowel elimination: ineffective function related to trauma and immobility. Potential alteration in bowel elimination: constipation related to immobility.	Short- and long-term goals: free of any gastrointestinal complications.	*Gastrointestinal* Teach abdominal exercises. Restrict oral fluids until there is a return of bowel sounds. Apply heating pad to abdomen. Utilize rectal tube. Encourage a well-balanced diet with plenty of fluids. Encourage exercises to activity level.	The patient should have normal peristalsis.

Assess the patient's ability to feed self. Assess the patient's knowledge of the basic four food groups.	Potential self-feeding deficit related to application of halo apparatus.	Short- and long-term goals: no deficit in nutritional intake.	*Nutrition* Assist patient in learning how to feed self without tilting the head. Utilize straws for liquids. Attach a mirror to the overhead frame to improve the patient's visual field and assist with eating. Encourage a well-balanced diet with plenty of fluids and roughage. Discuss measures to prevent weight gain.	The patient should have adequate nutritional intake with minimal assistance in eating.
4. Assess for level of understanding about the rehabilitation process and home care. Assess the patient's stage of adaptation to the disability.	4. Potential knowledge deficit related to the rehabilitation process and home care.	4. Short- and long-term goals: a decrease in anxiety through increased knowledge.	4. Patient Teaching Discuss rationale for halo apparatus. Discuss the rehabilitation process. Demonstrate to patient, family, and significant other methods of bathing, shampooing hair, sleeping and dressing. Discuss ways of riding in a car. Discuss the change in body image. Include family and/or significant other in teaching plan. Teach a family member or significant other how to do pin site care. Discuss potential complications.	4. The patient should have a decrease in the level of anxiety. The patient should be able to verbalize an understanding of the rehabilitation process and home care. The patient should be able to discuss changes in body image due to wearing the halo apparatus.

then be done once every shift. That assessment should include monitoring for signs of increasing intracranial pressure, any indication of cervical nerve impingement, and for vascular changes in the extremities.

The neurological assessment for increased intracranial pressure should include (1) vital signs (temperature, pulse, respiration, and blood pressure), (2) level of consciousness, (3) orientation, (4) speech quality, (5) strength of the grip in both hands, (6) patient's ability to raise the arms above the head, (7) presence of any numbness or tingling in the upper extremities or difficulties with jaw movements, such as an inability to bite down, open the mouth wide, or stick out the tongue, (8) extraocular movement and pupil reaction, (9) peripheral vision checks, and (10) checks for any visual difficulties, such as blurred vision, double vision, or nystagmus. Minor nystagmus is normal in the extreme lateral gaze, but all other nystagmus findings should be considered abnormal. If one of the patient's eyes deviates nasally, record the movement as esotropic (ET); if there is a deviation toward the temple, record it as extropic (XT); and record any upward deviation as hypertropic (HT). Readers are referred to the neurological nursing references in the bibliography at the end of this chapter for further details on neurological checks for increased intracranial pressure.

Observe the patient's body alignment and correct the positioning of the halo apparatus. Check for any loosening of pins or screws and note if the patient has any complaints of an unusual pulling sensation on the head or scalp. Check for any friction or wearing where the halo is attached to the rest of the apparatus. Determine the level of discomfort and the effectiveness of nursing measures and medications to relieve discomfort. Determine the level of anxiety as evidenced by the patient's verbalization and cooperation with the plan of care. Assess the effectiveness of interactions between the patient and the family or significant others. Assess pin sites for signs and symptoms of infection such as redness, edema, drainage, increased temperature, or pain. Assess the function of the respiratory and gastrointestinal systems by auscultating the chest and the abdomen.

Nursing Diagnosis and Goal Formulation

Nursing diagnoses for a typical patient in a halo apparatus following a cervical fracture are (1) alterations in comfort related to pain in the cervical region from trauma, (2) alterations in mobility related to instability in the cervical spine from trauma, (3) potential complications related to trauma and the halo apparatus, and (4) alterations in psychological well-being, related to anxiety and knowledge deficit of the injury and treatment methods.

Short-term goals are to have the patient experience (1) a decrease in the amount of pain through nursing measures and prescribed medications, (2) an increase in mobility through the use of the halo apparatus and exercises, (3) an absence of complications from decreased mobility and the halo apparatus, and (4) a decrease in anxiety through increased knowledge. Long-term goals are to have the patient free of pain with a return to full function after approximately 3 months in the halo apparatus.

Planning and Intervention

Alleviate Pain. If a patient in a halo apparatus has proper pin placement with a correct amount of force applied, there should be minimal to no cutaneous discomfort. For patients complaining of pain, first assess for the severity, duration, and location of the pain. Check that the patient is in correct alignment and that there is no pull or stress on the halo apparatus. For complaints of minor discomfort, analgesics are administered.

Careful placement of the pins is important to avoid the risk of cranial nerve damage. If the anterior pins are placed too far medially on the frontal bone, severe pain can result from supraorbital nerve irritation. Similarly, if the posterior pins are placed too far forward on the temporal bone, the patient will have pain when chewing or speaking as a result of impingement on a branch of the trigeminal nerve, which controls jaw muscle motion and sensation. If the patient complains of undue discomfort related to the sensory–motor pathways of the face or scalp, the physician must be notified. Depending on the severity of the symptoms, pin removal and replacement may be necessary.

Increase Mobility

Position. The patient in a halo apparatus following a cervical fracture will find that the only comfortable position in bed is lying supine. To help reduce the stress on the back, some patients use a pillow under the knees.

Halo Apparatus. The halo apparatus, first used for the immobilization of a cervical fracture in 1959, is now used for a number of severe cervical and upper thoracic spinal instabilities, including fractures that could cause spinal cord or nerve root damage, cervical fusions, tumors of the head or neck, and rheumatoid arthritis. Skeletal fixation is achieved by a stainless steel "halo ring" that fits around the patient's head and is attached to the skull by four pins (Fig. 5–7). The sharp pointed pins are placed approximately 0.5 mm deep into the outer portion of the skull. To prevent pin migration, bone erosion, and penetration of the dura, the pins are inserted in the frontal bones 1 cm above each eyebrow and in the temporal bones 1 cm above and behind the top of the ears. The insertion of the pins may be done under general anesthesia, but is usually done with local anesthesia at the pin sites. Traction on the skeletal system is maintained by threaded steel uprights that are attached to the halo ring and to the body jacket (or brace or cast) (Fig. 5–8).

Exercises. The patient in a halo apparatus has no movement of the cervical spine and the head, and will feel that the apparatus inhibits move-

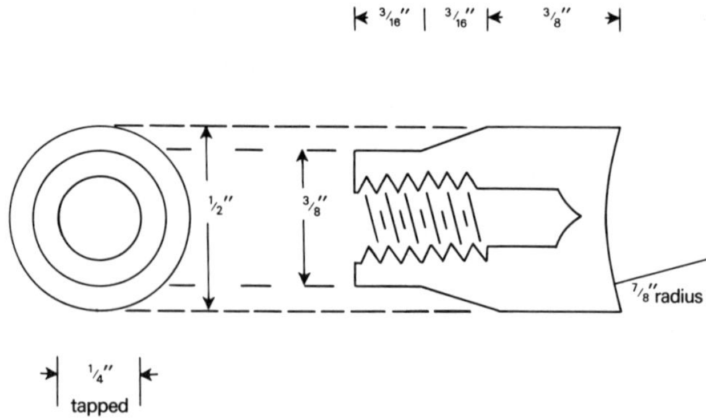

A

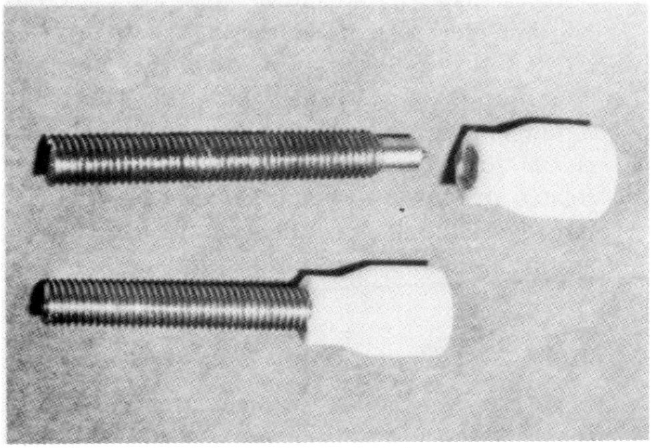

B

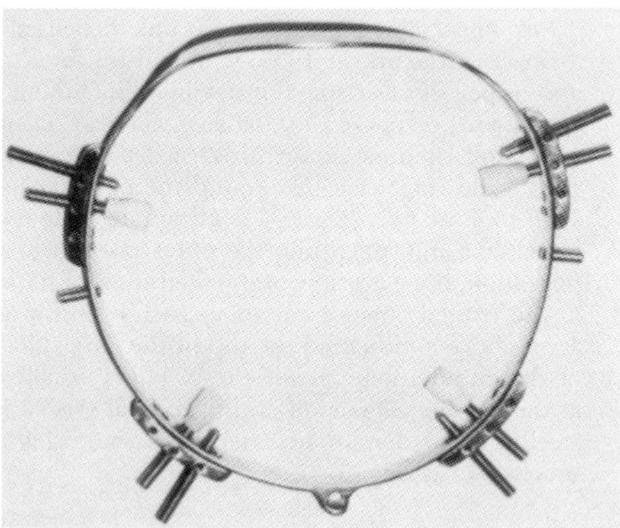

C

Figure 5–7. A. through **E.** Details of the halo-bound fittings. *(From Roaf, R., & Hodkinson, L.J., 1980, pp. 472–473, with permission.)*

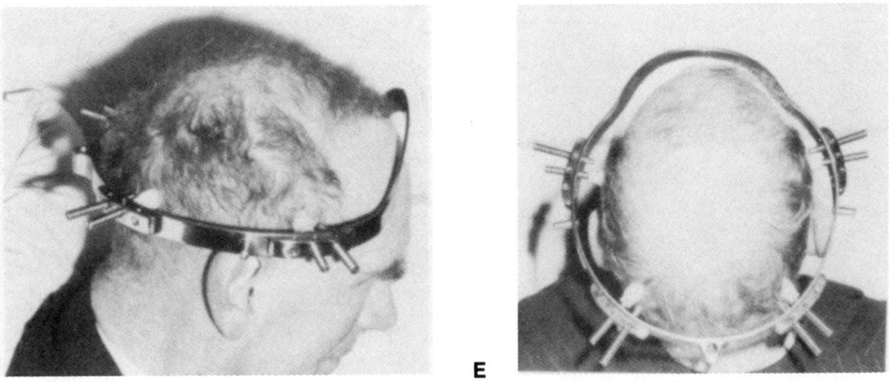

D E

Figure 5–7. *(continued)*

ment in the rest of the body. A program of active range-of-motion exercises is encouraged. If necessary, a program of passive range-of-motion exercises of the upper extremities should be done twice a day. For the lower extremities, the patient may be started on an exercise program utilizing a stationary bicycle twice a day for 15 to 20 minutes each time. The goal of the exercise program is to retain range of motion in the joints and to prevent decrease in muscle tone and strength.

Ambulation. It is important that the patient in a halo apparatus understand the need for safety. The patient should become as independent as possible, but realize that the field of vision is restricted, which could result in a fall or jars to the halo. The patient needs to learn to turn the body instead of the head to look to the side, and realize that it will become easier as peripheral vision improves. The patient will need assistance in learning how to get out of bed with the added weight of an approximately 7-pound apparatus. If the patient holds onto the steel uprights when getting up or lying down, he or she is usually able to move better with the apparatus. Once out of bed, the patient may have trouble with balance and stability, and initially will need to walk with someone. The patient must then learn how to get in and out of a chair and go up and down stairs. Going upstairs usually poses minimal difficulties, but going downstairs is more difficult because of the inability to look down to see the next step.

Prevent Complications. Complications that can occur with a halo apparatus include (1) infection of pin sites, (2) loosening of pins or screws; (3) increased anxiety or depression; (4) decreased muscle tone; (5) traction-induced cranial nerve lesion, (6) paralytic ileus, and (7) respiratory compli-

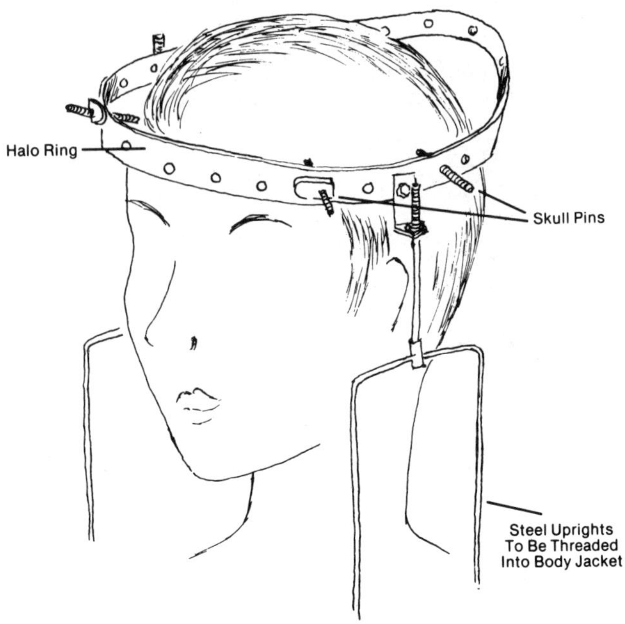

Figure 5–8. Halo apparatus. *(From Brantley, P., & Analla, M., 1980, p. 61. Courtesy of Howmedica.)*

cations. Other aspects of the patient's care to be monitored are hygiene and nutrition.

Pin Site Infections. With four pins inserted into the patient's skull, there is a chance of infection at the pin sites. Take the patient's temperature and assess for pain, tenderness, heat, swelling, redness, and drainage at least once every shift. If there is drainage, send a culture to the laboratory and notify the patient's physician. Measures that help to prevent or reduce pin site infections are washing the patient's hair on a regular basis and doing pin site care every shift.

Loosening of Screws. The screws can be loosened by jars to the apparatus, getting the apparatus caught on clothing while dressing, roughness in washing the patient's hair, and by the patient's coughing and sneezing. Loose screws need to be tightened or, in some instances, replaced. During pin care, check the pins and the screws for loosening. Listen for any complaints of an unusual pulling sensation on the head or scalp. Check the apparatus for any friction or wearing at sites of contact. Notify the patient's physician if there is any loosening of pins, and keep a wrench at the bedside.

Increased Anxiety and Depression. Patients in a halo apparatus commonly have periods of anxiety and depression. Look for decreased concentration, fatigue, increased restlessness, increased complaints, or withdrawal from staff and others. Measures that help to reduce anxiety and depression are to listen to the patient express feelings and to educate the patient about the apparatus and how to live with it (see patient education, pp. 139–146). Encourage the patient and family to verbalize questions, and introduce the patient to others who are wearing or have worn a halo. Allow the patient to participate in planning daily activities.

Decreased Muscle Tone. Because of decreased mobility, patients with a halo apparatus may develop decreased muscle tone. A program of exercise is essential (see increase mobility, pp. 133–135). Encourage active range-of-motion exercises and assist with passive range-of-motion exercises as indicated by the patient's condition.

Cranial Nerve Lesions. Stretching or kinking of cranial nerves can result from the traction force applied by the halo to immobilize the head and the neck and to reduce the cervical fracture. Those lesions are most likely to occur immediately after the halo is applied and attached to the extension bars. A stretching lesion, referred to as a neurapraxia, is a temporary injury that causes palsy or paralysis of the innervated area with anatomical degeneration. Damage may be caused by overextension, nerve fiber compression, or disruption of the nerve's blood supply (Sunderland, 1968). Similarly, cranial nerve deficits may be caused by a kinking of the cranial nerve root at the base of the brain (Wilkins & MacEwen, 1977). The most important principle is prevention, or should dysfunction occur, immediate detection. The prognosis for complete recovery is good, but the time it takes to recover is directly related to the amount of time the nerve was kinked or overextended. When the halo is initially applied, do cranial nerve checks every 15 minutes for the first hour. If the patient has any subjective complaints that may indicate cranial nerve deficit, do an assessment immediately and notify the physician. The only effective treatment for traction-induced cranial neurapraxia or kinking is a prompt and substantial decrease in the force of distraction.

Paralytic Ileus. The patient immobilized by a cervical fracture is prone to develop a paralytic ileus. (For further discussion, see pp. 79 and 84.)

Respiratory Complications. The combination of recumbency, the drugs used for pain relief that depress respirations, a decrease in the body's need for oxygen due to inactivity, and the resistance of the bed and halo apparatus against the patient's chest wall can lead to respiratory complications. Nursing measures are needed to prevent respiratory complications, but having the patient cough or causing the patient to sneeze tends to jar the apparatus, which causes the patient discomfort and leads to a loosening of the screws.

Nutrition. Because of the position and immobilization of the head and the neck, the patient may find that just getting a glass of water takes some effort. Once the glass is filled, the patient must learn to get the water to the lips and drink without tilting the head. Using a straw helps. With eating, there are problems getting the food from the plate to the mouth. A mirror attached to the overhead bedframe can improve the patient's visual field and help self-feeding.

The patient needs a well-balanced diet. Emphasis must be placed on preventing the patient from gaining weight as the halo apparatus does not allow for an increase in trunk size. Special care should be taken to prevent gastrointestinal problems that occur with decreased mobility.

Hygiene. Changing the lining of the vest may become necessary because of excessive perspiration, extended use of the halo apparatus, or wounds that drain and soil the liner. The posterior liner can be changed safely by the following steps:

1. Have the patient lie prone on a firm bed with a pillow under the chest and a pillow under the head to support and maintain alignment.
2. Remove the lower two bolts on the vest. If the crossbar snaps out of alignment, the patient is not balanced on the pillows evenly; resecure the bolts, readjust the pillows, and then proceed.
3. Release the side straps and the shoulder straps. Check that the neck is maintained in correct alignment.
4. Remove the posterior section of the vest and liner.
5. Cleanse the patient's back and dry well.
6. Replace the liner, which is held in place with velcro.
7. Replace the posterior section and resecure.

To change the anterior liner safely:

1. Have the patient lie supine with a small pillow behind the head.
2. Release the two bolts and four straps.
3. Remove the anterior section of the vest and liner.
4. Cleanse the patient's chest area and dry well.
5. Attach a new liner and replace the anterior section.
6. Refasten the straps and *then* replace the two bolts.

The total time for changing the liners and cleansing the patient's chest and back is usually about 15 minutes (Ace Orthopedics, 1982, p. 10).

Patient Teaching. In most instances there is very little time for the patient to learn about the halo apparatus before it is applied. Thus the patient must learn how to live with the apparatus and how to perform self-care while wearing it at the same time. Help the patient adjust by always explaining what you are going to do, how you are going to do it, and why it is necessary. Learning to eat and ambulate are some of the first activities a patient must learn. Others are how to bathe the body, shampoo the hair, sleep, dress, and ride in a car.

In bathing, sponge baths are easiest, but occasionally a tub bath is desired. Even though approximately 4 inches of water is allowed in the tub, a nonskid mat is recommended to prevent slipping. Someone may be able to assist the patient in cleansing under the brace with a damp (not wet) cloth and no soap. If permitted by the patient's physician, a family member or significant other can be taught to change the liner as discussed under hygiene.

Shampooing the patient's hair may not be done every day, but can be accomplished with little effort. One way is to have the patient kneel over the edge of a bathtub (or sink if the patient is tall enough) with a towel for padding at the tub edge. The patient will need to hold the sidebars of the apparatus and brace his or her elbows on the tub. The helper is then able to gently wash and rinse the patient's hair. A hose spray attached to the shower is a great help in moistening and rinsing. If this is not available, water can be poured from a plastic container. Three things to remember in washing a patient's hair are: (1) place a towel around the patient's neck to prevent water getting under the vest; (2) be very gentle in cleansing and rinsing; and (3) make sure all of the soap is rinsed out (Wells & Trostle, 1984). Short hair is easier to care for than long hair, so the patient may choose to have the hair cut. Changes in hair color are not recommended, as the patient has skin openings at the pin sites.

Getting into a comfortable position to sleep is a problem for most patients, because they must sleep on the back. Some ways to help the patient are to put a pillow under the knees (if allowed by the patient's physician) to reduce the stress on the back and to use a triangular pillow for a head rest. Most patients require more sleep than normal while they are wearing the halo apparatus, so plan for rest periods and naps during the day.

Learning what to wear and how to dress need not present a big problem. The patient will need clothing several sizes larger in the chest with a large neck opening to allow for the bars of the halo apparatus. The clothing could be a loose fitting shirt or blouse or, for women, a large dress with a front zipper or buttons, or even a muumuu. The only real requirement is the neck opening. Slacks or skirts can be worn as the apparatus does not extend below the waist. However, the patient needs to bend to put on shoes, socks, and stockings. Shoes should give support to the feet and help stabilize the patient during walking.

Traveling can be a problem, and getting into a car requires some thought. The easiest way is probably to have the patient ride in the front passenger seat. The patient can back up against the side of the seat, bend at the hips, and sit down. The patient can then bring the head inside the car, making sure that it clears the car frame, and then turn to the correct position. Reverse that procedure in getting out of the car. The patient can turn and lead out with the head. While riding, the patient should be advised to hold onto the side bars to prevent the jarring of the apparatus, especially when riding over railroad tracks or on bumpy roads. The use of seat belts is strongly recommended.

Patients must realize that people will stare at them because of the apparatus. They should also recognize that the apparatus is only temporary, and allows them to function while their fracture is healing.

Evaluation and Reassessment

Determine that the patient is free of pain and has only occasional headaches, which are relieved by analgesics. Make sure the patient knows who to contact if additional pain should occur after the patient is home. Discuss with the patient the signs and symptoms of potential complications and what should be done if any occur. Observe the patient closely to make sure that he or she knows how to get in and out of bed and is able to move about safely. Have the patient demonstrate going up and down stairs.

Go over the procedure for pin care with the patient and the person who will be helping the patient at home. Ask the person who will be helping the patient to demonstrate pin site care in the hospital before the patient is discharged. Allow the family or significant other to help with washing the patient's hair. Discuss with the patient the type of clothing to wear, and if possible have some clothing brought to the hospital so he or she can learn to dress.

Fractures and Dislocations of the C3 to C7 Vertebrae

An *extension* injury to the neck can produce tearing of the anterior longitudinal ligament with or without an avulsion fracture of the anterior aspect of one of the vertebral bodies. Fractures of the pedicles and posterior subluxation may also occur. This injury is commonly associated with a rear-end automobile accident. Subsequent symptoms may last for a prolonged period of time without objective documentation of any osseous or soft tissue abnormalities. With *flexion* injuries, a unilateral dislocation or fracture–dislocation of the facets on one side of the neck can occur, whereas the interarticular facets on the other side usually remain intact. If a fracture is present, it is usually of the dislocated facet. Unilateral dislocation and interlocking of the cervical facets usually affects the lower cervical spine. The patient with a C3 to C7 fracture–dislocation usually complains of tenderness over one or more spinous processes, and has limitation of movement and muscle spasms. There may also be motor or sensory neurological injuries including quadriplegia.

Whether or not neurological damage is present, reduction of any displacement is essential. Reduction of dislocations and fracture–dislocations is accomplished with skull tongs. The patient is usually placed in skull tong traction with 15 pounds of weight, which may be increased by 5 pounds every hour until reduction is accomplished. After reduction is accomplished, immobilization using light skull traction may be continued for several days. In the absence of significant neurological deficit, the patient may then be placed in a Minerva or halo cast. If the injuries are unstable, skull calipers from the Minerva or halo cast may be used to immobilize the neck.

Skeletal Traction

The application of skeletal traction and other conservative measures may be the only treatment necessary for many fractures of the cervical spine. Regardless of what additional treatment may be required later, skeletal traction is usually applied promptly.

Crutchfield tongs (Fig. 5–9) have frequently been used to maintain skeletal traction. To apply Crutchfield tongs, the patient's hair is shaved at the areas where the tongs are to be placed, and the points of contact are marked for the insertion of the tongs. The two areas are then injected with a local anesthetic, and an incision down to the skull just large enough to admit a drill is made in each area. The drill penetrates only the outer portion of the skull, some 4 mm in adults. The points of the tongs are then fit into the holes in the skull and held in position until the tongs have been locked in place. The tongs are checked daily to see that they are firmly in place, and are tightened if necessary. Movements of the head result in local irritation, enlargement of the holes, and eventually disengagement of the tongs. On the other hand, excessive tight-

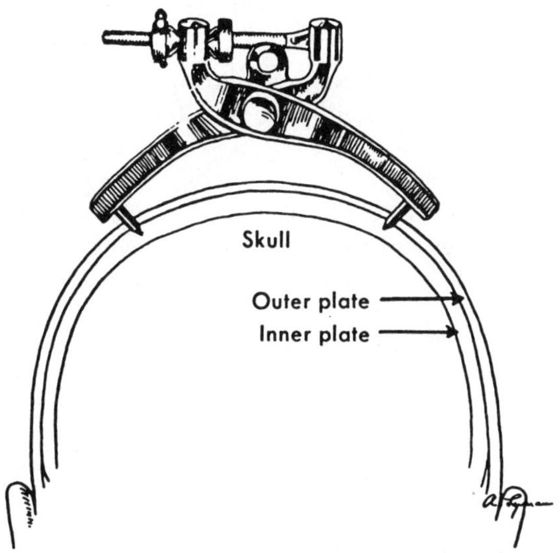

Figure 5–9. Crutchfield tongs apparatus. *(From Larson, C.B., & Gould, M.* Orthopedic nursing *(9th ed.). St. Louis, Mo.: C.V. Mosby, 1978, p. 199, with permission.)*

ening of the tongs may result in a perforation into the inner skull.

The recommended weight for each cervical vertebra is:

Level of Fracture	*Pounds of Weight*
1st cervical vertebra	5 to 10
2nd cervical vertebra	6 to 10–12
3rd cervical vertebra	8 to 10–15
4th cervical vertebra	10 to 15–20
5th cervical vertebra	12 to 20–25
6th cervical vertebra	15 to 20–30
7th cervical vertebra	18 to 25–35

Today, Crutchfield tongs are being replaced by Gardner-Wells tongs, which are easier to apply and have a self-contained tension device. The points of the Gardner-Wells tongs are needle sharp, and need to be cleansed with an antiseptic before insertion. The hair and scalp are sprayed with an aerosol antiseptic and then rubbed at the temple ridges where the tongs will be inserted. A local anesthetic is injected at the site of the insertion, and the area is sprayed again. The tongs are then applied and tightened until the depth indicator shows a penetration of 1 mm. The tongs are checked and tightened over the next few hours as needed. Stability is usually achieved within 24 hours, after which the tongs need no further adjustment.

□ NURSING PROCESS (Table 5–2)

Assessment

The initial nursing assessment of a typical patient following a fracture of a cervical vertebra and the application of skull–tong traction should include an in-depth neurological assessment in addition to a general evaluation of the patient. The assessment should include monitoring for signs of increasing intracranial pressure, for any indication of cervical nerve impingement, and for vascular changes in the extremities. (For specific details on neurological assessment, see pp. 126 and 132 and references in the bibliography to this chapter.)

Observe the patient's body alignment with respect to the traction. Check the placement of the tongs and make sure there is an equal pull on both sides. Assess the tong sites for signs and symptoms of infection. Check for any friction or rubbing on the rope. The weights should have the correct poundage and hang free of all obstacles. Determine the level of discomfort and the effectiveness of the traction and nursing measures used to relieve discomfort. Note if the patient has any complaints of unusual pulling sensations. Determine the level of anxiety as evidenced by the pa-

TABLE 5–2. NURSING PROCESS FOR FRACTURED CERVICAL VERTEBRA TREATED WITH SKULL-TONGS AND A TURNING FRAME

Assessment	Nursing Diagnosis	Goal Formulation	Planning and Intervention	Evaluation and Reassessment
1. Assess the location, duration and severity of pain. Observe for verbal and nonverbal cues of pain. Assess for signs of increasing intracranial pressure. Check for any signs of cranial nerve impingement.	1. Alteration in comfort: pain in the head and neck related to bone and soft tissue trauma.	1. Short-term goal: a decrease in pain through immobilization with traction. Long-term goal: freedom from pain.	1. Alleviate Pain Maintain continuous traction. Maintain correct body alignment. Discuss rationale for traction. Teach relaxation techniques. Administer prescribed pain medication as indicated. Notify physcian if patient experiences undue discomfort.	1. With proper placement of tongs and continuous traction, the patient should have only minimal pain which is relieved by medication.
2. Check body alignment with respect to traction. Check tong placement for equal pull on both sides. Check for any friction or rubbing on traction rope. Check for correct poundage and that the weights hang free of any obstacles.	2. Impaired physical mobility: a decrease in neck function related to bone and soft tissue trauma.	2. Short-term goal: an increase in mobility through traction and use of a turning frame. Long-term goal: regain full neck function with no residual effects.	2. Increase Mobility *Position* Keep patient either supine or prone on a turning frame. Utilize a footboard (when patient is supine). Place sandbags or trochanter rolls against the patient's hips. Attach arm boards to the turning frame.	2. Proper positioning and alignment should be maintained at all times. The patient should not develop signs of footdrop, external rotation at the hips, adduction contractures of the shoulders, or flexion contractures of the elbows.
			Turning Explain the procedure of turning. Remove arm and footboard and place pillow over lower legs (if patient is supine). Turn the patient on a turning frame every 2 hours during the day and every 4 hours at night.	The patient should be turned safely and without undue increase in the patient's anxiety.

(continued)

TABLE 5–2. *(Continued)*

Assessment	Nursing Diagnosis	Goal Formulation	Planning and Intervention	Evaluation and Reassessment
			Exercise Start passive range-of-motion exercises of the extremities 48 hours posttrauma if patient's condition allows; exercises should be done 4–5 times a day. Encourage active range-of-motion exercises (as patient's condition permits).	The exercises should preserve joint function and increase circulation.
3. Check vital signs. Assess for pain. Assess for signs of infection. Check for any drainage.	3. Potential for injury: infection related to skull tongs. Potential for injury: break in skin integrity related to pressure.	3. Short- and long-term goals: free of any integumentary complications.	3. Prevent Complications *Integumentary* Do pin site care every shift. Culture any drainage and notify physician. Administer antibiotics as prescribed. Turn every 2–4 hours. Wash patient with mild soap, rinse, and dry well. Keep areas over bony prominences soft and well-lubricated with an emollient lotion. Massage gently with a circular motion. Keep linen dry and wrinkle free.	3. The patient should remain free of any signs of pressure or infection. The patient should remain free of signs of anxiety or depression, decreased muscle tone, a traction-induced cranial nerve lesion, a paralytic ileus, constipation, or respiratory complications.

			Potential Complications Due to Immobility (See Table 5–1 and Chap. 3)	
4. Assess the patient's level of understanding about immobilization and the rehabilitation process.	4. Potential knowledge deficit related to immobilization and the rehabilitation process.	4. Short- and long-term goals: a decrease in anxiety through increased knowledge.	4. Patient Teaching Discuss the various steps in the rehabilitation process. Carefully answer all questions. Explain the purpose of the turning frame and traction. Make sure the patient is informed before each procedure. Explain to the patient the potential complications and related care. Encourage patient participation in scheduling the daily activities. Help patient develop activities which are enjoyable and stimulate interest in the world outside self and hospital. Include patient's family and significant other in teaching plan.	4. The patient should be able to verbalize an understanding of the rehabilitation process. The patient should not be anxious when turning or discussing the future. The patient should be able to help with as much self-care as possible, work out a schedule for activities, and spend time on activities of interest.

tient's verbalization and cooperation with the plan of care. Assess the effectiveness of interactions between the patient and the family or significant others. Determine the status of the respiratory and gastrointestinal systems.

Nursing Diagnosis and Goal Formulation

Nursing diagnoses for a typical patient in skeletal traction following a cervical fracture are (1) alterations in comfort related to pain in the cervical spine region related to trauma, (2) alterations in mobility related to instability in the cervical spine, (3) potential complications related to trauma and skeletal traction, and (4) alterations in psychological well-being related to anxiety and knowledge deficit about the injury and the treatment methods.

Short-term goals are to have the patient experience (1) a decrease in pain through nursing measures and prescribed medications, (2) an increase in mobility through exercise and skeletal traction, (3) an absence of complications from decreased mobility and skeletal traction, and (4) a decrease in anxiety through increased knowledge. Long-term goals are to have the patient free of pain with a return of full function.

Planning and Intervention

Alleviate Pain. If a patient in skeletal traction has the proper tong placement, the correct amount of force applied, and the correct body alignment, there will be a minimal amount of pain. For complaints of discomfort, analgesics are administered. (For further discussion of pain relief, see p. 133.)

Increase Mobility

Position. The patient in continuous skeletal traction must be maintained in proper alignment when he or she is either supine or prone on a turning frame. A footboard is generally attached to prevent footdrop when the patient is in the supine position. When the patient is prone, the feet should hang over the end of the canvas in a flexed position. A sandbag or trochanter roll should be placed against the patient's hips to prevent external rotation at the hip. Armboards are attached to position the patient's arms to prevent adduction contractures of the shoulders and flexion contractures of the elbows. The armboards should be attached slightly below the level of the turning frame when the patient is in the prone position and level with the frame when the patient is in the supine position. In the supine position the armboards may also be used as siderails.

Skeletal Traction. After skeletal tongs are inserted, the patient is placed supine on a turning frame and prepared for the application of traction. Adequate room should be left at the head of the frame for the traction apparatus. A rope is attached to the skeletal tong apparatus, threaded through the hole in the center of the disc at the head of the frame, and laid over the pulley. The rope is then attached to the weight carrier and all knots are taped. The weights should then be lowered gently to apply the traction to the cervical spine. The weights should be checked for correct poundage and hang free of the bed, wall, or other obstacles. The traction must be maintained without interruption until it is discontinued.

Stryker Wedge Turning Frame. Turning frames are a way to safely turn a patient from supine to prone, or vice versa, without torsion or abnormal flexion–extension. They facilitate the movement and care of patients who should not or cannot move voluntarily. The turning frame may be a Foster bed, a Circo-lectric bed, a Stryker parallel frame, or a Stryker wedge frame. Today, most patients are placed on a Stryker wedge turning frame.

Stryker and Foster frames consist of an anterior and a posterior rectangular metal frame to which canvas covers are attached. Thin, sponge rubber mattresses covered with sheets are placed over the canvases. The frames are fastened to each other by a metal attachment with a knurled nut at both the head and the foot. Narrow forehead and chin straps are provided to support the head. The bed is also equipped with armboard and footboard attachments. Three restraining straps are placed around both frames when turning the patient. They may also be fastened around the patient as a safety precaution either continuously or at night, because the bed is narrow. In the Stryker wedge turning frame, which requires only one nurse to turn the patient, the anterior and posterior frames are not parallel to one another. Instead, the upper frame is angled toward the lower frame on the side toward which the frame will turn, preventing the patient from sliding out between the frames during the turn.

Turning. The patient in skeletal traction on a Stryker wedge frame is usually turned every 2 hours. If the patient's condition permits, the patient is only turned every 4 hours at night. The turning schedule should accommodate meals and visiting hours. In preparation for turning, explain the procedure to the patient and ensure that the wheels of the turning frame are locked. When the patient is supine on the posterior frame, remove extra bed linen and place a sheepskin, pillow, or other comfort aids on top of the patient, before applying the anterior frame. Be sure to place a pillow lengthwise over the lower legs and remove any armboards or footboards. Open the turning circle and put the head end of the anterior frame on the securing bolt and fasten it with the nut. Next, fasten the bolt at the foot end of the anterior frame, making sure that the patient's legs and feet are correctly positioned. The patient may then clasp with the hands around the anterior frame or the patient's arms may be placed at the side and a safety strap placed around the whole frame at the elbow level to constrain the patient's arms during the turn. Close the turning circle until it locks automatically, and pull out the bed turning lock at the head of the bed and the red turning lock knob on the turning ring. Tell the patient you are about to make the turn, grasp the handle on the turning ring, and turn. The narrow side of the wedge (at the patient's right) will always turn down, and the frame will automatically lock when the bottom frame is horizontal. Push in the circular silver lock knob on the turning ring. Once the turn is complete, the turning circle can be opened and the knurled nuts unscrewed. The posterior (upper) frame can then be removed and the turning circle relocked for safety. To turn the patient on a Stryker wedge frame from prone to supine, reverse the procedure for turning from supine to prone. Remember that the narrow side of the wedge (on the patient's right) always turns down so the patient cannot slip out.

Exercises. Depending on the severity of the trauma, the patient may be started on passive range-of-motion exercises of the extremities within 48 hours after traction is applied. The goal of the exercises is to preserve joint motion and stimulate circulation. Toes, metatarsals, ankles, knees, and hips, as well as the joints of the upper extremities, should be put through full range of motion at least four and ideally five times daily. If the patient's condition permits, active range-of-motion exercises are also started.

Ambulation. After the lengthy period of absolute immobilization, the duration of which depends on the severity and mechanism of injury, the patient may be allowed to gradually assume an erect position. The patient usually requires a neck brace to reduce movement of the cervical spine and to allow continued bone healing. The commonly used orthoses (braces) are (1) a two-poster firm brace with chest extension, which gives support under the patient's chin and subocciput, and (2) a four-poster cervical brace with chest extension. For patients without neurological deficit, reduction in traction followed by rigid immobilization for approximately 16 weeks usually restores skeletal function.

Prevent Complications. Complications of skull–tong traction include (1) infection of tong sites, (2) increased anxiety or depression, (3) decreased muscle tone, (4) a traction-induced cranial nerve lesion, (5) a paralytic ileus, (6) constipation, (7) respiratory complications, and (8) pressure areas. (For a discussion of the first four complications, see pp. 133–135, 136–137, and 139–140; for paralytic ileus, see pp. 79 and 84; for constipation, see p. 84; and for respiratory complications, see pp. 79 and 137–138.)

Skin breakdown can develop in less than 6 hours. Because the patient is immobilized, areas of local tissue ischemia develop where there is continuous pressure, and that may be compounded by inadequate peripheral circulation due to spinal shock. Turning every 2 hours aids in the prevention of pressure areas and prevents the pooling of blood and tissue fluid in the dependent areas. Every few hours the patient's skin should be washed with a mild soap, rinsed well, and blotted dry. The sacrum, trochanter, ischia, iliac spines, knees, heels, scapula, and shoulders are especially susceptible to pressure. Those areas should be kept soft and well-lubricated with an emollient lotion. Massage should be done gently with a circular motion. Linen under the patient should be kept dry.

Patient Teaching. To help reduce anxiety, let the patient express fears and concerns. Carefully answer all questions in a way the patient can understand. Explain the purpose of the turning frame and how it works. Make sure the patient is informed before doing any procedure. Explain to the patient the potential problems and what nursing assessments and interventions are needed to prevent them. Let the patient participate in scheduling the daily activities, for example, procedures that can be done when the patient is either supine or prone.

The amount and kind of activities the patient can do depends on the amount and level of the trauma. Try to help the patient develop activities that are enjoyable and that stimulate an interest in the world outside the hospital. When the patient is prone reading may be possible, and when supine he or she can listen to music or to a "talking book." Prism glasses can help the patient watch television. At other times, the patient may be able to do some kind of handicraft, especially while lying prone.

Evaluation and Reassessment

Insure that the patient is always in correct alignment and free of pain. During turns check that the patient's body is held firmly between the frames and that traction is maintained. If the patient experiences an increase in pain during the turn, have the patient describe the pain in detail, assess the patient's neurological status and compare it to the preturn status, and consider the possibility of a psychological component to the pain. Notify the patient's physician if pain persists or if there is a change in neurological status. Evaluate the condition of the patient's skin. Check that there are no wrinkles in the pads, canvas, or linen. Check that the turning schedule is appropriate and that the patient does not remain in one position too long.

Evaluate the patient's understanding of the turning frame and the procedures performed. Observe for possible anxiety during interactions between the patient and the family or significant others.

Stable or Unstable C3 to C7 Fractures

Stable fractures are treated nonoperatively with a brace, whereas unstable injuries with ligamentous tearing are usually considered for surgical treatment. Unstable fractures are reduced by traction or surgical reduction of facet dislocations, followed by a posterior surgical wiring and fusion. Unilateral facet dislocations with nerve root impingement usually require early open reduction and fusion.

Posterior Cervical Fusion with Wire Fixation. A posterior cervical fusion is performed to relieve pain and provide stability in the cervical spine (Fig. 5–10). In

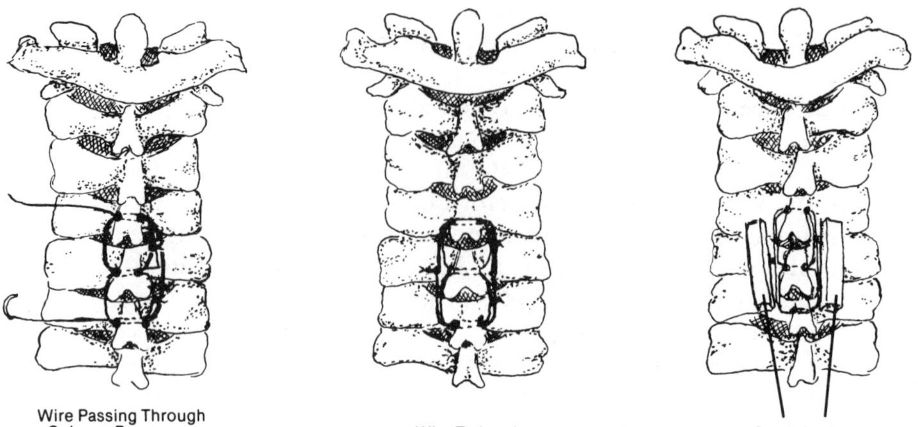

Figure 5–10. Posterior cervical fusion with wire fixation. *(From Brantley, P., & Analla, M., 1980, p. 53. Courtesy of Howmedica.)*

this procedure holes are drilled through the cortices of the spinous process in each cervical vertebra being fused. A wire is then passed through each hole and twisted into place. One additional wire is placed around all of the vertebrae being fused. Corticocancellous bone strips are taken from the iliac crest and laid along the vertebrae to aid in vertebral fusion. Postoperatively, a soft collar or brace is worn for 4 to 6 months until bony fusion occurs.

Soft Tissue Injuries With or Without Neurological Deficits

In soft tissue injuries with neurological deficits, the type of neurological deficit determines the surgical approach to be taken. For example, complete quadriplegics do poorly with immediate operative intervention, and are usually allowed to stabilize. In the absence of a bone lesion, an early myelogram or computed tomographic (CAT) scan is usually performed to identify the defect and relate it to the patient's clinical symptoms. When a patient develops quadriplegia with no damage to the posterior column, immediate anterior decompression of the spinal cord is essential (Edmondson & Crenshaw, 1980, p. 1956). Fractured facets, laminae, and pedicles with intact ligamentous structures and without neurological deficits usually heal with immobilization in a Minerva or halo cast. If an established pattern of chronic pain develops and persists for 12 months, however, an anterior cervical fusion may be indicated.

Anterior Interbody Cervical Fusion

In an anterior cervical fusion, the approach is commonly made through an anterolateral incision (Fig. 5–11). The cervical disc is removed, the interbody

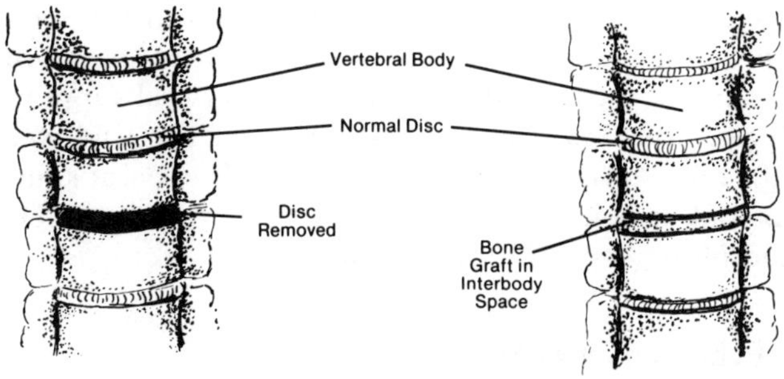

Figure 5–11. Anterior interbody cervical fusion. *(From Brantley, P., & Analla, M., 1980, p. 51. Courtesy of Howmedica.)*

space is curetted, and any osteophytes of the vertebral body are excised. A bone graft taken from the iliac crest is cut to fit into the space from which the disc was removed. The bone graft is put into place and the surgical incision closed. Following closure and the application of a dressing, the patient is placed in a soft cervical collar. At about the seventh to tenth day after surgery, the patient may be placed in a more rigid brace. Excessive extension of the neck is to be avoided to prevent unsatisfactory impaction of the graft or anterior displacement. Accurate and continous observation is essential to prevent respiratory distress, neurological deficits, and hematoma formation at the neck and at the donor site. Bony fusion is usually established in approximately 5 to 6 months. The wearing of the neck brace is gradually reduced as the fusion becomes complete.

Pathology

ARTHRITIS AND INFECTIONS

Rheumatoid Arthritis

Patients with rheumatoid arthritis of the cervical spine typically have a more generalized pattern of rheumatoid arthritis. Approximately 30 percent of patients having chronic rheumatoid arthritis with severe peripheral joint involvement show evidence of cervical spine subluxation on roentgenography. Often the patient with a cervical spine abnormality does not have associated neurological symptoms. Only about 5 percent of patients with significant cervical subluxation have signs of neurological involvement or spinal cord compression. These abnormal neurological findings vary from quadriplegia to minimal proprioceptive loss in either the upper or lower extremities.

When rheumatoid arthritis effects the upper levels of the cervical spine, it usually produces cervical spinal fusion in children and cervical spinal subluxation in adults. The most common subluxation is an anterior subluxation of C1 or C2. Patients with a significant C1–2 subluxation are usually at risk from falls, "whiplash" injuries, and excessive head movements, especially during anesthesia. When a cervical spine subluxation leads to neurological involvement or spinal cord compression, treatment includes the use of a firm cervical support, a halo cast apparatus (see pp. 133–135), or surgical fusion of the subluxed vertebrae (see pp. 149–150). Long-term studies of patients with cervical spine subluxations due to rheumatoid arthritis indicate that 25 percent will worsen, 25 percent will improve, and 50 percent will remain stable.

Degenerative Diseases of the Cervical Spine

Degenerative disease of the cervical spine is a fairly common problem, and usually involves one of three major pathological conditions. They are cervical disc degeneration, degenerative arthritis of the cervical spine, and herniation of a cervical disc. Although the basic causes of these conditions are not yet known, the pathological changes that occur in them are quite similar, differing only in degree. For example, cervical disc degeneration and degenerative arthritis of the cervical spine basically cause symptoms of pain and stiffness in the neck. Moreover, degenerative arthritis of the cervical spine and a herniated cervical disc may cause compression of the adjacent spinal nerve roots.

Cervical Disc Degeneration

Degeneration of a cervical intervertebral disc represents premature aging of the disc. The pathophysiology of disc degeneration involves the deterioration of the nucleus pulposus and annulus fibrosus and the lessening of the mechanical efficiency of the disc as a shock absorber or insulator between the adjacent vertebral bodies. The anterior margins of the involved vertebrae soon begin to show wear and osteophyte formation. With the decrease in the space between the vertebral bodies, the axis of motion shifts posteriorly to the apophyseal joints. Those joints cannot withstand the increased stress, and degenerative changes follow that alter the smooth contour of the apophyseal joints (Gartland, 1979, p. 367).

The patient with symptoms of cervical disc degeneration is generally younger than the patient with degenerative arthritis of the cervical spine, and women are more frequently affected than men. The patient with a cervical disc degeneration usually complains of an acute onset of neck pain, commonly localized to one side of the neck, with the pain extending into the interscapular area. The symptoms may come on spontaneously or may be the result of trauma. The neck pain can be reproduced or aggravated by motions of the head. Typically, the patient complains of neck pain being worse in the morning upon arising and usually associated with occipital headaches. At times, the patient may complain of pain radiating into the trapezius muscle and into the general area of the shoulder.

On examination, neck motion is usually restricted because of the pain. There is usually tenderness and palpation along the paracervical muscle masses and over the trapezius muscle. Tenderness over the spinous process and the interspinous ligaments of both the cervical and the upper thoracic spine is common. There is usually no neurological deficit.

The majority of patients gain relief with conservative treatment. Treatment involves relieving the pressure on the involved disc and resting the neck with the use of a soft cervical collar, especially during sleep. Moist heat applications to the neck through hot packs or hot showers are also helpful. Salicylates and anti-inflammatory drugs help to relieve the pain and the stiffness. Patients who do not respond to conservative treatment may require an anterior interbody cervical fusion (see pp. 150–151).

Degenerative Arthritis of the Cervical Spine

Degenerative arthritis of the cervical spine involves the simultaneous deterioration of intervertebral discs, vertebral bodies, ligamentous structures, and apophyseal joints. With multiple disc degeneration and a narrowing of multiple disc spaces, hypertrophic bone changes appear in the form of osteophytes or spurs. Those osteophytes form along the margins of the vertebral bodies, and are usually more prominent anteriorly than posteriorly. As the narrowing process continues, the apophyseal joints sublux, resulting in additional degeneration of those joints.

The typical patient with degenerative arthritis of the cervical spine is past middle age and complains of stiffness and neck pain. The stiffness is worse following periods of immobility of the head, and is partially relieved by slow and controlled motion. Characteristically the pain is aggravated by sudden or rapid movements of the head and certain sleeping positions (e.g., sleeping with arms above the head). The pain may be localized in the neck, but may also radiate to the head, the anterior chest, the thoracic spine region, and the shoulders. Motions of the cervical spine are restricted by the pain and stiffness and there is usually tenderness over the posterior neck and the trapezius muscles. If the patient complains of pain radiating to the arm or hand, it may be an indication of cervical nerve root compression by bony impingement on adjacent spinal nerve roots. The C4–5, C5–6, and C6–7 interspaces are the most frequently involved.

In most instances the symptoms caused by degenerative arthritis of the cervical spine can be alleviated by nonoperative measures, such as supporting the head in a cervical collar, particularly during periods of sleep, applying moist heat to the neck muscles, and using anti-inflammatory drugs to relieve pain and stiffness. Surgery is rarely required unless the patient develops an intractable cervical radiculitis. Spinal fusion may then be necessary to control chronic neck pain.

Herniation of a Cervical Disc

Herniation of a cervical disc characteristically occurs laterally where the annulus fibrosus is weakest and the posterior longitudinal ligament is thinner. Thus, on the herniated side there are symptoms of nerve root compression with radicular pain and parasthesia corresponding to the nerve root dermatome. Persistent pain in the neck and arm is usually caused by cervical nerve root compression at an intervertebral foramen.

There are two types of processes that lead to herniated cervical discs and that produce identical symptoms. The first process is the formation of osteophytes, which encroach on the intervertebral foramen and cause a narrowing of the intervertebral disc. The second process is an acute posterolateral rupture of a cervical disc with immediate compression of the nerve root in the foramen. These lesions usually occur at the site of maximum mobility of the cervical spine, i.e., the fifth and sixth cervical junction.

Ninety-five percent of all herniated cervical discs occur at the level of the fifth and sixth discs. The remainder occur at the level of the fourth and seventh cervical discs. About 5 percent of the time cervical discs herniate centrally rather than laterally. These ruptures usually develop suddenly and cause immediate paraplegia, constituting an acute surgical emergency.

Assessment. The patient with a herniated cervical disc usually complains of pain in the lower part of the neck radiating into one shoulder and arm and spreading anteriorly and posteriorly over the upper chest area. Abnormal sensations, such as numbness and tingling, are common over the radial aspect of the forearm, the hand, and the fingers. Pain is accentuated by movement of the neck and by coughing, sneezing, and straining. The discomfort is usually severe at night and interferes with the patient's sleep. Relief is often obtained by sitting up, standing, and even ambulating. When the patient moves the head either forward, backward, or toward the side of the pain, the discomfort increases. The patient usually is most comfortable with the head in neutral flexion and tilted away from the side of the lesion.

Upon examination, there are marked muscle spasms and limitations of active and passive motion, particularly toward the side of the lesion. The normal cervical lordosis is reduced or absent. When a forcible movement of the head is tried, it will reproduce the pain. When pressure is applied to the top of the patient's head, it accentuates the symptoms (Fig. 5–12). The patient usually complains of localized tenderness over the involved disc space (Hoppenfeld, 1976, p. 126).

When there is a herniation of the fifth cervical disc, the symptoms usually are (1) paresthesia in the thumb and the radial side of the hand, (2) hypesthesia in the sixth cervical dermatome on the dorsal and lateral aspects of the thumb and the radial side of the hand, (3) weakness and atrophy in the biceps, and (4) reduction of the biceps reflex, which is indicative of sixth cervical nerve root involvement (Turek, 1977, p. 744). With a herniation of the sixth cervical disc, the symptoms usually are (1) pain and paresthesia in the index and middle fingers and in the dorsum of the hand on compression testing, (2) hypesthesia in the seventh cervical dermatome, i.e., the index and middle fingers and the dorsum of the hand, (3) weakness and atrophy in the triceps, and (4) reduction of the triceps reflex, which is indicative of seventh cervical nerve root involvement.

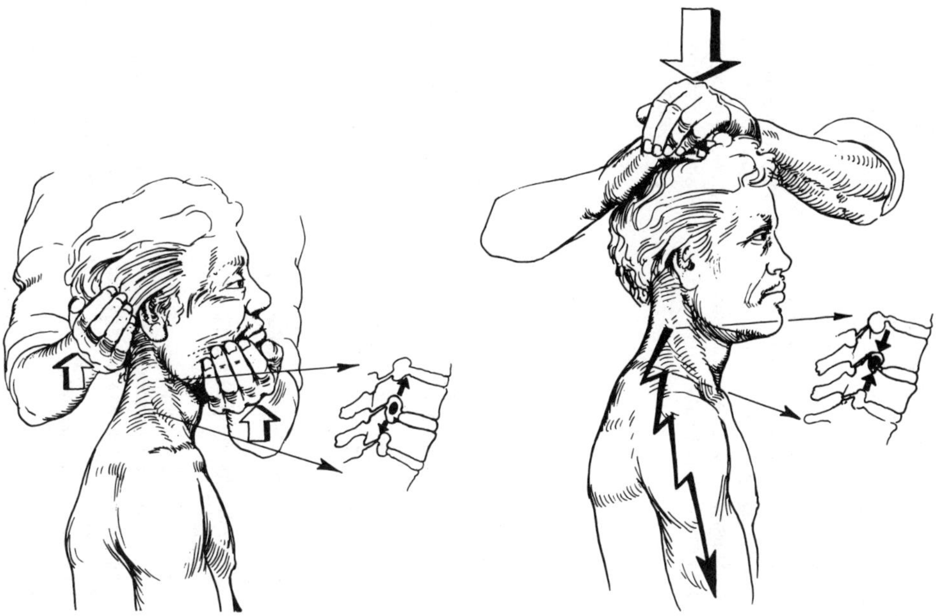

A B

Figure 5–12. A. The distraction text. **B.** The compression test. *(Figures 5–12, 5–14, 5–15, and 5–20 are reproduced from Hoppenfeld, S., 1976, with permission.)*

Conservative Treatment. Most of the patients with a herniated cervical disc obtain satisfactory relief from conservative treatment. The treatment includes the use of a cervical head halter or skeletal traction, complete bedrest, sedatives, hot packs applied to the neck at frequent intervals to reduce muscle spasms, and possibly the use of muscle relaxants. The patient needs to continue with the treatment for a long period of time, and may even be advised to set up a cervical skin traction apparatus at home. After the initial acute symptoms have subsided, a soft felt or foam rubber collar is usually applied and is worn continuously to keep neck movement at a minimum. A cervical plaster cast or brace affords maximum immobilization and may occasionally be indicated. Surgery is done only for persistent or frequently recurring pain and disability.

□ NURSING PROCESS (Table 5–3)

Assessment

The nursing assessment of a typical patient with a herniated cervical disc who is in cervical traction includes a comprehensive assessment of the total

TABLE 5–3. NURSING PROCESS FOR HERNIATED CERVICAL DISC TREATED WITH CERVICAL TRACTION

Assessment	Nursing Diagnosis	Goal Formulation	Planning and Intervention	Evaluation and Reassessment
1. Assess the location, duration, and severity of pain. Check the alignment and pull of the traction. Assess for any complaints of headache, increased neck pain, pressure on the ears or side of the face, or pain along the chin, jaw line or in the ears.	1. Alteration in comfort: pain in the cervical spine and upper extremities related to soft tissue trauma.	1. Short-term goal: a decrease in pain through use of traction. Long-term goal: free of pain.	1. Alleviate Pain Maintain traction. Keep traction pull evenly distributed between the chin and the occiput. Keep cervical spine straight. Teach relaxation techniques. Administer muscle relaxants and pain relief medications.	1. There should be a decrease in neck pain after application of traction. Correction of misalignment should help reduce headaches and pain in the temporomandibular joint.
2. Check the patient's position. Check the alignment of the traction pull. Check for any obstacles that may interfere with traction pull. Check poundage of traction.	2. Impaired physical mobility: a decrease in neck and arm function related to soft tissue trauma.	2. Short-term goal: an increase in neck and upper extremity function through traction. Long-term goal: regain full neck and upper extremity function.	2. Increase Mobility *Position* Keep patient supine, shoulders level and relaxed, and back flattened against the bed. Utilize a small pillow if necessary to maintain forward flexion of the head and neck. Elevate the head of the bed to a position of comfort (while maintaining traction). Assist with side lying at night.	2. The patient should be able to remain in traction, in the correct position, at all times. The patient should be able to lie on the side in a comfortable position for 30–60 minutes at a time.
			Traction Explain purpose of traction. Maintain continuous straight pull. Keep spreader bar and weights free of obstacles. Maintain correct poundage.	The traction should help reduce muscle spasms and pain. Correct poundage should prevent overpull of neck muscles.
			Ambulation Apply cervical collar when patient gets out of bed. Assist with ambulation.	The patient should be able to walk safely with assistance.

3. Assess for any signs of irritation on the chin. Check for any pressure on the sides of the patient's face or on frames of patient's glasses. Check for any pressure or redness at the nose bridge or behind the ears of the patient wearing glasses. Check that a man's long beard is smoothed over the chin. Assess ears for pressure due to the traction.	3. Potential for injury: a break in skin integrity related to pressure and friction.	3. Short- and long-term goals: free of any integumentary complication.	3. Prevent Complications *Integumentary* Keep traction pulling evenly between occiput and chin. Encourage men with fast-growing beards to shave twice a day. Apply traction smoothly over a man's long beard. Utilize a wide spreader bar to keep pressure off sides of face and ears. Ask individuals to remove earrings. Ask individuals with long hair to secure their hair on the top of their head.	3. The patient should not develop any injury to a facial nerve, breakdown of skin, or irritation and trauma to the temporomandibular joint.
4. Assess the patient's level of understanding about the rehabilitation process and home care. Assess the patient's level of anxiety.	4. Potential knowledge deficit related to the rehabilitation process and home care.	4. Short- and long-term goals: a decrease in anxiety through increased knowledge.	4. Patient Teaching Discuss the stages of the rehabilitation process. Teach the patient the purpose of the traction Demonstrate how to set up traction at home. Discuss methods of applying heat to the cervical neck in the home setting. Demonstrate a home exercise program. Discuss methods of preventing undue stress or strain to the cervical area (for example, while sitting or sleeping). Include patient's family and significant other in the teaching plan.	4. The patient should feel confident in continuing with the rehabilitation program at home.

patient with a focus on pain and the neurovascular status of the upper extremities. The neurovascular assessment of the upper extremity is described in Chapter 2. Assess the patient for any increased neck pain, pressure on the ears, and pain along the chin, jaw line, or ears. Assess for complaints of headaches as they could be an indication of venous pressure, venous stasis, or overpull on cervical muscles. Inspect the skin surfaces under the traction for possible irritation or pressure areas.

Determine that the patient is in correct alignment. The pull of the cervical traction should be equal on both sides, and be evenly distributed between the chin and the occiput. Check that the patient's head is tilted slightly forward so that the pull is on a straight cervical spinal column. The patient may or may not require a small pillow to obtain the desired neck flexion. The direction of the traction pull must cause the chin to be tucked in toward the chest, not drawn upward or backward. Check that the weights have the correct poundage, and that the weights and the pulleys hang free of the wall, bed, or other obstructions. The weights are usually only 2–5 pounds, but may be more in some instances. Most authorities agree that the weights should not exceed 10 pounds.

Nursing Diagnosis and Goal Formulation

Nursing diagnoses for a typical patient in cervical skin traction for a herniated cervical disc are (1) alterations in comfort related to pain in the soft tissue trauma of the cervical spine, (2) alterations in mobility related to neck and arm pain and muscle spasms, (3) potential complications due to soft tissue trauma in the cervical spine, and (4) alterations in psychological well-being related to anxiety and knowledge deficit about injury and treatment methods.

Short-term goals are to have the patient experience (1) a decrease in the amount of pain through nursing measures and prescribed medications, (2) an increase in mobility through increased muscle and nerve function, (3) an absence of complications from decreased activity and traction, and (4) a decrease in anxiety through increased knowledge. The long-term goals are to have the patient free of pain with a return of full function.

Planning and Intervention

Alleviate Pain. The patient with a herniated cervical disc will have pain. If there is an increase in neck and head pain after the application of the traction, determine whether the traction has an even pull between the occiput and the chin. Too much pull on the occiput will interfere with circulation and cause increased pain in the neck and especially the head. Adjust by raising the chin and tilting the head backward. If the patient complains of jaw or ear discomfort, the pull may be too much on the chin, causing pressure on the temporomandibular joint, which in turn causes irritation and pain. Adjust by tilting the head forward. If there is pressure on the ears, or discomfort along one side of the chin or jaw line, the traction may be pulling on that side more than the other. Correct the patient's positioning. Check to make sure the straps on the cervical traction are not pressing too tightly against the side of the patient's face, causing pressure on the facial nerve (cranial nerve VII). Such pressure on the patient's ears, jaw line, or glasses may be caused by a spreader bar that is too narrrow. Replace the spreader bar with a wider one. Make sure the head halter is not pressing on the patient's ears, and have the patient remove any earrings that interfere with the traction.

For chin discomfort when the alignment is correct, look for redness or irritation. If they are present, some authorities feel that a soft pad should be placed between the halter and the patient's chin. Others disagree, saying that the padding only increases pressure on the chin, and advocate that the traction should be removed to relieve the pressure. Which method to follow depends on established procedures. If no inflammation is present, alcohol rubs may also be used to toughen the skin on the chin. If the patient has a beard, make sure the beard is brought down flat under the chin as the halter is applied. If the halter is readjusted, the beard needs to be smoothed again. Men who are prone to a "5 o'clock shadow" may have to shave twice a day to reduce discomfort from the head halter rubbing against their whiskers. Individuals with long hair wearing the two-strap type of halter may need to keep their hair on the top of the head to reduce slipping of the posterior strap.

Increase Mobility

Position. The patient in cervical skin traction should be in a comfortable position on the back with the body in good alignment. The shoulders should be level and relaxed, and the back flattened against the bed. No pillow is generally used, although if the patient needs an increase in forward flexion of the head, a cervical or other small pillow may be allowed. The patient must be down far enough in bed to allow room for the spreader bar when it is attached to the head halter. The traction equipment is attached to the head of the bed unless the head board is too high. In that case, the head of the bed may be elevated, or the patient's head and traction equipment may be placed at the foot of the bed. Today, with the variety of bed and traction equipment available, such adjustments are usually not necessary.

During the day, some patients may be able to have the traction reattached higher on the bed frame so they can be in a sitting position, or even have the traction equipment set up on a geri chair so they can sit in the chair. Many patients have problems sleeping, as lying on the back is not comfortable. If allowed, nursing measures can permit patients to sleep on the side. Fold a regular pillow and tape the pillow so that it stays folded. Disconnect the traction and allow the patient to turn to the side, placing the folded pillow under the head so that the cervical spinal column is still straight. Reattach the traction so the pull is correct, the patient is in correct alignment, and the spreader bar is free of the pillow.

Cervical Skin Traction. Skin traction is applied to the patient's cervical spine by means of a head halter (Fig. 5–13). Various types of head halters may be obtained from orthopaedic and surgical supply houses, including soft disposable head halters, leather or canvas halters, and disposable two-strap halters. Cervical traction may be applied to relieve muscle spasms and pain caused by an injured cervical disc, arthritic radicular pain (i.e., radiated pain from nerve pressure), and conditions involving displaced (dislocated or subluxated) cervical vertebrae. Skin traction is rarely used for cervical vertebral fractures except as a preliminary immobilization prior to the insertion of skeletal tongs for long-term immobilization. Head halter skin traction may also be used at home by some patients for relief of cervical pain. In addition to the head halter, a spreader bar, rope (traction cord), weight carrier, and pulley attachment are needed to apply the traction. The kinds of bars and pulleys used will vary with the type of equipment.

Before applying the traction, explain to the patient the purpose of the traction and what it should do. Set up the traction equipment on the bed. Make sure the patient is comfortable and correctly positioned in bed. Because cervical neck injuries cause muscle spasms and headaches, the patient should not be asked to hold the head up during the application of the traction. Support the patient's head by placing your left hand under the patient's head if you are on the patient's left or your right hand if you are on the patient's right. With your other hand, put the head halter over the patient's face and under the chin. You may have to bring the posterior portion of the halter down the back of the patient's head to get the halter completely under the chin. Adjust the posterior portion to the level of the occiput. For the halter with side adjustments, attach the side closures and adjust the straps so that the halter feels comfortable. The straps do not have to be tight, just secure enough to hold the halter in correct position. If the cervical traction is being applied with a disposable two-strap halter, make sure the straps are in place and the ropes that connect them are applying equal pull. Connect the head halter to the spreader bar. Apply a few pounds of pull manually to check the adjustment of the head halter before applying the weights. Put the correct amount of weight on the weight carrier and gradually, smoothly let go of the traction. The direction of the pull of the traction must cause the chin to be tucked in toward the chest and not drawn upward or backward. The patient should be instructed to maintain proper body alignment. With cervical skin traction, countertraction is provided by the patient's body weight and position in bed.

Heat and Massage. Heat is applied to the cervical area for its analgesic and muscle-relaxing properties, and it tends to improve circulation to the

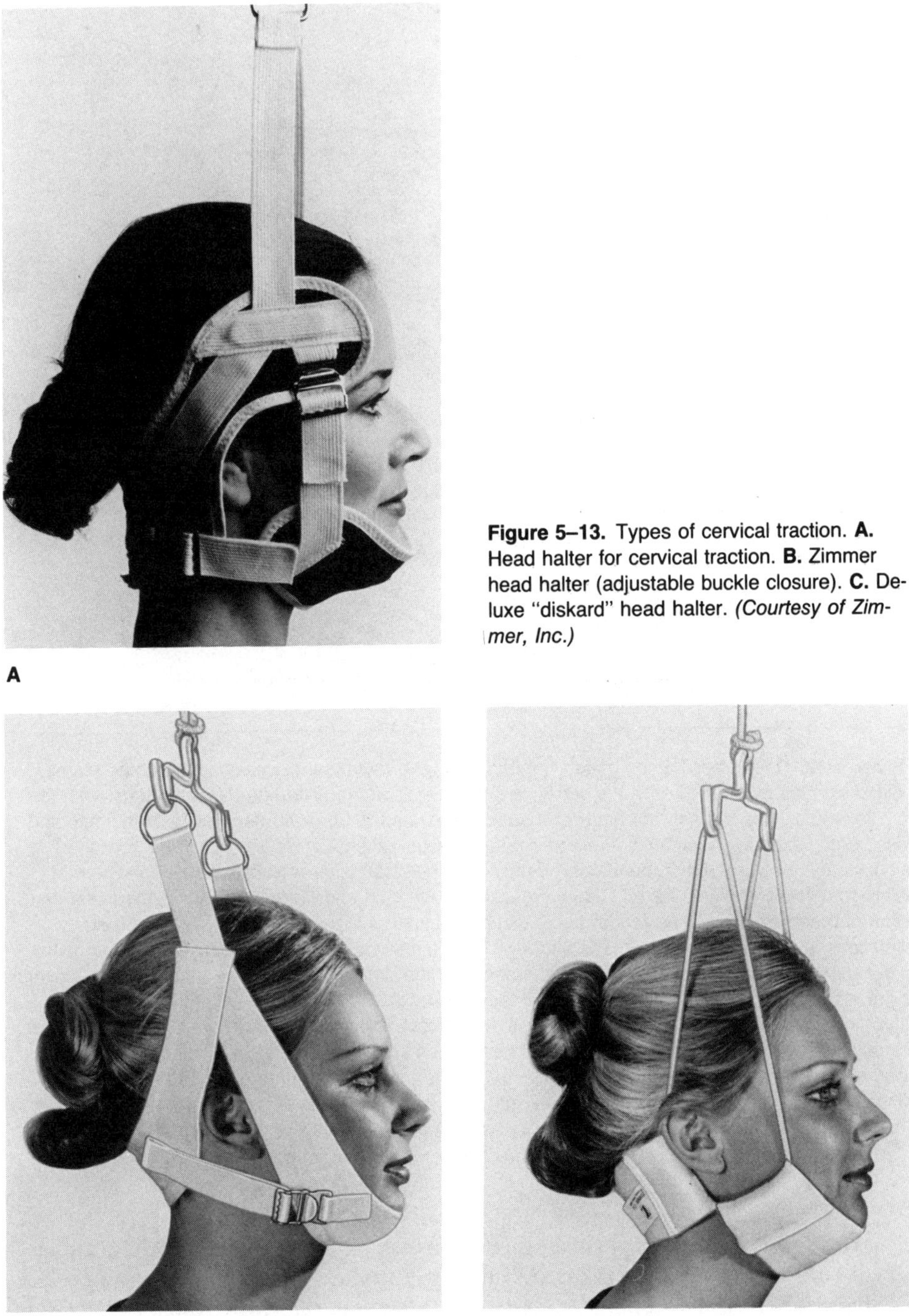

A

B

C

Figure 5–13. Types of cervical traction. **A.** Head halter for cervical traction. **B.** Zimmer head halter (adjustable buckle closure). **C.** Deluxe "diskard" head halter. *(Courtesy of Zimmer, Inc.)*

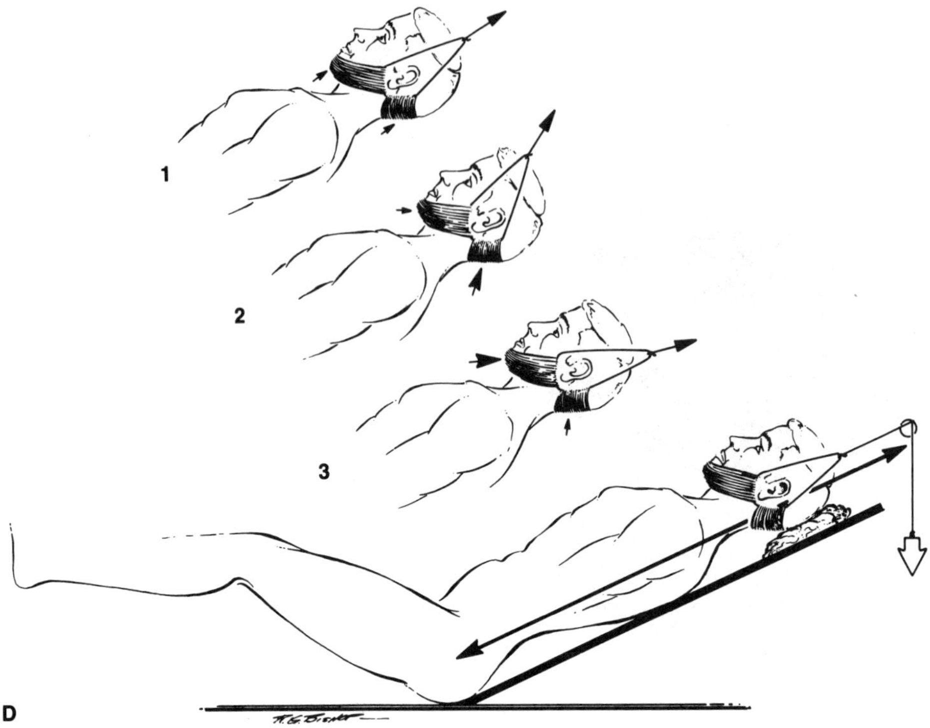

Figure 5–13. D. The application of cervical traction in the recumbent position is generally accomplished with the patient flat or in the semiflexed position *(bottom).* With the patient in traction in the semiflexed position, the head of the bed should be elevated to 30 or 40 degrees, with the hips and knees both flexed approximately 45 degrees. The line of pull should be a straight line from the buttocks to the pulley. Attachment to the head with a cervical halter is shown *(top). (1)* When the pull is completely straight, there is equal pressure on the chin and on the occiput. In the event that either of these areas become tender because of continued pull, the pressure may be altered by alterations in the direction of pull. The alteration of pull may be accomplished by leaving the pulley in the same place and raising or lowering the head of the bed, so that the line of pull, in relationship to the long axis of the trunk, is altered. *(2)* If the head of the bed is lowered slightly, the pull is in a more anterior direction, causing less pressure on the chin and more pressure on the occiput. *(3)* If the occiput has become tender and occipital headaches have occurred as a result of the pull, the head of the bed can be raised slightly. This causes the pull to be in a more posterior direction, which causes a greater amount of pressure on the chin and a lesser amount on the occiput. *(From Lewis, R. C.* Handbook of traction, casting and splinting techniques. *Philadelphia: Lippincott, 1977, p. 21, with permission.)*

skin and the more superficial muscle layers. Having the patient recumbent during heat applications further adds to muscle and psychic relaxation and pain relief. (For further details on heat therapy, see pp. 192–193.) Massage also helps to increase circulation to the area and relax the muscles.

Ambulation. Most patients are allowed out of cervical skin traction for activities of daily living, though they are encouraged to keep the traction on as much as possible. When patients have bathroom privileges, they will need assistance in getting out of bed as well as getting out of the traction. Many patients need to wear a cervical collar to help support the head during ambulation. If the patient has been on muscle relaxants, it is best to walk with the patient to ensure safety.

Prevent Complications. The major complications for a patient with a herniated cervical disc being treated with cervical skin traction are injury to the facial nerve, breakdown of skin on the chin, irritation and trauma to the temporomandibular joint, and overpull of muscles of the neck. Nursing measures to prevent those complications have been discussed under how to alleviate pain and increase mobility.

Potential nonphysical complications are depression and the acceptance of the sick role by the patient. Nursing measures to help prevent those complications are one-to-one therapeutic discussions with the patient, giving the patient realistic information on the treatment and prognosis, and encouraging the patient to be as actively involved in self-care as physically possible.

Patient Teaching. The patient must know the purpose of the traction and how it works, to decrease the anxiety and fear of the equipment and to enable performance of self-care without undue stress. If home traction is indicated, explain its purpose, how it is to be set up, and how often it is to be used. Pictures are a great help. Most patients need to wear a cervical collar for a period of time. Tell them whether the collar is to be worn with the higher or lower portion in front, and why. They should be told to report to their physician any increase in pain or pressure that may develop after they start to wear the collar. Most individuals with a cervical collar have no problems bathing, because they can remove the collar and shower.

At home, heat should be applied using an electric heating pad set on low or medium. After the traction is removed, the patient needs to begin an exercise program for the cervical area. Isometric exercises come first. They provide small changes of stress to the ligaments, bones, and joints to strengthen those structures as well as muscles. Each set of exercises should be done approximately 15 minutes per day unless otherwise instructed. The amount of force the patient actually applies depends on a number of factors, including the patient's strength before the injury, level of pain, pain tolerance, and body build. Each repetition of the exercise should cause either slight discomfort or a pulling sensation. If the patient remains comfortable, the exercises are probably not beneficial. If they are painful, they will not be tolerated.

The neck exercises can be done in a standing, sitting, or reclining position. They can be done all at once or spread out over the day. The following neck exercises are to be done:

1. With the head held erect and face squarely forward, the patient places the base of the right palm (the part of the palm nearest the forearm) against the head, just above the right ear. The patient then pushes the head toward the right while resisting with the palm so there is no appreciable motion. The exercise is held for the count of ten.
2. The patient then repeats the same exercise on the left side.
3. With the patient's head held erect and face squarely forward, the patient places the right palm on the right side of the forehead, and left palm on the left side of the forehead with the hands touching each other. The patient then pushes the head in a forward direction while resisting with the palms so there is no appreciable motion. The exercise is held for the count of ten.
4. With the patient's head held erect and face squarely forward, the patient places the right palm on the right side of the back of the head and the left palm on the left side of the back of the head, interwining the fingers. The patient then pushes the head in a backward direction while resisting with the palms so there is no appreciable motion. The exercise is held for the count of ten.

The number of times each exercise is repeated gradually increases, and active exercises are also added as the patient's condition improves (Carle Clinic Association, Orthopedic Department).

Patients need to know how to prevent any undue stress or strain to the cervical area. *Do Nots* include (1) sleeping with an arm under the face or over the head, (2) sleeping with a high pillow, (3) sleeping on the abdomen, as it forces the head to the side, (4) lying on the sofa while watching television, (5) lying in bed to read, and (6) sleeping in a chair. All of the above can cause severe strain to the neck.

Evaluation and Reassessment

Determine whether the pain decreased in severity after the application of traction and the administration of pain medications and muscle relaxants. Evaluate the effectiveness of the traction to relieve muscle spasms by how well the patient tolerates the traction and continues to utilize it. Check for any possible complications from the traction. To evaluate the status of the patient's facial nerve (cranial nerve VII), observe the patient's face for symmetry. Then ask the patient to raise and lower the eyebrows, again observing for symmetry. Next, ask the patient to close the eyes tightly while you try to raise the lids. Finally, ask the patient to smile, show the teeth, and puff out the cheeks, so you can assess facial muscle strength. If signs of decreased nerve function are observed, remove the traction and notify the physician. Evaluate how well the patient, family, or significant other understands home care by asking them to tell you how the patient should carry out the activities of a normal day. Have the patient explain to you the side effects of the medications.

Surgery (Cervical Laminectomy). A cervical laminectomy is a surgical procedure to remove a herniated nucleus pulposus. A midline incision is usually made from the spinous process of the fourth cervical vertebra to the first thoracic, and the posterior muscles are separated at the midline by blunt dissection. The laminae of the fifth, sixth, and seventh cervical vertebrae are then denuded, and the attachment of the ligamentum is separated from the anterior surface of the laminae above. The caudal third of the lamina above the lesion and the cephalic third of the lamina below the lesion are then removed laterally. If a herniated disc is present, the adjacent nerve root has probably been flattened and displaced posteriorly. The nerve root is retracted upward and the herniated disc is removed. The removal of the disc is usually easy unless there are bone spurs from osteoarthritis that displace the nerve root backward. The surgical wound is then closed, and in many instances a wound drain is put into place.

Cervical Nerve Root Compression Syndrome (Cervical Radiculitis, Cervical Root Syndrome)

Any condition of the neck that causes impingement or entrapment of a cervical nerve root or encroachment on its intervertebral foramen may cause cervical nerve root compression syndrome. The most frequent causes are degenerative arthritis and a herniated intervertebral disc, although in the cervical spine, degenerative changes with accompanying posterior spur formation are the most common. Less frequent causes include cervical subluxations and dislocations, cervical fractures with backward displacement of the fragments, congenital anomalies of the cervical spine, and tumors.

The major complaints of a patient with cervical nerve root compression (or cervical radiculitis) is shoulder and arm pain associated with numbness and tingling in the hand and the fingers The pain is usually described as severe and sharp, and commonly radiates from the shoulder to the arm and frequently into the forearm and the fingers. The pain may also radiate to the anterior chest or subscapular area. Pain is aggravated by certain motions of the head, particularly turning toward the side of the pain. It is also intensified by coughing, sneezing, straining, jarring the neck, or applying pressure to the top of the head. In general, the pain is related to movement of the head and the neck, and is not produced by movements of the shoulder and the arm. The most common areas of involvement are C5–6 and C6–7, with entrapment of the sixth and seventh cervical nerve roots (to distinguish between those nerve roots, see p. 154).

Treatment of cervical nerve root compression syndrome depends on the cause of the compression. If there is arthritic spur impingement or a herniated intervertebral disc, the patient is usually treated using a head halter cervical traction. Several weeks in traction may be needed to relieve the nerve compression. Heat applications, muscle relaxant drugs, and analgesics may also be required, and a cervical collar is used when the patient is allowed out of bed. Surgical treatment is reserved for those patients who fail to respond to conservative treatment, have a significant neurological deficit, or have compression from a tumor, cervical dislocation, or displaced cervical fracture.

THORACIC SPINAL COLUMN

Trauma

FRACTURES

The most common injury to the thoracic region of the back is a compression fracture of a vertebral body. This injury can arise in many ways, including a fall from a height, the effects of an explosion, or a hyperflexion of the spine. The most frequent kind is a wedge compression fracture of a vertebral body. In that injury, one or more vertebral bodies collapse anteriorly, become wedge-shaped, and create a prominence of the spinous process posteriorly. Neurological deficits may occur, depending on the severity of the injury. The fracture is basically stable in that no further deformity is likely to occur. The usual treatment is a short period of bedrest, followed by the redevelopment of the spinal muscles. Hyperextension jackets and posterior spinal supports are usually contraindicated, as they cause stiffness of the uninjured parts of the spine and thus may do more harm than good (Gartland, 1979, p. 327; Iversen & Clawson, 1977, p. 117–118; Roaf & Hodkinson, 1975, p. 151).

There are other types of compression fractures of the thoracolumbar spine. One is when a vertebral body is invaded by both of its adjacent discs, and a biconcave prominence is produced; that *codfish* is seen in advanced cases of osteoporosis, and the bone deformity is caused by chronic compressive stress. A *burst* or *explosion* fracture is caused by extreme compression on a vertebral body that produces a vertical fracture that splits the body in two. The fracture is stable unless the posterior portion displaces posteriorly into the spinal canal, causing a neurological deficit. There is normally little stress on ligamentous structures. If a large compressive force is applied to the spine with degenerated and extensively fibrosed intervertebral discs, the most likely result is a uniform flattening of a vertebral body.

The other compression fractures of the thoracolumbar spine are usually treated with bedrest on a firm mattress followed by early mobilization. While on bedrest, sitting is not permitted. The head of the bed should not be elevated more than 20 to 30 degrees, and turning the patient from side to side must be done by log rolling. Analgesics are usually given for pain relief if there is no complication from head injuries. When the initial pain subsides, progressive muscle strengthening exercises for the spine are started. When the patient begins to ambulate, a reinforced thoracolumbar garment (corset) or orthosis is usually worn for 6 to 8 weeks for comfort. For patients with severe pain after a period of bedrest, a body cast is applied while the spine is extended by traction. After approximately 6 weeks in the cast, the patient wears a corset for another 4 to 6 weeks. During that time, exercises to strengthen the spinal extensor muscles are encouraged to permit the later discontinuation of the external support. Exercises that involve spinal flexion, such as sit-ups, are discouraged. If the spinal deformity involves a loss of more than 50 percent of the height of the fractured vertebral body, a substantial spine support, such as a molded plaster jacket, may be applied for 12 to 16 weeks to prevent progressive deformity and protect against spinal instability. The support is followed by a corset that is worn for 2 more months.

Fracture–dislocations of the thoracolumbar spine are usually caused by automobile accidents. Either the spinal cord or the cauda equina is frequently damaged, causing sudden traumatic paraplegia. A rotory or lateral force, superimposed upon a flexion force, is the mechanism of injury. Pathologically, the spine and the posterior longitudinal ligaments are torn, the posterior facet joints may be fractured, the upper part of the vertebral body is sheared off, and the spinal column dislocated and completely unstable. In the thoracic region the spinal cord may be injured and is frequently transected, whereas in the lumbar region the cauda equina is usually damaged but the nerves are not necessarily transected. With incomplete paraplegia of sudden traumatic onset, some spinal nerve tracts at the level of the injury may escape damage, and some recovery may be possible.

In fracture–dislocations of the thoracolumbar spine that do not involve paraplegia, open reduction and fusion by means of plating the spinous processes and bone grafting are indicated to prevent subsequent neurological damage. With incomplete paraplegia of sudden traumatic onset, treatment is usually bedrest on a turning frame for 12 weeks. If the fracture is still unstable, spinal fusion is done. Even with complete paraplegia, early open reduction, plating, and bone grafting are necessary to reduce the risk of subsequent injury to nerve roots that have been spared, to facilitate nursing care, and to get the individual up safely.

Pathology

TUBERCULOSIS OF THE SPINE

Tuberculosis should be considered when there is a spinal infection. A tubercular infection of the spine, by far the most common form of skeletal tuberculosis, is known as Pott's disease. It commonly affects the segment from the tenth thoracic to the first lumbar vertebra, the segment of the spine that possesses the greatest mobility. Although spinal tuberculosis may strike any age group, about half of the patients are between 3 and 5 years of age at the time of onset. In general, spinal infections tend to be more serious than those in the peripheral joints, because the spinal cord may become involved. Pott's disease is more serious in instances where there are tubercular lesions elsewhere in the body, where the primary focus of infection is virulent, where the patient is very old or very young, and where associated debilitating conditions, such as diabetes, nephritis, and anemia are present (Cailliet, 1981, pp. 202–203).

A spinal infection usually begins in the vertebral body along the anterior aspect of the bone, causing bone destruction that leads to the collapse of the vertebral body. Necrotic material is then forced out into the soft tissues forming paravertebral abscesses, and the infection may spread beneath the anterior longitudinal spinal ligament to involve several vertebrae (Gartland, 1979, pp. 187–188).

The collapse of one or more vertebral bodies can lead to compression of the spinal cord at any level from the foramen magnum to the upper lumbar region. It occurs most often in the thoracic spine where the spinal canal is narrow and the cord occupies most of the space, so that even a small abscess or bone sequestrum may produce cord pressure and paraplegia. Spinal cord compression is less likely in the cervical region, as the infected material can follow the fascial plane, or in the lumbar region where it can go along the psoas muscle sheath toward the groin.

The patient with Pott's disease complains of back pain that restricts spinal movement. He or she tends to squat rather than bend to retrieve an object from the floor. Because of pain, the spinal movements are guarded and the patient tends to walk with a protective gait. If there is a marked anterior collapse of several vertebral bodies in the thoracic region, the patient develops a pointed protuberance of the spine called a *gibbus* (Fig. 5–14). In the days when spinal tuberculosis was common, it was the chief cause of the "hunchback" deformity.

The major complications of spinal tuberculosis are psoas abscess, paraplegia, and tuberculous meningitis. A psoas abscess is a paravertebral abscess composed of necrotic debris that pushes out against the psoas muscle. The abscess may spread down tissue planes to a point in the thigh or spread backward through the lumbar triangle to form a lumbar abscess. If the abscesses drain to the skin surface, a tuberculous sinus is formed.

Paraplegia, one of the most disabling complications of spinal tuberculosis, is a result of cord compression and occurs in about 10 percent of patients. The impairment may vary from a slightly spastic gait to complete paralysis. Partial or complete paralysis is more common with involvement of the posterior aspect of the vertebral bodies, the laminae, the pedicles, or the transverse processes, because of their close proximity to the spinal cord.

Tuberculous meningitis is the result of a rupture of a tuberculous abscess through the dura mater. Before the development of antituberculin drugs, tuberculous meningitis was frequently fatal.

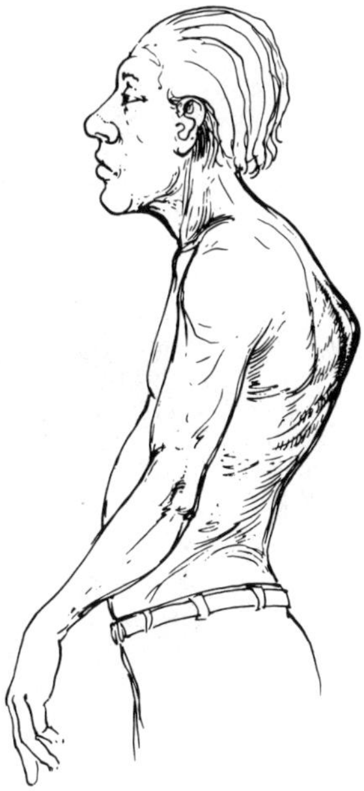

Figure 5–14. Gibbus deformity.

Immobilization of the spine by bedrest and a plaster cast or spinal brace, coupled with prolonged drug therapy, is usually considered the best treatment for spinal tuberculosis. At times, posterior spinal fusion of the involved vertebrae may be required to obtain complete immobilization of the spinal column.

SCOLIOSIS

Scoliosis is a lateral curvature of the spine that can result from either a specific pathology or from unknown causes (Fig. 5–15). It may develop in a localized area or involve the entire spinal column, and the degree of curvature may be mild, moderate, or severe. Scoliosis is classified by the nature of the lateral curvature produced, specifically (1) functional curvature, where there are no structural alterations within the vertebral column, (2) structural curvature, where there are structural alterations within the vertebral column, (3) S-shaped curvature, a double curvature comprised of a major curve and a compensatory curve, (4) C-shaped curvature, where the lateral curvature involves all or most of the lumbar and thoracic areas, and (5) double major curvature, where there are two primary curves of equal or almost equal size. For a more in-depth discussion of pediatric scoliosis, see references at the end of the chapter.

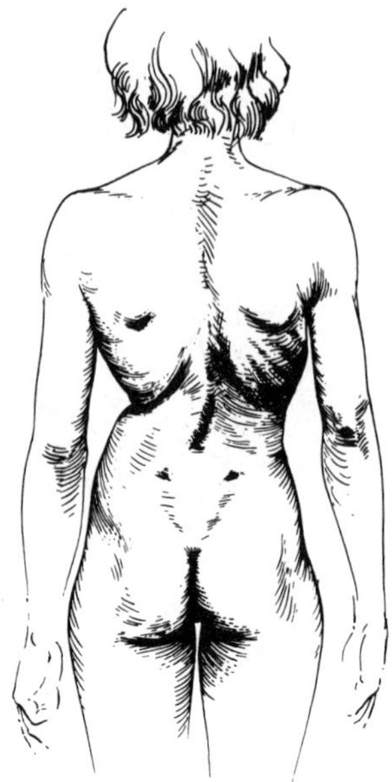

Figure 5–15. Lateral curvature of the spine (scoliosis).

Adult Scoliosis

After vertebral growth is completed (at approximately age 15 for women and age 17 for men), an existing scoliosis persists into adult life. The major impairment from scoliosis is the cosmetic deformity. The involved vertebrae may rotate, however, producing rib cage deformities and decreasing pulmonary capacity. In severe scoliosis, when the curvature exceeds 50 degrees in the thoracic region, cardiopulmonary complications are possible. Patients with a large curvature in the lumbar region may experience considerable pain. Confirmation of adult scoliosis is based on clinical examination and roentgenograms.

Treatment of adult scoliosis is different from that of the childhood disease. The adult spine is less flexible and thus less correctable by flexibility exercises, bracing, casting, or use of a scolio-tron. The progress of adult scoliosis is not a result of vertebral epiphyseal deformation, but of asymmetrical intervertebral disc compression and degeneration on the concave side of the curves. In adult scoliosis, the increase in spinal curvature due to disc deterioration may be 1 degree per year. A scoliotic curve of 45 degrees in a patient aged 17 might be considered acceptable, but 20 years later, when the patient would be 37, the curvature could approach 65 degrees (Cailliet, 1981, pp. 99–105).

Treatment consists of weight reduction, active and passive exercises, and bracing or corsetting to support the spine if pain occurs. Such conservative treatment is rarely effective for adults. Advances in the past few decades have improved surgical methods of correcting the curvature in adult scoliosis and preventing the progression of the deformity. Even with surgical intervention, however, it is impossible to totally correct the curvature or alleviate the deformity. The three major surgical methods currently utilized are the Harrington rod instrumentation, the Dwyer cable instrumentation, and the Luque rod instrumentation.

Harrington Rod Instrumentation Procedure

The Harrington rod instrumentation procedure (Fig. 5–16) is used when there is a desire to correct and fuse a large portion of the spinal column. The patient is placed on the operating table in the prone position, and a midline incision is made down the center of the patient's back. All soft tissue and cortical bone are denuded from the spinous processes laterally to the transverse processes

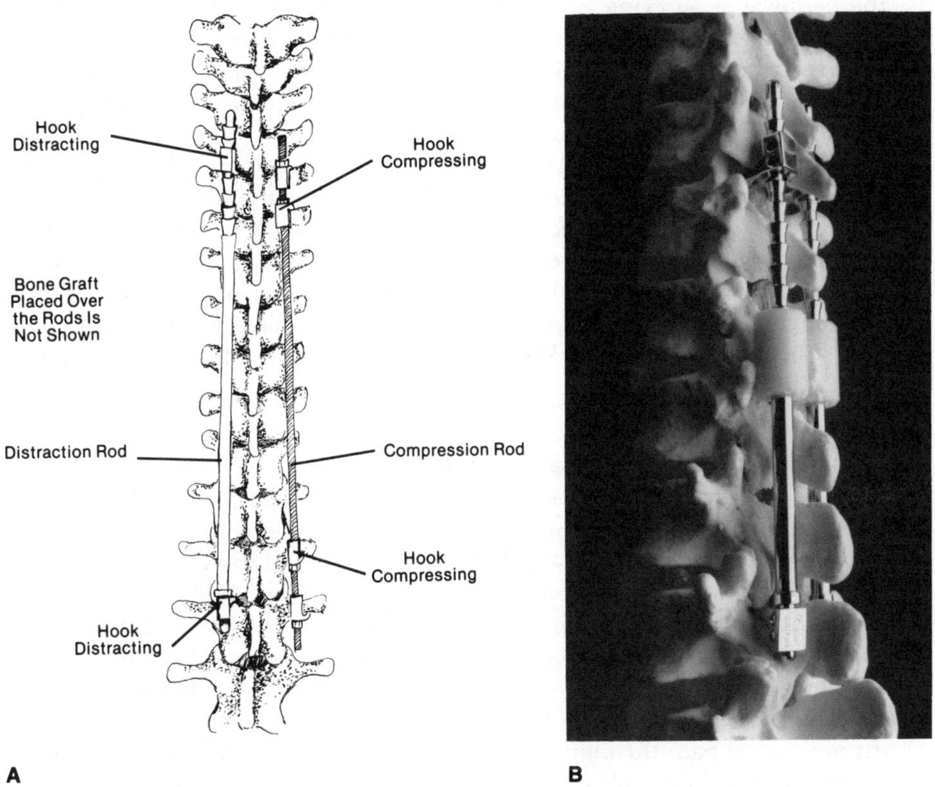

Figure 5–16. A. Harrington rod instrumentation. *(From Brantley, P., & Analla, M., 1980, p. 58. Courtesy of Howmedica.)* **B.** Edwards rod sleeves and Edwards anatomic spinal hooks. *(Courtesy of Zimmer, Inc.)*

on both sides of the spine. Hooks are then placed in vertebrae at the upper and lower portions of the curve, and the Harrington rod attached. Distraction forces are exerted as the rod is extended, which reduces the spinal curvature. Large amounts of cortical and cancellous bone are then placed over the rods and the denuded area. Some bone for the graft may have been obtained from the iliac crest. The incision is closed with wound catheters in place.

□ NURSING PROCESS (Table 5–4)

Assessment

The initial assessment of a typical patient following a posterior spinal fusion with Harrington rod instrumentation should emphasize the neurovascular status of both lower extremities (Chap. 2). Assess neurovascular status every 15 minutes for 2 hours, every 30 minutes for 2 hours, every 2 hours for 24 hours, and then at the beginning of every shift. Check that the hemovac is working properly and determine the amount of drainage in the hemovac. The patient's bed should be flat and the patient should be in correct body alignment with no elevation of the shoulders. Assess for the severity, location, and duration of pain. Determine if the patient has any signs of nausea.

Continuing assessment should include an assessment of the patient's understanding of postoperative care. Monitor the patient's intake and output, and check the specific gravity of the patient's urine. Assess anal sphincter control by digital examination and assess urinary sphincter control after the Foley catheter is discontinued. Continue to assess the amount of pain, and be especially alert for sudden onset of pain between the shoulders. Check bowel sounds. Assess the patient's anxiety level and note any signs of depression.

Nursing Diagnosis and Goal Formulation

Nursing diagnoses for a typical patient following a posterior spinal fusion with Harrington rod instrumentation are (1) alterations in comfort related to pain in the posterior spinal column (thoracic through lumbar) from surgery, (2) alterations in mobility related to spinal instability, (3) potential complications related to surgical procedure and enforced encumbency, and (4) alterations in psychological well-being related to anxiety and knowledge deficit about the surgical procedure and rehabilitation process.

Short-term goals are to have the patient experience (1) a decrease in the amount of pain through nursing measures and prescribed medications, (2) an increase in mobility through the use of a body cast and body brace and through controlled ambulation, (3) an absence of complications from surgery and decreased activity, and (4) a decrease in anxiety through increased knowledge. Long-term goals are to have the patient free of pain and to have return of function and activities.

TABLE 5–4. NURSING PROCESS FOR POSTERIOR SPINAL FUSION WITH HARRINGTON ROD INSTRUMENTATION

Assessment	Nursing Diagnosis	Goal Formulation	Planning and Intervention	Evaluation and Reassessment
1. Assess the location, duration, and severity of pain. Observe for verbal and nonverbal cues of pain. Assess the neurovascular status of both legs. Check for correct body alignment. Check vital signs.	1. Alteration in comfort: pain in the back related to bone and soft tissue trauma.	1. Short-term goal: a decrease in pain through positioning and medications. Long-term goal: free of pain.	1. Alleviate Pain Place patient in correct body alignment. Utilize noninvasive nursing measures for pain relief. Teach relaxation techniques. Administer prescribed pain medications as indicated.	1. Morphine sulfate (with or without Vistaril) every 3–4 hours should help keep the patient relatively comfortable.
2. Assess for spinal column alignment when patient is turned to one side. Assess neurovascular status of both legs. Check for correct body alignment. Assess patient's ability to do exercises. Assess patient's willingness to follow restrictions. Assess muscle tone and strength.	2. Impaired physical mobility: a decrease in spinal flexibility related to surgical instrumentation.	2. Short-term goal: an increase in mobility through immobilization and controlled exercises. Long-term goal: regain as much spinal flexibility as possible.	2. Increase Mobility *Position* Utilize an extra firm mattress or place a board under the patient's mattress. Keep patient's bed flat. Keep patient supine for the first 8 hours. Avoid turning the patient prone. Some patients may have their knee gatch raised or pillows placed under their knee when supine.	2. Flexion of the knees should help reduce stress on the patient's back.
			Turning Log roll every 2–4 hours. To log roll, place pillows between the patient's legs. Utilize two persons (with or without a turning sheet) and turn the patient as a unit while keeping the spinal column straight.	Turning should be done without twisting or stressing the spinal column.

(continued)

TABLE 5–4. *(Continued)*

Assessment	Nursing Diagnosis	Goal Formulation	Planning and Intervention	Evaluation and Reassessment
			Maintain straight alignment of the hips and shoulders at all times. Place pillows to support the back when the patient is lying on the side.	
			Exercises Teach muscle setting exercises (quadriceps and gluteal setting). Teach mild active exercises to the lower extremities (plantar and dorsiflexion and active range of motion of the ankles). Encourage active range of motion of the upper extremities. Encourage patient to help with activities of daily living.	The patient should be able to do the exercises without applying stress to the back.
			Ambulation Utilize a tilt table for helping patient stand for the first time. Assist with ambulation when patient has a body jacket on.	The patient should be able to ambulate with assistance.
3. Assess the neurovascular status of both legs. Listen for complaints of "heaviness," "tingling" or "pins and needles." Assess for any complaints of a headache.	3. Potential for injury: neurovascular deficit related to surgery and soft tissue swelling.	3. Short- and long-term goals: free of any injury related to neurovascular deficit.	3. Prevent Complications *Neurological* Do neurovascular checks to both lower extremities every 15 minutes for the first 2 hours after surgery, every 30 minutes for the next 2 hours, every hour for the next 2 hours, every 2 hours for the next 18 hours, and then at the beginning of every shift.	3. The patient should not develop any neurovascular deficiency such as a muscle weakness or paresthesia.

			Notify physician of any abnormal responses.	
Assess for bowel sounds. Check for expulsion of flatus. Check for any abdominal distention. Measure abdominal girth. Check for nausea and vomiting. Assess for pain.	Potential alteration in bowl elimination: ineffective bowel function related to immobility and surgical procedure.	Short- and long-term goals: return of a functioning bowel without complications.	*Gastrointestinal* Restrict oral fluids until bowel sounds are heard for several hours. Administer sips of clear liquids with a syringe. Slowly increase fluid oral intake as bowel sounds return. Apply heating pad to abdomen. Utilize rectal tube.	The patient should have good bowel sounds and be expelling flatus by the third postoperative day. Using a syringe for liquids should help the patient take oral fluids without swallowing air and thus avoid excessive belching.
Check wound catheter suction. Assess incisional line for any signs of infection (redness, swelling or hardness). Check the incision line for approximation. Check vital signs.	Potential for injury: hematoma related to surgical procedure. Potential for injury: infection related to surgical procedure.	Short- and long-term goals: free of any integumentary complications.	*Integumentary* Maintain wound catheter suction. Keep dressing clean and dry. Encourage a well-balanced diet with plenty of fluids. Administer antibiotics as prescribed.	The patient should not have any signs of infection or hematoma.
Check intravenous flow rate. Check intake and output. Assess vital signs. Observe patient's color, skin turgor, and mucous membrane texture.	Potential alteration in fluid volume: deficit related to decreased intake and lack of muscle tone.	Short-term goal: have fluid volume maintained within normal limits. Long-term goal: free of any circulatory complications.	*Circulatory* Maintain hydration. Offer oral fluids (based on bowel sounds). Explain the need for fluid intake. Apply elastic stockings. Turn and position patient every 2 hours.	The patient should not have more than 500 cc of drainage within 8 hours. The patient's urine output should not be less than 150 cc every 8 hours.

(continued)

TABLE 5–4. *(Continued)*

Assessment	Nursing Diagnosis	Goal Formulation	Planning and Intervention	Evaluation and Reassessment
Check specific gravity of urine. Assess amount of drainage from wound catheters. Assess muscle tone and strength.				
Assess for shortness of breath, pulmonary congestion, abnormal breath sounds, and a change in respiratory rate. Note any jugular venous distention. Check for any increased pulse volume or blood pressure. Assess if fluid intake is greater than output. Note any change in mental status. Note any restlessness or anxiety. Assess for fatigue. Check for taut, shiny skin.	Potential alteration in fluid volume: excess related to parental fluid intake.	Short-term goal: have fluid volume maintained within normal limits. Long-term goal: free of any circulatory complications.	Give fluids with caution (set up a 24-hour schedule). Monitor vital signs and urine output every 2 hours. Observe for signs of congestive heart failure. Turn and position every 2 hours. Administer skin and mouth care. Restrict sodium intake. Take safety precautions against periods of confusion.	After restricting fluids, the patient should start diuresing within 2–3 days.

Assess for any increase in pain. Assess for level of comfort after activity. Assess for correct alignment during activities.	Potential for injury: loosening of instrumentation related to stress and strain on spinal column.	Short- and long-term goals: free of any complications.	*Dislocation of Hooks and Rod(s)* Encourage deep breathing exercises but no coughing. Utilize measures to prevent vomiting. Hold the patient's shoulders against the bed should vomiting occur. Assist with turning and ambulation. Educate the patient on proper techniques for movement.	The patient should be able to avoid twisting or stressing the spinal column when turning, ambulating, sneezing, coughing, or vomiting.
4. Assess patient's level of understanding about rehabilitation process and home care. Assess patient's level of anxiety.	4. Potential knowledge deficit related to immobilization and rehabilitation process.	4. Short- and long-term goals: a decrease in anxiety through increased knowledge.	4. Patient Teaching Discuss the surgical procedure and the various steps in the rehabilitation process. Review how to turn, get in and out of bed, get in and out of a chair, and how to do activities of daily living. Reinforce proper body mechanics. Instruct patient, family, and significant other on cast care. Review signs and symptoms of potential complications.	4. The patient, family, and significant other should feel confident about home care. The patient should verbalize an understanding of the rehabilitation process and the importance of own role. The patient should be able to demonstrate proper body mechanics.

Planning and Intervention

Alleviate Pain. Following a posterior spinal fusion with Harrington rod instrumentation the patient will usually have a fair amount of back pain from the surgery. Injections of narcotics, such as morphine sulfate (subcutaneous) every 3 to 4 hours PRN, are usually necessary for the first several days after surgery, and then oral narcotics are usually sufficient. For anxious patients, hydroxyzine (Vistaril) in addition to the morphine provides an additional analgesic effect. Pain at the graft site on the iliac crest is also common. Movement always produces pain in the beginning, though medications for muscle spasms are not usually needed. The use of noninvasive measures such as conveying a sense of concern by talking softly to the patient, using therapeutic touch, distraction, relaxation techniques, and visual imagery are also effective in reducing the degree of pain.

Increase Mobility

Position. Following spinal surgery the patient's bed should be kept flat and have a solid bottom or a board under the mattress. The patient is usually kept on the back for the first 8 hours to keep compression on the operative site, and is tilted only briefly to assess the dressing. After the first 8 hours, the patient is usually turned every 2 to 3 hours as ordered. Some physicians restrict the patient's turn to only 20 to 30 degrees on either side. Patients should not lift the shoulders off the bed. If the patient should start to sneeze or vomit, hold the patient's shoulders to keep stress off the spine. While the patient is supine, some physicians allow the knee gatch to be raised or pillows placed under the knees to reduce stress on the back.

Turning. The patient must be turned by logrolling. In logrolling, the patient is turned by using a turning sheet. Ideally, the turning sheet should be about 78 inches long and 65 inches wide, so it will extend from the patient's shoulders to the knees. A draw sheet is usually not adequate, but a folded top sheet generally works.

Two persons are needed to move and turn a patient lying on a turning sheet. They should stand on opposite sides of the bed. If the patient is very heavy, or is unconscious, a third person is usually needed to support the head and neck or the legs. Before starting to move the patient, the patient's arms should be crossed over the chest and one or two pillows should be placed between the patient's legs. Take hold of the turning sheet at the level of the patient's buttocks and shoulders. Using an overhand grasp, both persons should roll or gather the sheet until their hands touch the patient's body, and then pull the draw sheet taut.

The person on the side of the patient that is raised calls the signals. The first step is move the patient to the signal caller's side of the bed. Grasp the turning sheet and stand facing the patient with one foot closer to the bed than the other. The person who will move the patient toward them (the signal caller) has the weight on the forward foot. The other person has the weight on the back foot.

Both movers should flex the hips and knees. The signal caller gives the count, and the movers shift their weight from one foot to the other as they move the patient to the side of the bed. To turn the patient, the signal caller grasps the turning sheet at the level of the patient's shoulders and buttocks. The other person reaches across the patient and grasps the turning sheet at the level of the patient's knees and waist. That positioning makes it possible to turn the patient's trunk, hips, and knees simultaneously, thus reducing the chances of twisting the patient's spine. The movers should flex their hips and knees, and turn at the signal callers count.

Once the turn is completed, the person on the side the patient is turned toward helps the patient maintain that position, while the signal caller places pillows for support. The pillow under the head is replaced, and two pillows may be used to support the patient's back and buttocks. Reposition the pillow or pillows between the patient's legs. A pillow can be placed in front of the patient's chest to support the patient's uppermost arm.

To turn a patient to the left side, without a turning sheet, both persons should stand on the right side of the bed. Each person has the same foot forward and that leg is braced against the bed. The movers bend at the hips and knees, and place their arms under the patient. One person places the hands and forearms all the way under the patient's upper trunk. The other person places the hands and forearms under the patient's buttocks, keeping the arms close together so the patient's buttocks will not sag and make lifting the patient difficult. The person who is lifting the buttocks calls the signals. Turning the patient is done in approximately the same manner as with a turning sheet. Follow the procedure as described above, moving the patient with your arms instead of the sheet.

Once the patient is able to help to some extent, log rolling the patient can be accomplished by one person with or without a turning sheet. Eventually the patient may feel able to turn on his or her own, but patients with Harrington rod instrumentation should not do so. Other patients may be allowed to turn themselves, but not until after proper instructions so that they will be able to keep the spine straight.

Body Jacket. Some physicians apply a body jacket cast immediately after surgery, whereas others do not apply a cast until some 10 to 14 days after surgery. A body cast is used to immobilize the spine and promote the healing of the surgical fusion. The body jacket extends from the suprasternal notch of the upper chest to the symphysis pubis in front and from the tip of the coccyx to the scapulae behind so as to prevent the smallest degree of spinal flexion. Some body jackets may include the thighs and the pelvis or even the cervical spine. After the cast is applied, repeat the assessment and nursing measures used immediately after the patient's surgery.

Exercises. Check with the patient's physician on the type of exercises allowed. Most patients do muscle setting exercises (such as quadriceps and gluteal setting exercises) and some mild active exercises to the lower extremities (such as plantar and dorsiflexion, and active range of motion of the ankles). Some institutions utilize a footboard or flexion pillow at the foot of the bed to support the patient during the exercises. Exercises for the upper extremities involve muscle setting exercises, activities of daily living (such as bathing the face and the arms, and other mild range-of-motion exercises to help maintain muscle strength).

Ambulation. Patients are not usually allowed out of bed until the body jacket cast is applied (or a second cast applied if one was put on immediately after surgery). The rationale for ambulation at that time is that loading the spine helps to lay down new bone and thus facilitates the calcification of the fusion. In the beginning, a tilt table may be used to get the patient up, because patients frequently have symptoms of orthostatic hypotension. Even though the patient may be highly motivated, it may take several days before he or she can stand upright without symptoms. Patients will need assistance in ambulating until they learn to maintain balance in the body cast.

Prevent Complications. Following a posterior spinal fusion with a Harrington rod instrumentation, the patient is a potential candidate for all of the complications of immobility (especially respiratory, integumentary, and musculoskeletal problems), and nursing measures should be instituted to prevent those difficulties (see Chap. 3). There are also potential surgical complications, however, including neurological impairment, altered gastrointestinal status, wound complications, fluid and electrolyte imbalance, and dislocation of the hooks and rod(s).

Neurological Complications. Potential neurological complications are muscle weakness, paresthesias, and dural lacerations. Neurovascular checks help in the early detection of potential problems. Subjective data presented by the patient may be complaints of "heaviness' in the legs indicating muscle weakness, or of "tingling" or "pins and needles" in the legs indicating sensory nerve impairment. Lacerations of the dura are usually detected and corrected in surgery. If the laceration was undetected, however, the patient may complain of a headache similar to that experienced after a spinal tap.

Gastrointestinal Complications. The patient will probably have decreased to absent bowel activity for at least 1 day after surgery, and then have hypoactive bowel activity on the following day. The patient should receive no oral fluids until bowel sounds are heard for several hours or until the patient expels flatus, usually on the second or third day postoperatively. Start fluids with a teaspoon of ice chips every hour. When no nausea or abdominal distention occurs, "sips" of clear liquids may be given with a syringe. This prevents the patient from swallowing air, which usually occurs when drinking through a straw. Gradually increase the amount of liquids as bowel sounds and the feeling of hunger return. The slow increase in liquid intake is absolutely necessary because patients with midthoracic or lower spine surgery are predisposed to develop a paralytic ileus. The sudden correction of the spinal curve by internal fixation may narrow the angle at which the superior mesenteric artery leaves the aorta, thereby partially or completely obstructing the blood flow to the duodenum.

Wound Complications. Two potential problems that can occur at the wound site are infection and the development of a hematoma. Each time the patient is turned, check the wound site for edema, redness, hardness, warmth, drainage, and the presence of an odor. Most patients have wound catheters inserted, but they may be obstructed, work ineffectively, or be removed too soon, and thus a hematoma may develop. A body temperature of 102 degrees that persists for a couple of days after surgery is not uncommon due to the patient's reaction to surgery, stress, and dehydration, but it should be reported and recorded.

Fluid and Electrolyte Disturbance. Because of the stress and the large amount of blood and fluid loss during surgery, fluid and electrolyte disturbances, such as sodium and water retention, potassium excretion, and a negative nitrogen balance can occur. The amount and kind of fluid replacement the patient has received, the amount of urine output and its specific gravity, and other clinical conditions determine the fluid replacement therapy.

Water intoxication can develop secondary to an inappropriate release of antidiuretic hormone (SIADH). The symptoms are usually headache, weight gain, weakness, mental confusion, lethargy, and progressive central nervous system deterioration. Urinary output diminishes and urine concentrates to a specific gravity of 1.025 or more. Treatment is usually the restriction of fluid intake to establish a negative water balance, and diuresis usually begins after 2 or 3 days.

Dislocation of Hooks and Rod(s). Dislocation of the hooks and rods is not common. Predisposing factors are twisting or stressing the spinal column when turning, ambulating, sneezing, coughing, or vomiting. The patient must understand that the back needs to be kept straight, especially once the immobilizing device is removed.

Patient Teaching. Patient teaching for a patient having a posterior spinal fusion with a Harrington rod instrumentation begins preoperatively. Review how to properly turn, how to get out of bed, how to get in and out of a chair, and how to do activities of daily living. Reinforce proper body mechanics, especially the use of the legs instead of the back.

Instruct the patient, family, and significant other on cast care. Discuss methods of doing activities of daily living with the cast on. It is essential to have therapeutic communication to determine the patient's understanding of the rehabilitation process and to reinforce any weak points. Make sure the patient knows the signs and symptoms of potential problems, such as infection, paralytic ileus, or problems with the cast that may develop after the patient returns home.

Evaluation and Reassessment

Determine that the patient is obtaining adequate relief from pain. Use indicators such as irritability, restlessness, elevated systolic blood pressure, and increased heart rate to help determine the presence of pain. If nausea or vomiting occur after those signs are exhibited, pain is usually extreme. Evaluate how well the patient does muscle setting and range-of-motion exercises. Check muscle tone and strength. The patient should not turn or be turned prone.

The patient should be free of complications from immobility or surgery. Check that the patient does not have more than 500 cc of drainage within 8 hours. Urinary output should not be less than 150 cc in 8 hours. In monitoring vital signs, the patient's blood pressure should not be below 90/50, pulse should not be above 120, and the oral temperature should not be above 102°F. The patient should be free of any signs of infection or neurological impairment. Evaluate the patient's ability to ambulate with the cast on, to demonstrate proper body mechanics, and to verbalize cast care.

Anterior Dwyer Instrumentation Procedure

The anterior Dwyer procedure (Fig. 5–17) is done for idiopathic thoracolumbar and lumbar scoliosis and lordosis, especially when there are spinal deficiencies. In surgery, the patient is placed on the table in a lateral decubitus position with the convex side of the curve in the upward position. An intercostal incision is made and a rib is removed to provide exposure of the spinal column. The rib is saved for use as a bone graft. After the spinal column is exposed, the intervertebral discs along the curve are removed. A staple and a screw are then placed laterally into each vertebral body, and bone grafts are placed into each vertebral space. A heavy wire cable is passed through the heads of the vertebral screws and tightened. The screw heads are then crimped to the cable, and the incision is closed with chest tube drainage in place. Postoperatively, the care of a patient with anterior Dwyer instrumentation focuses on immobilizing the spinal column and promoting the return of lung function.

Luque Rod Instrumentation Procedure

The Luque rod instrumentation procedure is usually reserved for patients with neuromuscular conditions who cannot tolerate the reduced respiratory capacity associated with the application of a cast. However, some physicians utilize Luque rod instrumentation for all surgical conditions of the spine. Relative to the Harrington rod instrumentation, the advantages of the Luque rod instrumentation are tempered by intraoperative factors. The procedure involves inserting a large amount of instrumentation near the spinal cord, requires a longer period under general anesthesia, increases the risk of neurological problems, and increases blood loss. Blood loss is especially great for patients with neuromuscular problems due to poor muscle tone.

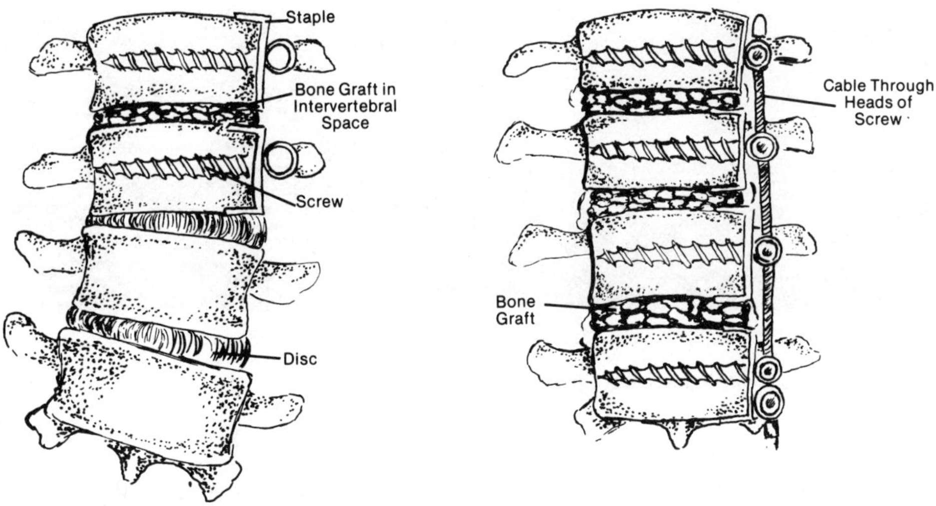

Figure 5–17. Anterior view, Dwyer instrumentation. *(From Brantley, P., & Analla, M., 1980, p. 57. Courtesy of Howmedica.)*

In surgery, the patient is intubated, transferred to a scoliosis frame, and a midline incision is made down the back, usually from the high thoracic area to the sacral area. A subperiosteal exposure of the spinous processes and posterior elements is carried out. The posterior elements in the thoracic area are exposed laterally to the facet joints, in the lumbar area to the transverse processes, and at the lumbosacral junction to the sacral alae. The facet joints are removed and packed with bone graft from the iliac crest. The spinous processes are then removed and the ligamentum flava is detached between each lamina to expose the neural canal. Loops of 16-gauge stainless steel wire are passed under and around each lamina. The L-shaped aspect of the Luque rod is then driven through the iliac wing along the superior border of the sacral alae (Fig. 5–18). The first rod is placed on the convex side of the curve. The wires are then sequentially tightened by twisting distally to proximally. The second Luque rod is then placed on the concave side, and wires tightened. Finally, the Luque rods are wired together transversely in two or three places with double wire loops. The posterior elements are decorticated, and the bone graft placed along the entire area for fusion. The wound is then closed and a compression dressing applied (Bowen, 1983).

Postoperatively, the patient with Luque instrumentation is cared for very much like a patient with Harrington rod instrumentation. Potential postoperative complications are atelectasis, retention of secretions in the lung, decreased circulatory volume, and neurovascular deficit.

The patient with Luque rod instrumentation is more active after surgery.

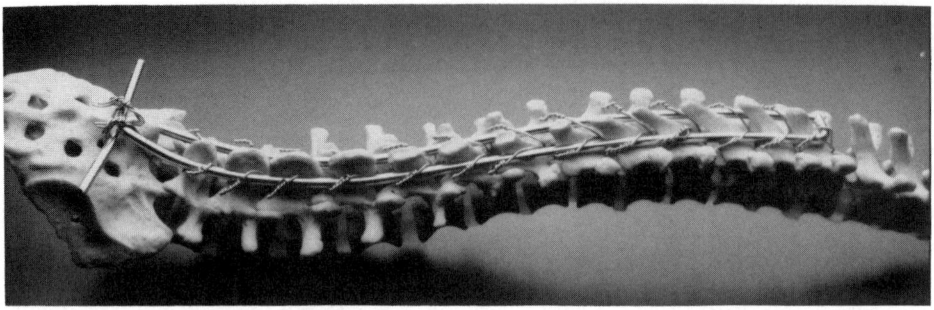

Figure 5–18. Luque instrumentation. *(Courtesy of Zimmer, Inc.)*

The physician may assist the patient to sit up in bed the evening of surgery, but most patients will not sit up until the second or third postoperative day. Some patients will not sit up until the third or fourth postoperative day, and will need to wear a corset or orthoplast jacket as a protective body splint. By the fifth to tenth postoperative day, most patients begin to return to their moderate preoperative activity levels.

LUMBAR SPINAL COLUMN

Trauma

The lumbar spine connects the upper portion of the skeleton with the lower, furnishes support for the torso, and transmits weight from the torso to the pelvis. As there are no ribs attached to the lumbar spine, it has a relatively wide range of motion.

LOW BACK PAIN

Low back pain has always been a human problem. Today, possibly because of obesity and a sedentary life-style, backache is second only to headache as the most common complaint of pain. Data from the National Center for Health Statistics indicate that in the United States chronic impairments of the back and the spine are the most common cause of activity limitations for persons under age 45. Back and spine impairment ranks third, after heart conditions and arthritis, as a cause of activity limitation for persons 45 to 64. Although numerous theories, techniques, and treatments have been advocated, low back pain remains a great dilemma for the health professions. Many patients with low back pain seem to improve regardless of what treatment is rendered, whereas a significant percentage never seem to improve (Lucas, 1983, p. 515).

Low back pain affects both men and women, and usually begins in the late twenties with the highest incidence among persons between the ages of 30 and 50. It has been estimated that up to 80 percent of the population will have at least one episode of low back pain during their adult years. Most of the time the pain spontaneously remits, with no residual disabilities or impairments. Approximately 70 percent of persons experiencing an episode of low back pain recover within a month, 90 percent recover within 3 months, and only 4 percent will have pain longer than 6 months (Cailliet, 1981, p. v).

There is often a problem in precisely locating the site of lower back pain. The patient's complaints may be vague or obscure and may even refer to the wrong organ, such as when pain in the lumbosacral area is referred to as "kidney pain," or when pain in the sacroiliac region is described as "hip pain." In some instances the pain may be extrinsic, that is, arising from a pathology in the genitourinary, gastrointestinal, reproductive, or nervous systems. In others, the cause may be intrinsic, that is, a pathology that involves the vertebrae directly or indirectly, such as a congenital anomaly, neoplasm, infection, or degenerative disease (Edmondson & Crenshaw, 1980, p. 2106).

Acute Back Pain

There are normally three types of injuries to the back. They are (1) injury to the disc or endplate of a vertebra from hyperflexion, (2) disruption or sprain of the ligaments of the posterior elements, particularly the posterior facets, following twisting, and (3) a herniated intervertebral disc. A flexion injury is about half as common as a twisting injury, and most often occurs at the L5–S1 level. A flexion injury is more likely to cause a disruption or a fracture of the endplate than an injury to the ligaments. The healing of a flexion injury is generally rapid, and the patient responds well initially to bedrest and then to gradual activity. However, a later sequela may be an invasion of the disc by fibroblasts that can lead to disc degeneration and subsequent subluxation of the posterior facet joints.

The second type of injury is caused by torsion or twisting, and accounts for approximately 70 percent of all causes of acute low back pain. Twisting injuries usually occur at the L4–5 level. Frequently, there is a ligamentous injury to the posterior facets, with a sprain of the posterior facet capsule. If severe enough, the torsion injury may actually cause a fracture of the facet joint or a tearing of the annulus of the disc. Patients with twisting injuries usually have pain on hyperextension and rotation of the spine, and are initially treated with bedrest and then placed in a back brace. A plastic, molded spinal orthosis usually works well. If a brace is not worn continuously during healing, posterior facet syndrome, i.e., instability of the facets and chronic low back pain, may develop. Patients with twisting injuries generally heal more slowly than patients with flexion injuries.

An acute herniated disc may be the result of natural degeneration with age or repeated torsional stress to the annulus. For that reason, a patient may sustain a herniated disc without any definite acute injury, although the nucleus pulposus may rupture and cause an acute injury to the disc. Initially the major complaint may be back pain, but severe leg pain develops when the nerve root becomes inflamed. Not all patients with an acute herniated disc need surgery, as most will respond to bedrest. Surgery is considered if the patient has a marked neurological deficit, such as bowel or bladder symptoms, or a marked motor weakness, such as dropped foot or severe, unrelenting leg pain. (For further information on herniated intervertebral discs, see pp. 187–202.)

When a patient has a first episode of sudden low back pain or leg pain, he or she may or may not report a precipitating factor as the cause of injury. For treatment, it is important to try to determine the mechanism of injury, that is whether the injury occurred with flexion, extension, or a twisting of the spine, and whether there is radiating pain to the legs.

Pain radiating from the back to the knee is characteristic of a disruption of a posterior facet or of an intervertebral disc without nerve root compression. Pain that radiates into the calf, ankle, or foot is more typical of a compression of a ventral nerve root, usually secondary to a herniated disc. Note whether the patient complains of discomfort with forward flexion or extension of the spine. When hyperextension and rotation causes more pain, the injury is typically a facet injury although neurological examination of the lower extremity should be performed to rule out nerve root compression and the possibility of a herniated disc. Straight leg raising is always painful in the acutely injured back, but if nerve root compression is present, the pain radiates into the calf and the foot.

Chronic Back Pain

Chronic back pain refers to pain lasting more than 3 months or repeated episodes of incapacitating back pain. Its most common cause is a chronic instability of the posterior facets together with a degeneration of the intervertebral disc. Those changes in the facet joint and disc may result from aging and the effects of normal daily activities. The instability and degeneration may be accentuated by weakness in the extrinsic stabilizing systems, i.e., the abdominal and back muscles. Weak abdominal and back muscles also increase the chance for injury to discs and facet joints. Chronic back pain may also come about through nerve root compression, due to either a long-standing herniated disc or a bony impingement. The reason certain persons experience back pain and others with similar body structures and life-styles do not still remains an unanswered question.

The patient with chronic recurrent back pain must be checked for previous injuries. Determine whether the patient is more comfortable standing, sitting, or lying and whether pain is radiating into the legs or is localized to the back. Once a diagnosis of chronic back pain is made, treatment consists of a thorough explanation of the cause of the pain and a recommendation of pain relief measures. Many patients seem to be able to function well with the back pain after the back problem has been diagnosed and the mechanism of pain explained to them. On the other hand, patients who have only been told that nothing was wrong, or that they have "arthritis," tend to have increased pain and considerable anxiety. Lucas (1983) felt that in the absence of a clear explanation, patients feel that they will soon be crippled by arthritis or that there is some serious condition that has not been detected. A diagnosis of a mechanical facet problem or disc narrowing, and an explanation of why pain occurs, will often produce a patient response of, "If that's all that is wrong, I can live with it."

To enhance the patient's understanding, reduce the pain associated with daily activities, and increase compliance with the rehabilitation program, some physicians advocate a "back school." The school program usually consists of a series of lectures by physicians, physical therapists, and psychologists, who discuss the influence of stress on daily life and its effect on pain, how to do activities with reduced pain, and how to develop and maintain an exercise program. Some patients need more than an explanation and an exercise program to reduce their pain. Other methods for possible pain relief are (1) transcutaneous electrical nerve stimulation, which works by blocking pain sensations, (2) injections of cortisone into a facet joint, which provides temporary relief, and occasionally (3) a percutaneous rhizotomy, which is a neurectomy of the posterior dorsal rami. Surgery for chronic back pain is usually a last resort, but may be indicated for patients with long-standing leg pain secondary to nerve root compression from either a herniated disc or stenosis of the spinal canal.

Herniated Intervertebral Disc

A herniated intervertebral disc is a rupture or herniation of the nucleus pulposus (the center of an intervertebral disc) into the posterior longitudinal spinal ligament or spinal canal, causing pressure on the adjacent spinal nerve root (Fig. 5–19). Ninety-five percent of herniations in the lumbar region occur at the vertebral interspaces L4–5 and L5–S1. They are seen mostly in men between the ages of 20 and 45 years.

Ordinarily the nucleus pulposus is maintained in place by a thick fibrous band called the annulus fibrosus. Stresses that suddenly or continually increase intervertebral pressure can eventually cause the posterior fibers of the annulus to give way. Examples of stressful activities include lifting, a fall on the buttocks, direct trauma to the back, twisting movements, or repeated flexion and lifting motions. Ruptures are particularly likely when the annulus has been weakened or has gone through degenerative changes. The annulus is notably softened and liable to rupture during pregnancy and labor, and after prolonged confinement to bed. Disc rupture can also occur without apparent cause, indicating that the degenerative process alone is sufficient to cause the annulus to yield to mere weight bearing (Turek, 1977, p. 1328).

An acute episode of pain from a herniated intervertebral disc usually subsides within a few days. For the typical patient, many such episodes mark the course of the condition, starting with a lesser amount of trauma, being pro-

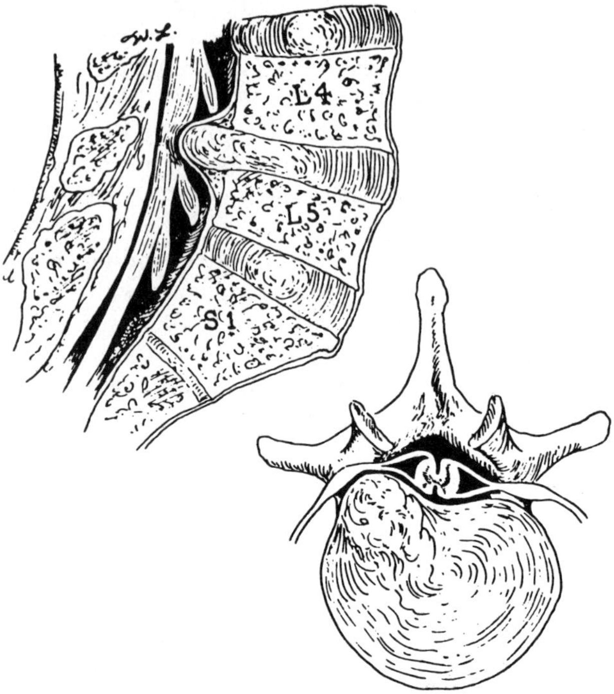

Figure 5–19. Diagram shows herniation of the nucleus pulposus. The upper drawing shows how such herniation presses upon the structures of the spinal cord. The lower drawing shows how such herniation may press upon the exit of the spinal nerve and produce pain and other symptoms. *(From Chaffee, E. E., & Lytle, I.* Basic physiology and anatomy. *Philadelphia: Lippincott, 1980, p. 130, with permission.)*

gressively more intense, lasting a longer time, and coming on after a shorter interval. Such repeated acute strains of the lumbosacral junction lead, sooner or later, to sciatic pain. Clinical manifestations of a herniated intervertebral disc are (1) sciatic pain, (2) paresthesia and numbness, (3) listing of the trunk, (4) decreased mobility, (5) tenderness in the lower back, (6) abnormal results in straight-leg raising tests (Fig. 5–20), and (7) decreased motor and sensory function in the legs. Sciatic pain may occur during the initial episode, but it usually appears gradually over subsequent episodes. The first appearance is usually as an ache in the buttocks. In later episodes, pain tends to radiate to the posterior thigh area, the popliteal area, the calf or anterolateral aspect of the leg, and even into the heel, the ankle, and the foot. The sciatic pain is generally unilateral, and is aggravated by coughing, sneezing, and straining while having a stool. A common complaint by the patient with a herniated intervertebral disc is the sensation of muscle cramping in the posterior thigh or calf. As the sciatic pain increases in intensity and extent, the back pain diminishes and occasionally may even disappear entirely.

Seventy percent of patients with herniated discs have sensations of paresthesia and numbness referred to the involved dermatome of the spinal nerve. An L5–S1 lesion causes pain and paresthesia in the sole and outer border of the foot; and L4–5 lesion causes referred sensations to the dorsum of the foot and big toe; and an L2–3 or L3–4 lesion causes referred sensations to the

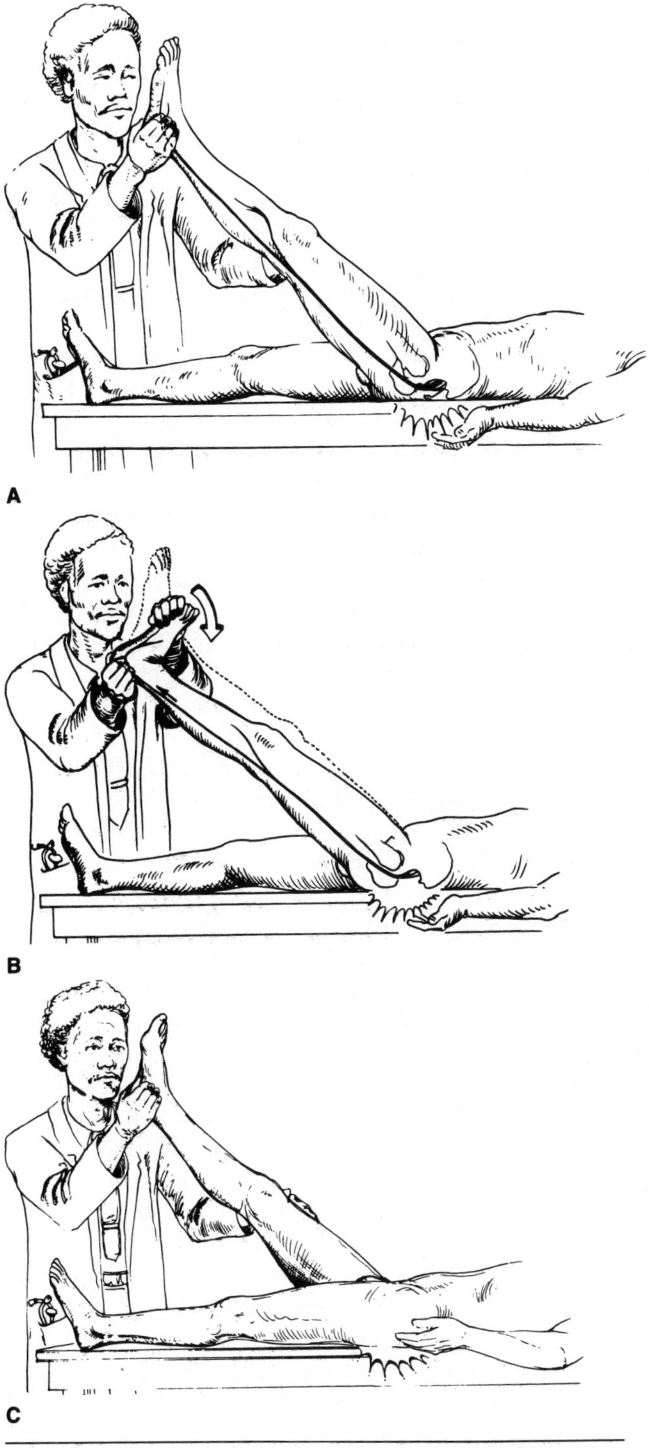

A

B

C

Figure 5–20. A. Straight leg raising. **B.** In this position, dorsiflexion of the foot reproduces sciatic pain. **C.** A positive straight-leg raising test: back pain on the involved side induced by straight leg raising the noninvolved leg.

anterior thigh, radiating to the anteromedial aspect of the leg (Turek, 1977, pp. 1328–1329).

Patients with herniated discs tend to tilt or list away from the affected side. The herniated disc is usually lateral to a nerve root, and the tilt of the spine away from the affected side may be an attempt to relieve pressure on the nerve. The list is often accentuated when bending forward. Any attempt to correct that lateral tilt often increases pain in the affected leg. Should the disc protrude medial to the nerve root, a less common occurrence, the list will be to the painful side.

Patients with herniated discs frequently have decreased mobility due to lateral tilting and forward bending. During an acute episode involving marked muscle spasms, mobility may be severely restricted.

Tenderness in the lower back around the affected area is very common. When pressure or percussion is applied over the interspace on the affected side of the spinal column, either local or sciatic pain is elicited. Sciatic pain is usually indicative of a herniated disc.

The straight-leg raising or La Segue test (see Fig. 5–20), in which the hip is flexed and the knee kept extended, is positive when pain in the sciatic area is reproduced. The well-leg raising test, which is performed by elevating the extended unaffected leg, is positive when sciatic pain is elicited in the opposite leg. It is a strong indicator of a herniated disc, often medial to the nerve root. Another test involves raising the extended affected leg to a point just short of producing pain, and then dorsiflexing the foot. If sciatic pain is elicited, that tends to confirm the presence of a herniated intervertebral disc.

Neurological evaluation of the patient is essential as 96 percent have abnormal motor signs. Those signs include atrophy of the leg muscles, which can be determined by measuring leg circumferences, and muscle weakness. Indications of muscle weakness are weakness on dorsiflexion of the large toe, an inability to walk on one's heels (which indicates fifth lumbar nerve root involvement), and an inability to walk on one's toes (which indicates calf muscle paresis and first sacral root involvement). Eighty percent of patients have sensory deficits. The third lumbar disc affects the fourth lumbar dermatome, and can cause a sensory deficit on the anteromedial aspect of the leg, the inner ankle, and the foot. The fourth lumbar disc affects the fifth lumbar dermatome, and can cause a sensory deficit on the anterolateral aspect of the leg, the medial aspect of the dorsum of the foot, the dorsum of the great toe, and occasionally the dorsum of the second toe. The fifth lumbar disc affects the first sacral dermatome, and can cause a sensory deficit on the posterolateral aspect of the lower leg, the outer foot, and the outer two or three toes. Ankle and knee reflexes are reduced when the first sacral and the fourth lumbar nerve roots, respectively, are involved.

Other diagnostic measures are roentgenograms of the spine, myelograms, epidural venograms, and CAT scans. Anteroposterior, lateral, and oblique roentgenographic views are usually taken. A newly herniated disc does not show any narrowing of the disc space, but degenerative changes in the posterior articulations, a predisposing factor, are visible. After a period of time, a herniated disc may be seen as the underlying cause if an upper vertebra settles downward and slightly backward, or if there is a marked narrowing of a disc space.

Myelogram. The diagnosis of a herniated disc can usually be confirmed and the position of the herniated disc accurately defined by injecting a radiopaque fluid into the dural space and taking roentgenograms. A defect, with rare exceptions, indicates a disc protrusion. A small disc protrusion, particularly in the spacious lower lumbar canal, however, may fail to indent the dura and thus may go undetected. In addition, the dura may not extend sufficiently caudally to allow the column of fluid to reach the level of the disc.

Epidural Venogram. A epidural venogram uses the veins of the epidura to allow the contrast medium to extend beyond the spinal canal and caudally to the L5–S1 level. The venogram demonstrates impingement upon an epidural plexus, a neural foramen, or a radicular vein.

Treatment

Ninety percent of the episodes subside with conservative treatment (Turek, 1977, p. 1333). Removal of pressure on the nerve root relieves the symptoms, allowing protruded disc tissue to be reabsorbed by the body and the defect in the annulus repaired by fibrous tissue. The healed area of the posterior annulus is thinner, more fragile, and less resistant to pressure, and fibrosis may engulf the dura and the nerve root and cause persistent low-grade symptoms. In most instances, the patient becomes less responsive to conservative treatment with each subsequent episode. Repeated dissolutions of a small portion of the disc may lead, however, to complete loss of the disc and a permanent cure.

Conservative Treatment

Conservative treatment may vary, but usually involves some combination of bedrest, traction, muscle relaxants, analgesics, local heat or cold therapy, radiant therapy, massage, topical medications, exercises, and supportive back brace or corset.

Bedrest. Bedrest is an important aspect of conservative treatment as it relieves stress on the inflamed tissue. The patient's position in bed is one in which the hips and the knees are flexed, which relaxes the sciatic nerve and reduces the lumbar lordotic curve, thereby opening the posterior disc interspaces. The period of bedrest varies with the length of the acute symptoms, which usually last from several days to a few weeks.

Bedrest does have some risks and limitations. It predisposes patients to venous stasis and can lead to progressive muscle weakness or even atrophy. Elderly patients are also prone to develop pulmonary congestion, osteoporosis, and urinary retention.

Traction. The two main types of traction used in the treatment and management of painful back disorders are pelvic traction and bilateral Buck's traction.

Hanging traction, although much less common, is utilized in some pain clinics and by some professional athletic trainers.

The rationale for traction in the treatment of painful back disorders is twofold. First, traction tends to separate vertebral bodies and to open the neuroforamina, which reduces the pressure on the protruding discs and thus helps decompress the nerve roots. Second, traction applies countertension against back muscles that are tense and in spasm. Some say there is a third reason, traction helps keep the patient in bed. Traction therapy is not always beneficial, and some patients find that traction aggravates their pain.

PELVIC TRACTION. Pelvic traction is accomplished by using a wide lumbar belt or a lumbar band that resembles an oversized garter belt. Ropes or straps on each side of the belt or band extend toward the foot of the bed and are attached to a spreader bar. From the center of the spreader bar, a rope is attached to the pulley and weights at the foot of the bed. The amount of weight utilized usually ranges from 20 to 40 pounds. With some patients, it may be necessary to raise the foot of the bed. For lighter-weight patients, the foot is elevated to prevent the patient from being pulled out of bed. For heavier patients, the elevation assists with countertraction.

BUCK'S TRACTION. Buck's leg traction is applied bilaterally with one weight per leg or one weight applied to both legs by means of a spreader bar. The weights employed commonly range from 10 to 15 pounds per leg. (For further discussion of Buck's traction, see pp. 272–273.)

HANGING TRACTION. Hanging (or gravitational) traction can be applied with the patient erect or inverted, and uses the weight of the patient's own body to provide the pulling force (Fig. 5–21). Hanging traction with the patient's head elevated can be done with either the patient lying on a tilting table (or frame) or with the patient ambulating on crutches. When a patient is on a tilting table, a chest harness or underarm straps are attached to the top of the table, which is then elevated 45 to 60 degrees, or occasionally as high as 90 degrees. Ambulatory hanging traction can be accomplished by having the patient use crutches to support the upper torso and allowing the pelvis and lower limbs to hang dependent during at least a portion of the time spent in ambulation. In inverted hanging traction, the bed it tilted 30 to 70 degrees, and the lumbar area is stretched by the weight of the patient's head and torso. The inverted method may be contraindicated in elderly patients (Wilkensen, 1983, pp. 148–151).

Heat and Cold Therapy. Heat applications provide soothing warmth and improved circulation in the skin and superficial muscles, and can be extremely effective in reducing local muscle spasm or tension. However, repetitive applications of heat may lead to a local impairment of thermal sensitivity. Some patients seem to welcome the pain associated with excessive heat because it provides a stimulating counterirritation, but cutaneous burns can easily result.

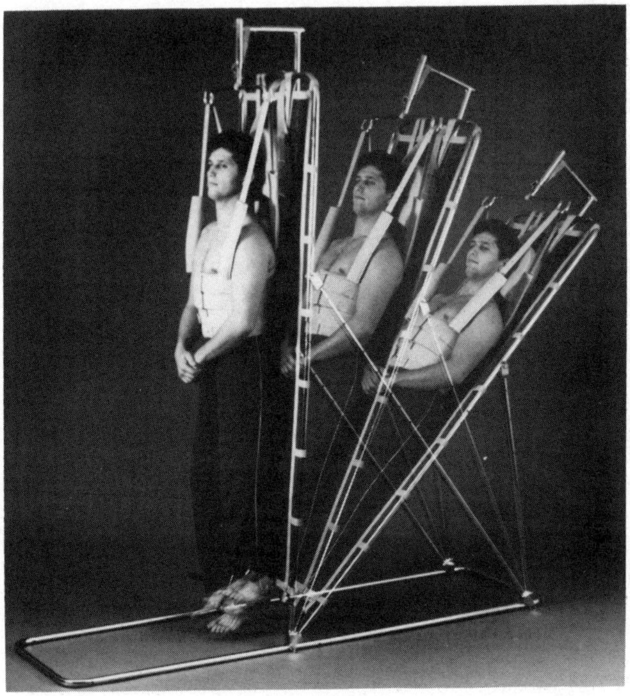

Figure 5–21. Hanging traction. The gravity lumbar reduction therapy program. *(Courtesy of Camp International, Inc.)*

Even if damaging heat levels are not reached, repetitive applications may lead to brownish skin discolorations. At home, heat can be applied to the lower back through the use of an electric heating pad set on low or medium heat. The pad will provide a continuous source of heat at a safe temperature.

Cold applications are useful for their analgesic or counterirritating effects. They are particularly beneficial in acute trauma situations or for the first 24 hours after an invasive needle procedure (e.g., myelograms, epidural venograms, or chemonucleolysis). The local, numbing cold produces hypalgesia in the skin and the tissues just below the skin. Like applications of heat, applications of cold must be made with caution to prevent thermal injury or frostbite. Cold applications can be in the form of cold compresses, crushed ice in a waterproof sack with a cloth between the ice and the patient, or sprayed-on applications of ethyl chloride. Occasionally, cold applications are followed by local massage.

Radiant Energy. Radiant energy, usually applied in the form of ultrasound or diathermy, can penetrate deeper into the body than topical heat or cold applications and heat deep as well as superficial tissues. Like topical heat applications they also produce local soothing and muscle relaxation.

Massage. Rolling, rubbing, pressing, kneading, and gently pounding tender areas helps to relax tight muscles and improve local circulation. The psychological support inherent in body contact and personalized therapeutic attention also helps bring relief. Massage is often facilitated by ointments or liquids, such as rubbing alcohol, which help protect the skin by reducing friction.

Topical Medications. Liniments may be applied independently or in conjunction with massage. Many include salicylates to provide a local analgesic effect, and other ingredients that create a sensation of warmth or heat. If care is taken to avoid skin blistering or allergic reactions, liniments may be a helpful adjunct to the treatment of painful backs and extremities.

Exercises. Exercises should be tailored to the patient's condition and should minimize painful exertion. Initially supervision is needed to insure that the exercises are performed properly, but patients must be encouraged to continue the activity program on their own. Low back exercises are designed to increase abdominal strength and endurance, stretch the low back, and develop and maintain the correct pelvic tilt. Back exercises should be done twice a day for the first 3 months, and once a day thereafter. Each exercise should be done every day, as it builds on the day before to increase strength and endurance.

Examples of low back exercises are:

1. Pelvic Tilt. Lying supine, the patient tightens the stomach muscles and then rocks the pelvis, flattening the low back, holding that position for 5 seconds.
2. Sit Up. Lying supine with the abdominal muscles tightened, the patient raises the head and the shoulders and reaches toward the knees, holding the position for 5 seconds. As the patient's muscles become stronger, they may fold the arms across the chest, and even advance to putting the hands behind the head.
3. Knee Chest. Lying supine with the abdominal muscles tightened, the patient raises the head and the shoulders and brings one knee up toward the nose, holding the position for 5 seconds.
4. Double Knee. The same as (3), except that the patient brings both knees up at the same time.
5. Straight Leg Raises. The patient lies supine with one knee bent and held to the chest with the hands. The patient then lifts the other leg, keeping the knee straight and ankle flexed.

The number of repetitions of each exercise depends on the patient's condition.

Back Supports. Corsets, braces, and belts afford another means to enforce inactivity for back pain relief. The simplest type of back support is the lumbar or lumbosacral belt, a 4- to 6-inch band of elastic material that fits around the patient's waist. It does little to impede back flexion and extension but helps to remind the patient to limit the back activities and provides some comforting pressure or counterirritation.

Corsets and girdles provide more back support than belts. Corsets are available in a variety of lengths, with or without plastic or steel stays. Corsets restrict a moderate amount of back motion in addition to providing comforting and reassuring pressure. The stays add additional support. The steel back braces provide the greatest stability. The shorter stay braces, such as chair back or Norton-Brown braces, permit upper trunk mobility. Full length bracing devices, such as the Taylor brace or a molded fiberglass or plaster bivalved body jacket, provide the most complete conservative immobilization for an ambulatory patient.

Back supports can be useful during acute episodes of back pain. The type of back support selected must be tailored to the patient's condition. Back supports, like enforced bedrest, however, have limitations in that they may aggravate arthritic stiffness and lead to progressive muscle weakness.

□ NURSING PROCESS (Table 5–5)

Assessment

The initial assessment of the typical patient with a herniated disc being treated by pelvic traction emphasizes the correct positioning and pull of the traction. Determine that the pull of the pelvic traction is correct (equal on both sides if the belt has two straps or in the center of the back if there is one strap). Check that the weights are of correct poundage, and that they hang free. Observe the patient's body for correct alignment, and check that the patient is in Williams' or contour position. Note any increased pain or discomfort, any tightness of the pelvic belt over the pelvis or bladder area, and any pain or discomfort over any bony prominences.

Nursing Diagnosis and Goal Formulation

Nursing diagnoses for a typical patient with a herniated disc being treated by pelvic traction are (1) alterations in comfort related to pain from soft tissue trauma in the low back, (2) alterations in mobility related to lack of muscle and disc integrity in the low back, (3) potential complications related to decreased activity and traction, and (4) alterations in psychological well-being related to anxiety and knowledge deficit about the injury and future rehabilitation.

Short-term goals are to have the patient experience (1) a decrease in the amount of pain through nursing measures, traction, and prescribed medications, (2) an increase in mobility through the use of traction and controlled exercises, (3) an absence of complications from bedrest and traction, and (4) a decrease in anxiety through increased knowledge. Long-term goals are to have the patient free of pain and to have return of full function without assistive devices.

TABLE 5–5. NURSING PROCESS FOR HERNIATED LUMBAR DISC TREATED WITH PELVIC TRACTION

Assessment	Nursing Diagnosis	Goal Formulation	Planning and Intervention	Evaluation and Reassessment
1. Assess the location, duration, and severity of pain. Observe for verbal and nonverbal cues of pain. Check for correct alignment and positioning. Check for tightness of traction belt.	1. Alteration in comfort: pain in the back related to soft tissue trauma.	1. Short-term goal: a decrease in low back pain through traction and positioning. Long-term goal: free of any pain.	1. Alleviate Pain Maintain pelvic traction. Keep patient in contour or Williams' position. Teach relaxation techniques. Utilize noninvasive nursing measures to reduce pain. Administer analgesics and muscle relaxants as indicated.	1. Staying in contour position should help relieve sciatic nerve pain. Traction and muscle relaxants should help relieve muscle spasms.
2. Assess patient for correct positioning. Assess for correct application of traction. Check for correct poundage. Assess patient's ability to do exercises. Assess patient's willingness to follow directions concerning positioning and exercises. Assess patient's ability to ambulate safely.	2. Impaired physical mobility: a decrease in spinal flexibility related to soft tissue trauma and muscle spasms.	2. Short-term goal: an increase in mobility through traction and controlled exercises. Long-term goal: regain full back motion.	2. Increase Mobility *Position* Keep patient supine. Keep patient in contour or Williams' position at all times. *Pelvic Traction* Maintain traction at all times. Keep the traction belt over pelvis (no higher than umbilicus) and directly on patient's skin. Apply correct amount of poundage.	2. The patient should be able to maintain correct positioning and traction at all times.

			Turning Allow patient to log roll to either side (with bed flat) to use bed pan. Do not allow patient to lie on the side with traction in place. Do not allow patient to lie prone.	The patient should be able to follow the back exercise program without supervision.
			Exercises Teach how to do back exercises. Instruct patient not to use trapeze.	
			Ambulation Remove traction belt before getting patient up. Assist with ambulation.	The patient should be able to ambulate with minimal assistance.
3. Assess for correct position of traction belt. Check the tightness of traction belt. Check for correct amount of poundage. Assess for any signs of redness or pressure over bony prominences.	3. Potential alteration in skin integrity: skin breakdown related to pressure and friction.	3. Short- and long-term goals: free of any break in skin integrity.	3. Prevent Complications *Integumentary* Do alcohol rubs and massage bony prominences. Apply traction tight enough to prevent rubbing. Apply padding around bony prominences. Apply traction to skin (make sure traction is the correct size).	3. The patient should remain free of any signs of skin breakdown.
Assess patient's ability to do exercises. Assess the patient's muscle tone and strength. Assess patient's understanding of the purposes of the exercises.	Potential impairment in physical mobility related to loss of muscle tone and strength.	Short- and long-term goals: free of any musculoskeletal complications.	*Musculoskeletal* Demonstrate back exercises. Encourage exercising even while in traction. Encourage active range of motion to all uninvolved joints. Discuss rationale for exercises. Encourage participation in activities of daily living.	The patient should maintain good muscle tone and strength.

(continued)

TABLE 5–5. *(Continued)*

Assessment	Nursing Diagnosis	Goal Formulation	Planning and Intervention	Evaluation and Reassessment
			Potential Complications Due to Immobility (Chap. 3)	The patient should not develop complications due to immobility.
4. Assess patient's level of understanding about the rehabilitation process. Assess anxiety level. Assess understanding of the role of exercise in rehabilitation process.	4. Potential knowledge deficit related to rehabilitation process and exercise program.	4. Short- and long-term goals: a decrease in anxiety through increased knowledge.	4. Patient Teaching Discuss the rehabilitation process. Discuss the mechanism of injury and how to prevent further injury. Discuss goals and purposes of the exercise program. Encourage patient to take a hot shower before doing exercises at home. Demonstrate proper body mechanics. Discuss ways of relieving stress on the back when standing, sitting, or lying. Discuss ways to reduce stress on the back during intercourse.	4. The patient should be able to verbalize an understanding of the rehabilitation process and the need to continue the exercise program. The patient should be able to demonstrate correct body mechanics.

Planning and Intervention

Alleviate Pain. The patient with low back pain should gain relief from muscle spasms with correct positioning and the application of traction. The correct position in bed helps relax the sciatic nerve and relieve sciatic nerve pain. Analgesics and muscle relaxants are also administered to relieve discomfort.

Tightness of the traction over the pelvis and the bladder may make the patient feel the need to void when he or she only has a small amount of urine in the bladder. This can be corrected by adjusting the tightness of the pelvic belt. The belt need only be tight enough to keep it from moving or slipping, which can cause skin irritation and reduce the traction pull.

Increase Mobility

Position. The correct position for a patient in pelvis skin traction is supine with the bed in contour or Williams' position. The patient needs to stay in that position at all times, including while asleep.

Pelvic Traction. Pelvic traction is used primarily in conservative management of low back pain to reduce muscle spasms and to immobilize the patient. It is applied to the lower back by means of a pelvic belt. Pelvic belts are adjustable and may come in several sizes or one universal size, depending on the manufacturer. They may have one strap down the center of the back or two straps, one down the lateral side of each leg.

Before applying traction, explain to the patient the purpose of the traction, what you are going to do, and the patient's role in maintaining the effectiveness of the treatment. If the pelvic belt comes in more than one size, measure the patient's hips at the pelvis to obtain the correct size. It is necessary to measure because most patients do not know the size of their pelvis. To apply the traction, have the patient lie flat in bed in correct alignment. Help the patient log roll to one side (see pp. 178–179). With the patient facing away, fold the pelvic belt in half and place the division line of the belt along the patient's spinal column. Holding the belt in place, fan fold the lower portion of the belt and tuck it under the patient's lower hip, as is done when changing the bottom sheet of an occupied bed. This method helps assure that when the patient log rolls back the traction will be symmetrical about the spinal column. Secure the pelvic belt across the patient's lower abdomen, making sure it is on the pelvis and that it does not go above the iliac crest or umbilicus. Do not pull the pelvic belt so tight that it interferes with comfort. With the patient remaining supine, put the bed in contour or Williams' position (i.e., 15 to 20 degrees of elevation of the knees or foot of the bed, and 30 to 45 degrees of elevation of the head of the bed). This position tilts the patient's pelvis, reduces the lordotic curve, and allows the pull to be applied to a straight lumbar spinal column. The straps from the belt should be attached to the spreader bar, and a rope from the center of the spreader bar should be threaded through the pulley and tied to the weight carrier. Apply manual traction to the spreader bar to check the pull before applying the weights. Connect the traction equipment to the spreader bar, apply the correct amount of weight to the carrier (probably 15 to 40 pounds), release the traction smoothly.

Turning. The patient in pelvic traction is not allowed to turn or to lie on the side or abdomen. However, if the patient needs to use the fracture pan, the bed may be flattened and the patient log rolled to the side.

Exercises. The patient is encouraged to do back exercises while in traction (see p. 194).

Ambulation. If the patient is allowed bathroom privileges, remove the weights and then the pelvic belt. Stay with the patient while he or she walks to the bathroom, as some patients may become dizzy, especially if they are receiving pain medications or muscle relaxants. The pelvic belt should be removed so that the patient does not trip or fall, and the patient should not reapply their own traction as that will apply stress to the injured back.

Prevent Complications. The most frequent complications are skin breakdown over bony prominences and muscle weakness. Other potential complications are related to bedrest, e.g., orthostatic hypotension, venous stasis, constipation, depression, and respiratory complications.

The pelvic skin traction should be applied directly to the skin to be most effective. Some patients object because they feel exposed, because the top linen cannot come over the traction apparatus. However, the linen can be brought up between the two traction straps and then carefully spread over the patient. If the patient still insists on clothing, women may be allowed to wear cotton panties and men cotton shorts. Gowns and pajamas of silk, rayon, or blended fabrics should not be worn as they allow the traction to slide and thus reduce the amount of pull.

Sometimes a patient will develop pressure areas over the iliac crests or coccyx. Special padding helps relieve the pressure. To prevent skin breakdown, alcohol rub can be used to toughen the skin.

Muscle weakness and even atrophy can develop if the patient does not follow the prescribed exercise program. The importance of the exercises should be emphasized, and they should be continued after the traction is no longer needed.

Patient Teaching. Patient teaching is an important, sometimes the most important, part of the treatment for the patient with low back pain. Patient education needs to focus on the mechanisms of injury, methods to prevent further injury, and how those methods work. (For a discussion of the mechanism of injury and methods of treatment, see pp. 187–190.)

Exercise and good body mechanics are the keys to preventing further injury. Teach the patient the goals and the purposes of the exercise program. Make sure the patient does the complete program correctly, and help the patient work out a routine he or she can use at home. A warm or hot shower before exercising may help relax the back muscles and make exercising easier and more effective.

Instruct the patient on proper body mechanics. The patient must learn to keep the back straight and use the leg muscles, not the back muscles, when picking up something from the floor or lifting a heavy object. When standing for any period of time (e.g., at the sink doing dishes), he or she should use a small stool or other means to elevate one foot to take the stress off the back. The best and easiest position for sleeping is to lie on one side with knees and hips slightly flexed. Persons with back pain should not sleep prone. If the patient sleeps supine, the knees need to be elevated. Some patients place a couple of pillows under the knees, whereas others use a box that has been padded and covered. The box should be of sufficient size so the patient can flex the hips and knees and have the lower portion of the legs horizontal on top of the padded box.

While sitting, the patient must keep the knees higher than the hips, even when driving a car. If necessary the patient should pull the car seat forward to raise and flex the knees.

For some patients sexual intercourse increases back discomfort. In particular the standard "missionary" position, with its basic to-and-fro pelvic thrusts, may aggravate a compromised spine. Coitus is generally not advisable for persons requiring substantial pain medications or who cannot walk without considerable pain. For others, a change of position may be enough to reduce or prevent pain and enable the patient to obtain sexual satisfaction. Patients should avoid lying prone, lying supine with hips extended, or bending forward with the knees straight.

For the man or woman in more acute stages of low back pain, the "side lie position" is likely to minimize discomfort. In the side lie position, the sexual partners lie on their sides with their hips and knees flexed and with the man facing the woman's back. In that position each person only supports their own body weight, not that of their partner, and the psoas muscle is not stressed. If the woman has chronic back pain, two possible positions are (1) the woman supine with hips flexed, upper torso supported by pillows, and thighs supported by the man's thighs and arms, as he is on his knees facing her and (2) the man supine and the woman astride. The latter position is also appropriate when the man has low back pain, though in that case the man's upper torso should be slightly raised on pillows. A number of other coital positions, as well as noncoital activities, can be explored if care is taken to avoid stressful positions (White, 1983, Ch. 8). As many patients are reluctant to ask questions about sexual matters, nurses should not hesitate to volunteer information on the subject.

Evaluation and Reassessment

Evaluate the effectiveness of medications, positioning, and traction in relieving pain. Evaluate how well the patient tolerates the traction and cooperates in maintaining it. Observe the patient exercising, evaluate the patient's compliance with the exercise program, and note whether the patient utilizes proper body mechanics. Ask the patient how he or she will incorporate the exercise program into daily activities.

Surgical Treatment

Laminectomy

When symptoms are persistent and intolerable, the disc is removed by a laminectomy. A surgical incision is made down the midline of the back over the affected disc (Fig. 5–22). The lamina over the involved nerve root and the underlying ligamentum flavum are excised. The nerve root is gently retracted, and the herniated nucleus pulposus is removed. The incision is then closed with wound catheters in place.

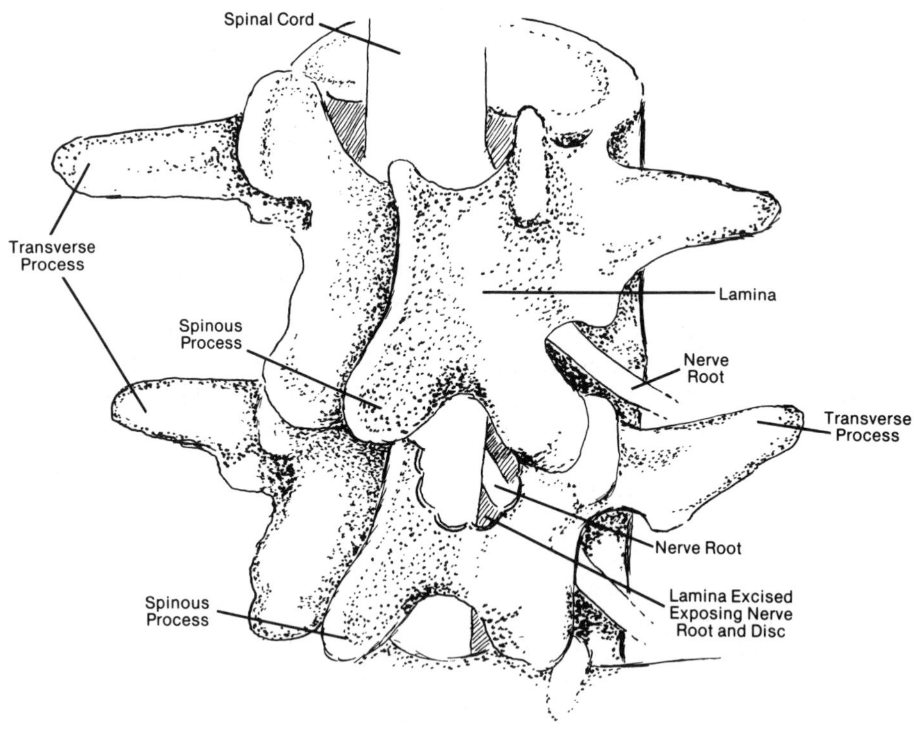

Figure 5–22. Lumbar laminectomy, posterior oblique view. *(From Brantley, P., & Analla, M., 1980, p. 54. Courtesy of Howmedica.)*

☐ NURSING PROCESS (Table 5–6)

Assessment

The initial nursing assessment of a typical patient following a posterior lumbar laminectomy should include a general assessment of the patient and emphasize the neurovascular status of both lower extremities (Chap. 2). Assess the neurovascular status every 15 minutes for the first 2 hours after surgery, and then every 30 minutes for 2 hours, every 2 hours for 18 hours, and subsequently at the beginning of every shift. Check that the hemovac is working properly and determine the amount of drainage in the hemovac. The patient's bed should be flat and the patient should be in correct body alignment. Assess for the severity, location, and duration of pain. Determine if the patient has any signs of nausea.

Continuing assessment should include exploring the patient's understanding of postoperative care. Check for bowel sounds and monitor the patient's intake and output. Continue to assess for pain, the patient's anxiety level, and signs of depression.

Nursing Diagnosis and Goal Formulation

Nursing diagnoses for a typical patient following a laminectomy are (1) alterations in comfort, pain and muscle spasms in the lumbar area and legs related to trauma and surgery, (2) alterations in mobility related to spinal instability, (3) potential complications related to the surgical procedure and trauma, and (4) alterations in psychological well-being related to anxiety and knowledge deficit about the surgical procedure and rehabilitation process.

Short-term goals are to have the patient experience (1) a decrease in the amount of pain through nursing measures and prescribed medications, (2) an increase in mobility through controlled ambulation and correct body mechanics, (3) an absence of complications from surgery and decreased activity, and (4) a decrease in anxiety through increased knowledge. Long-term goals are to have the patient free of pain with full return of function.

Planning and Intervention

Alleviate Pain. The amount of pain following a laminectomy varies with each patient. Intramuscular narcotic medications are usually needed to relieve pain during the first 48 to 72 hours. After that period, oral medications are usually sufficient to relieve discomfort. For some patients, however, additional medication for pain and the relaxation of muscle spasms is needed, as they experience those difficulties throughout their postoperative period in the hospital. Noninvasive measures, such as conveying a sense of concern by talking softly to the patient, using therapeutic touch, distraction, relaxation techniques, and visual imagery, are also effective in reducing the degree of pain.

TABLE 5–6. NURSING PROCESS FOR HERNIATED LUMBAR DISC TREATED BY LAMINECTOMY

Assessment	Nursing Diagnosis	Goal Formulation	Planning and Intervention	Evaluation and Reassessment
1. Assess the location, duration, and severity of pain. Observe for verbal and nonverbal cues of pain. Assess the neurovascular status of both legs. Check for correct body alignment. Check vital signs.	1. Alteration in comfort: pain in the back related to bone and soft tissue trauma.	1. Short-term goal: a decrease in pain through positioning and medications Long-term goal: free of any pain.	1. Alleviate Pain Place patient in correct body alignment. Utilize noninvasive nursing measures for pain relief. Teach relaxation techniques. Administer prescribed pain medications as indicated.	1. After 48–72 hours most patients should only require oral medications for pain. Muscle relaxants should relieve muscle spasms.
2. Assess for spinal column alignment when the patient is turned. Assess neurovascular status of both legs. Check for correct body alignment. Assess patient's ability to do exercises. Assess patient's willingness to follow restrictions on activity. Assess muscle tone and strength.	2. Impaired physical mobility: a decrease in spinal flexibility related to surgical procedure.	2. Short-term goal: an increase in mobility through immobilization and controlled exercises. Long-term goal: regain spinal flexibility.	2. Increase Mobility *Position* Utilize an extra firm mattress or place a bedboard under the patient's mattress. Keep the patient's bed flat. (Some patients have the head of the bed elevated if their hips are at the flex of the bed, or their knee gatch raised, or pillows placed under their knees when supine.) *Turning* Log roll every 2–4 hours. Avoid turning the patient prone. *Exercises* Teach muscle setting exercises (quadriceps and gluteal setting). Teach mild active exercises to the lower extremities (plantar and dorsi-	2. Flexion of the knees should help reduce stress on the patient's back. Turning should be done without twisting or stressing the spinal column. The patient should be able to do the exercises without applying stress to the back.

			flexion and active range of motion of the ankles). Encourage active range of motion of the upper extremities. Encourage patient to help with activities of daily living.	
			Ambulation Assist with ambulation.	The patient should be able to ambulate with only minimal assistance after the first couple of times.
3. Assess the neurovascular status of both legs. Listen for complaints of "heaviness," "tingling," "pins and needles," or "numbness" in the legs. Assess for any complaints of headache.	3. Potential for injury: neurovascular deficit related to surgery and soft tissue swelling.	3. Short- and long-term goals: free of any injury related to neurovascular deficit.	3. Prevent Complications *Neurological* Do neurovascular checks to both lower extremities every 15 minutes for the first 2 hours after surgery, every 30 minutes for the next 2 hours, every hour for the next 2 hours, every 2 hours for the next 18 hours, and then at the beginning of every shift. Notify the physician of any abnormal response.	3. The patient should not develop any neurovascular deficiency (e.g., muscle weakness or paresthesia).
Check wound catheter suction. Assess incision line for any signs of infection. Check incision line for approximation. Check vital signs.	Potential for injury: hematoma related to surgical procedure. Potential for injury: infection related to surgical procedure.	Short- and long-term goals: free of any integumentary complications.	*Integumentary* Maintain wound catheter suction. Keep dressing clean and dry. Encourage a well-balanced diet with plenty of fluids. Administer antibiotics as prescribed.	The patient should not have any signs of infection or hematoma.

(continued)

TABLE 5–6. *(Continued)*

Assessment	Nursing Diagnosis	Goal Formulation	Planning and Intervention	Evaluation and Reassessment
Assess for bowel sounds. Check for expulsion of flatus. Check for any abdominal distention. Measure abdominal girth. Check for nausea and vomiting. Assess for pain.	Potential alteration in bowel elimination: ineffective bowel function related to immobility and surgical procedure.	Short- and long-term goals: return of a functioning bowel without complications.	*Gastrointestinal* Restrict oral fluids until bowel sounds are heard for several hours. Slowly increase oral fluid intake and food as bowel sounds return. Apply heating pad to abdomen. Utilize rectal tube.	The patient should have good bowel sounds and be expelling flatus.
4. Assess the patient's level of understanding about the rehabilitation process and home care. Assess patient's level of anxiety.	4. Potential knowledge deficit related to immobilization and the rehabilitation process.	4. Short- and long-term goals: a decrease in anxiety through increased knowledge.	4. Patient Teaching Discuss the surgical procedure and the various steps in the rehabilitation process. Review how to turn, get in and out of bed, get in and out of a chair, and do activities of daily living. Reinforce proper body mechanics. Review signs and symptoms of potential complications.	4. The patient, family, and significant other should feel confident about home care. The patient should verbalize an understanding of the rehabilitation process and the importance of own role. The patient should be able to demonstrate proper body mechanics.

Increase Mobility

Position. Following a laminectomy the patient needs to be kept in correct body alignment to maintain a straight spinal column. The patient's bed needs to have a firm mattress or a bedboard under the mattress. Immediately after surgery the patient may be kept supine for a number of hours before being allowed to turn. Many physicians require that the patient's bed remain flat at all times. However, some will allow the head of the bed to be elevated a few degrees if the patient's hips are positioned at the flex of the bed, so that when the head of the bed is elevated the patient's spinal column remains straight and in good alignment. Other physicians allow only the knee gatch to be raised or pillows to be placed under the patient's knees to reduce stress on the back. The nurse should remind the patient not to keep the pillows under the knees at all times as that promotes venous stasis in the lower extremities.

Turning. Once the patient is allowed to turn, he or she is turned on a regular schedule. The patient should be turned by log rolling (see pp. 178–179) to prevent twisting the body. The patient may be log rolled with or without the use of a turning sheet, but whatever method is used, perfect alignment of the body should be maintained at all times. Gradually, patients become able to move and turn themselves.

Exercises. Check with the patient's physician regarding the type of exercises allowed. Most patients do muscle setting exercises (such as quadriceps and gluteal setting exercises) and some mild active exercises of the lower extremities (such as plantar and dorsiflexion, and active range of motion of the ankles). Some institutions utilize a footboard or flexion pillow at the foot of the bed to support the patient during the exercises. Exercises for the upper extremities involve muscle setting exercises, activities of daily living (such as bathing the face and arms), and other mild range of motion exercises to help maintain muscle strength.

Ambulation. Some physicians allow the patient to dangle on the side of the bed as early as the evening after a morning surgery. To dangle the patient, explain the procedure to the patient, administer pain medication, and let enough time elapse for the medication to take effect. Then log roll the patient onto one side, as close to the edge of the bed as safety permits. Have the patient flex their hips and knees, and make sure the pillow is still between the patient's legs. Raising the patient requires coordinated movement. The patient pushes up with one hand, as one nurse supports the patient's shoulders and the other nurse brings the patient's legs over the edge of the bed. In this way, the patient is brought to a sitting position on the side of the bed without twisting the body. If the patient's bed has upper and lower side rails, the upper rail can be left up so the patient can use it to help push up. Once the patient is sitting on the side of the bed, support the patient's back and shoulders to prevent slumping. Have the patient take deep breathes and move the feet up and down to exercise the ankles and increase circulation. To put the patient back to bed, reverse the procedure.

Within 24 hours, the patient is allowed out of bed and encouraged to walk. Get the patient up by using the above technique. Once the patient is sitting on the side of the bed, wait a few moments before helping the patient stand. It is usually better to have two persons assist the patient in ambulating for the first time. The patient will have discomfort when standing and will need to be encouraged to move. Walking helps to relieve the pain by making it intermittent rather than continuous, and promotes venous return from the lower extremities.

Once the patient is out of bed, he or she may be allowed to sit for a short period of time in a firm chair with good back support and arm rests. To ease the process of getting into and out of the chair, the patient should use the arm and leg muscles and keep the back straight.

Prevent Complications. Potential complications following a laminectomy are infection (see p. 181), neurological deficit (see p. 180), gastrointestinal complications (see pp. 180–181), spinal instability requiring spinal fusion (see p. 181), and residual leg and back pain.

Patient Teaching. Patient teaching for a patient with a posterior lumbar laminectomy should begin preoperatively. An important aspect of care is psychological support, including an explanation of the procedure and the expected results. Demonstrate the proper way to turn, get in and out of bed, get in and out of a chair, and do activities of daily living. Have a male patient practice voiding while lying supine or on one side. After surgery, reinforce proper body mechanics, especially the use of the legs instead of the back. Discuss positions for sleeping such as (1) sleeping in a side-lying position with knees bent, (2) not sleeping on the back unless the knees are supported by a pillow, (3) using flat pillows under the head and neck to avoid straining the neck and shoulders, and (4) never sleeping on the abdomen as that leads to lordosis and puts stress on the shoulders. The patient should be advised to rest the back when he or she feels tired, avoid riding in a car unless absolutely necessary, and make sure the knees are higher than the hips when in a sitting position.

The patient should not undertake any exercise or activity that has not been permitted by the physician. Ask the patient to write down questions or concerns at the time they occur so the patient will remember to ask about them. In particular, patients are often concerned about when they can resume sexual activities but may be reluctant to ask the physician. The nurse may need to remind the patient to do so, or ask the physician to discuss the matter with the patient.

Evaluation and Reassessment

Determine that the patient is obtaining adequate relief from pain, using the indicators discussed on p. 184. After 48 to 72 hours, most patients require only oral pain medications. The patient should be able to walk for increasingly longer periods of time without fatigue and should remain free of any complications from immobility or surgery. Through therapeutic discussions, evaluate how well the patient understands the rehabilitation process and his or her capacities and limitations. Have the patient discuss the activities of a typical day at home.

Chemonucleolysis

Chemonucleolysis is defined as the dissolution of the nucleus pulposus of the intervertebral disc by the injection of the enzyme chymopapain. Chymopapain, which is derived from the crude latex of the *Carica papaya,* is a proteolytic enzyme that changes the chemical composition of the nucleus pulposus. It breaks down the sulfhydryl bonds of the mucopolysaccharides of the nucleus pulposus without affecting the collagen of the annulus fibrosis (Dunn et al., 1976).

Chemonucleolysis offers an additional option in the treatment of a herniated nucleus pulposus. It is generally administered only to patients who have a herniated nucleus pulposus demonstrated through physical examination, history, myelography, and/or tomography and who have failed to respond to conservative treatment. Since 1964 chymopapain has been used in more than 17,000 patients in the United States and Canada. It has been widely reported as effective, with a success rate of 75 percent (Javid, 1980; Wiltse et al., 1975). In 1975, however, chymopapain was taken off the market when the results of a double-blind study on 104 patients showed no difference between the drug and a placebo. In November 1982, based on new clinical studies, chymopapain was again approved by the Food and Drug Administration.

Contraindications for the use of chymopapain include (1) rapidly progressing neurological deficit, (2) bladder and bowel dysfunction, (3) previous use of chymopapain, (4) allergy to papaya or meat tenderizers, (5) a complete block of cerebrospinal fluid circulation demonstrated on myelogram (i.e., a possible tumor), and (6) pregnancy. Chymopapain action is specific for the nucleus pulposus and thus is not useful in treating bony deformities such as spinal stenosis and spondylolisthesis.

The chemonucleolysis injection procedure is done in the operating room under fluoroscopy. The patient may receive a local or general anesthetic. A posterior–lateral approach is used to avoid damaging the nerve roots. Six-inch, 18-gauge needles are employed, and are usually centered 8 cm to the right of the midline at a 55-degree angle, using fluoroscopy to guide needle placement. The iliac crest is a general guide for L4–5 placement, with L3–4 placement approximately 1 inch cephalad from that, and L5–S1 placement angled 30 degrees caudad from the L4–5 insertion site. The L5–S1 space may be extremely difficult to inject due to the location of spinal facets and the elevation of the iliac crest.

Some physicians use a controversial procedure called a discogram to visualize the disc. In a discogram, a water soluble dye is injected into the disc space, and roentgenograms are taken to confirm needle placement and disc herniation. The dye stays in a small round form if the disc is normal and takes other forms if the disc is herniated. After 15 minutes, the abnormal disc is injected with 3000 units of chymopapain. The needle(s) are then removed and small dressing(s) applied (Pellino, 1983).

□ NURSING PROCESS (Table 5–7)

Assessment

The first step in the assessment for a typical patient following a chemonucleolysis is to check the neurovascular status of the lower extremities (Chap. 2). Assess the amount, severity, and location of the patient's pain. Assess for the presence of muscle spasms, especially in the area of the injection. Check that the patient is in a semi-Fowler's or a side-lying position with good body alignment.

Nursing Diagnosis and Goal Formulation

Nursing diagnoses for a typical patient following a chemonucleolysis are (1) alteration in comfort from pain in the lumbar spine related to soft tissue trauma, (2) alterations in mobility related to lack of muscle and disc integrity, (3) potential complications related to the procedure and decreased activities, and (4) alterations in psychological well-being related to anxiety and knowledge deficit of the procedure and rehabilitation process.

Short-term goals are to have the patient experience (1) a decrease in the amount of pain through nursing measures and prescribed medications, (2) an increase in mobility through positioning and controlled ambulation, (3) an absence of complications from bedrest, and (4) a decrease in anxiety through increased knowledge. Long-term goals are to have the patient free of pain and to have return of full function without a supportive device.

Planning and Intervention

Alleviate Pain. Patient reactions to chemonucleolysis vary widely. Some patients obtain pain relief almost immediately. Others may notice an immediate increase in pain before a gradual decrease sets in, and require days, weeks, or even months to obtain complete pain relief. Intramuscular narcotics are usually needed for the first 24 to 48 hours, after which oral medications may be used. Muscle spasms in the back area are common. Muscle relaxants are needed immediately and are continued as long as the patient experiences spasms. The use of ice massages or heating pads is helpful to relieve both pain and muscle spasms.

TABLE 5–7. NURSING PROCESS FOR HERNIATED LUMBAR DISC TREATED BY CHEMONUCLEOLYSIS

Assessment	Nursing Diagnosis	Goal Formulation	Planning and Intervention	Evaluation and Reassessment
1. Assess the location, duration, and severity of pain. Observe for verbal and nonverbal cues of pain. Assess neurovascular status in both legs.	1. Alteration in comfort: pain in the back related to soft tissue trauma.	1. Short-term goal: a decrease in the amount of low back and leg pain. Long-term goal: free of pain.	1. Alleviate Pain Utilize noninvasive nursing measures to reduce pain. Teach relaxation techniques. Do an ice massage. Apply a heating pad. Administer pain medications and muscle relaxants as indicated.	1. Forty-eight to 72 hours after injection, the patient should only need oral medications and muscle relaxants to keep pain and muscle spasms under control.
2. Check for correct body alignment. Assess the patient's ability to turn while keeping the trunk of the body straight. Assess the patient's ability to ambulate safely. Assess neurovascular status in both legs.	2. Impaired physical mobility: a decrease in spinal flexibility related to pain and muscle spasms.	2. Short-term goal: an increase in mobility in the low back. Long-term goal: regain complete back function.	2. Increase Mobility *Position* Keep patient on bedrest for the first 4–48 hours. Place patient in semi-Fowler's or a side-lying position with pillows between the legs, and with the hips and knees flexed. *Turning* Log roll to turn patient. Teach patient how to turn while maintaining correct body alignment.	2. Immediately postinjection, patients may not be able to turn by themselves.
			Exercises Instruct patient to avoid bending, lifting or doing exercises for 3 weeks. After 3 weeks, back exercises should be resumed.	Patients should verbalize an understanding of the restrictions placed on exercising.

(continued)

TABLE 5–7. *(Continued)*

Assessment	Nursing Diagnosis	Goal Formulation	Planning and Intervention	Evaluation and Reassessment
			Ambulation Assist patient in getting out of bed. Reinforce proper body mechanics. Teach patient to reduce weight on the involved side as much as possible when standing. Some patients may need a lumbosacral corset to ambulate	
3. Preinjection: ask patient about possible allergies to papaya, meat tenderizer, medications, or anesthetics. Postinjection: observe for hives, rashes and/or periorbital edema.	3. Potential for injury: allergic reaction to drugs.	3. Short- and long-term goals: free of any allergic reaction.	3. Prevent Complications Preinjection: check for patient allergies. Postinjection: observe for allergic reaction. If there is an allergic reaction, maintain a patient airway and notify the physician.	3. The patient should remain free of any signs of an allergic reaction.
4. Assess for the patient's level of understanding about the rehabilitation process and home care. Assess the patient's anxiety level.	4. Potential knowledge deficit related to the rehabilitation process and home care.	4. Short- and long-term goals: a decrease in anxiety through increased knowledge.	4. Patient Teaching Reinforce preoperative instructions about the procedure. Discuss realistic expectations from the procedure. Review the stages of the rehabilitation process. Discuss the need for rest period during the rehabilitation period. Instruct patient to resume normal activities gradually. Include patient's family and significant other in teaching plan.	4. The patient should feel confident about home care and continuing the rehabilitation at home. The patient should be able to verbalize an understanding of the appropriate activity level.

Increase Mobility

Position. Postinjection, the patient is usually kept on bedrest for 4 to 48 hours (typically 24 hours), depending on the patient's level of comfort. The most comfortable positions in bed are a semi-Fowler's or a side-lying position with pillows between the legs, and with the hips and knees flexed.

Turning. When turning, the patient must maintain correct body alignment and prevent any twisting movement of the lower back. Immediately postinjection, a patient with severe pain and muscle spasms may need to be log rolled.

Exercises. Exercises are not usually prescribed for at least 3 weeks, as bending and lifting are to be avoided. (For a discussion of back exercises, see p. 194.)

Ambulation. When the patient is allowed out of bed (usually within 24 hours) it is important to reinforce proper body mechanics. The best way for the patient to get out of bed is from a side-lying position with knees together. When standing, the patient should reduce the weight on the affected leg as much as possible. Sitting is usually an uncomfortable position, and should be limited at first to 5 to 10 minutes, with the time gradually increased to 20 to 30 minutes over the next few days. Some patients may need a lumbosacral corset for 3 to 6 weeks after they begin ambulating.

Prevent Complications. Potential complications following chemonucleolysis are allergic reactions to the chymopapain, discogram, and anesthesia; increased muscle spasms; and failure to obtain relief from pain. To prevent allergic reactions, ask the patient about allergies: (1) for chymopapain, to papaya or meat tenderizer; (2) for the discogram, to shellfish or iodine; and (3) to any medications or anesthetics taken in the past. Postinjection, observe the patient for allergic reactions, usually manifested by hives, rashes, and periorbital edema. Maintain a patent airway if the patient has difficulty breathing and immediately report any allergic reaction to the physician.

For a discussion of increased muscle spasms, see nursing measures for the alleviation of pain. Some patients do not receive any relief from chemonucleolysis, for reasons yet to be determined. Those patients may later need a laminectomy for pain relief.

Patient Teaching. Probably the most important aspect of nursing care for a patient having a chemonucleolysis is psychological support, including an explanation of the procedure and the results to be expected. Many patients expect to gain immediate pain relief, but back and leg pain may increase immediately after the procedure before decreasing over the next several weeks. During the period of recovery, patients often become discouraged with the slow pace of the recovery and need encouragement and emotional support from health care personnel and family members.

Because patients do not have a surgical incision and are usually released from the hospital within 72 hours, many do not realize that they will need a period of recovery and thus some restrictions on physical activities. Common guidelines are similar to those following a surgical incision, e.g., a laminectomy. Patients need several hours of rest a day. They are encouraged to resume normal activities gradually, beginning with walking short distances and standing or sitting for short periods. They should not return to an exercise program where there is bending, lifting, or twisting of the torso for several weeks. The patient will usually not be able to return to work for 6 weeks to 3 months, depending on the type of work and level of discomfort. Patients will usually return to full function in 6 to 12 months. Proper body mechanics should be emphasized to ensure that the patient does not apply stress to the back.

Evaluation and Reassessment

After 48 to 72 hours following a chemonucleolysis, the patient should require only oral pain medications and muscle relaxants to keep the pain and the muscle spasms under control. The patient will still need to spend several hours a day in bed, but should gradually begin resuming activities

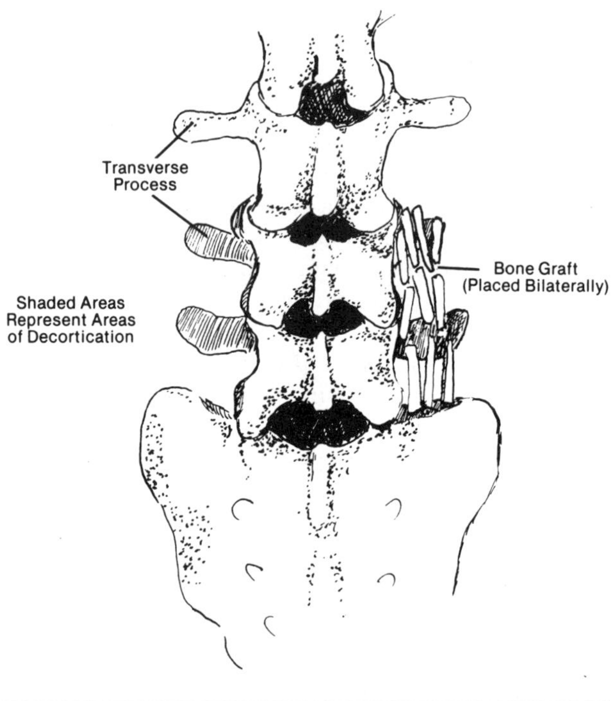

Figure 5–23. Lumbar spinal fusion, transverse process fusion. *(From Brantley, P., & Analla, M., 1980, p. 55. Courtesy of Howmedica.)*

such as sitting and walking. The patient should be able to walk short distances without assistance.

Through therapeutic discussions, evaluate how well the patient is adjusting to the rehabilitation process and how familiar the patient is with capacities and limitations. Explore the patient's understanding by encouraging discussion of how he or she will go through a typical day at home.

Spinal Fusion

Loss of a disc through a laminectomy may cause increased stresses on the posterior articulations leading to degenerative changes. These changes may produce disabling symptoms and instability requiring a spinal fusion. A spinal fusion may also be done in conjunction with a laminectomy to provide spinal stability for patients who will engage in heavy lifting.

In a lumbar spinal fusion (Fig. 5–23), the transverse process of the sacrum, and the fifth, fourth, and a portion of the third lumbar vertebrae are decorticated. The lateral portion of the pedicle and the lateral portion of the superior articular facets are also decorticated. Large amounts of cortical and cancellous bone are taken from the iliac crest and placed over the decorticated areas. The procedure may be carried out on both sides of the lumbar spine. The incision is closed with wound catheters in place.

Pathology

ARTHRITIS AND INFECTIONS

Degenerative Arthritis (Osteoarthritis)

The lumbar spine is a common site for degenerative arthritis or osteoarthritis (lumbago) in patients over age 50. In younger patients degenerative arthritis may involve the thoracic or lumbar spine, particularly as a complication of a malalignment of the vertebrae, such as from Scheuermann's disease or scoliosis (Gartland, 1979, p. 343). Degenerative arthritis may affect a number of vertebrae as part of a generalized disease process or be localized to one spinal segment as a result of trauma or repeated stress. Patients may remain pain free for long periods only to have symptoms reappear after a trauma to the back. Degenerative arthritis, discogenic degenerative disease, and spondylosis are morbidly and mechanically similar as sequelae to intervertebral disc degeneration (Cailliet, 1981, p. 176).

In general as an intervertebral disc degenerates, the elastic fibers of the annulus decrease and are replaced by fibrous tissue. A loss of elasticity ensues, and the flexibility of movement between the two adjacent vertebrae is diminished. The intradiscal pressure that normally helps keep the vertebrae apart is decreased, and the shock-absorbing capacity of the disc is diminished. The fibrous capsule and its ligaments become slack, and an anterior–posterior shearing movement can then occur. The vertebral periosteal attachment of the ligaments also weakens, and pressure that is exerted on the ligament may cause it to detach. As the pressure increases the annulus fragments, the disc ruptures, and disc material is extruded. Once begun, the degenerative process becomes a vicious cycle. The extruded material evokes an irritation reaction as a foreign body, becoming at first fibrous and then calcified. That calcified extruded tissue is the "arthritic spur" seen on roentgenography.

Characteristically, patients with osteoarthritis of the lumbar spine have stiffness and an ache in the low back area. Stiffness following periods of inactivity is common, particularly first thing in the morning or after long periods of sitting. The sensation of stiffness may be somewhat relieved by activity, but prolonged activity will bring back the pain. Discomfort is usually aggravated by cold damp weather and is frequently relieved by rest and local heat. Many patients have associated muscular and ligamentous radiation of pain into the buttocks, anterior thigh area, pelvis, and along the tensor fasciae latae to the lateral aspect of the knee. If spurs impinge on the lower spinal nerve roots in the root canals, the patient will have sciatic symptoms of lumbosacral nerve root compression syndrome. Often a trochanteric bursitis may be associated with osteoarthritis of the lumbar spine.

Effective relief of pain and stiffness requires treatment of the underlying osteoarthritis. Salicylates and anti-inflammatory drugs are beneficial, though oral steroids have had little positive effect. In addition to medication, conservative treatment includes weight reduction (if indicated), adequate rest, the use of local heat, and exercises to maintain muscle tone and joint mobility. Brace and corset use are usually contraindicated, as these patients benefit more if kept flexible. Various physical therapeutic measures such as diathermy and massage may also be helpful.

Surgery has a limited role in the treatment of osteoarthritis. However, surgical decompression of a spinal nerve root is occasionally necessary if osteoarthritis spurs impinge on it and cause sciatica.

Infection

Infection of the spine, although rare, is considered in the differential diagnosis of low back pain. Infection of the spine may affect the vertebral body, causing osteomyelitis, or it may affect the intervertebral disc.

Vertebral Body Infections

Pyogenic infection of the spine is called vertebral osteomyelitis or pyogenic spondylitis. The infecting organism, often a *Staphylococcus,* is usually bloodborne to the spine from some primary focus of infection elsewhere in the body, such as a pelvic inflammatory disease or a genitourinary tract infection. The condition rarely develops following spinal surgery or a spinal puncture. The onset is insidious and a chronic infection usually develops. Diabetics are especially susceptible. In most cases, two adjacent vertebrae and their intervening disc are involved. An abscess may be formed as the result of the infection and there may be neurological involvement (Cailliet, 1981, pp. 201–202).

The patient with an infection may initially complain of a "nonspecific" backache. The pain may or may not be associated with systemic signs of infection. The back pain is usually moderate to severe, with more severe pain at night, and is frequently associated with functional disability. All movement may be painful with marked guarding of the paravertebral and hamstring muscles. The involved vertebrae are usually exquisitely sensitive to percussion. Roentgenography usually shows evidence of bone destruction involving one or more vertebral bodies, accompanied by a narrowing or loss of intervertebral disc space (Gartland, 1979, p. 343). Diagnostic tests that may be indicative if performed early in the disease process are white blood counts, sedimentation rates, and blood cultures.

Before treatment begins the organism is usually isolated by a biopsy or needle aspiration. Antibiotic treatment is then dependent on sensitivity studies. Bedrest with or without a body cast or brace may be necessary for as long as 3 to 6 months. Fusion occurs in about 50 percent of the patients. If an abscess forms, surgery may be needed to drain it (Cailliet, 1981, p. 202).

Tuberculous infection (Pott's disease) is also a possibility. It is often secondary to tuberculosis elsewhere in the body, and is most common in the thoracolumbar junction (Gartland, 1979, p. 343). (For a more detailed discussion of the tuberculosis of the spine, see pp. 167–168.)

Intervertebral Disc Space Infection

Intervertebral disc space infection or "discitis" may occur following a discectomy and is the primary cause for the development of severe low back pain, marked rigidity, and local tenderness 2 or 8 weeks after surgery. The pain is usually "excruciating," restricting any movement and occurring at night as well as during the day. The patient's sedimentation rate is usually markedly elevated. Discitis can also occur following bacteremia secondary to urinary tract infection, with or without a catheterization or cystoscopy. Drug abusers frequently develop infectious discitis from self-administered infections with improper sterile technique (Cailliet, 1981, pp. 202–203).

With discitis there is a narrowing of the disc space and a sclerosing of the vertebral endplates. The vertebral bodies gradually undergo destruction. Biopsy or needle aspiration may be required to culture the organism for antibiotic therapy. Treatment is usually similar to that indicated for vertebral osteomyelitis.

NEOPLASMS

Benign

Benign tumors involving the vertebrae are unusual. A *hemangioma* is an uncommon benign bone tumor composed of vascular channels of varied patterns occuring in a vertebral body. It weakens the structure of the bone, leading to a pathological fracture. A hemangioma is most often seen in the skull, the vertebrae, and the long bones of patients over age 40. When seen in the spine, the hemangioma usually occurs in two or more contiguous vertebral bodies. The lesion tends to cause symptoms by applying direct pressure on the spinal cord or on spinal nerve roots. Hemangiomas are not believed to undergo malignant transformations, and radiation therapy is usually the treatment of choice (Turek, 1977, pp. 578–579).

An *aneurysmal bone cyst* is a benign, solitary lesion of bone occuring most often in the metaphysis of long bones, flat bones, and vertebrae. The growth of the lesion causes a ballooning of the overlying cortex, which tends to expand the host bone and destroy the overlying periosteum.

The bone cyst occurs most commonly during the second and third decades of life. The patient's chief complaints are usually pain and a mass on the spine. Extensive bleeding may result if the overlying cortical bone shell is broken and a pathological fracture occurs. Cysts of a vertebral body are usually treated by radiation to sclerose the blood vessels of the tumor.

Malignant

Except for plasma cell myeloma, primary malignant bone tumors of the vertebral column are quite rare. More frequently, the spine is the site of metastatic cancer from primary tumors in the breast, prostate, thyroid, kidney, and lungs. Secondary involvement of the vertebral column may also accompany leukemia, Hodgkin's disease, and malignant lymphoma.

A *chordoma* is an uncommon tumor that occurs in bone primarily at either end of the vertebral column. It develops from remnants of the embryonic notochord, such as the nucleus pulposus or abnormal "rests" of notochordal tissue, and affects most patients in the middle years of life. More than half of the tumors occur in the sacrococcygeal region. The tumor is slow growing, and is considered malignant because it is locally invasive. Treatment is usually surgical excision.

Intraspinal tumors may give rise to back and leg pain similar to that from radiculitis or a herniated lumbar disc. Approximately 1 percent of the patients operated on for herniated lumbar disc are found to have an intraspinal tumor (Gartland, 1979, p. 345).

In general, two types of intraspinal tumors may occur: extradural and intradural. Extradural tumors are usually secondary and represent metastatic carcinoma from lymphatic system tumors, such as Hodgkin's disease, lymphosarcoma, and reticulum cell sarcoma. Intradural tumors are most often primary and include meningioma, neurofibroma, glioma, medulloblastoma, and ependymoma (Gartland, 1979, p. 345).

The existence of an intraspinal tumor, rather than a herniated lumbar disc, is suspected when (1) there is a failure to respond to conservative treatment and the pain remains intractable, or there is an unusual progression of the neurological signs; (2) a neurogenic type of bladder or bowel dysfunction exists; (3) nocturnal pain awakens the patient and such pain is essentially unrelated to movement, position, or activity; (4) patient's complaints cannot be localized to a single nerve rest; or (5) there is upper motor neuron dysfunction. For example, the presence of spasticity, hyperactive reflexes, clonus, and positive Babinski signs all indicate a tumor in the central nervous system and not the lower neuron type of involvement found in herniated disc disease. The presence of a spinal cord tumor can be confirmed by lumbar puncture, cystometric test of bladder function, myelogram, or CAT scan. In some instances, however, surgical exploration is necessary.

OTHER COMMON CONDITIONS

Spondylolisthesis

In spondylolisthesis, there is a forward subluxation of the body of one vertebra on the vertebra below it. The term is derived from "spondylo" meaning vertebra and "olisthesis" meaning slipping, sliding, or falling. The body and pedicles of the affected vertebra tend to slip forward, whereas the laminae and spinous process remain in approximately the correct position (Gartland, 1979, pp. 335–338). Normally sliding is prevented by the mechanical relationship of the articular facets and the ligaments (Cailliet, 1981, p. 188).

Spondylolisthesis occurs because of the development of a defect or break in the pars interarticularis, giving rise to a bony discontinuity between the anterior and posterior halves of the neural arch. Most causes of spondylolisthesis are undetected fatigue fractures occurring in an elongated and mechanically weak portion of the pars interarticularis of the fifth lumbar vertebra. Another type seen frequently in the lumbosacral joint is due to a congenital anomaly. A third type, which is degenerative, occurs at the fourth lumbar vertebra, usually in women over 50. Degenerative spondylolisthesis is not associated with a neural arch defect, but frequently produces spinal stenosis at the level of the vertebral slipping.

Patients with spondylolisthesis usually have chronic low back pain. If there is lumbosacral nerve root involvement, the patient may have pain that radiates into the hips, the thighs, and even the feet, but usually there is only numbness or "tingling" noted in the legs. The patient typically complains of back stiffness, limited forward flexion of the lumbar spine, muscle spasm, and discomfort when lifting or bending.

The vast majority of patients with spondylolisthesis are treated conservatively. The back pain can best be controlled by the use of a back support such as a corset, brace, or cast (see pp. 179 and 194–195), combined with back strengthening exercises (p. 194), and the avoidance of bending and lifting. Spinal fusion of the involved vertebrae is indicated in patients who fail to respond to conservative methods or who are likely to experience further slippage. The fusion usually involves L4 to S1 or L5 to the sacrum. It is most commonly done using a posterior approach, but may be accomplished by an anterior interbody fusion.

Spinal Stenosis

Spinal stenosis is the narrowing of any region of the spinal canal or nerve root foramina, and usually involves pressure on spinal nerves or the vessels supplying those nerves. Spinal stenosis may be caused by a congenital anomaly such as achondroplasia, or it may develop following severe degenerative spinal changes, spondylolisthesis, spinal surgeries such as laminectomy or spinal fusion, trauma to the spine, or Paget's disease.

Pain may be caused by ischemia and compression from a blockage or restriction to the flow of cerebrospinal fluid due to the stenosis (Cailliet, 1981, 180–183). The onset of the discomfort may be tingling, weakness, or clumsiness, and the "pain" may be only minimal. As the condition progresses, pain develops in the back and buttocks, and there is often intermittent claudication, i.e., severe pain in the calf muscles during walking that subsides with rest. The leg pain is not relieved by standing. In many instances, the patient can obtain pain relief by sitting down and assuming a flexed back posture.

The first step is conservative treatment to decrease the lumbar lordosis and relieve pain (see the conservative treatment for herniated disc, pp. 191–195). Emphasis should be placed on the importance of good body mechanics and the need to reduce stress on the spinal column.

Surgical intervention is considered when the patient has (1) daily activities unacceptably restricted or intolerable pain in spite of conservative treatment, e.g., the patient has difficulty walking 50 yards or sitting for 30 minutes, or has recurrent leg cramps that interfere with sleep, (2) a progressive neurological deficit, such as a motor weakness of the quadriceps, that causes one knee to "buckle" or an ankle dorsiflexion paresis, or (3) a bladder dysfunction from a neurogenic cause. Prevention of further disabilities, lessening of pain, and improvement in daily function are the major objectives of the surgery. Complete relief from pain is not assured, nor is marked improvement in functional activities predictable following surgical decompression.

Ankylosing Spondylitis

Ankylosing spondylitis (or Marie-Strümpell arthritis or Bechterew disease) is a disease of the spinal column that occurs predominately in men in late adolescence or early adulthood. It is characterized by a slow, progressive inflammation of the spine, the sacroiliac, and the larger joints of the extremities (particularly the hips, knees, and shoulders), leading to a fibrous or bony ankylosis and deformity. The cause is unknown, and it is not clear whether it is a variant of rheumatoid arthritis or a totally different entity. The pathological joint changes are undistinguishable in the two diseases (see rheumatoid arthritis,

Chap. 4), but the majority of patients with ankylosing spondyloitis have a negative rheumatoid factor.

The condition usually starts insidiously. The first symptoms are most often vague and poorly localized. The patient complains of aching and stiffness about both sacroiliac joints, which usually occur as a morning backache. The pain subsides with activity but returns after sitting in one position for a long period of time. The patient commonly has a sciatic radiating pain, either unilateral or bilateral. Initially, the patient rarely has discomfort in the lumbothoracic or the cervicothoracic area. After 6 months to a year, the pain and the stiffness become progressively worse and slowly spread to the rest of the spine. There are severe spasms in the paraspinal muscles, with the flexors predominating and pulling the entire spine into forward flexion, so that the cervical and lumbar curves are obliterated. The thoracic curve is exaggerated, and the end result is a single kyphotic rounding of the entire back. Although the deformity is occurring in the spine, the hips, the knees, and the shoulders become painfully distended with increased synovial fluid. The muscles around the joints develop painful spasms that produce flexion adduction deformities of the hips, flexion of the knees, and adduction and internal rotation of the shoulders. At that stage, the typical "stooped-over" position is usually evident. The patient faces downward, as the entire back is rounded, the hips and the knees are semiflexed, and the arms cannot be raised more than a limited amount. Complaints include radicular pain in the upper extremities, in the intercostal and anterior abdominal areas, in the groin, and in the lower extremities.

On clinical examination in the early stages, when the sacroiliac joints are involved, tenderness can be elicited over the joints either externally or on rectal examination. As the disease progresses, there is limitation of motion, first in the lower spine and then throughout the entire spine. As the condition progresses, chest expansion is restricted by the increasing spinal kyphosis.

Treatment

At present, no treatment effectively cures or arrests the progression of ankylosing spondylitis. Treatment is directed toward relieving the pain and keeping the spine erect. The overall prognosis for pain relief and maintenance of function is generally good. Despite serious activity limitations, about 75 percent of patients manage to work full time (Gartland, 1979, p. 147).

Conservative Treatment. Conservative treatment consists of drugs, positioning, exercises, and physical therapy. Drugs used in the treatment of rheumatoid arthritis are helpful in the treatment of ankylosing spondylitis, especially cortisone which has been effective in reducing inflammation and relieving pain in the early stages. In addition, roentgen therapy may relieve pain quickly, apparently by lessening the muscle spasms. Although it has been very effective, it is not curative and only lasts for approximately 6 months (Türek, 1977, p. 1389).

Positioning means keeping the back in correct alignment. During the acute stage the patient may need to be flat in bed, possibly with the back in slight hyperextension to help the spine straighten. In some instances, cervical traction or a cervical collar may be used. Other patients may have traction to the lower extremities to overcome flexion deformities. A well-molded plaster jacket may be applied to maintain a slight lumbar lordosis and a straight thoracic spine.

Hot moist therapies (e.g., Hubbard tanks) are used to help reduce muscle spasms and permit strengthening of antagonist (extensor) muscles. Exercises are needed to keep the back as mobile as possible. The exercises, best done immediately after heat has been applied, are directed toward specific muscles, especially the back extensors, hip abductors and extensors, shoulder abductors and external rotators, and knee extensors. However, the patient also needs to do deep breathing exercises to maintain maximum vital capacity.

Surgical Treatment. Hip surgery generally precedes back surgery, with hip flexion contractures corrected by bilateral total hip replacements (see pp. 285–288). These procedures may obviate the need for further surgery.

The most common back surgery is an osteotomy of the spine introduced by Smith-Petersen in 1945. A wedge of bone is removed from the posterior portion of the spinal column, usually at the lumbar level (L2–3 or L3–4). That area is usually selected because the thoracic spine is fixed by rib attachments, the lumbar canal is wider, and that level is below the level of the cord. With the patient positioned laterally (to facilitate breathing), a midline incision is made along the spinous processes of four vertebrae, two above and two below the osteotomy site. The ossified ligamentum flavum and parts of the adjacent laminae are excised. The wedge of bone is then removed from the superior and inferior articular processes and the intervening vertebral joint, which is usually ankylosed. The point of the wedge is directed toward the front of the intervertebral foramen, and the angle of the wedge is equal to the amount of the correction. An adequate amount of bone is removed to preclude the nerve root from being compressed when the spine is hyperextended by pressure on the manubrium sterni, the symphysis pubis, and about the osteotomy site. The straightening of the spine is done slowly to avoid sudden stretching of abdominal structures. When the wedge is closed, slivers of cancellous bone are added to promote fusion. After the wound is closed, posterior and anterior plaster shells are constructed to provide support for the patient's back and chest. The patient is placed on a Stryker frame and is not allowed up for 8 to 10 weeks. A body cast or brace is worn when the patient begins ambulation.

THORAX

The thoracic cage protects the heart and the lungs. Rigidity is provided by the sternum, the ribs, and the thoracic vertebrae, whereas flexibility is supplied by the muscles of respiration. The thorax may be injured or deformed directly, or it may be involved secondarily to malformations or curvatures of the spine. The main topics of interest for adult orthopaedics are fractures of the ribs and sternum and, occasionally, tumors involving the ribs.

Trauma

FRACTURES OF THE RIBS AND STERNUM

Trauma to the chest wall may cause fractures of the sternum or of one or more ribs. The fourth, fifth, sixth, seventh, and eighth ribs are the most commonly fractured, usually by blows, crushing injuries, or strains caused by severe coughing or sneezing. Rib fractures cause pain with movement of the thoracic cage, especially during inspiration. The area is very tender to the touch, and the patient protectively guards the chest and takes very shallow breaths. If there is no displacement of the fragments, the fractures usually heal without complications if the chest is immobilized by strapping the chest with adhesive tape from the affected side to the unaffected side or by applying a circular strapping using an elastic bandage, chest binder, or rib belt. When the pain is severe and is not relieved by strapping and analgesic medications, a regional nerve block may be used for pain relief. That procedure involves infiltrating the intercostal spaces above and below the fractured rib with 1 percent procaine. If there is displacement, the bone fragments may penetrate the pleural cavity and pierce a lung or intercostal artery. When that occurs, the fracture is complicated by a pneumothorax or a hemathorax, and the respiratory problem takes priority over the repair of the fracture.

Severe trauma to the chest wall may cause multiple fractures of the ribs and the sternum, with the subsequent development of a flail chest, i.e., a condition where the chest wall no longer provides the rigid bony support necessary for normal ventilation. This causes paradoxical breathing, where the portion of the lung underlying the unstable chest wall moves opposite to the remainder of the lung. On inspiration that portion of the lung sucks in while the remaining lung expands. On expiration it balloons out as the remaining lung contracts. It can result in a vicious cycle of events leading to hypoxia. Internal stabilization of the chest is best obtained by the use of a volume-controlled ventilator attached to a cuffed tracheostomy tube.

External stabilization of a flail chest due to multiple rib fractures was common prior to the introduction of modern ventilators, and was achieved using skeletal traction. Under local anesthesia, stainless steel wires were attached to the ribs or sternum to pull the chest wall outward. The wires were then connected to a rope and pulley with about 5 pounds of weight. It usually took 14 to 21 days for the chest to be rigid enough to permit removal of the traction. In some instances towel clips were used instead of the stainless steel wire.

Pathology

NEOPLASMS

A variety of bone tumors may affect the bony thorax, particularly the ribs. In some instances the tumor may cause pain, and occasionally a pathological fracture of the rib may occur. In other instances, patients may first become aware of the tumor when they notice a lump on their rib cage. Roentgenography and histological interpretation of the tissue obtained at biopsy are usually needed to confirm the diagnosis.

The tumors may be benign, malignant, or metastatic. Benign tumors most commonly affecting the ribs are enchondroma and fibrous dysplasia. Primary malignant bone tumors affecting the ribs include chondrosarcoma, osteosarcoma, and Ewing's tumor. Involvement of the ribs with metastatic carcinoma from the breast, lung, kidney, thyroid, and prostate is relatively frequent.

PELVIS

Trauma

SACROILIAC STRAIN

Sacroiliac strain is a painful stretching of the ligaments about one or both sacroiliac joints. The condition is uncommon because the sacroiliac ligaments are very strong, and the movements of bending, lifting, or hyperextending the back, which are likely to produce a torsion strain on the sacroiliac joints, will probably first cause a strain on the smaller lumbosacral ligaments. Individuals are most prone to sacroiliac strain when the ligaments are softened and elongated by pregnancy, prolonged periods of bending and lifting, or degenerative arthritis. The injury usually occurs in the act of straightening up from a stooped position. The hip flexors may hold the ilium forward while the sacrum is rotated backward, or the hamstrings and the gluteus maximus may extend the hip, rotating the ilium backward, while the sacrum is held forward by the weight of the trunk.

Sacroiliac Subluxation

Sacroiliac subluxation implies that ligamentous stretching has been sufficient to permit the ilium to slip on the sacrum. Typically, an irregular prominence on one articulating surface becomes wedged on another prominence of the opposite articulating surface. The ligaments become taut, reflex muscle spasms are intense, and pain is severe and continuous until reduction is effected. The displacement may be so slight that it cannot be recognized in roentgenograms. The condition is differentiated from sacroiliac strain in that pain is more intense and is not relieved by sitting, recumbency, or a tight encircling bandage. The pain is often relieved dramatically and suddenly by manipulation.

PELVIC FRACTURES

Pelvic, sacral, and coccygeal fractures usually occur from vehicular accidents, crush injuries, or falls that cause trauma to the pelvis directly or indirectly through the femur. After head injuries, pelvic fractures have been reported as the most common cause of traumatic death. The life-threatening nature of pelvic fractures arises from the multiple fractures, soft tissue injuries, hemorrhages, and shock that typically accompany them. About two-thirds of pelvic fractures have one more of those complications, and a fatality rate as high as 30 percent has been reported for pelvic hemorrhage (Iversen & Clawson, 1977, p. 1983). Pelvic hemorrhages are especially serious because of the rich blood supply to the pelvis, the possibility of massive and hidden bleeding in the cancellous surfaces of the fracture fragments, and the laceration of veins and arteries (including the iliac artery) by bone spicules (fragments).

Pelvic fractures are suspected in trauma patients who manifest pain, crepitus, or tenderness over the symphysis pubis, anterior spines of the ilium, iliac crest, sacrum, or coccyx. A good roentgenogram is essential for diagnosis. Ongoing and continuing nursing assessment for injuries to the bladder, rectum, intestines, and intra-abdominal organs is vital.

All patients, except those with minimal trauma, need an indwelling urinary catheter to measure urine output relative to shock and to collect urine to examine for evidence of bladder damage. For a period after the injury, the urine of patients with minimal trauma should also be measured and examined for blood. If there is any evidence of possible urinary tract trauma, a cystometrogram, cystourethrogram, or intravenous pyelogram is done. Those tests are also helpful to delineate the size of any pelvic or retroperitoneal hematoma. Despite the difficulties involved and the possible pain to the patient, a pelvic and rectal examination is usually done to check for fresh blood, perineal sensation, and sphincter control. All stools are saved for a period of time and examined for blood. An extensive intra-abdominal or retroperitoneal hemorrhage is indicated by abdominal distention or a mass palpated during the pelvic or rectal examination. Severe back pain indicates retroperitoneal bleeding, rather than intra-abdominal bleeding. The peripheral pulses of both lower extremities are palpated, because absence of peripheral pulses may indicate a tear in the iliac artery or one of its branches. A neurological evaluation is essential as pelvic fractures are frequently associated with neurological damage. The patient should be handled as carefully as possible to minimize further bleeding and shock.

Treatment

If there is evidence of bleeding, the immediate objective is to restore the circulating volume and initiate emergency treatment for intrathoracic, intra-abdominal, and intracranial injuries. Hemorrhage is first treated by extenders to replace circulating volume, and second by reducing and immobilizing the fractures. Immediate measures for blood replacement are essential as blood losses of 2500 ml are common. The effectiveness of the treatment is best monitored by the patient's pulse, blood pressure, central venous pressure, and urine output. An external compression suit (Medical Anti-Shock Trousers or MAST) may be applied to the body below the diaphragm to help control hemorrhaging and combat shock. The suit is deflated at intervals to evaluate whether hemorrhaging has recurred and to inspect the skin. Pulmonary support, e.g., humidified oxygen, endotracheal intubation, and mechanical ventilation, such as PEEP, may be required. Bleeding from the bones and the veins may stop spontaneously if the fractures are immobilized. Surgery is usually required for ruptured abdominal or pelvic viscera, and occasionally for hemorrhage.

Most fractures of the pelvis heal rapidly because the innominate bones are mostly cancellous bone, which has a rich blood supply. Nonoperative treatment consists of immobilization through bedrest, skeletal traction with a pelvic sling, or a double hip spica cast. The type of immobilization depends on the nature and location of the fractures.

Fractures of the pelvis (Fig. 5–24) are usually treated successfully by closed methods. Even after extensive injuries, such as a separation of the symphysis pubis with fractures of the ilium or a dislocation of the sacroiliac joint, a satisfactory closed reduction can usually be obtained. Disability is usually slight even with rather gross displacement or nonunion of one or more rami of the pubis and ischium. Replacement and realignment of the pelvis by surgery (Fig. 5–25) is rarely necessary (Edmondson & Crenshaw, 1980, p. 659).

Avulsion fractures of the apophyses of the iliac crest, anterosuperior iliac spine, or ischial tuberosities are not uncommon in teenage athletes and are usually the result of vigorous activities such as running or dancing. Closed treatment usually yields excellent results without surgery. When an avulsion of the ischial apophysis heals, however, it may produce a florid callus or myositis. This excess reactive bone may be misdiagnosed as it causes local irritation and pain when the patient sits. Surgery to remove the callus is usually delayed until the fracture has fully healed (Edmondson & Crenshaw, 1980, p. 659).

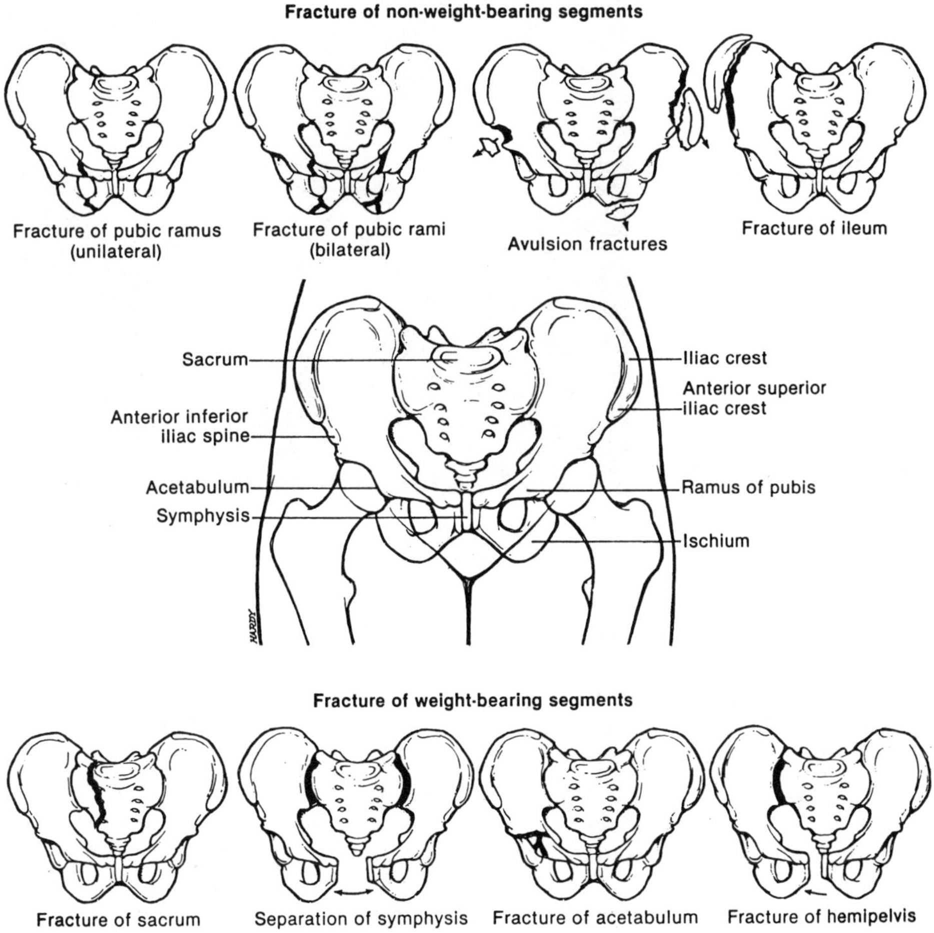

Figure 5–24. Pelvic fractures. *(From Brunner, L. S., & Suddarth, D. S.* Textbook of medical-surgical nursing *(5th ed.). Philadelphia: Lippincott, 1984, p. 1443, with permission.)*

Fractures of the sacrum and pelvis without disruption of the pelvic ring, and fractures not involving the weight-bearing portion of the pelvis, are treated symptomatically. The patient should be turned by log rolling or treated on a turning frame until the severe pain subsides. As soon as the patient can move comfortably in bed, he or she may begin to ambulate with a walker or crutches. Well-stabilized fractures through cancellous bone usually present signs of healing within 3 to 6 weeks, with excellent healing expected within 2 months. However, because of the dense plexus of nerves about the sacrum and the coccyx, injuries to that area may lead to chronic pain, especially if the patient is not encouraged to accept some pain and start an early active exercise program.

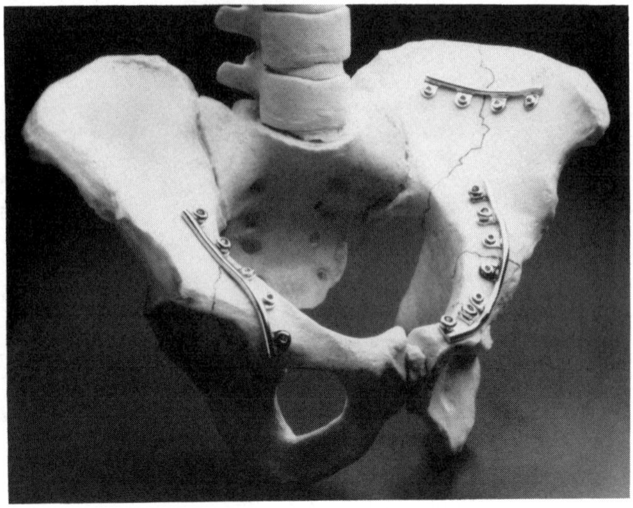

Figure 5–25. Zimmer pelvic plates. *(Courtesy of Zimmer, Inc.)*

Fractures that disrupt the pelvic ring and those that involve weight-bearing areas are especially likely to damage visceral organs and major nerves and blood vessels. After the patient's condition has stabilized, those fractures are usually reduced with skeletal traction, but manipulative reduction under general anesthesia and the application of a double hip spica cast may be necessary. A pelvic sling may be used, but is not usually the treatment of choice because it has a high rate of complications and is uncomfortable. A spica cast, skeletal traction, or an external fixation device is usually recommended instead because each provides much greater comfort, better control of the fracture, and easier administration of nursing care. Immobilization must be maintained for 6 weeks, after which active exercises in bed may be instituted. Patients are not allowed to bear weight for at least 12 weeks.

REFERENCES

Bowen, M. R. Operative technique: Posterior spinal fusion with Luque instrumentation. *Orthopaedic Nursing,* 1983, *2* (3), 16.

Cailliet, R. *Scoliosis, diagnosis and management.* Philadelphia: F. A. Davis, 1981.

Cailliet, R. *Low back pain syndrome* (3rd ed.). Philadelphia: F. A. Davis, 1981.

Cailliet, R. *Neck and arm pain* (2nd ed.). Philadelphia: F. A. Davis, 1981.

Dunn, J. E., Johnson, C. L., & Cox, W. Treatment of lumbar disks with chymopapain. *Physical Therapy,* 1976, *56* (4), 399–402.

Edmondson, A. S., & Crenshaw, A. H. (Eds.). *Campbell's operative orthopaedics* (6th ed.). St. Louis: C. V Mosby, 1980.

Gartland, J. J. *Fundamentals of orthopaedics* (3rd ed.). Philadelphia: W. B. Saunders, 1979.

Hoppenfeld, S. *Physical examination of spine and extremities.* New York: Appleton-Century-Crofts, 1976.

Iversen, L. D., & Clawson, D. K. *Manual of acute orthopaedic therapeutics.* Boston: Little, Brown, 1977.

Javid, M. J. Treatment of herniated lumbar disc syndrome with chymopapain. *Journal of the American Medical Association,* 1980, *243* (20), 2043–2048.

Lucas, P. R. Low back pain. *Surgical Clinics of North America,* 1983, *63* (3), 515–528.

Pellino, T. A. Chymopapain: Alternative to laminectomy for herniated lumbar discs. *Orthopaedic Nursing,* 1983, *2* (2), 14–21.

Roaf, R., & Hodkinson, L. J. *Textbook of orthopaedic nursing* (2nd ed.). Oxford: Blackwell Scientific, 1975.

Sunderland, S. *Nerves and nerve injuries.* Edinburgh: Livingstone, 1968.

Turek, S. L. *Orthopaedics, principles and their applications* (3rd ed.). Philadelphia: Lippincott, 1977.

Wells, R., & Trostle, K. Creative hairwashing technique for immobilized patients. *Nursing 84,* 1984, *14* (1), 47–51.

White A. A. *Your aching back, a doctor's guide to relief.* New York: Bantam, 1983.

Wilkensen, H. A. *The failed back syndrome, etiology and theory.* Philadelphia: Harper & Row, 1983.

Wilkins, C., & MacEwen, G. D. Cranial nerve injury from halo traction. *Clinical Orthopaedics and Related Research,* 1977, *126* (4), 106–110.

Wiltse, L. L., Widell, E. H., & Yuan, H. A. Chymopapain: Chemonucleolysis in lumbar disk disease. *Journal of the American Medical Association,* 1975, *231* (5), 474–479.

BIBLIOGRAPHY

Agee, B. L., & Herman, C. Cervical log rolling on a standard bed. *American Journal of Nursing,* 1984, *84* (3), 314–318.

Allard, J. L., & Dibble, S. L. A look at Luque rods. *American Journal of Nursing,* 1984, *84* (5), 609–614.

Beeson, P. B. & McDermott, W. *Cecil-Loeb textbook of medicine.* Philadelphia: W. B. Saunders, 1971.

Blount, W. P., & Mallancamp, D. D. The effect of pregnancy on idiopathic scoliosis. *Journal of Bone and Joint Surgery,* 1980, *62A* (7), 1083–1087.

Bodnar, L. M. Sports medicine with references to back and neck injuries. *Current Practice in Orthopaedic Surgery 1977,* 1977, *7,* 116–154.

Bohlman, H. H. Acute fractures and dislocations of the cervical spine. *Journal of Bone and Joint Surgery,* 1979, *61A* (8), 1119–1142.

Bosacco, S. J., & Love-Mignogna, S. Complications of lumbar disc surgery. *Orthopedic Nurses' Association Journal,* 1978, *5* (11), 13–16.

Boyd, R. J. Low back pain: Assessment and management. *Current Practice in Orthopaedic Surgery 1979,* 1979, *8,* 1–12.

Bradford, D. S. Treatment of severe spondylolisthesis: A combined approach for reduction and stabilization. *Spine,* 1979, *4* (5), 423–429.

Bradford, D. S. Spondylosis and spondylolisthesis. *Current Practice in Orthopaedic Surgery 1979,* 1979, *8,* 12–38.

Bradley, G. W., King, H. A., & Dunn, H. K. Surgical stabilization of spine fractures: A community experience. *Orthopedics,* 1980, *3,* 38–43.

Branson, K. A. Patient management following amipaque myelography. *Orthopaedic Nursing,* 1982, *1* (6), 38–40.

Brantly, P., & Analla, M. *The nurse and orthopedic surgery.* Rutherford, NJ: The Orthopedic Nurses' Association, Inc. in cooperation with Howmedica, Inc., 1980.

Burton, C. V. High resolution CT scanning: The present and future. *Orthopaedic Clinics of North America,* 1983, *14* (3), 539–552.

Calliet, R. *Soft tissue pain and disability* (5th ed.), Philadelphia: F. A. Davis, 1981.

Clissold, G. *The body's response to trauma: Fractures.* New York: Springer, 1973.

Cochran, G. Van B. *A primer of orthopaedic biomechanics.* New York: Churchill Livingstone, 1982.

Colletti, R. B., Moreland, M. S., Peters, R. F., & Young, P. C. Primary sternal osteomyelitis with a negative bone scan. *Orthopedics,* 1980, *3,* 209–212.

Cozen, L. Closed needle biopsy of the lumbar spine: A safe and easy method. *Orthopedics,* 1980, *3,* 321–322.

Cummine, J. L., Lonstein, J. E., Mac, J. H., et al. Reconstructive surgery in the adult for failed scoliosis fusion. *Journal of Bone and Joint Surgery,* 1979, *61A* (8), 1151–1161.

Curtis, R. S., Dickson, J. H., Harrington, P. R., & Erwin, W. D. Results of Harrington instrumentation in the treatment for severe scoliosis. *Clinical Orthopedics,* 1979, *144,* 128–134.

DeOliveria, J. C. The new type of fracture–dislocation of the thoracolumbar spine. *Journal of Bone and Joint Surgery,* 1978, *60A* (4), 481–488.

Diekmann, E. Understanding your scoliosis surgery: A preoperative teaching booklet for Harrington instrumentation and spinal fusion patients. *Orthopedic Nurses' Association Journal,* 1978, *5* (10), 24–27.

Drennan, J. C., & King, E. W. Cervical dislocation following fusion of the upper thoracic spine for scoliosis. *Journal of Bone and Joint Surgery,* 1978, *60A* (7), 1003–1005.

Eismont, F. J., & Bohlman, H. H. Posterior atlanto-occipital dislocation with fractures of the atlas and adontoid process. *Journal of Bone and Joint Surgery,* 1978, *60A* (3), 397–399.

Farrell, J. Caring for the laminectomy patient: How to strengthen your support. *Nursing 78,* 1978, *8* (5), 65–69.

Faut, M. M. Spondylolisthesis in the adolescent. *Orthopedic Nurses' Association Journal,* 1979, *6* (5), 195–202.

Fielding, J. W., Pyle, R. N., & Fietti, V. G. Anterior cervical vertebral body resection and bone-grafting for benign and malignant tumors. *Journal of Bone and Joint Surgery,* 1979, *61A* (2), 251–253.

Ford, L. T. Chemonucleolysis by chymopapain. *Current Practice in Orthopaedic Surgery 1979,* 1979, *8,* 38–58.

Fries, J. F. *Arthritis, A comprehensive guide.* Menlo Park, Calif.: Addison-Wesley, 1982.

Griffin, J. B. Benign osteoblastoma of the thoracic spine. *Journal of Bone and Joint Surgery,* 1978, *60A* (6), 833–835.

Hausman, D., Gates, S. J., & Peters, R. G. Percutaneous lateral discectomy: Another approach for the treatment of a herniated nucleus pulposus. *Orthopaedic Nursing,* 1984, *3* (6), 9–17.

Henning, J. H., Allard-Paliembo, J., Pellino, T. A., et al. Preparation for the Luque procedure: Patient education booklet. *Orthopaedic Nursing,* 1984, *3* (5), 50–51.

Hitch, M. Nursing assessment of a patient with low back pain. *Orthopedic Nurses' Association Journal,* 1979, *6* (12), 484–488.

Ho, K., & Pak, M. Glomus tumor of the coccygeal region. *Journal of Bone and Joint Surgery,* 1980, *62A* (1), 141–142.

Hoppenfeld, S. *Physical examination of the spine and extremities.* New York: Appleton-Century-Crofts, 1976.

Hudgins, W. R. The role of microdiscectomy. *Orthopaedic Clinics of North America,* 1983, *14* (3), 589–604.

Keene, G., et al. Atlas fracture: Demonstration using computerized tomography. *Journal of Bone and Joint Surgery,* 1978, *60A* (8), 1106–1107.

Koch, R. A., & Nickel, V. L. The halo vest: An evaluation of motion and forces across the neck. *Spine,* 1978, *3* (2), 103–107.

Lawlis, G. F., & McCoy, C. E. Psychological evaluation: Patients with chronic pain. *Orthopaedic Clinics of North America,* 1983, *14* (3), 527–538.

Lundeen, M. A., & Herring, J. A. Osteoid-osteoma of the spine: Sclerosis in two levels. *Journal of Bone and Joint Surgery,* 1980, *62A* (3), 476–479.

Macnab, I. *Backache.* Baltimore: Williams & Wilkins, 1977.

Mansour, A. L., Nabos, J. F., & Taddonio, R. F. Psoas abcess: Thirty-four years after pyogenic osteomyelitis of the spine. *Orthopedics,* 1979, *2* (3), 262–264.

Mayer, T. G. Rehabilitation of the patient with spinal pain. *Orthopaedic Clinics of North America,* 1983, *14* (3), 623–638.

McCarthy, R. E. Coping with low back pain through behavioral change. *Orthopaedic Nursing,* 1984, *3* (3), 30–35.

Mooney, V. The syndromes of low back disease. *Orthopaedic Clinics of North America,* 1983, *14* (3), 505–516.

Morrey, B. F., Kelly, P., & Nickols, D. R. Viridans streptococcal osteomyelitis of the spine. *Journal of Bone and Joint Surgery,* 1980, *62A* (6), 1009–1010.

Musolf, J. Chemonucleolysis: A new approach to herniated intervertebral disks. *American Journal of Nursing,* 1983, *83* (6), 882–886.

O'Brien, J. P. The role of fusion for chronic low back pain. *Orthopaedic Clinics of North America,* 1983, *14* (3), 639–648.

O'Keefe, T. J. Retroperitoneal abcess: A potentially fatal complication of closed fracture of the pelvis. *Journal of Bone and Joint Surgery,* 1978, *60A* (8), 1117–1121.

Owen, B. Q. How to avoid that aching back. *American Journal of Nursing,* 1980, *80* (5), 894–897.

Patterson, D. Case study: Fractured pelvis multiple trauma. *Orthopedic Nurses' Association Journal,* 1978, *5* (6), 25–31.

Pheasant, H. C. The problem back. *Current Practice of Orthopaedic Surgery 1977,* 1977, 7, 89–116.

Pinzur, M. S., Mayer, P. R., Lautenschlager, E. P., et al. Measurement of internal fixation device support in experimentally produced fractures of the dorsalumbar spine. *Orthopedics,* 1979, *2* (1), 28–34.

Ransford, A. O. Halo-pelvic apparatus: Peritoneal penetration by pelvic pins. *Journal of Bone and Joint Surgery,* 1978, *60B* (3), 404–405.

Reeder, J. M. Adult scoliosis: A personal experience. *AORN Journal,* 1981, *33* (1), 35–50.

Rinsky, L. A., Guris, M., Bleck, E. E., et al. Intraoperative skeletal scintigraphy for localization of osteoid-osteoma in the spine. *Journal of Bone and Joint Surgery,* 1980, *62A* (1), 143–144.

Riseborough, E. J. Scoliosis in adults. *Current Practice in Orthopaedic Surgery 1977,* 1977, 7, 36–56.

Rutecki, B., & Saligson, D. Caring for the patient in a halo apparatus. *Nursing 80,* 1980, *10* (18), 73–77.

Sawyer, M. W. The role of the physical therapist before and after lumbar spine surgery. *Orthopaedic Clinics of North America,* 1983, *14* (3), 539–552.

Sahlstrand, T. Disruption of the pelvic ring treated by external skeletal fixation. *Journal of Bone and Joint Surgery,* 1979, *61A* (3), 433–444.

Selby, D. K. When to operate and what to operate upon. *Orthopaedic Clinics of North America,* 1983, *14* (3), 577–588.

Shahriarie, H., Sajadi, K., & Roohslamini, S. A. A family with spondylolisthesis. *Journal of Bone and Joint Surgery,* 1979, *61A* (8), 1256–1258.

Sigmon, H. D. Helping your long-term trauma patient travel the road to recovery. *Nursing 84,* 1984, *14* (1), 58–63.

Steinberg, G. G. Osteomyelitis of the rib presenting as painful torticollis. *Journal of Bone and Joint Surgery,* 1979, *61A* (4), 614–615.

Swinson, D. R., & Swinburn, W. R. *Rheumatology.* New York: Wiley, 1980.

Taylor, S. L. Musculoskeletal assessment: Low back pain assessment: Part 1—History-taking. *Orthopaedic Nursing,* 1983, *2* (4), 11–17.

The traction handbook. Wawsaw, Ind.: Zimmer, USA, 1975.

Wang, G. J., et al. The treatment of fracture dislocation of the thoracolumbar spine with halofemoral traction and Harrington rod instrumentation. *Clinical Orthopedics,* 1979, *142,* 168–175.

Wells, R., & Trostle, K. Creative hairwashing techniques for immobilized patients. *Nursing 84,* 1984, *14* (1), 47–51.

White, A. H. Injection techniques for the diagnosis and treatment of low back pain. *Orthopaedic Clinics of North America,* 1983, *14* (3), 553–568.

Wiltse, L. L. Chemonucleolysis in the treatment of lumbar disc diseases. *Orthopaedic Clinics of North America,* 1983, *14* (3), 605–622.

Winter, R. B. Combined Dwyer and Harrington instrumentation and fusion in the treatment of selected patients with painful adult idiopathic scoliosis. *Spine,* 1978, *3* (2), 135–141.

Yong-Hing, K., & Kirkaldy-Willis, W. H. The pathophysiology of degenerative disease of the lumbar-spine. *Orthopaedic Clinics of North America,* 1983, *14* (3), 491–504.

6

THE HIP AND UPPER LEG

Chapter 6 focuses on the care of patients with traumatic and pathological conditions of the hip, including the proximal third of the femur. Surgical procedures that correct hip deformities, and their associated nursing care, are discussed, from minor hip dislocations to hip disarticulations due to neoplasms. The chapter begins with a review of the anatomy of the hip.

ANATOMY

The hip joint is a ball and socket joint with movements of flexion–extension, adduction–abduction, and a combination of circumduction and medial and lateral rotation. The head of the femur articulates with the cup-shaped fossa of the acetabulum. The head of the femur is completely covered with articular cartilage, except over the small, roughened pit to which the ligament of the head of the femur is attached. The articular surface of the acetabulum forms an incomplete ring, termed the lunate surface, broadest at its upper part where the pressure of the body weight falls in the erect position and narrowest where it covers the pubic constituent. The ligamentous structures of the joint are the fibrous capsule, the acetabular labrum, the ligament of the head of the femur, and the iliofemoral, ischiofemoral, pubofemoral, and transverse acetabular ligaments. The capsule is surrounded by muscles on all sides. Different muscles produce different movements. Flexion is accomplished by the psoas major and the iliacus, assisted by the pectineus, the rectus femoris, and the sartorius with the adductor longus assisting in the early stages. Extension is accomplished by the gluteus maximus and the hamstring muscles. Abduction is achieved by the glutei medius and minimus, assisted by the tensor fasciae latae and the sartorius. Adduction is achieved by the adductors longus, brevis, and magnus, assisted by the pectineus and the gracilis. Medial rotation is accomplished by the tensor fasciae latae and the anterior fibers of the glutei minimus and medius.

Lateral rotation is accomplished by the obturator muscles, the gemellus, and the quadratus femoris, assisted by the piriformis, the gluteus maximus, and the sartorius. The arteries that supply the joint are derived from the obturator, the medial circumflex femoral, and the superior and inferior gluteal arteries. The nerves are derived from the femoral nerve, directly or through its muscular branches, the obturator, the accessory obturator, the nerve to the quadratus femoris, and the superior gluteal (Warwick & Williams, 1973, pp. 446–449).

THE HIP

Trauma

DISLOCATIONS OF THE HIP JOINT

A dislocation occurs when the bones that make up a joint are out of anatomical alignment. Adult hip dislocations are most commonly traumatic, following such events as difficult deliveries, athletic injuries, and vehicular accidents, or are postoperative complications of a hip arthroplasty (Gartland, 1979, p. 384).

Types of Dislocations

Posterior Dislocations
Most frequently, the dislocation is posterior and occurs when the patient is sitting. A blow on the knee drives the femoral head posteriorly out of its socket, frequently fracturing the rim of the acetabulum. In other instances, the dislocation may be due to abduction, in which case the head of the femur dislocates inferiorly and then assumes the posterior position (Roaf & Hodkinson, 1975, p. 116). When that occurs, the hip internally rotates and is locked in a position of adduction and flexion, and the leg is shortened up to 5 cm (2 inches) (Fig. 6–1). Only the foot can be actively moved. The greater trochanter is abnormally prominent, whereas palpation beneath the inguinal ligament for the femoral head yields only an indentation. Passive rotation of the femur is absent. The pain is severe and constant in the inguinal region and thigh.

Anterior Dislocations
Anterior dislocations of the hip are rare but can occur, for example, when a person lands on the feet after a fall. The femur is forcefully externally rotated and abducted, causing the femoral head to dislocate through a ruptured anterior capsule of the hip. The lower extremity is held in a position of abduction and external rotation, slight flexion, and often the femoral head can be palpated beneath the inguinal ligament in the anterior part of the thigh. There is no shortening of the limb, because the head is impaled anteriorly in the iliofe-

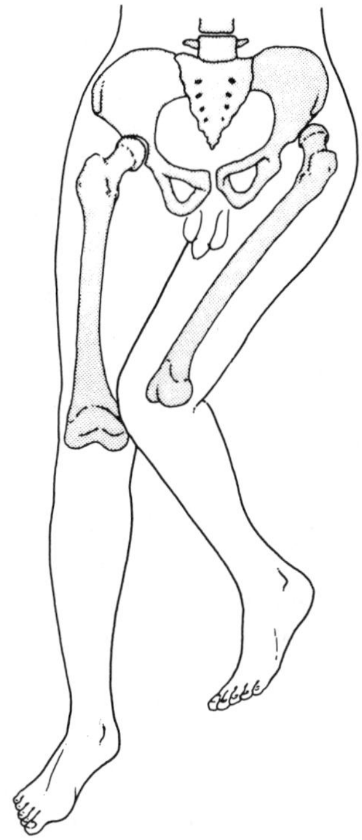

Figure 6–1. Posterior dislocation of the hip. *(From Roaf, R., & Hodkinson, L. J., 1980, p. 114, with permission.)*

moral ligament. The femoral artery and nerve, which run in that area, can be compromised at that point.

Central Dislocations
A central dislocation of the hip can occur with a central fracture of the acetabulum, the mechanism of injury being a direct blow to the trochanteric area (Donahoo & Dimon, 1977, p. 72).

Methods of Repair

The treatment of a posterior dislocation is reduction within 24 hours following injury (Gartland, 1979, p. 384), done by anesthetizing the patient, lying the patient flat on the back, and then flexing the knee and the hip to right angles. With one assistant holding the pelvis, the physician lifts the hip gently forward until the head of the femur is felt to enter the acetabulum, at which time the leg can be extended and externally rotated (Roaf & Hodkinson, 1975, pp. 116–117) (Fig. 6–2). Most reductions can be accomplished without open surgery, but occasionally the iliopsoas, the capsule, or both, may prevent nonsurgical reduction (Donahoo & Dimon, 1977, p. 72).

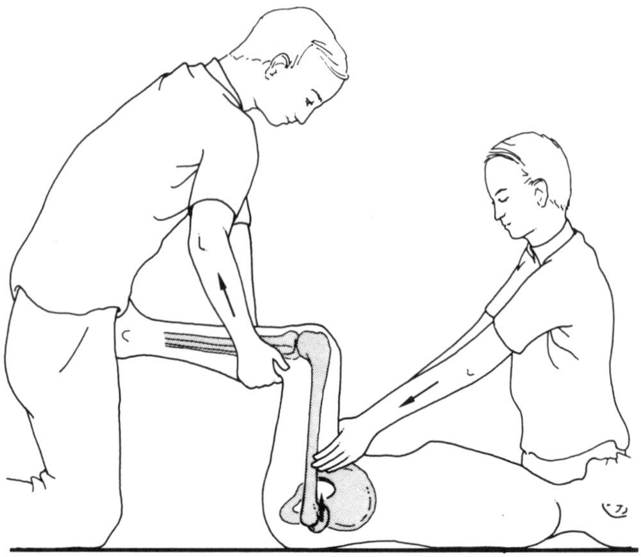

Figure 6–2. Reduction of a dislocated hip. *(From Roaf, R., & Hodkinson, L. J., 1980, p. 117, with permission.)*

Postoperatively, the hip is kept in a stable position until the capsule and the soft tissue can heal. Because of the instability of the joint, skeletal traction may be used for an extended period of time. Gradual mobilization is then allowed.

There is a difference of opinion on what is the best medical care following a successful reduction. It is well recognized that after a dislocation of the hip, some 25 to 30 percent of the patients develop avascular necrosis of the head of the femur due to interference with the blood supply. Most surgeons, however, believe that no treatment can alter the incidence of that condition. Therefore, after 10 days or so of traction in recumbency, they see no reason why the patient should not start gentle nonweight-bearing exercises, and as soon as muscle tone has been restored, resume partial weight bearing, perhaps within 3 to 4 weeks after injury. On the other hand, some surgeons believe that prolonged recumbency for 3 months diminishes the incidence of avascular necrosis. To date, there are no available figures concerning that contention. If there is no associated injury about the hip joint, the majority of the patients make a full recovery.

☐ NURSING PROCESS (Table 6–1)

Assessment

The initial assessment of a typical patient admitted with a dislocated hip includes an evaluation of the physical and emotional status with an emphasis on a complete description of what happened to cause the injury as well as a physical assessment of the hip. The physical position of the involved leg is important. For a posterior hip dislocation, the leg is in adduction and flexion, and may be shortened by up to 5 cm (2 inches). The greater trochanter is abnormally prominent and only the foot can actually be moved. Pain is usually severe and constant in the inguinal region and the thigh. Because of the nature of the injury there will usually be an abrasion on the knee. For anterior dislocations, the leg is in abduction and external rotation, slight flexion, and sometimes the femoral head is palpable beneath the inguinal ligament in the anterior part of the thigh. There is no shortening of the leg, but, because of the position of the dislocated femoral head, the femoral artery and nerve can be compromised. Their function should be assessed quickly.

Postoperatively, the assessment is the same as for a patient recovering from general anesthesia and in skeletal traction. Special considerations include neurovascular checks (Chap. 2) of the affected leg and checks of the traction apparatus (Appendix A).

Nursing Diagnosis and Goal Formulation

For a typical patient recovering from surgery for a dislocated hip, nursing diagnoses are (1) alterations in comfort related to hip pain from trauma, (2) alterations in mobility related to lack of joint stability in the hip, (3) alterations in psychological well-being related to anxiety and knowledge deficit, and (4) potential complications related to surgical procedure and immobility.

Short-term goals are to have the patient experience (1) a decrease in pain through the use of correct positioning, traction, and prescribed medications, (2) an increase in mobility by maintaining immobilization of the involved leg through traction, exercises, and crutches, (3) a decrease in anxiety through increased knowledge, and (4) an absence of complications from surgery and decreased activity. Long-term goals are to have the patient free of pain in the involved joint with complete restoration of function.

Planning and Intervention

Alleviate Pain. For pain management, see the nursing care of a patient with an internal fixation. A large amount of pain in a patient with a hip dislocation is from muscle spasm and soft tissue trauma. Traction, by applying a continuous pull, helps to reduce the pain by reducing muscle spasms. When patients are first removed from traction, the pain may temporarily increase somewhat.

Increase Mobility

Position. Immediately after reduction, the involved leg is placed in traction until the joint capsule and soft tissue can heal. In most instances this

TABLE 6–1. NURSING PROCESS FOR HIP DISLOCATION TREATED WITH SKELETAL TRACTION

Assessment	Nursing Diagnosis	Goal Formulation	Planning and Intervention	Evaluation and Reassessment
1. Assess the duration, location, and severity of pain. Assess neurovascular status. Observe for verbal and nonverbal cues of pain. Check for correct positioning of the leg. Check vital signs.	1. Alteration in comfort: pain in the hip related to soft tissue trauma.	1. Short-term goal: a decrease in hip pain through nursing measures and immobilization. Long-term goal: free of pain.	1. Alleviate Pain Maintain traction. Maintain correct positioning of the leg. Discuss the effect of traction on muscle spasms. Utilize noninvasive nursing measures. Teach relaxation techniques. Administer prescribed medications.	1. The patient should have a decrease in pain as determined by verbal responses and outward appearance. Inquire as to what aggravates and intensifies pain, and what seems to relieve it.
2. Check the position of the involved leg. Check the line of pull of the traction. Assess the patient's ability to do exercises. Check for correct body alignment.	2. Impaired physical mobility: decreased leg movement related to lack of joint stability.	2. Short-term goal: an increase in mobility by immobilizing the involved leg with traction. Long-term goal: regain full mobility.	2. Increase Mobility *Position* Keep patient supine. Maintain skeletal traction at all times. Discuss purposes and rationale for traction. *Exercises* Teach quadriceps and gluteal setting exercises.	2. The patient should be doing the exercise program even while in traction. The patient should maintain the supine position even when asleep. If allowed, flexion and

			Teach active range of motion for the ankle of the involved leg and all uninvolved joints. *Ambulation* Teach exercises to prepare for crutch walking.	extension of the involved leg may be started.
3. Assess for any redness, swelling, or drainage. Assess for pain at the pin sites. Check vital signs.	3. Potential for injury: infection at the pin sites related to skeletal traction.	3. Short- and long-term goals: free of any signs of infection.	3. Prevent Complications *Integumentary* Keep dressing clean and dry. If appropriate, do pin care. *Potential Complications Due to Immobility* (See Chap. 3 and Table 6–2)	3. The patient should remain free of any complications due to traction or immobility.
4. Assess patient's understanding about injury and rehabilitation process.	4. Potential knowledge deficit related to injury and rehabilitation process.	4. Short- and long-term goals: a decrease in anxiety through increased knowledge.	4. Patient Teaching Discuss mechanism of injury. Discuss the various stages in the rehabilitation process. Discuss the prognosis.	4. The patient should have a decrease in anxiety with explanation and discussion of rehabilitation and prognosis.

will be a form of skeletal traction with a pin through the tibia. Skeletal traction is used because of the length of time the patient will be in traction and the amount of weight necessary to immobilize the leg, keep the hip in anatomical alignment, and reduce muscle spasm. More specific details on traction and the care of patients in traction is discussed on pp. 278–279 and Appendix A.

Ambulation. The basic nursing measures to increase ambulation are to have the patient do active bed exercises using all unaffected joints. If allowed by the physician, flexion and extension of the involved leg may be used to prevent stiffness. If the patient will be using crutches, exercises should be used to prepare the arms and the shoulders for weight bearing. Even if flexion or movement of the leg are not allowed, quadriceps and gluteal setting exercises are usually allowed. The objective of those exercises is to help restore muscle tone, to help develop muscle strength, and to help prevent the hip from dislocating again.

Patient Teaching. Most of patients are healthy individuals with no other major medical problem. Once the hip is back in anatomical position, the patient, family, and significant others need to understand the necessity for immobilization and the plan of treatment. Some may find it harder to understand immobilization and restriction for a dislocation, whereas with a fracture it is perfectly understandable.

Prevent Complications. The major potential complications are those related to infection at the skeletal pin site and the effects of bedrest (Chap 3).

Evaluation and Reassessment

The considerations discussed for the patient who has had an internal fixation apply here as well (see pp. 262–263). Special emphasis should be given to evaluating the patient's response to immobilization.

FRACTURES OF THE HIP

A fracture of the hip refers to a fracture of the proximal one-third of the femur, which extends up to 5 cm (2 inches) below the lesser trochanter. It occurs most commonly through the neck or the intertrochanteric region of the femur. Fractures of the hip are classified as either intracapsular or extracapsular. Intracapsular fractures are those occurring within the hip joint capsule, that is, within the fibrous tissues that enclose the hip joint. The intracapsular fractures are (1) capital fractures (fractures of the head of the femur), (2) subcapital (fractures just below the head of the femur), and (3) transcervical (fractures of the neck of the femur). Extracapsular fractures are those outside of the joint capsule through the femur's greater or lesser trochanter, in the intertrochanteric area, or in the subtrochanteric area.

□ NURSING PROCESS

Preoperative Assessment

The patient admitted with a chief complaint of hip injury generally arrives on a stretcher. The first step in assessment is usually a visual inspection of the affected extremity. The classical features of the patient with a fractured hip are that the patient is usually elderly, has fallen, and has pain in the hip, with shortening, adduction, external rotation, and slight flexion of the affected leg. However, different types of hip fractures may cause a slightly different positioning of the affected extremity. With extracapsular fractures, the leg rests in external rotation of 90 degrees and there is shortening and a lot of bruising, but with intracapsular fractures, the joint capsule restrains rotation to about 45 degrees and there is considerable swelling of the upper thigh. In patients having displaced intracapsular fractures, the extremity usually assumes a position of shortening and external rotation due to displacement at the fracture site and muscle spasm, which shortens and externally rotates the involved leg. When the femur separates at the time of the fracture, the strong gluteus medius muscle pulls the distal portion upward. The iliopsoas tends to rotate the leg outward, as does the gluteus maximus.

The major exception to the above picture is that patients with impacted intracapsular fractures are usually relatively pain free at first. The patient may have walked into the hospital after having walked on the fractured hip for a week or more, before the discomfort increased enough to require medical attention. Upon observation of the affected leg, the nurse may notice that there is no shortening and the leg is in good alignment. The patient will limp only minimally. There is usually no deformity to the leg, but there may be marked valgus, that is, the patient will display a knocked knee. Pain can be elicited by slightly forcing the hip into internal rotation. A way to distinguish an impacted fracture from a displaced fracture is that the patient with an impacted fracture can lift the foot off the bed.

Subtrochanteric fractures usually involve younger patients, with the fracture produced by severe trauma. The fracture may be open or closed, and typically there is extensive hemorrhage into the soft tissue. The affected leg appears shortened and there may be an anterior and lateral rotation. The line of pull and the great strength of the muscles of the hip and the thigh tend to produce marked displacement of bone fragments. Many powerful short muscles pull on the neck fragment, especially the iliopsoas, and tend to flex and rotate the proximal fragment.

An assessment of the injured hip must include a neurovascular check of the area distal to the injury. The neurovascular check must include capillary filling, color, temperature, edema, pulse, sensory nerve function, and motor nerve function (Chap 2). An adequate assessment of the entire extremity is imperative to guard against permanent neurovascular damage.

The complete assessment of the patient must include not only the assessment of the obvious injury, but also an assessment of the patient's general status. That must be accomplished quickly, but thoroughly, before proceeding with nursing actions concerning the obvious injury. An open subtrochanteric fracture of the femur may appear to be the most serious injury but in many instances may in fact not be the most urgent. Pertinent observations of the patient can be made while personal clothing is being exchanged for a hospital gown and the patient is helped into a position of comfort. The injury may have just occurred, or the patient may have fallen at home and was unable to get help for several hours. Some patients may have abrasions or other skin lesions from dragging themselves trying to get help if they live alone. The major points in the general assessment are to assess for (1) chest pain or difficulty breathing, (2) possible internal bleeding at the fracture site, shock, or dehydration (e.g., vital signs, swelling at the site of the fracture, ecchymosis if the fracture occurred some hours before, skin turgor, and condition of the mucous membranes), (3) level of consciousness, orientation to time, place, and person, and ability to communicate, (4) the condition of other extremities (e.g., perhaps the patient has previously had a stroke, or just suffered one that caused the fall), (5) pain, (6) the presence of other health problems, and (7) anxiety level. Find out who the patient's significant others are, if they are there, or whether they have been notified. If those persons cannot come to the hospital before surgery, it may be possible to have them talk directly to the patient by phone. If the family or significant others of the patient are available, it is a good time to give information about the patient's condition, but also to gain knowledge about the patient. Information needed may be on the mental alertness of the patient, the patient's ability to care for and feed self, ambulatory status before injury, and other health problems, as well as the patient's likes and dislikes on food, fluids, and daily routines. Depending on the patient's condition and the time of the surgery, the nurse can do a more complete assessment and nursing history at that time (Chap. 2).

Preoperative Nursing Diagnosis and Goal Formulation

Specific nursing diagnoses and goals are derived from the assessment of each patient. In a typical patient, however, nursing diagnoses might be (1) alterations in comfort related to hip pain from trauma, (2) alterations in mobility related to lack of bone integrity in the affected hip, and (3) alterations in psychological well-being related to anxiety and lack of knowledge about the injury and method of treatment. In such instances, goals should be formulated to (1) alleviate pain so that the patient can obtain physical and emotional rest, (2) prevent further damage to soft tissues, nerves, and blood vessels, through immobilization of the leg, and (3) provide health education about injury and care.

Preoperative Planning and Intervention

Preoperative planning to accomplish the above formulated goals might be (1) to alleviate pain, by talking to the patient about the nature of the pain, repositioning the patient for improved comfort, and administering pain medications under appropriate medical orders, (2) to achieve immobilization, through the use of pillows, sandbags, trochanter rolls and/or skin traction, and (3) to provide health education, by explaining the nature of the injury, the procedures to be done, and the follow-up care that will be provided. The plans should be implemented in priority order as indicated above.

Preoperative Evaluation and Reassessment

The reaction of the patient to the nursing interventions should be carefully evaluated to see if the goals are being met, that is, whether pain is being relieved, immobility achieved, and the patient brought to awareness of the situation. If the evaluation shows that the goals are not being met, or that a change has occurred in the patient's condition, the reassessment will indicate a need to reinitiate the nursing process.

Methods of Surgical Repair

The choice of procedure in the treatment of a hip fracture depends primarily upon the type of fracture and secondarily upon the patient's general physical and emotional condition, the length of time since the fracture was sustained, and the surgeon's preference and judgment. Most patients with hip fractures, being elderly, have chronic health problems. The hip fracture is complicated by or perhaps has complicated an existing cardiac condition, diabetic problem, or other health deficit that frequently accompanies the aging process. In view of modern surgical techniques, many surgeons feel that the sooner operative fixation is done the better, but in some instances, reduction and fixation of the fracture must be delayed 24, 48, or even more hours to permit the complete medical evaluation and treatment of an existing health problem. The primary consideration in delaying surgery is the patient's general condition. If surgery is delayed for intracapsular or extracapsular fractures, the application of skin traction (Buck's extension, Russell's traction, or a similiar apparatus) will help to immobilize the fracture and lessen muscle spasms, thus making the patient more comfortable. Patients with impacted intracapsular fractures will probably not need to be placed in traction because the fracture site is stabilized by the impaction itself. In the case of a subtrochanteric fracture, the flexion pull of the iliopsoas muscle makes 90-90 traction effective in aligning the distal fragment with the proximal fragment (Fig. 6–3).

Treatment of hip fractures usually consists of realigning the fragments by either closed or open methods, followed by operative insertion of some metallic internal fixation device, such as a compression screw or multiple threaded pins, to fasten the broken fragments together until healing occurs. In selected frail or aged patients, in those few patients for whom the head fragment cannot be reduced, or in some fractures of the proximal neck of the femur, the femoral head may be removed and a metallic femoral head prosthesis inserted. All things considered, however, it is usually better for the patient to obtain healing

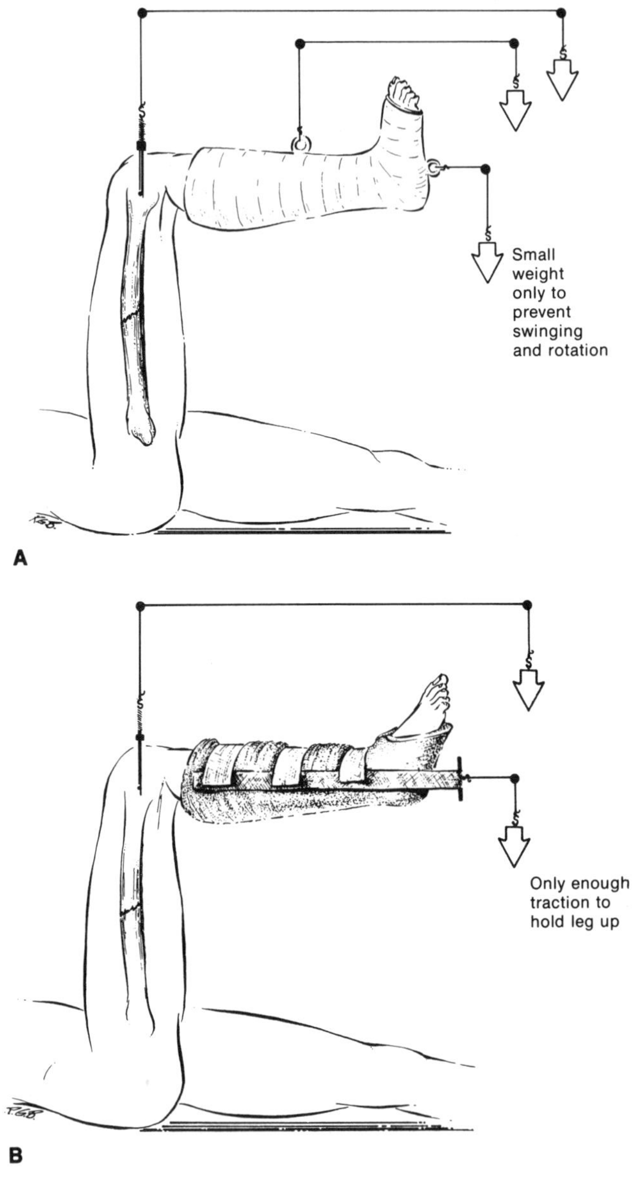

Figure 6–3. A. and **B.** 90-90 traction. Various methods of 90-90 traction used in treatment of femoral fractures. The traction is applied through a skeletal pin through the distal femur. The femur is held perpendicular to the bed so that the effect of muscle pull and the effect of gravity can be simultaneously corrected. *(From Lewis, R. C.* Handbook of traction, casting and splinting techniques. *Philadelphia: Lippincott, 1977, p. 43, with permission.)*

of the fracture by means of internal fixation than to have prosthetic replacement of the femoral head (Gartland, 1979, p. 389–390).

Intracapsular Fractures

An intracapsular fracture is a serious orthopaedic problem because the fracture may severely restrict the blood supply to the femoral head. The restriction or destruction of the blood supply may occur at the time of fracture or any time prior to internal fixation. The proximal fragment of the femur, being inside the joint, is almost devoid of soft tissue attachments. Its major blood supply (the retinacular or epiphyseal arteries) runs along the femoral neck in a distal to proximal direction to enter the base of the head of the femur. All interosseous vessels are interrupted by the fracture, leaving the femoral head dependent on the ligament of the head of the femur, which carries little or no circulation. For that reason, a femoral neck fracture is a vascular emergency that demands immediate attention. The blood supply is disturbed in some 25 percent (Gartland, 1979, p. 89) to 40 percent (Roaf & Hodkinson, 1975, p. 117) of the patients, and at the present time there is no known method whereby avascular necrosis can be avoided. It is believed that the more efficient the internal fixation, the less the chance of avascular necrosis. In contrast, for fractures of the intertrochanter or below, the blood supply to both portions of the femur is almost always satisfactory.

An impacted intracapsular fracture of the femur usually is in a position that allows for fairly good function, as even in the acute injury phase the patient may be able to walk on the affected leg. Usually that type of fracture is stabilized without manipulation and can be treated with success conservatively (i.e., by bedrest without internal fixation). Because the fracture usually occurs in persons for whom prolonged bedrest would be unsuitable, such patients are usually treated by internal fixation in the form of threaded pins (i.e., 4 or 5 Knowles or Hagie pins or Deyerle nails or compression screws) (Fig. 6–4) to prevent further displacement of the femoral head (Donahoo & Dimon, 1977, p. 72). A Smith-Peterson nail or other three-flanged or flat-ended devices (see Fig. 6–4) are not used in the treatment of impacted fractures because the impaction should be preserved. If a three-flanged nail is pounded into the compact bone of the femoral head, the impaction may be broken up and the head distracted from the neck, which could produce nonunion or avasuclar necrosis (Compere, 1974, p. 128).

On the other hand, the treatment of displaced intracapsular fractures is either reduction and internal fixation of the femoral head or replacement by a prosthesis. The procedure is to use a three-flanged device with plate (typically a Smith-Peterson or Jewett nail with plate) followed by impaction of the fracture or employment of a sliding device (Ken nail or Massie nail) (see Fig. 6–4), which allows the fracture to impact (Ghista & Roaf, 1978, p. 212). Because these fractures frequently occur in elderly patients with other serious health problems, mortality within a year of the accident is considerable and residual disability is common among those who survive. Some surgeons believe that the results of internal fixation are so poor that an immediate replacement endo-

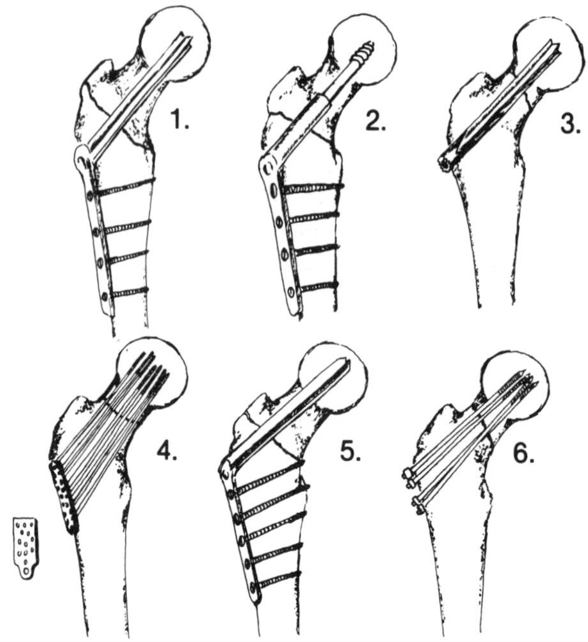

Figure 6–4. Variety of hip internal fixations. **(1)** Jewett nail; intertrochanteric fracture. **(2)** Compression hip screw; intertrochanteric tracture. **(3)** Smith Peterson nail; femoral neck fracture. **(4)** Deyerle nail; femoral neck fracture. **(5)** I-Beam nail (Sarmenito); intertrochanteric fracture. **(6)** Knowles or Hagie pins; femoral neck fracture. *(From Brantley, P., & Analla, M., 1980, p. 74. Courtesy of Howmedica.)*

prosthesis is the correct treatment (Tronzo, 1973, p. 531). The problems are particularly severe for the displaced subcapital intracapsular fracture, which has been named "the unsolved fracture" (Compere, 1974, p. 130; Roaf & Hodkinson, 1975, p. 118).

Extracapsular Fractures

Intertrochanteric. Intertrochanteric fractures of the femur occur most commonly in women. As a general rule, these patients are older than those fracturing the neck of the femur but healing at that location is more favorable because of the blood-rich cancellous bone. Treatment of the fracture usually consists of an open reduction and internal fixation by means of a metallic, nail-plate device with or without a compression element (Gartland, 1979, p. 389). Some of the devices may be the Ken nail, Jewett nail with plate, I-Beam nail, Massie nail with plate, or the Ender nail (Fig. 6–5).

Subtrochanteric. A subtrochanteric fracture of the femur, one just below the trochanteric region, has been viewed by physicians as being difficult to manage either surgically or conservatively. These fractures usually occur with other body trauma and may be either open or closed fractures (Tronzo, 1973, p. 576). The muscle forces in that area cause problems with the maintenance of

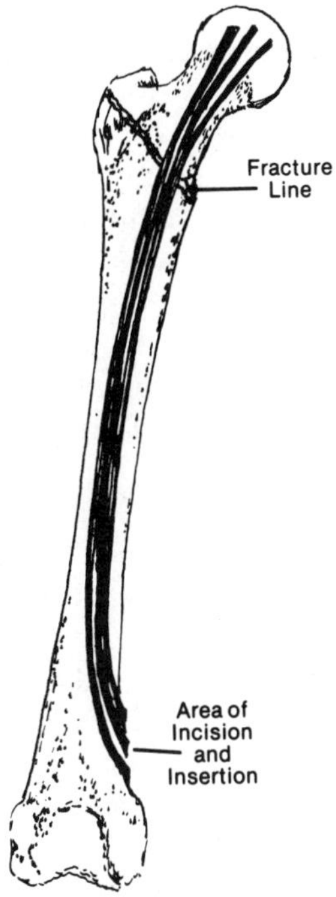

Figure 6–5. Ender nail. *(From Brantley, P., & Analla, M., 1980, p. 75. Courtesy of Howmedica.)*

reduction by closed or open methods. Treatment is by immediate surgery, if possible, with either a side plate with or without a nail, by a standard intramedullary rod (Donahoo and Dimon, 1977, p. 75; Roaf & Hodkinson, 1975, p. 119), or by a nonstandard intramedullary rod with special nail attachments such as the Küntscher or Ziekel rods (Tronzo, 1973, p. 579). Bone grafting is sometimes necessary, depending on the type of fracture (Tronzo, 1973, p. 580). If conservative treatment is done, it is usually with skeletal traction or Russell's traction modified for skeletal application. During traction, it is necessary to keep the patient's leg in slight adduction and moderate flexion because the proximal fragment is pulled in the upward direction (toward the body) by the iliopsoas muscle (Tronzo, 1973, p. 577).

Lesser Trochanteric. Isolated avulsion fractures of the lesser trochanter, usually occurring in young athletes, can usually be treated symptomatically with excellent return of function. Open reduction is usually not necessary. Fractures of the greater trochanter, also avulsion injuries, are generally essentially undisplaced. They can usually be treated symptomatically with bedrest for a few days with the leg held slightly abducted. Healing is usually complete in about 6 weeks (Tronzo, 1973, p. 514).

Surgical Complications

The most serious complication of (intracapsular) fractures of the femoral neck is avascular necrosis. The second is nonunion. It has been estimated that one out of four patients sustaining a fracture through the neck of the femur fails to obtain a successful union (Gartland, 1979, p. 389). Because of those two problems, some physicians prefer endoprosthesis surgery to internal fixation. Loss of reduction of the fracture usually occurs only if the fixation is not good, because of too few pins, poor pin placement, or inadequate impaction of the fractured fragments (Tronzo, 1973, p. 522). Infection occurs in older patients because of poor subcutaneous tissues, but even in those patients the infection rate can be reduced to as low as 2 percent with prophylactic antibiotics (Tronzo, 1973, p. 522).

Avascular necrosis and nonunion are rarely encountered following intertrochanteric fractures of the hip because of the relative abundance of the blood supply in the cancellous segment of the femur. An intertrochanteric fracture is a more severe injury than an intracapsular fracture, however, because of the high incidence of complications involving blood loss, shock, fat embolisms, pulmonary embolisms, and pneumonia (Ghista & Roaf, 1978, p. 210). Shortening of the affected leg is common. Some patients will have a shortening of one-half to three-fourths of an inch because of the collapse of the fragments at the fracture site, which frequently occurs during the healing phase (Tronzo, 1973, p. 574). Those fractures commonly unite with considerable varus because the lesser trochanter has usually been avulsed from the femur. For that reason, there is no effective action of the psoas muscle and the uncompensated action of the gluteal muscles produces a coxa vara deformity (Roaf & Hodkinson, 1975, p. 119). Attempts have been made by physicians to overcome that by weakening the abductor muscles at the time of surgery by dividing them at their point of insertion into the greater trochanter (Roaf & Hodkinson, 1975, p. 119).

Other complications that can occur in patients with hip fractures are nail or pin penetration into the acetabulum, breakage of the fixation device, deep infection around the implant, thrombophlebitis, and pulmonary embolism. Deep infection around the implant often develops slowly. The patient usually complains of increased pain in the hip. Roentgenograms in the early stage of the infection are generally negative but the sedimentation rate is usually elevated. With deep infections, the physician usually tries to keep the implant in place, at least until the fracture has healed. If that is not possible, the implant is removed and irrigation with large amounts of antibiotics is usually done by means of closed-tube drainage. Patients with fractures of the hip repaired by internal fixation are usually elderly and the implant can easily remain in place without difficulty. Younger patients whose life span can be expected to be many years should have the device removed about 1 year after healing has occurred. That will avoid weakening the bone from any reaction to the implant.

A high incidence of thrombophlebitis and pulmonary embolism occurs in injured patients. Patients with fractured hips are in particular jeopardy, as about 30 percent develop thrombophlebitis and about 2 percent die of pulmonary embolism (Tronzo, 1973, p. 586). Several drugs have been used to try to prevent these problems, including heparin, warfarin, low-molecular-weight dextran, and aspirin. With heparin and warfarin, some patients, especially the elderly, developed sensitivities to the drug, whereas dextran has the complications of congestive heart failure, allergic reaction, renal failure, and anemia. Aspirin, also a drug with anticoagulent properties, has been used with various amounts of enthusiasm, because it can be difficult to determine the optimal dosage. Nonetheless, it has been the drug of choice to treat and prevent the problems of thrombophlebitis and pulmonary embolism for a large number of physicians (Chap. 3).

□ NURSING PROCESS (Table 6–2)

Postoperative Assessment

The immediate postoperative assessment for a typical patient following the repair of a fractured hip involves taking vital signs (e.g., pulse, respiration, and blood pressure), and observing the patient's general color and warmth. A neurovascular assessment of the affected leg (pulse, temperature, color, capillary filling, edema, sensory and motor nerve function) should be made (Chap. 2) and the position of the leg checked for proper alignment. The patient's level of consciousness and orientation should be determined. The incisional dressing and the area posterior to the dressing should be checked for drainage. If the patient has wound catheters in place, note the color and amount of drainage and whether the suction is working. Assess the type, severity, and location of pain, the patient's verbal and nonverbal expressions of pain, and note whether the patient received medication in surgery or in the postanesthesia room. Have the patient cough and deep breathe and auscultate the chest for clearness of the lungs and any cardiac abnormalities. Note the type of intravenous solution, the rate of flow, and the amount left in the bottle or bag. Obtain from the anesthesia and postanesthesia room records or personnel the amount of blood loss in surgery and the amount of fluid replacement. Check the patient for bladder distention, urgency, or the need to void.

Frequent assessment of the patient should be made during the postoperative period. Auscultation of the patient's chest should be done at least once a shift. For the first few postoperative days the nurse will also need to assess for bowel sounds. Neurovascular assessments of the affected extremity are usually done every 15 mintues for 2 hours, then every 30 minutes for 2 hours, then every hour for 2 hours, then every 2 hours for 18 hours, then at the beginning of every shift.

Postoperative Nursing Diagnosis and Goal Formulation

In a typical patient, postoperative diagnoses might be (1) alterations in comfort related to hip pain from trauma and surgery, (2) alterations in

TABLE 6–2. NURSING PROCESS FOR FRACTURED HIP TREATED WITH AN OPEN REDUCTION AND INTERNAL FIXATION

Assessment	Nursing Diagnosis	Goal Formulation	Planning and Intervention	Evaluation and Reassessment
1. Assess the duration, location, and severity of pain. Assess verbal and nonverbal expressions of pain. Check when the last pain medication was received. Check vital signs.	1. Alteration in comfort: pain in the hip related to bone and soft tissue trauma.	1. Short-term goal: a decrease in hip pain through nursing measures and prescribed medications. Long-term goal: free of pain.	1. Alleviate Pain Talk about the pain. Explain the patient's need to ask for assistance in dealing with pain. Reposition the patient. Teach muscle setting exercises, giving the patient an opportunity to demonstrate comprehension. Teach relaxation technique. Administer pain medication as indicated.	1. The patient should have a decrease in pain as determined by verbal responses and outward appearance. Inquire as to what aggravates and intensifies it, and what seems to relieve it.
2. Assess the neurovascular status. Check the position and alignment of the leg. Assess the patient's general muscular development and strength. Assess the patient's range of motion in uninvolved joints. Assess the patient's ability to understand and follow simple directions.	2. Impaired physical mobility: no weight bearing on involved leg related to lack of bone stability in the leg.	2. Short-term goal: an increase in mobility through the use of exercises and assistive devices. Long-term goal: able to walk without discomfort using a 3-point gait for the first 6 to 12 months and without supportive devices thereafter.	2. Increase Mobility *Position* Position the patient supine with the affected leg in slight abduction and no rotation. Explain the need for correctly positioning the leg. Elevate the head of the bed 45 degrees for meals. *Turning* Teach turning to either side with pillows between the legs. *Exercises* Teach resistive and isometric exercises (e.g., quadriceps and gluteal setting, plantar and dorsiflexion, active range of motion of the ankle and exercises for the upper extremities). Give the patient an opportunity to demonstrate comprehension.	2. The patient should follow the exercise routine and be able to utilize assistive devices. Evaluate the degree to which the patient has maintained or regained activities of daily living. The patient should be able to ambulate with a steady gait.

			Trapeze Teach correct method of using the trapeze. Explain rationale for trapeze use. Give the patient an opportunity to demonstrate ability to use the trapeze. *Ambulation* Teach proper method of getting out of bed. Explain the rationale and give the patient an opportunity to demonstrate comprehension. Demonstrate the correct nonweight bearing gait. Allow the patient an opportunity to ask questions and demonstrate comprehension. Demonstrate the correct method of sitting and allow the patient an opportunity to demonstrate comprehension.	
3. Auscultate the chest for clearness of lungs and cardiac abnormalities. Check respirations for depth and rate. Assess the patient's ability to cough and deep breathe. Assess for the use of accessory muscles. Note any nasal flaring.	3. Potential alterations in respiratory function: ineffective airway clearance related to improper positioning and immobility.	3. Short-term goal: no respiratory problems due to immobility. Long-term goal: free of respiratory complications.	3. Prevent Complications *Respiratory* Explain rationale for preventing respiratory complications. Teach coughing and deep breathing exercises. Encourage good oral hygiene. Teach use of assistive equipment. Encourage the patient to turn and move in bed. Facilitate early ambulation. Increase fluid intake as indicated. Provide for the proper level of environmental humidity.	3. Determine that the patient is well hydrated and has no confusion. Breathing should be deep and regular with no shortness of breath or nasal flaring. The patient should have good color and normal temperature.

(continued)

TABLE 6–2. *(Continued)*

Assessment	Nursing Diagnosis	Goal Formulation	Planning and Intervention	Evaluation and Reassessment
Check whether patient is coughing up sputum. Assess for signs of confusion.			Elevate the head of the bed. Give back rubs with clapping and vibration.	
Assess vital signs. Observe the patient's color and temperature. Check for any increased pulse volume or increase in blood pressure. Check skin turgor and mucus membrane texture. Assess muscle tone and strength. Assess fluid intake and output. Note any jugular venous distention. Note any restlessness, anxiety, or change in mental status. Assess for shortness of breath, pulmonary congestion, abnormal breath sounds and change in respiratory pattern.	Potential fluid volume excess related to parenteral fluid intake. Potential fluid volume deficit related to decreased intake, lack of muscle tone, and volume loss in surgery.	Short-term goal: fluid volume within normal limits. Long-term goal: free of circulatory complications.	*Circulatory* Maintain hydration. Teach patient to change position slowly and resume a standing position gradually. Teach exercises for turning, lifting, and moving. Facilitate early ambulation. Teach use of elastic stockings. Administer prescribed anticoagulant drugs.	The patient should have no signs of congestive heart failure. Output should be within normal range when compared to intake. The patient should be well hydrated with good skin turgor. Vital signs should be within normal limits with no signs of confusion.

Auscultate for bowel sounds. Check for expulsion of flatus. Check fluid intake and output. Assess for nausea or anorexia. Check frequency and consistency of stools. Assess for abdominal softness. Assess for abdominal distention by measuring abdominal girth. Note pain medications and stool softners utilized. Check for any complaints of pressure in the rectum or pain on defecation. By manual examination, palpate for possible impaction.	Potential alteration in bowel elimination: constipation related to immobility and pain medications. Potential alteration in bowel elimination: ineffective bowel function related to immobility secondary to surgery and trauma.	Short-term goal: normal peristalsis and regular elimination without pain or discomfort. Long-term goal: free of gastrointestinal complications.	*Gastrointestinal* Teach exercises for movement and early ambulation. Maintain fluid and electrolyte balance. Discuss the need for diet with sufficient bulk, fluids, and roughage. Explain the effect of pain medication on elimination. Assist with proper physiological position for defecation. Explain rationale for stool softner and laxatives. Offer bedpan on a daily schedule.	Determine that the patient's abdomen is soft with no increase in abdominal girth. The patient should have no complaints of nausea or vomiting. Determine that the patient has return of normal bowel sounds and elimination pattern.
Assess for bladder distention. Note frequency, amount, color, and odor of urine, and whether urination is accompanied by pain. Check fluid intake and output.	Potential alteration in urinary elimination: infection due to urinary stasis related to immobility.	Short-term goal: urination without pain or discomfort. Long-term goal: free of any urinary complications.	*Genitourinary* Allow privacy. Offer bedpan on schedule. Assist patient into a comfortable physiological position for voiding. Maintain fluid and electrolyte balance. Explain rationale for drinking liquids that alter the acidity of the urine. Teach perineal care.	There should be no bladder distention or urinary incontinence. Determine if there is any pain or discomfort on voiding.

(continued)

TABLE 6–2. ***(Continued)***

Assessment	Nursing Diagnosis	Goal Formulation	Planning and Intervention	Evaluation and Reassessment
Assess range of motion of unaffected joints. Note the patient's ability to move and change position independently. Assess the patient's general muscular development and strength.	Potential alteration in mobility: contracture related to immobility.	Short-term goal: able to move freely without any joint impediment. Long-term goal: free of any mobility complications.	*Musculoskeletal* Teach correct positioning, and how to change position. Teach range-of-motion exercises. Teach exercises for muscle setting. Encourage independent movement. Make sure joints actually change position (re: flexion and extension).	The patient should have no decrease in joint mobility. Evaluate how well the patient is able to perform the exercise program and activities of daily living.
Assess for reddened areas over bony prominences and under traction apparatus. Note complaints of pain or discomfort on the heel, coccyx, etc.	Potential impairment of skin integrity: pressure areas related to immobility. Potential for injury: infection related to surgical incision.	Short-term goal: free of pain or discomfort from pressure. Long-term goal: free of any integumentary complications.	*Integumentary* Teach how a shearing force affects the skin. Explain rationale for use of sheepskin, eggcrate, etc. Schedule changes of position. Encourage fluids and a well-balanced diet. Maintain dry dressing.	The patient should not have any reddened areas. The patient should be free of any integumentary complications.

Assess for pain, hardness, heat, discoloration, and exudation in the area of the incision. Assess nutritional intake and hydration.			Use proper aseptic technique during wound care and dressing changes.	
4. Assess the patient's understanding of the surgical procedure and method of treatment and general ability to comprehend. Inquire about the patient's family and significant others. Assess the patient's home care resources. Observe for manifestations of anxiety.	4. Potential knowledge deficit related to injury and treatment methods.	4. Short- and long-term goals: a decrease in anxiety through increased knowledge.	4. Patient Teaching Explain expected postoperative course. Allow expression of feelings. Provide information to counter myths and misinformation related to surgery. Allow patients to participate in planning own care. Work with patient, family, and significant others in discharge planning. Discuss the restriction of no weight bearing on the involved foot. Stress "can do" activities.	4. The patient, family, and significant others should understand the rehabilitation regime. The home care resources available to the patient should be adequate. The patient, family, and significant others should understand what the patient can and cannot do. There should be a decrease in the patient's anxiety level about future ambulation.

mobility related to a lack of bone stability in the affected leg, (3) potential complications related to the surgical procedure and immobility, and (4) alterations in psychological well-being related to anxiety and knowledge deficit of treatment methods and rehabilitation process.

Short-term goals are to have the patient experience (1) a decrease in amount of pain in the hip through the use of nursing measures and prescribed medications, (2) an increase in mobility through the use of exercises and assistive devices, (3) an absence of complications from surgery and decreased activities, and (4) a decrease in anxiety through increased knowledge. Long-term goals are to have the patient free of pain and able to walk without discomfort using a three-point gait for the first 6 months to a year, and eventually able to walk without needing supportive devices.

Postoperative Planning and Intervention

Alleviate Pain. The first step is to assess for the location, severity, and degree of physical and emotional pain. Do not hesitate to give pain medications during the first 24 hours following surgery if the patient's condition allows. Talk to the patient and reassure the patient while trying physical nursing measures for pain relief. Sometimes the patient becomes anxious and tense, and tightens the muscles to prevent any movement. This increases the discomfort, but leads the patient to tighten the muscles even more. After reassuring the patient and getting the patient to relax the affected leg in your hands, use both hands and gently lift the leg and move it through its range of motion several times before repositioning it. Frequently the pain will go away or at least be greatly reduced. In general, muscle setting exercises, which increase circulation, help to relieve pain.

With the pain due to muscle tension eased by exercise, it is much easier to determine the amount of pain medication needed for the patient's underlying condition. Caution should be exercised to prevent oversedation or excessive doses of pain medication. Especially among the elderly, there is great variability in the absorption, distribution, metabolism, and excretion of drugs, and these factors may effect the patient's immediate and long-term responses to medications. Be alert for physical, behavioral, and mental changes that may be drug induced. Elderly patients on the whole do not tolerate sedatives well, particularly barbiturates, because they tend to produce drowsiness and a "hangover" the next day.

Do give medications for pain relief, but assess pain, try nursing measures for pain relief, note the dosage of all medications given, and definitely observe for physical and mental reactions to the drugs.

Increase Mobility

Position. Following hip surgery, efforts to increase the patient's mobility involve turning, exercise, and ambulation. Immediately after surgery, when the patient is supine, the affected leg should be in correct alignment (which for some patients, may mean being in slight abduction), but often the leg will have a tendency to move toward slight external rotation. To prevent external rotation, place a trochanter roll beside the lateral aspect of the thigh or, if need be, place a sandbag or trochanter roll along the lateral aspect of the lower leg. Make sure that it is not placed in a position that will apply pressure against the proximal portion of the fibula (near the location of the peroneal nerve) or the external malleolus. Teach the patient where the support should be positioned and why it is necessary. Another way to prevent external rotation is to teach the patient to keep the toes straight up toward the ceiling when lying supine.

Check to see if there are any specific restrictions in positions or activities for the patient. In general, the patient can have the head of the bed elevated for meals and activities of daily living. Most patients will not want the head elevated more than 30 to 40 degrees because of the stress that it places on the muscles of the hip and the fracture site. The patient should not have the head of the bed elevated at all times (unless medically warranted) because of the possibility of developing hip flexion contractures and the shearing effect on the skin at the coccyx.

Turning. When the patient returns to the unit from the postanesthesia room and the initial assessment is satisfactory, one of the first things to do is turn the patient to the unaffected side. The patient may have been lying supine for several hours on a variety of firm surfaces, and hence have some stiffness and discomfort. Turning immediately also lets the patient know that he or she is able to move. Movement helps the patient in expelling respiratory secretions and in improving circulation, and turning is usually done every 2 to 3 hours.

When helping a patient with a hip fracture turn following insertion of an internal fixation, avoid extremes of motion, prevent strain on the hip, maintain alignment of the affected leg and hip, and handle the operated leg gently. At first, the patient may be somewhat uncooperative because of pain and apprehension, but that usually passes after a few turns. Nurses usually work with the assumption of not turning a patient to the affected side unless there are specific orders. Most patients with internal fixations, however, are allowed to turn to the operated side because the bed acts as a splint for the injured hip. Sometimes patients cannot tolerate being turned completely onto the side, especially to the affected side. In those instances, turn the patient at least 45 degrees. If the patient is not allowed to turn for some reason, he or she may be able to lift straight up periodically with the use of the trapeze for back care and linen changes.

When turning the patient onto the unoperated side, place one pillow between the patient's thighs and another one or possibly two pillows, depending on the amount of abduction and the size of the patient, between the lower legs and the feet. The pillows help keep the operated leg aligned with the trunk, or in slight abduction when warranted, and prevent a twisting movement of the leg. A slight abduction reduces the stress to the incisional area and fracture site. In the beginning, at least two persons are necessary to turn the patient. In turning a patient with a fractured right hip onto the unaffected left side, one person gently places the hands under the patient's right side, with one hand under the patient's right shoulder and the other near the buttocks under the upper right thigh. The second person, on the left side of the bed, reaches across the patient, places one hand in the patient's lumbar area and the other under the right upper thigh distal to the first person's hand. The person on the left side of the bed is in a position to support the affected leg during the turn. The patient is then rolled toward the left side of the bed onto the unaffected side. The side rails should be up on the left side of the bed before the turn is started, and the patient should be encouraged to breathe out or at least breathe normally during the turning. Once the patient is turned to the side, the patient can use the side rails for support until complete positioning is done. The pillows prevent the operated leg from dropping down into adduction. While the patient is turned to the side, the knee of the affected leg may be flexed, and a slight flexion of the hip is also allowed. To foster mobility, make sure that the position of the patient's hip actually changes in the turn. Before leaving the patient, insure that the upper leg is securely positioned on the pillows.

If a patient takes a deep breath and holds it during the turn, it evokes the Valsalva maneuver. The Valsalva maneuver (filling the lungs, closing the glottis, and forcibly attempting to exhale) raises intrathoracic pressure and resists venous blood from entering the large veins. When the glottis is released and the lungs are allowed to exhale, the intrathoracic pressure falls, causing a large volume of blood to enter the heart. This may pose a serious problem for patients with cardiac conditions and for the elderly, because of the stress it places on the heart. Prevent the problem by having the patient breathe with the mouth open during the turn.

Exercises. Exercises should be started as soon as possible to restore normal joint function and muscle tone. If time and conditions allow, the patient may be taught some of the exercises before surgery, doing leg exercises with the unaffected leg. Exercises for the patient having hip surgery include breathing exercises, abdominal exercises, gluteal setting, quadriceps setting, plantar and dorsiflexion exercises (which exercise the muscle of the calf and foreleg), active range of motion of the ankle on the affected side, exercises for the upper extremities, and active range of motion for all unaffected joints. Most exercises are started on the first postoperative day.

At first, the patient should not be left alone to do the exercises. In assessing the degree of supervision required, consider the age of the patient, motivation, and understanding of what is being asked. Most patients need some assistance, probably need to have the instructions for the exercises gone over several times, possibly even every exercise time. Some of the exercises can be incorporated into self-care activities, which makes the patient more independent. Observe the patient for signs of fatigue, weakness, or stiffness. Encourage quadriceps and gluteal setting exercises hourly for the first 2 to 3 days.

To begin quadriceps setting exercises, the patient should sit or lie in a comfortable position and have the exercise demonstrated on the unaffected leg. Place a hand behind the knee and instruct the patient to press the knee down against the hand or have the patient pretend he or she is pushing the knee into the bed. A strong contraction of the quadriceps should occur when the patient presses. This tightening should be followed by complete relaxation. The patient should be taught to press for a slow count of three and then to relax for a slow count of three. The alternate contractions and relaxations of the muscle should be built up so that it can be performed 20 times an hour. The quadriceps femoris muscle extends the leg and is one of the major muscles necessary for ambulation.

The abdominal exercises (discussed under gastrointestinal complications), the breathing exercises (discussed under respiratory complications), and the gluteal setting exercises are isometric exercises that strengthen the muscle but do not move any joint. Gluteal setting exercises, which simply tighten and relax the gluteal muscles on a slow count of three, help to increase circulation to the gluteal area and preserve muscle tone.

Performing arm exercises (flexion and extension of the arms) strengthens the muscles in the shoulder girdle and upper extremities, which must be strong enough to bear the patient's weight so that the patient can use an assistive device for walking. The use of the trapeze, which strengthens the biceps of the arm, helps, but the major muscle in the arm that needs strengthening is the triceps. Strengthening of the triceps can be accomplished by the following exercises. The patient, in a sitting position, takes a weight in each hand and flexes both arms and then extends the hands above the head toward the ceiling. Another exercise uses sawed off crutches or books placed in the bed on each side of the patient. The patient pushes down on the books or crutches and lifts the buttocks off the bed.

Trapeze. Teach patients how to use the trapeze correctly. It will greatly help patients reposition themselves while supine, help them get out of bed, and enable them to assist when nurses have to reposition them in bed, give them the bedpan, administer skin care, and change the linen. Use of the trapeze helps maintain muscle tone and builds up strength in the arms and shoulders as well as helping to improve the functioning of the respiratory and circulatory systems. In using the trapeze, the patient should grasp it with both hands, and, flexing the unaffected knee and hip, bring the unaffected foot up and place it flat on the bed at least to the level of the knee of the affected leg. Next, the patient should pull on the trapeze and push down on the unaffected foot, lifting the buttocks off the bed. If the patient needs to move up in bed after lifting the buttocks, the patient should push with the unaffected foot to move the body toward the head of the bed. In the beginning, the nurse may have to assist because the patient lacks strength in the arms.

Ambulation. In some instances, patients who have had an internal fixation for a hip fracture may be allowed out of bed on the first postoperative day to sit in a chair. Before attempting to get the patient up, explain every step of the procedure. Tell the patient how he or she can be of help, and make sure the patient is informed about weight bearing on the affected leg. Commonly, patients with internal fixation devices are not allowed weight bearing on the affected leg in the early postoperative period. Depending on the size and age of the individual, weight bearing before bone union may exert too much stress to the fracture site and thus cause bending, breaking, or displacement of the implant, crushing of bone at the fracture site, or loss of fixation due to the device's cutting through the bone. Do not rush or try to hurry the patient through the transfer. First, move the patient so that the unaffected hip is at the side of the bed, and bring the patient to a sitting position on the edge of the bed. Let the patient sit there for a few mintues to prevent orthostatic hypotension. Next, pivot the patient into a chair, insuring that there is no weight bearing on the affected leg. The first time, the assistance of another person may be advisable. Talk to and reassure the patient during the activity. The patient can assume a normal sitting position, and encourage the patient to do exercises such as deep breathing, abdominal, gluteal, quadriceps setting, and ankle exercises while in the chair. If a chair that allows a rocking motion is available, it will help the patient to flex and extend the knees and ankles. After the patient gains confidence, and if the chair has arm rests, encourage the patient to periodically push down on the chair arms and raise the buttocks off the chair. The raising allows circulation to the buttocks and also helps build up muscles in the upper extremity for crutch walking.

Most patients start ambulation by first pivoting to a chair as described above. The time up in the chair may be gradually increased but not so that the patient becomes fatigued. Next, the patient will be able to use a walker. After developing a safe steady gait, most patients will progress to crutches, using a three-point gait. Crutches allow for more and easier mobility, and the patient should be encouraged to use them even if he or she feels less sure at first. Patients should also be taught how to get in and out of a chair and on and off the toilet, how to go up and down stairs with or without arm rails, and how to get in and out of a car. How to do these movements is discussed in Appendix C.

Prevent Complications. Most postoperative complications are related to imposed immobility, and are discussed in Chapter 3. Patients having internal fixations for fractured hips are particularly susceptible to pulmonary emboli, one of the leading causes of death following hip surgery. Fat emboli are especially likely in patients with fractures of the intratrochanteric or subtrochanteric regions. A paralytic ileus can occur. The most common musculoskeletal complications are flexion contractures of the hip and the knee and equinus contractures of the foot ("footdrop"). (For a discussion of these potential complications, see Chap. 3.)

Wound Infection. To enhance wound healing and avoid or control infection, physicians may place wound catheters (usually two) into the wound before closing the incision line. The wound catheters are generally inserted through the skin a few inches from the incision line. They may be connected to a Hemovac, J Vac, or Gomco for continuous suction. The placement of the catheters and the continuous suction is to prevent pooling of blood within muscle layers, which can be a source of infection. The catheters are usually in place 36 to 48 hours.

The initial dressing is usually removed the same day that the wound catheters are removed. The best procedure is to remove the wound catheters first and leave a pressure dressing on for an hour or so before changing the dressing. Reinforce a dressing if it becomes soiled or loosened. Once the initial dressing is removed, a variety of methods to care for the incision may be employed. One is to leave the incision open to the air. A second is to use alcohol swabs and do a daily cleansing of the incision, which toughens the skin. A third is to do a daily betadine scrub of the incision.

Nurses should recognize that most patients are not only weak from the trauma and shock of the injury and surgery, but are elderly. In preventing complications, therefore, it is frequently necessary to consider both orthopaedic and gerontological nursing concepts. Elderly patients are more likely to be affected by circulatory overload, skin breakdown, and constipation. Lower tract urinary infections are of special concern. Elderly men usually have an enlarged prostate and an atonic decompensated bladder. Elderly women may have interstitial cystitis, a contracted bladder, stress incontinency due to a prolapsed uterus, and urine collecting in the vagina because of their unaccustomed position during voiding.

Patient Teaching. Patients have rights whether they are coherent or confused, and one of those rights is the right to considerate and respectful care. For the patients who are confused, the first step is orientation to self, place, and time. Call them by name instead of using terms such as grandma unless the patient requests otherwise. Once the person is oriented, explain what has happened and what is being done. Patients have a right to receive information concerning diagnosis, treatment, and prognosis in terms they can be reasonably expected to understand. Most of that information is usually provided by the physician, but the nurse may need to go over it several times before the patient is able to comprehend what it means. Remember, having a fractured hip is very traumatic psychologically as well as physiologically. Most patients are elderly. Some have a fear of death, because many remember when an elderly person taken to the hospital with a fractured hip died. Most fear a fractured hip because it means not being able to walk and care for themselves.

The nurse must gain the confidence and trust of the patient. Spend time with the patient talking with the realistic assurance of someone who cares and wants to help. Use a lot of touch and direct eye contact. Let the patient have a say in decisions being made about care when possible. Encourage as much self-care as possible within medical limits.

A knowledgeable patient is a much more cooperative patient. Education begins when the patient is first seen on admission, in the emergency room, or on the unit. When the patient understands the rationale for specific exercises and positioning, he or she is much more willing to cooperate.

In general, adults learn better when working at their own pace. When the pace is determined by someone else, performance typically declines. Older individuals can and do learn. They just do it a little slower. It should be remembered that if one can simplify the demands of the task and make it meaningful, older people will do relatively well, though caution seems to increase with age.

Teaching the patient should be as well planned as the other aspects of care and follow the steps of the nursing process. Teaching sessions should be scheduled for when the nurse is unhurried and the time is right for the patient to learn. Patients under stress tend not to hear or comprehend all that is being said, and adults want to know how the information is relevant to them. Teaching materials can be collected from numerous sources. Many orthopaedic supply companies have educational materials available on request, either from their representative in the area or from the home office. You may create your own, individualized to the patient. Once you, the plan, the materials, and the patient are all ready, go over the material in simple steps, allowing time for the patient to comprehend and ask questions. If necessary have the patient demonstrate understanding by, for example, actually putting on those elastic stockings with an assistive device, and evaluate how well the patient understands the procedure.

Discharge planning should begin when the patient is admitted. Spend time with the patient discussing the realistic options for care once he or she leaves the hospital. The anticipated date of discharge to home, an extended care facility, or a nursing home is usually about 6 to 21 days, depending on the patient's medical condition. The patient, the family, and significant others need to be aware of approximate length of stay. Utilize the assistance of a social worker when warranted.

If the patient is to return to his or her own home or to the home of a family member or significant other, the home must be made safe. The patient will be using a walker or crutches, and should be able to safely go up and down stairs. Pets, such as cats and dogs, can cause an unsteady person to fall. Loose rugs should be removed and a comfortable chair should be available. Those who will be living with the patient should be aware of the extent to which the patient will not be self-sufficient, and know how to provide the nursing care, but do so without making an invalid out of the patient.

Evaluation and Reassessment

For a typical patient recovering from surgery with an internal fixation for a fractured hip, the evaluation would cover the following areas. In evaluating the goal of alleviating pain in the hip, determine whether the individual is having any pain by verbal responses and by the patient's outward appearance, including facial grimacing during movement, the positions assumed, restlessness, walking in a stooped position, and keeping the affected leg in a particularly stiff position. Sympathoadrenal signs signifying pain might be changes in pulse, blood pressure, and respiration, diaphoresis, depression and mood swings. If pain still exists, determine the location, duration, and intensity of the pain, what aggravates and intensifies it, and what measures have been able to relieve it. Inadequate reduction or avascular necrosis of the head of the femur may produce pain or muscle spasm beyond the normal pain associated with the healing of soft tissue and the beginning of bone calcification.

When evaluating care to increase mobility, determine the patient's compliance with the exercise routine and utilization of assistive devices such as the trapeze and walker or crutches. To what degree has the patient maintained or regained activities of daily living and range of motion? How steady is the nonweight-bearing gait with assistive device? Is the patient able to use crutches or is the walker still necessary? Determine whether or not the patient, the family, and significant others have been able to follow a rehabilitation regime, how well the family is managing with home care, and how useful the discharge plan appears to be. How well does the patient, the family, and significant others understand what the patient can and cannot do?

Prevention of complications should be evaluated. Look for the absence of contractures, pressure areas and decubiti, the absence of an elevated temperature, and other signs that complications are absent. If the goals have not been met, both the goals and the plan of care must be reassessed and the nursing process begun again.

Pathology

ARTHRITIS AND INFECTIOUS DISEASES

Rheumatoid Arthritis

Rheumatoid arthritis (RA) is a chronic, systemic disease in which inflammatory changes occur throughout the body's connective tissues. The articular and periarticular structures are progressively destroyed by chronic proliferative inflammation. The proliferating connective tissue tends to overgrow and erode the joint cartilage and to invade the supporting cancellous bone, leading to severe disability and deformity, often with ankylosis of the joint. As the disease destroys the joints internally, the patient suffers pain, stiffness, and swelling. Small joints, such as the joints in the hands, wrists, elbows, feet, and ankles, are usually involved before weight-bearing joints such as the hips and knees (Luckmann & Sorenson, 1980, p. 1705). (For further information on RA, see Chap. 4.)

Surgery plays an important role in the treatment and rehabilitation of patients with RA of the hip who do not respond adequately to nonoperative measures. Operations on the joints can be effective in preventing some deformities, in relieving pain, and in improving overall function. Many types of operations have proved successful in the past, and new procedures have been developed that promise success in the future. It is no longer necessary to wait until the disease has run its course in the hip if it is believed surgery can help the patient.

For patients with RA, persistent pain unrelieved by conservative methods is the most demanding reason for surgery. Pain during activities can be controlled by the patient through restricting those activities, but pain at rest and at night may convince the patient and the physician of the need for surgical intervention. A second important indicator is the restriction of movement in the hip.

Surgical Procedures

Over the years, many surgical procedures have been used for RA of the hip, but few have been very successful:

1. Synovectomy (removal of the synovial membrane), effective on a number of other joints, was found to be unsuitable for the hip joint.
2. Arthrodesis (surgical fusion of a joint) of the hip was found to be an excellent procedure if the other hip, lumbar spine, and knees work well. Because this is rarely the case, arthrodesis is usually contraindicated.
3. The Girdlestone procedure (removal of the lip of the acetabulum, the greater trochanter, the neck and head of the femur, and creating a gliding surface between the two bones), originally introduced for tuberculosis of the hip, requires a long convalescence, and active control of the joint is slow to develop. After recovery, passive range of motion is good and pain at rest is relieved, but discomfort persists on activity. More importantly, the hip joint is unstable, and the patient must use crutches or canes to ambulate, a serious problem for patients with upper extremity RA.
4. A subtrochanteric or femoral osteotomy (cutting a wedge into the femur to allow a change in the position of weight bearing in the joint) does not materially improve the stability of the hip either, and the femoral head has been known to collapse after such procedures.
5. An Austin-Moore, Bateman, or Thompson endoprosthesis (removal of the head and neck of the femur and replacement with a metallic component with the metallic head the same size as the one removed) is of value only if the acetabulum is healthy, so for patients with RA this procedure is not useful because the acetabulum is always involved.
6. Some patients who cannot withstand extensive surgery can benefit from an operation that severs the muscles that move the hip joint. This

"hanging hip" procedure permits some limited ambulation while providing symptomatic relief.

7. The cup arthroplasty or mold arthroplasty (where the acetabulum is reamed down to untraumatized surface and a metal cup is fitted over the head of the femur), which has been used since 1943, has a long rehabilitative period, with 12 or more months or non- or partial-weight bearing. It is still considered in adolescents or young adults where the disease has not progressed to the stage of severe bone involvement, and where symptoms with disability persist despite a full and fair trial of conservative treatment.

A total hip arthroplasty (removing the head and neck of the femur, reaming out the femoral canal and acetabulum, and implanting a polyethylene acetabular cup and a metallic femoral component) has become the surgery of choice for most adult RA patients. For patients considered too young for a total hip replacement, a total joint surface replacement, which involves only the joint surfaces and not the joint itself, is indicated. The joint surface of the femoral head is capped by a metallic shell held in place by methyl methacrylate, and a plastic cup is cemented into the acetabular cavity. The main advantage of this technique is that the femoral head and neck are preserved rather than resected. It allows the retention of adequate bone stock for further reconstructive hip surgery should these implants fail.

Osteoarthritis

Osteoarthritis (also known as degenerative joint disease or hypertrophic arthritis) is a "wear and tear" type of degenerative disease process of joints affecting most weight-bearing joints. The noninflammatory disease is characterized by deterioration and abrasion of articular cartilage with formation of new bone at the joint surfaces. These outgrowths are called osteophytes or spurs. Nearly all individuals over 45 years of age have some degeneration, but symptoms occur only in a small number of individuals. The onset is insidious and gradual, with aching pain the most common symptom. Other symptoms are limitation of motion, contractures, and muscle spasms. Pain is not pronounced after exercise, and pain at rest may be caused by muscle spasm. Osteoarthritis of the hip may occur as a complication of other hip disorders, such as fractures and fracture–dislocations involving the femoral neck, the femoral head, or the acetabulum.

Osteoarthritis of the hip produces pain, limp, limited joint motion, and deformity of the affected leg. Pain is usually felt in the region of the groin and may be referred along the anterior surface of the thigh to the knee, along the lateral aspect of the thigh, or posteriorly to the buttock or low back area. Pain is invariably associated with a sensation of stiffness. In severe hip joint involvement, the affected leg tends to shorten and turn into external rotation. The leg is usually flexed and adducted at the hip joint. Limp may be due to pain, stiffness, shortening of the leg, or disturbance in gluteus medius function. Often several of these factors operate to produce an abnormal gait in a patient with an externally rotated leg.

The presence of flexion contractures of the hip and limited joint motion is detected by comparing the passive range of motion obtained in both hips, as patients with osteoarthritis of the hip joint usually lose hip joint motion sequentially. The ability to rotate the hip joint internally or externally is always lost first. The motion of abduction and adduction are lost next, with hip flexion maintained longest. (For more information on osteoarthritis, see Chap. 4.)

Surgical Procedure

Surgical procedures are becoming more important as part of the treatment program for patients with osteoarthritis of the hip. A variety of different procedures may be performed to relieve general symptoms, decrease pain, improve function, and correct deformities. For example, an osteotomy of the femoral neck may relieve symptoms by changing the position of the head of the femur when it is being subjected to impact stress against the acetabulum. Persons with advanced joint destruction and intractable pain may benefit from surgical procedures such as arthrodesis or arthroplasty. Arthrodesis sacrifices function of the joint but relieves pain in severely damaged joints. The "hanging hip" procedure, which permits some limited ambulation while providing symptomatic relief, has been effective in some elderly persons. Arthroplasty, (total hip replacement) is used when the destructive process has involved both the acetabulum and the femoral head.

Osteomyelitis

Osteomyelitis is an infection in or around bone. It is caused by *Staphylococcus aureus* in 70 to 80 percent of the cases, but can also be caused by *Streptococcus* and *Pneumococcus*. The condition can be either acute or chronic, though the acute form is rare in adults. The infection is most often bloodborne from another infected area, but it can develop directly as a result of an open fracture, a surgical procedure, a puncture, or a gun shot wound. Osteomyelitis can cause the nonunion of fractures (Gartland, 1979, p. 176), and both the infection and the nonunion of the fracture may follow unsuccessful open reduction of the fracture. In most instances, the infection tends to remain medullary, progressing to cancellous and cortical bone. When the suppurative process reaches the periosteum, erosion occurs and a soft-tissue abscess forms. If the infection invades the bone itself, the bone undergoes necrosis and has a tendency to retain the infection, resulting in retardation of the healing process. The necrotic area can become a potential focal point for reinfection. The sequestrum or necrotic bone can be surgically separated from normal bone, and following that procedure, new bone begins to form as the body attempts to repair itself. However, some remaining sequestrum may be covered by new bone although healing seems to occur, the remaining sequestrum becomes chronically infected and is prone to repeated abscess formation. In the hip joint this may lead to resecting the joint and the surrounding tissue. Prevention is the most critical factor in eliminating osteomyelitis (Armstrong et al., 1979, p. 1043). (For more information on osteomyelitis, see Chap. 4.)

Surgical Procedure

Most adults with osteomyelitis of the hip, who are candidates for surgery, have had the infection for some time, and medical management with antibiotics, even by the closed irrigation method, has been ineffective. These patients have been having pain for some time, and may even appear physically debilitated because the pain has caused loss of appetite. They tend to hold the affected leg in a position of hip flexion because it reduces the strain on the hip and thus they may have a hip flexion contracture. They are usually extremely apprehensive, especially of having the affected leg moved. If moving the leg is necessary, handle it gently, but securely and slowly. Another realistic fear the patient has is the uncertainty of the outcome. Their self-image is impaired by the prospect of scars, deformity, and limitation of motion. The most common surgery, the Girdlestone procedure, generally does leave the patient with some degree of limited mobility. At best, the recovery and rehabilitation from surgery will be prolonged, difficult for the patient to adjust to, and probably expensive.

Tuberculosis

Tuberculosis of the hip is the second most common form of skeletal tuberculosis, and the majority of patients with turberculosis of the hip are young children. In most cases, a previous infection in the lung acts as the source, although genitourinary or intrapelvic tuberculosis abscesses can extend directly into the hip or reach it through the lymphatic system. Because there does not have to be a pulmonary focus for tuberculosis to exist in the hip, its diagnosis is sometimes difficult.

When tuberculosis is diagnosed early, before joint destruction, immobilization and chemotherapy may induce healing and preserve joint mobility. Bedrest with traction can then be done to counteract muscle spasm and pain. For irreparable joint destruction, operative fusion for control of infection and relief of pain is necessary. The joint is surgically cleaned of all tubercular tissues and articular cartilage, and the denuded cancellous bone of the femoral head and acetabulum are placed in contact. An iliac bone graft is usually placed between the ilium and the femur to promote osteogenesis. If an abscess or draining skin sinuses are present, some physicians will do an extra-articular fusion, that is, bypass the hip joint and run the iliac graft from the trochanteric area of the femur to the ischium.

Surgical Procedures

Osteotomy. A femoral osteotomy involves surgery on the femur, which changes its alignment, altering weight bearing in the hip joint, and transferring a greater part of the body's weight to healthier parts of the joint (Fig. 6–6). The

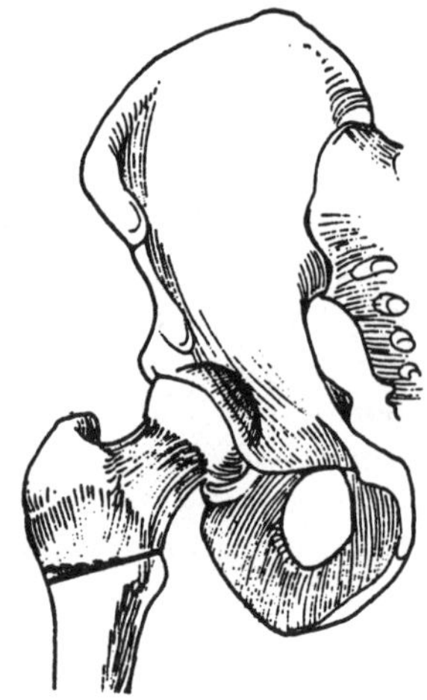

Figure 6–6. Intertrochanteric osteotomy is done to relieve pain early in the course of degenerative joint disease, when hip motion is still good. Weight is shifted from bad cartilage onto good cartilage, either by an opening-wedge (shown here) or closing-wedge osteotomy. *(Reproduced with permission of* Patient Care, *March 15, 1972, p. 88. Copyright © 1972, Patient Care Communications, Inc., Darien, Conn. All rights reserved.)*

procedure, which has a number of variations, may also be used to correct angulation or deformities. Postoperatively the femur is immobilized in some manner, and the care of the patient is the same as that of a patient who has had a hip fracture. The time when weight bearing may begin and the amount of weight bearing that will be allowed depend on the specific type of surgical procedure used.

Hanging Hip. The "hanging hip" operation, developed by Voss, releases the fascia lata and the adductor muscles in an attempt to decrease pressure on the articular cartilage of the hip (Fig. 6–7).Many versions of this procedure have

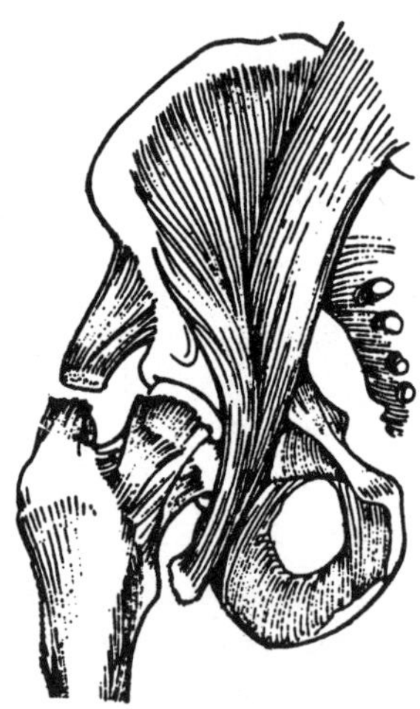

Figure 6–7. Hanging hip operation candidates are old patients who may never walk again, but whose pain can be relieved if the tight structures about the hip are cut to allow articular surfaces to separate. *(Reproduced with permission of* Patient Care, *March 15, 1972, p. 88. Copyright © 1972, Patient Care Communications, Inc., Darien, Conn. All rights reserved.)*

been developed. Some physicians release different muscles, others do the muscle release in combination with another procedure, such as an osteotomy, and still other physicians do a closed adductor tenotomy. The effect of the muscle-release operation is muscular decompression, correction of contractures, and improvement of weight-bearing surfaces. The main goals of the muscle-release operation are the relief of pain and the correction of harmful soft tissue contractures. The degree of joint motion does not usually increase postoperatively, but the correction of contractures places it into a more useful range. The main complications are thrombophlebitis and pulmonary embolism. Other complications, such as anterior subluxation of the femoral head and marked and prolonged abductor limp, can be prevented with proper surgical technique and adequate postoperative muscle reeducation.

□ NURSING PROCESS (Table 6–3)

Assessment

In general, the preoperative physical assessment focuses on pain in the hip, contractures of the hip, and patient mobility. Patients with osteoarthritis tend to be older, but patients with RA may be of any age. It is essential to assess the patient's strength in the upper extremities for mobility with assistive devices, and the ability to do self-care. If the patient with RA is having hip problems, he or she probably also has advanced problems with the smaller joints, which may impede other activities. It is especially important to assess the emotional reaction of the patient toward the pathology and the impending surgery. (For a more detailed assessment of a patient with arthritis, see Chapter 4, and for a more complete assessment of orthopaedic patients, see Chapter 2.)

Following the "hanging hip" procedure, the patient is assessed following the format discussed in the postoperative care of patients undergoing an internal fixation for a fractured hip. Specifically, the nurse should observe the amount of drainage from the wound catheters, the alignment and positioning of the involved leg, and the amount of weight, fit, and position of the Buck's traction, and do neurovascular checks of the affected leg.

Nursing Diagnosis and Goal Formulation

Typically, nursing diagnoses and goals, which are derived from the assessment are (1) alterations in comfort related to hip pain from pathology and surgery, (2) alterations in mobility related to decreased muscle integrity, (3) alterations in psychological well-being related to anxiety and knowledge deficit about future mobility with or without the use of an assistive device, and (4) potential complications due to the surgical procedure and decreased activity.

Short-term goals are to have the patient experience (1) a decrease in pain through the use of nursing measures and prescribed medications, (2)

TABLE 6–3. NURSING PROCESS FOR HANGING HIP PROCEDURE WITH BUCK'S TRACTION

Assessment	Nursing Diagnosis	Goal Formulation	Planning and Intervention	Evaluation and Reassessment
1. Check vital signs. Assess neurovascular status. Assess the duration, location and severity of pain. Assess tightness of the traction boot.	1. Alteration in comfort: hip pain related to soft tissue and bone trauma.	1. Short-term goal: a reduction in pain through the use of nursing measures and prescribed medications. Long-term goal: regain optimal hip function.	1. Alleviate Pain Maintain Buck's traction. Move leg carefully when repositioning. Teach relaxation techniques. Utilize noninvasive nursing measures to relieve pain. Administer prescribed pain medications.	1. Positioning and other nursing measures should keep the patient fairly comfortable. Medication should relieve severe pain.
2. Check for correct positioning of leg. Check for correct maintenance of traction. Assess for correct body alignment. Assess ability to do exercises. Check for safety when crutch walking.	2. Impaired physical mobility: reduced hip function related to a decrease in muscle integrity.	2. Short-term goal: an increase in mobility by muscle reeducation through the use of exercises and ambulation techniques. Long-term goal: regain optimal hip function.	2. Increase Mobility *Position* Keep patient supine. Teach patient how to use trapeze. *Exercises* Teach bed exercises (quadriceps, gluteal setting and active range of motion of the ankle). Explain rationale for muscle reeducation and Hubbard-Tank done by PT. Teach upper extremity exercises for crutch walking. *Traction* Maintain 5–7 pounds of Buck's traction while in bed. Discuss rationale and purpose of traction. *Ambulation* Assist patient to wheelchair (usually third day after surgery). Demonstrate transfer to wheelchair. Demonstrate crutch walking with no weight bearing.	2. The patient should be able to stay supine, keep traction in place, and do the required exercises. The patient should accept responsibility for exercising without supervision. With practice, the patient should be able to transfer to a wheelchair without help.

3. Assess for pain in the affected leg. Check for a positive Homan's sign. Assess for any redness in the leg or increased temperature.	3. Potential alteration in peripheral tissue perfusion: thrombus related to immobility.	3. Short- and long-term goals: free of any circulatory complications.	3. Prevent Complications *Circulatory* Maintain patient hydration. Teach exercises and frequent changes in position. Facilitate early ambulation. Apply elastic stockings. Administer prescribed anticoagulant drugs.	3. The patient should remain free of complications due to surgery and immobility.
Auscultate the chest for lung clearance. Check respiratory rate, depth, and rhythm. Assess patient's color. Check for any shortness of breath or chest pain. Check for any petechiae.	Potential alterations in respiratory function: impaired gas exchange related to pulmonary and fat emboli.	Short- and long-term goals: free of any respiratory complications.	*Respiratory* Keep patient well hydrated. Administer anticoagulant drugs. Teach muscle setting exercises. *Occurrence of Emboli* Immobilize patient. Elevate head of bed. Start oxygen. Notify physician. *Potential Complications Due to Immobility* (See Table 6–2 and Chap. 3)	The patient should remain free of respiratory problems.
4. Assess the patient's level of understanding concerning the rehabilitation process and home care.	4. Potential knowledge deficit related to the rehabilitation process and home care.	4. Short- and long-term goals: a decrease in anxiety through increased knowledge.	4. Patient Teaching Discuss the various steps in the rehabilitation process. Help in setting realistic goals. Discuss ways of implementing care at home. Demonstrate techniques of bathing and dressing.	4. The patient should be able to discuss rehabilitaion and prognosis. The patient should be able to implement ways of bathing, dressing and continuing the rehabilitation exercise program at home.

an increase in mobility by muscle reeducation through the use of exercises and the help of a physical therapist, (3) a decrease in anxiety through increased knowledge about the surgical procedure, muscle reeducation, postoperative care, and prognosis, and (4) an absence of complications from surgery and decreased activity. Long-term goals are to have the patient (1) free of pain or with only minimal pain in the hip, (2) mobile without even an abductor limp within 6 months to 1 year, and (3) able to accept physical conditions with a realistic, positive outlook.

Planning and Intervention

Alleviate Pain. While talking with the patient, try physical measures for pain relief. Then, if necessary, use prescribed medication. Handle the affected extremity carefully when repositioning or moving for any reason. The Buck's traction also helps to relieve pain by decreasing muscle spasms. See the nursing care of a patient with an internal fixation for further details on measures for pain relief (p. 256).

Increase Mobility

Exercises. Patients need a positive attitude toward exercises as they will have to continue them long after leaving the hospital. Teach patients how to use the overhead trapeze to change position and assist in their own care. Bed exercises, which usually begin with muscle setting (isometric) exercises such as quadriceps, gluteal setting, and active range of motion of the ankle, are discussed in more detail for the patient with an internal fixation. Physical therapy, including Hubbard-tank treatments and muscle reeducation, is usually begun 2 weeks after surgery.

Buck's Traction. Postoperatively, intermittent Buck's traction (approximately 5 to 7 pounds) is usually used for a period of 2 weeks. Buck's traction (Fig. 6–8) is a means to maintain a steady pull on the involved leg, to alleviate or eliminate muscle spasm and pain, and to keep the leg in correct position and alignment. (For further details see Appendix A.)

Ambulation. Beginning about the third postoperative day, the patient is allowed up in a wheelchair for increasing periods of time. Exercises to assist with crutch walking should be encouraged if the patient was not using crutches before surgery. Note patient safety, especially if the gait is different from the preoperative gait. Crutch walking without weight bearing on the involved leg is started after 1 week, and with partial weight bearing after 2 weeks. Crutches can usually be discarded after 3 months, but a cane may be used for several months or even the rest of the patient's life. The abductor limp often disappears between 6 months and a year with effective physical therapy.

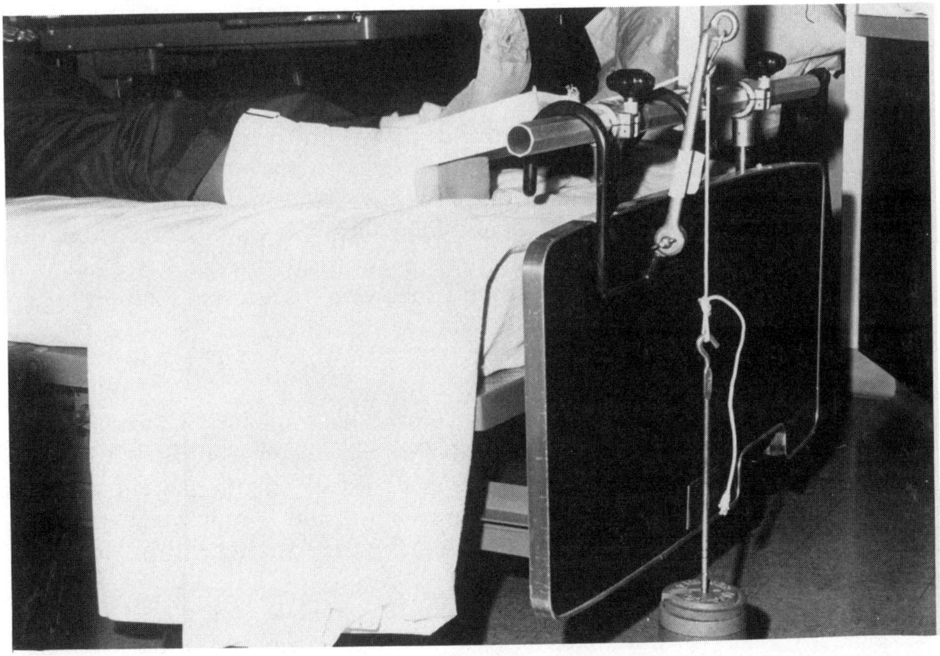

A

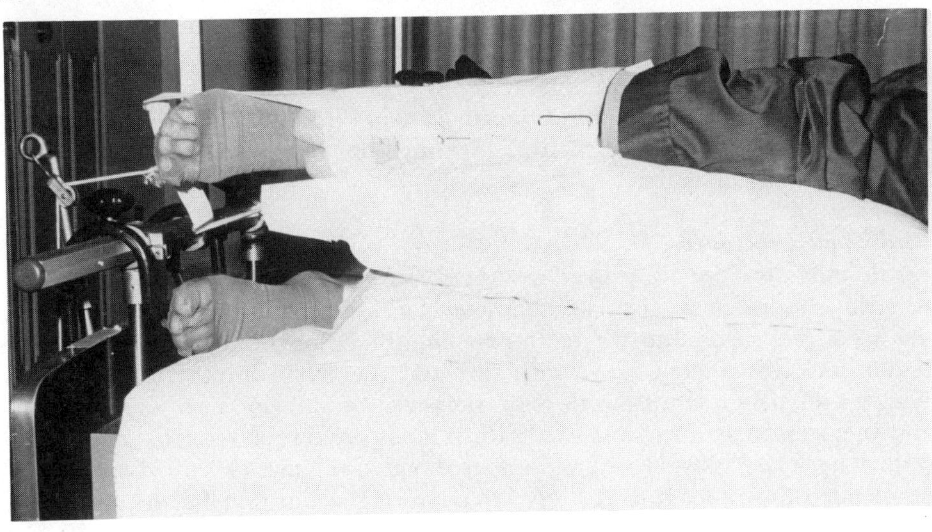

B

Figure 6–8. A. Buck's traction. **B.** Buck's traction (side lying). *(Courtesy of Carle Foundation Hospital and Clinic.)*

Patient Teaching. Allocate time for therapeutic communication with the patient, the family, and significant others. Discuss realistic short- and long-term goals, the safety of the home environment, and coping with restricted mobility.

Prevent Complications. The patient has undergone a major surgical procedure; therefore, nursing measures must focus on preventing complications common to all surgical patients. In particular, following a hanging hip procedure patients are prone to thrombophlebitis and pulmonary embolism. (For a more detailed plan of care to prevent these problems, see Chap. 3 and for the nursing care of a patient following an internal fixation of the hip, see Table 6–2.)

Evaluation and Reassessment

For the typical patient recovering from a "hanging hip" procedure, the evaluation would cover the four goals that have been identified. The evaluation of pain is essentially the same as described for the patient who has had an internal fixation. Usually the level of pain is much below what it was preoperatively, as the major reason for the hanging hip procedure is the reduction of pain.

Evaluate whether the patient is able to ambulate with a safe gait. The patient's ability to ambulate largely depends on how well and how diligently exercises have been done to reeducate the muscles. Does the patient have a positive attitude toward and an understanding of the exercises? Continually check for the presence of potential complications such as thrombophlebitis and pulmonary embolism.

If the evaluation should find that the desired goals are not being met, both the goals and the plan of care must be reassessed and the nursing process begun again.

Girdlestone Procedure

Girdlestone developed a procedure to cut away the lip of the acetabulum and trim the femoral neck to create gliding surfaces between the bones. By leaving the lip of the acetabulum alone and keeping much of the inferior neck of the femur, a cleft is created between the greater trochanter and the inferior neck. A new articulation can then develop between the inferior neck of the femur and the acetabular lip (Amstutz, 1973, p. 684). Different versions of the procedure have been developed, and one is shown in Figure 6–9. Girdlestone recommended the procedure for any infection of the hip that failed to respond to conservative treatment, but at present most physicians do not agree. The Girdlestone operation is so extensive that it produces a marked shortening of the leg, and can result in an ankylosis or in a nearly useless pseudoarthrosis (i.e., false joint) on which weight bearing is virtually impossible. For those reasons, most physicians consider the procedure a last resort (Edmondson & Crenshaw, 1980, p. 1070). It is mainly used for patients with pyogenic infection after hip surgery, or a chronic infection secondary to infectious arthritis or

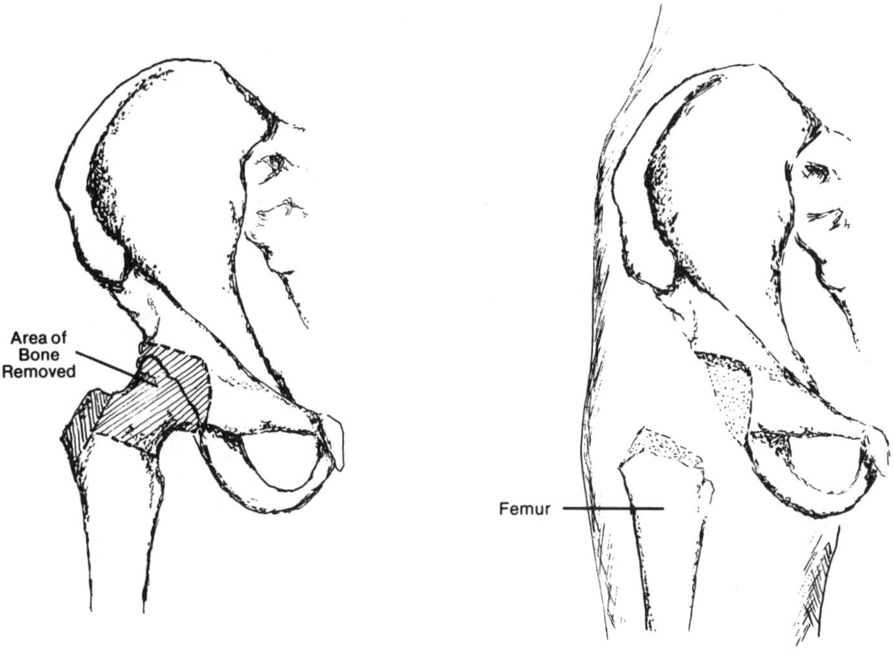

Figure 6–9. Girdlestone procedure. *(From Brantley, P., & Analla, M., 1980, p. 69. Courtesy of Howmedica.)*

tuberculosis, or in instances involving osteomyelitis of the hip joint with surrounding muscle infection (Edmondson & Crenshaw, 1980, p. 1070; Gartland, 1979, p. 69).

□ NURSING PROCESS (Table 6–4)

Assessment

Because the typical patient undergoing the Girdlestone procedure has a history of chronic hip infection, pain, and decreased mobility, the general physical and emotional condition may be weak. Postoperatively, most patients have some kind of traction applied to the involved leg, which should be in neutral rotation and slight abduction. In some instances, the patient may be immobilized in a hip spica cast.

Nursing Diagnosis and Goal Formulation

The nursing diagnoses for a typical patient following a Girdlestone procedure are (1) alterations in comfort related to hip pain from muscle and bone surgery, (2) alterations in mobility related to lack of joint integrity in

TABLE 6–4. NURSING PROCESS FOR GIRDLESTONE PROCEDURE WITH SKELETAL TRACTION

Assessment	Nursing Diagnosis	Goal Formulation	Planning and Intervention	Evaluation and Reassessment
1. Assess the location, duration, and severity of pain. Observe for verbal and nonverbal cues of pain. Check vital signs. Assess neurovascular status.	1. Alteration in comfort: hip pain related to soft tissue and bone trauma.	1. Short-term goal: a decrease in hip pain through nursing measures, traction, and prescribed medications. Long-term goal: free of hip pain.	1. Alleviate Pain Maintain traction. Keep leg in correct alignment. Utilize noninvasive pain relief measures. Utilize distraction. Teach relaxation techniques. Administer pain medications as needed.	1. The level of pain should diminish with healing of soft tissue and the development of a pseudoarthrosis.
2. Assess the position of the leg and the positioning of the traction. Check for correct body alignment. Assess the patient's ability to do the exercise regime. Check muscle strength.	2. Impaired physical mobility: decreased hip function related to lack of joint integrity in the involved hip.	2. Short-term goal: an increase in mobility by doing bed exercises and utilizing traction. Long-term goal: regain optimal function.	2. Increase Mobility *Position* Keep patient supine. Keep leg in a neutral position with slight abduction. Discuss rationale of traction. Maintain hip in 20–30 degrees of flexion. *Exercises* Demonstrate isometric exercises. Teach upper extremity exercises for crutch walking. Demonstrate knee and hip exercises.	2. Correct leg position should be accomplished with traction. The patient should be able to do the exercise regime without supervision.

			Ambulation Demonstrate the nonweight-bearing crutch gait. Allow time for patient's return demonstration.	
3. Assess for any redness, hardness, increased temperature, or pain in the incisional area. Check vital signs.	3. Potential for injury: infection related to breaks in skin integrity.	3. Short- and long-term goals: free of any complications.	3. Prevent Complications *Integumentary* Keep dressing clean and dry. Do pin care. Encourage a well-balanced diet with plenty of fluids. *Potential Complications Due to Immobility* (See Chap. 3 and Table 6–2)	3. The patient should remain free of any complications.
4. Assess level of understanding of the rehabilitation process and prognosis. Assess for stages of adjustment to a disability.	4. Potential knowledge deficit related to surgical procedure and rehabilitation.	4. Short- and long-term goals: a decrease in anxiety through increased knowledge.	4. Patient Teaching Allow time for therapeutic communication. Have open discussion about prognosis. Discuss the various stages of the rehabilitation process. Discuss home care with patient, family, or significant other. Include family or significant other in teaching plan.	4. The patient, family, and significant other should have a decrease in anxiety level with increased knowledge. The patient should be able to start discussing future ambulation and help in planning home care.

the involved hip, (3) alterations in the psychological well-being related to anxiety and knowledge deficit about the surgical procedure and future mobility, and (4) potential complications related to preoperative infection and decreased activity.

Short-term goals are to have the patient experience (1) a decrease in the amount if not all of the hip pain through nursing measures and prescribed medications, (2) an increase in the potential for mobility by doing bed exercises and utilizing traction, (3) a decrease in anxiety through increased knowledge, and (4) an absence of complications related to preoperative infection and decreased activity. Long-term goals are to have the patient (1) free of pain or with only minimal pain in the hip, (2) able to ambulate, though probably with an abductor lurch gait using a shoe with an elevated sole and heel, and (3) positive toward future ambulation with an elevated shoe, with or without additional assistive devices.

Planning and Intervention

Alleviate Pain. While talking with the patient, try physical measures for pain relief. Then, if necessary, use pain medication. Traction helps to relieve muscle spasm and to immobilize the joint space.

Increase Mobility

Skeletal Traction. Traction is used to insure that the leg is in neutral rotation and slight abduction so that the greater trochanter is kept snug against the acetabular lip. This position encourages the development of a pseudoarthrosis. If an adductor contracture develops, the neck of the femur will slip past the acetabular edge and the joint will be unstable. Many physicians use 10 pounds of skeletal traction for 6 weeks, with a pin through the tibia and the hip in 20 to 30 degrees of flexion (Fig. 6–10). This procedure is generally used in combination with a Thomas splint and a Pearson attachment. During that time the patient should do knee and hip exercises in a sling–suspension apparatus. Other physicians use a balanced suspension and skin traction with 7 pounds for 4 weeks, followed with intermittent traction for an additional 4 weeks and physiotherapy to mobilize the hip and strengthen the hip muscles. Still other physicians immobilize the hip using a hip spica cast.

Ambulation. During the 4 to 6 weeks of immobilization, the patient should do bed exercises and exercises to help with ambulation, especially to build strength in the arms. In the beginning, ambulation may be started on parallel bars with no weight bearing on the involved leg. Partial weight bearing with crutches usually begins after 8 weeks. Usually braces are not used, but the patient will be fitted with a shoe that has the temporary sole and heel elevated to partially compensate for the 3/4- to 1 1/4-inch shortening of the involved leg. The shoe is usually not elevated to make the legs

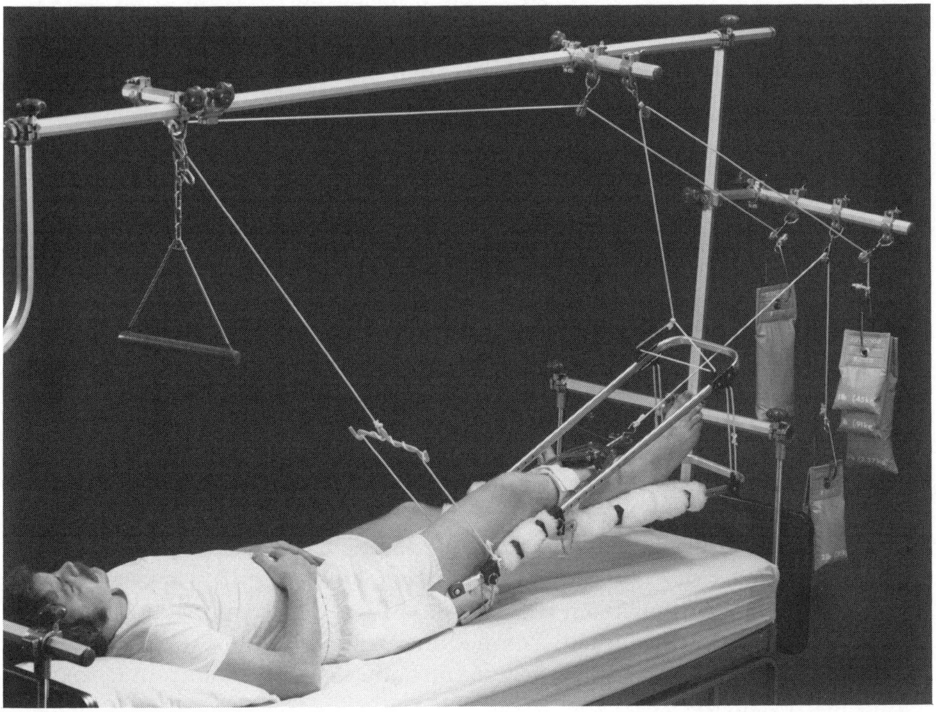

Figure 6–10. Balanced traction and suspension with Thomas leg splint (utilizing skeletal traction). *(Courtesy of Zimmer, Inc.)*

of equal length, forcing the patient into an abductor lurch gait, and thereby prevent an adduction contracture. The patient may be able to walk with one or two canes 4 to 6 months after surgery. Some patients, however, will never be able to walk without crutches.

Patient Teaching. Allocate time for therapeutic communication with the patient, the family, and significant others. Keep in mind the stages of adjustment to a disability. Let the patient know that the pain in the hip will diminish gradually with the healing of the soft tissue surrounding the hip joint and the formation of a pseudoarthrosis. For a more detailed plan of care to prevent these problems, see the nursing care of a patient following an internal fixation of the hip (pp. 261–262).

Prevent Complications. To deal with problems of infection, antibiotics are usually given for 6 weeks or more. See Table 6–2 and Chapter 3 for further measures on how to prevent complications.

Evaluation and Reassessment

The considerations discussed for the patient who has had an internal fixation apply here as well. Special emphasis should be given to problems of immobility in the initial stage of recovery and to the patient's attitude and ability to ambulate in the latter stage.

Arthrodesis

A hip arthrodesis is the surgical fusion of a hip joint (Fig. 6–11). Its purpose is to halt the disease process, provide stability, and relieve pain. Some physicians feel that it is the best type of surgery for young men with chronic hip joint infection, for with a good spinal column and no problems with the other hip, fusing the infected hip gives it stability and allows the patient to do heavy manual labor (Gartland, 1979, p. 396). With the present extensive use of the total hip replacement procedure, however, there is a decreased use of hip arthrodesis. It is most strongly indicated for tuberculosis of the hip, a pyogenic hip joint, and osteoarthritis (especially of a traumatic nature in a young patient). There are major complications with the hip arthrodesis. Specifically, (1) there is a high rate of nonunion, especially in infected hips; (2) in hip fusions where internal fixation is used, fatigue fractures may develop at the level where the metallic implants end; (3) because 4 or more months of bedrest typically follow surgery, there is a danger from the disabilities that develop during immobility; and (4) the femur may be malpositioned in surgery. The most obvious disadvantage for the patient is that there is no motion in the joint, and, for that reason many patients avoid the procedure.

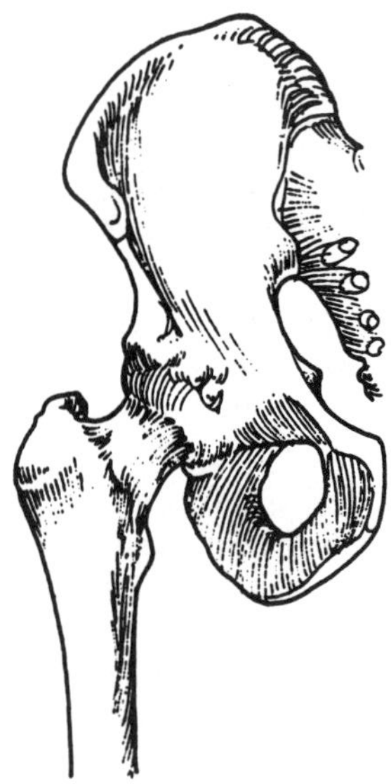

Figure 6–11. Arthrodesis is an ideal operation for the young, vigorous male. The joint is fused, becoming very stable, enabling patients to do heavy work. *(Reproduced with permission of* Patient Care, *March 15, 1972, p. 88. Copyright © 1972, Patient Care Communications, Inc., Darien, Conn. All rights reserved.)*

□ NURSING PROCESS (Table 6–5)

Assessment

Because most of the patients undergoing hip arthrodesis have a history of infection, look for systemic infection and for pain in the soft tissue and bone of the hip. If the hip was securely fixed internally and no femoral osteotomy was done, immobilization in a cast may or may not be used. However, if the hip arthrodesis did not utilize an internal fixation device, or if an intertrochanteric or subtrochanteric osteotomy was done, the patient will be in a hip spica cast from the nipple line to the toes on the affected side and to just above the knee on the other side. Assess for physical discomfort from the cast and for emotional reactions such as feelings of claustrophobia, tightness, or being unable to breathe. Assessment of the respiratory and gastrointestinal system is an ongoing need during the time the patient is in the cast.

Nursing Diagnosis and Goal Formulation

The nursing diagnoses for a typical patient following a hip arthrodesis are (1) alterations in comfort related to hip pain from muscle and bone surgery, (2) alterations in mobility related to lack of joint mobility due to surgery and an immobilizing device, (3) alterations in psychological well-being related to anxiety and knowledge deficit from surgical procedure, immobilization, and future ambulation, and (4) potential complications related to preoperative infection and decreased activity.

The short-term goals are to have the patient experience (1) a decrease in the amount, if not all, of the pain in the hip, (2) an increase in the potential for ambulation by doing bed exercises and keeping the hip joint immobile, (3) a decrease in anxiety through increased knowledge and a positive attitude toward months of immobilization, and (4) an absence of complications related to infection and decreased activity. Long-term goals are to have the patient free of pain or with only minimal pain in the hip and to ultimately be able to ambulate without an assistive device.

Planning and Intervention

Alleviate Pain. While talking with the patient, try physical measures for pain relief such as turning the patient, and encourage diversions such as reading, watching television, and doing handicrafts, as well as providing prescribed medications. The hip spica cast prevents some discomfort by immobilizing the hip joint.

Increase Mobility

Hip Spica Cast. If the surgical procedure did not use an internal fixation, or femoral osteotomy was also done, most patients will be in a one and one-half hip spica cast. (Fig. 6–12). The cast may be changed at 8-week intervals, but roentgenographic studies of the hip will determine the

TABLE 6–5. NURSING PROCESS FOR HIP ARTHORODESIS WITH A HIP SPICA

Assessment	Nursing Diagnosis	Goal Formulation	Planning and Intervention	Evaluation and Reassessment
1. Check vital signs. Assess location, duration, and severity of pain. Observe for verbal and nonverbal signs of pain. Check for any tightness of the cast.	1. Alteration in comfort: hip pain related to soft tissue and bone trauma.	1. Short-term goal: a decrease in pain through immobilization. Long-term goal: free of hip pain.	1. Alleviate Pain Teach muscle setting exercises. Teach relaxation techniques. Turn and reposition patient. Encourage diversional activities. Utilize noninvasive nursing. Administer prescribed medications.	1. Pain in the early postoperative stage usually requires medication to make the patient comfortable.
2. Assess for emotional reaction to cast. Check ability to breathe comfortably. Assess for any physical discomfort from the cast. Observe the patient's ability to do exercises and help care for self.	2. Impaired physical mobility: decreased hip function related to lack of joint mobility.	2. Short-term goal: an increase in mobility through bed exercises and hip joint immobilization. Long-term goal: regain optimal mobility.	2. Increase Mobility Explain rationale for hip spica cast. Keep bed flat. Teach bed exercises. Turn from back to unaffected side to abdomen; to return, reverse the procedure. Active range-of-motion exercises for all uninvolved joints.	2. The patient should be able to exercise all uninvolved joints and help with some activities of daily living.
3. Assess for signs and symptoms of infection. Check vital signs. Assess for pain.	3. Potential for injury: infection related to a break in skin integrity.	3. Short- and long-term goals: free of any complication.	3. Prevent Complications *Integumentary* Teach the signs and symptoms of infection. Encourage a well-balanced diet with plenty of fluids.	3. The patient should remain free of complications.

			Encourage as much exercise as possible. Investigate any complaint of pain. Administer antibiotics as prescribed.	
Auscultate the chest for lung clearance. Check respiratory rate, depth, and rhythm. Assess patient's color. Check for any shortness of breath or chest pain. Check for any petechiae.	Potential alteration in respiratory function: impaired gas exchange related to pulmonary and fat emboli.	Short- and long-term goals: free of any respiratory complications.	*Respiratory* Keep patient well hydrated. Administer anticoagulant drugs. Teach muscle setting exercises. *Occurrence of Emboli* Immobilize patient. Elevate head of bed. Start exercise. Notify physician. *Potential Complications Due to Immobility* (See Chap. 3 and Table 6–2)	
4. Assess level of understanding about surgical procedure, immobilization, and prognosis.	4. Potential knowledge deficit related to surgical procedure, immobilization and future ambulation.	4. Short- and long-term goals: a decrease in anxiety through increased knowledge.	4. Patient Teaching Allocate time for therapeutic communication. Have open discussion on the possible effect of hip fusion on personal, social, vocational, and economic status. Discuss safety factors in hospital and home care. Demonstrate to the patient, and to individuals caring for the patient at home, how to turn and care for a patient in a hip spica cast.	4. With increased knowledge, the patient should be able to help formulate a plan for home care. The patient should be able to discuss future goals for personal and professional life.

length of immobilization. When the fusion is far advanced, some physicians may apply a single spica walking cast, which will usually be from the nipple line to above the ankle on the affected side. Partial weight bearing in the cast with crutches is then allowed to a limited extent. If the hip has not fused after 4 months, a short spica cast is applied until the fusion becomes solid.

If the hip was fused with an internal fixation and no femoral osteotomy was done, the hip spica cast may or may not be used. Some physicians apply no cast for 2 weeks and then a short spica cast, which allows knee motion, for 8 to 10 weeks, gradually beginning weight bearing after the removal of the cast. Other physicians never apply a cast. In these instances, partial weight bearing on crutches may be allowed a few days or weeks after surgery. Crutches must be used until the fusion is solid (Edmondson & Crenshaw, 1980, p. 1199).

Turning. Turning is a primary concern following an arthrodesis of the hip. The schedule is every 2 to 3 hours during the day and every 4 hours during the night. Place pillows between the patient's legs and with ample help turn the patient to the uninvolved side. If the patient has a hip spica cast (Fig. 6–12), no pillows are necessary for the turn and the patient may be left on the unaffected side with the involved leg supported by at least two slings connected to the overhead frame and with pillows to support the trunk. The next time, the patient may be turned onto the abdomen. Make sure that there is ample help and that the patient is positioned so the feet will be off the end of the mattress. To turn to the back, reverse the procedure.

Exercises. Bed exercises, such as muscle setting exercises, are encouraged. That will lessen atrophy in the muscles that are immobilized by the cast. Some patients may be able to use the trapeze, but most will have very restricted use because the cast begins at the nipple line. At that level, the cast also prevents raising the head of the bed unless the entire bed is tilted using 4- to 8-inch blocks. If the bed is flat some patients have a feeling that their head is actually lower than their body.

Patient Teaching. Allocate time for therapeutic communication with the patient, the family, and significant others. Special points of concern are most likely to be (1) the adjustment to the long period of immobility and what that means to the patient's personal, social, vocational, and economic status, (2) whether the patient has to stay in the hospital during the complete recovery, go to a nursing home, or return home with a hip spica cast, and (3) that the patient must be extremely careful about stumbling or falling, which could easily result in a fracture of the femur. In patients with internal fixation the fracture usually occurs just below the fixation device. Work closely with a social worker in making arrangements for accommodations, and with the family, significant others, and possibly public health workers or home health nurses concerning the specifics of care.

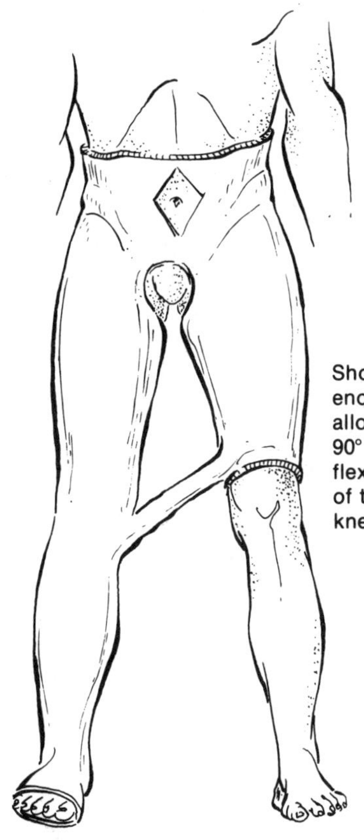

Figure 6–12. Hip spica cast. A one and one-half spica cast, extending from the lower rib margin to the tips of the toes on the involved side, and to the knee on the opposite side. Generally, the hip is held in slight abduction in order to separate the legs enough to allow for peroneal care. A support is necessary between the short segment and the major segment of the cast. *(From Lewis R.C.* Handbook of traction, casting and splinting techniques. *Philadelphia: Lippincott, 1977, p. 82, with permission.)*

Prevent Complications. The patient has undergone a major surgical procedure and is immobilized; therefore, nursing measures must focus on preventing complications common to all surgical and immobilized patients. For a more detailed plan of care, see the nursing care of a patient following an internal fixation of the hip, Table 6–2 and Chapter 3. A special concern following arthrodesis is infection, because most patients have a history of hip infection.

Evaluation and Reassessment

The considerations discussed for the patient who has had an internal fixation apply here as well. Special emphasis should be given to evaluating the patient's response to long-term immobilization in the initial stage and ability to walk and sit in the latter stage.

Arthroplasty

An arthroplasty is the surgical formulation or reformation of a joint. The goals of a hip arthroplasty are to relieve pain and deformity and to restore joint mobility. Three common types of hip arthroplasty are the cup or mold arthroplasty (Fig. 6–13), the total hip arthroplasty (Fig. 6–14), and the total hip surface replacement arthroplasty (Fig. 6–15). With the cup arthroplasty, the acetabulum and the head of the femur are reamed down to an untraumatized surface, and an appropriate size metal cup is fitted over the head of the femur. Presently, that kind of arthroplasty surgery is largely being replaced by the other two. The procedure for a total hip arthroplasty is to remove the femoral head and neck, and ream the femoral canal to accept the metal femoral component, which includes the head, the neck, and a stem that is implanted in the femoral shaft. The acetabulum is reamed to accept a polyethylene acetabular cup. The total hip surface replacement arthroplasty, the newest of the three procedures, consists of reaming out the acetabulum and implanting an acetabular cup while the femoral head is only reamed down to accept a metal femoral cup.

Another procedure discussed previously, the insertion of an Austin-Moore, Bateman, or Thompson endoprosthesis (Fig. 6–16), is sometimes referred to as a hemiarthroplasty. It is used in the treatment of some intracapsular fractures of the femur and involves replacing the patient's femoral head and neck with a metal component the same size as the patient's original femoral head. Because the principles of care for a hemiarthroplasty are very similar to those for a hip arthroplasty, the nursing care of both kinds of patients are discussed together. Care specific to one or the other procedure is indicated. It

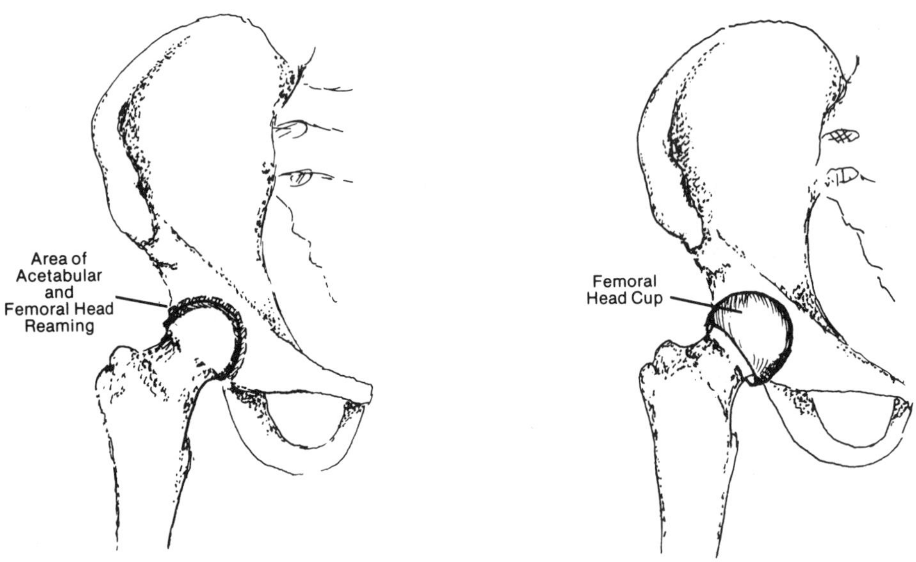

Figure 6–13. Cup arthroplasty. *(From Brantley, P., & Analla, M., 1980, p. 65. Courtesy of Howmedica.)*

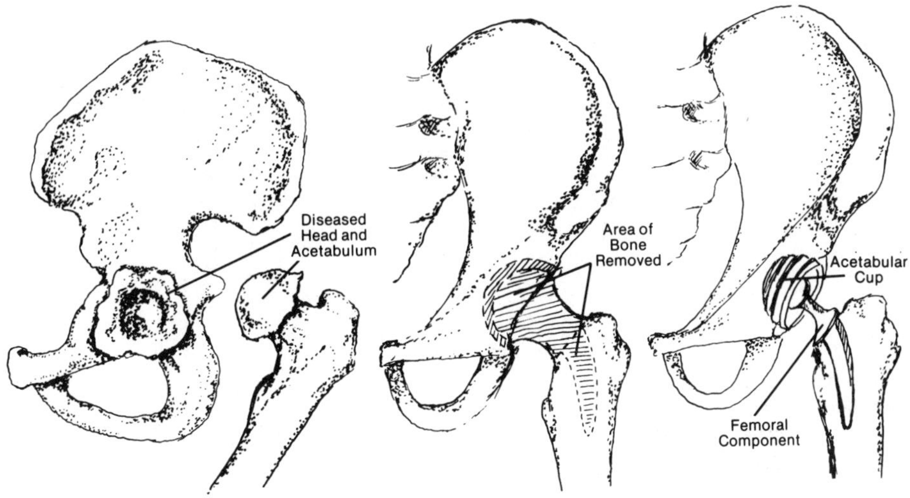

Figure 6–14. Total hip arthroplasty. *(From Brantley, P., & Analla, M., 1980, p. 66. Courtesy of Howmedica.)*

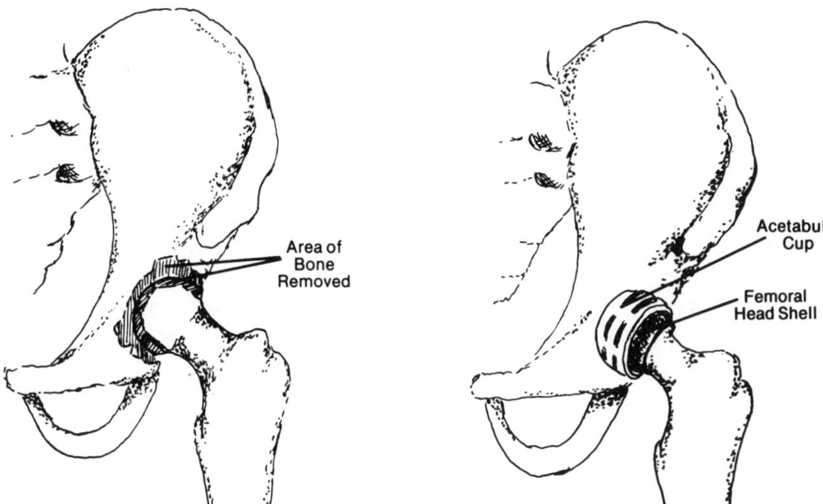

Figure 6–15. Total hip surface replacement arthroplasty. *(From Brantley, P., & Analla, M., 1980, p. 68. Courtesy of Howmedica.)*

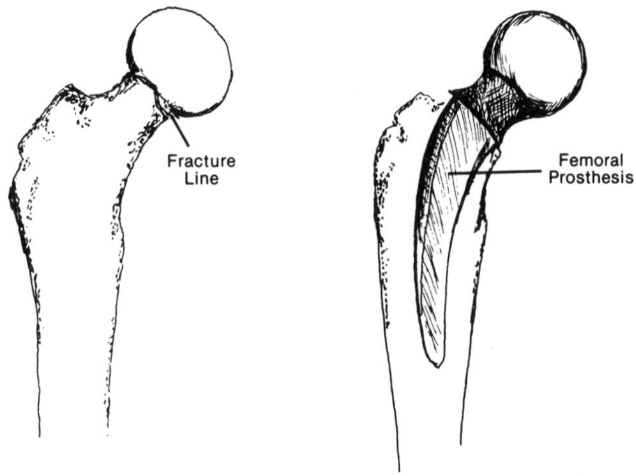

Figure 6–16. Hip prosthesis or hemiarthroplasty. *(From Brantley, P., & Analla, M., 1980, p. 76. Courtesy of Howmedica.)*

should be understood that the postoperative care required depends on the operative procedure and the condition of the patient.

In general, the nursing care for a hip arthroplasty patient is the same as the care for a patient with an internal fixation of the hip. Only measures that relate specially to a patient with a hip arthroplasty are discussed below.

□ NURSING PROCESS (Table 6–6)

Assessment

Immediately after surgery, the patient should be observed closely for any evidence of shock or cardiopulmonary abnormality. The chief cause of hypotension in postoperative shock is a failure to maintain blood volume, but it could result from cardiac abnormalities. Some hip arthroplasties can be performd without giving blood in surgery, but blood may be necessary postoperatively. Monitor central venous pressure, especially to avoid overhydration in the elderly, and record urinary output. Patients who were on steroids preoperatively may need them intravenously after surgery. Assess the neurovascular status in the involved leg (Chap. 2), which should be in abduction and neutral rotation. The leg may be held in abduction by splints, pillows, traction, or casts. The age of the patient undergoing a hip arthroplasty ranges from the late teens to over 80. Assess physical and emotional needs specific for age. (For a more detailed assessment, see the care of a patient having an internal fixation of the hip and Chap. 2.)

Nursing Diagnosis and Goal Formulation

Typically, the nursing diagnoses for a patient following a hip arthroplasty are (1) alterations in comfort related to pain in the hip from bone and soft

TABLE 6–6. NURSING PROCESS FOR HIP ARTHROPLASTY WITH BUCK'S TRACTION

Assessment	Nursing Diagnosis	Goal Formulation	Planning and Intervention	Evaluation and Reassessment
1. Assess the location, duration, and severity of pain. Assess neurovascular status. Check positioning of the involved leg and tightness of the traction.	1. Alteration in comfort: hip pain related to bone and soft tissue trauma.	1. Short-term goal: a decrease in pain through positioning and traction. Long-term goal: free of pain.	1. Alleviate Pain Position involved leg in abduction. Maintain Buck's traction. Teach muscle setting exercises. Utilize distraction. Teach relaxation techniques. Administer pain medications as indicated.	1. The patient's pain should be relieved by nursing measures and prescribed medications. Lifting the leg and changing position should greatly help in relieving pain.
2. Assess the patient's ability to utilize the trapeze and do the exercise program.	2. Impaired physical mobility: decreased hip function related to lack of joint and muscle integrity.	2. Short-term goal: an increase in mobility through exercises and positioning. Long-term goal: regain optimal hip function.	2. Increase Mobility *Position* Keep patient supine or lying on uninvolved side. Keep the involved leg in abduction. Maintain Buck's traction. Explain purpose and rationale for traction. *Exercises* Instruct on quadriceps and gluteal setting exercises, plantar and dorsiflexion exercises, and active range of motion of the involved ankle to be done 5 minutes every hour while awake. Instruct on active range of motion of all uninvolved joints.	2. Preoperative patient teaching should greatly reduce the need for in-depth instruction after surgery. The patient should be able to do the exercises easily. The patient should follow the exercise program without supervision. Evaluate crutch walking gait and amount of weight bearing.

(continued)

TABLE 6–6. *(Continued)*

Assessment	Nursing Diagnosis	Goal Formulation	Planning and Intervention	Evaluation and Reassessment
			Medicate patient before starting exercise program. Demonstrate skateboard and knee flexion exercises (30 minutes bid). Teach how to use a stationary bicycle (when utilized). *Turning* Turn patient to back and uninvolved leg. Keep the leg in abduction even when patient is lying on uninvolved side. *Ambulation* Demonstrate how to use trapeze. Demonstrate exercises to strengthen upper extremities for crutch walking. Demonstrate how to get out of and return to bed with less than 90 degrees of hip flexion. Demonstrate walker and crutch walking (4-point gait). Demonstrate method of sitting with less than 90 degrees of hip flexion.	

3. Assess the neurovascular status of the involved leg and compare it with the uninvolved leg. Assess for any pain or discomfort below the knee.	3. Potential for injury: neurovascular deficit related to application of traction.	3. Short- and long-term goals: free of any neurovascular deficit.	3. Prevent Complications *Circulatory* Apply traction correctly. Make sure traction straps are not too tight. Check neurovascular status after changing patient's position or reapplying traction.	3. The patient should remain free of any neurovascular deficit.
Auscultate the chest for lung clearance. Check respiratory rate, depth, and rhythm. Assess patient's color. Check for shortness of breath or chest pain. Check for any signs of petechiae.	Potential alteration in respiratory function: impaired gas exchange related to pulmonary and fat emboli.	Short- and long-term goals: free of respiratory complications.	*Respiratory* Keep patient well hydrated. Administer anticoagulant drugs. Teach coughing and deep breathing exercises. Teach muscle setting exercises. *Occurrence of Emboli* Immobilize patient. Elevate head of bed. Start oxygen. Notify physician.	The patient should remain free of any respiratory complications.
Assess vital signs. Assess pain level at incision site. Check incision for any redness, swelling, hardness, or drainage.	Potential for injury: infection related to surgical incision.	Short- and long-term goals: free of any signs of infection.	*Integumentary* Keep dressing clean and dry. Do daily wound care. Encourage a well-balanced diet with plenty of fluids. Administer antibiotics as prescribed.	The patient should remain free of any sign of infection.

(continued)

TABLE 6–6. *(Continued)*

Assessment	Nursing Diagnosis	Goal Formulation	Planning and Intervention	Evaluation and Reassessment
Assess for adduction and internal rotation of the involved leg. Assess gluteal area. Assess duration, location, and severity of pain. Obtain history of recent activity. Assess ability to move leg.	Potential for injury: dislocation of hip related to turning or position		*Musculoskeletal* Teach patient how to keep the leg in abduction, turn to unaffected side, prevent 90 degrees of hip flexion, and get in and out of bed and chair. *Potential Complications Due to Immobility* (See Chap. 3 and Table 6–2).	The patient's total hip replacement should remain intact.
4. Assess level of understanding about the rehabilitation process and home care. Assess home environment and the need for assistive devices in the home.	4. Potential knowledge deficit related to rehabilitation process and home care.	4. Short- and long-term goals: a decrease in anxiety through increased knowledge.	4. Patient Teaching Discuss safety procedures to prevent dislocation. Suggest methods of dressing and bathing. Demonstrate home exercises. Discuss use of assistive devices at home. Discuss methods of travel and chairs for sitting in at home. Demonstrate how to apply elastic stockings.	4. The patient, family, or significant other should feel confident about home care and the continuation of the rehabilitation process.

tissue trauma, (2) alterations in mobility related to joint and muscle integrity, (3) alterations in psychological well-being related to anxiety and knowledge deficit about the surgical procedure and future ambulation, and (4) potential complications related to surgical procedure and immobility.

Short-term goals are to have the patient experience (1) a decrease in hip pain through the use of nursing measures and prescribed medications, (2) an increase in mobility through exercise, (3) a decrease in anxiety through knowledge and a positive attitude toward future daily activities, and (4) an absence of complications from surgery and immobility. Long-term goals are to have the patient free of pain in the hip and able to walk without an assistive device.

Planning and Intervention

Alleviate Pain. Some patients will not complain of pain after a hip arthroplasty, saying that the postoperative pain is so much less than what they were suffering that they do not want anything for pain. Those patients need to be encouraged to take pain medications for the first 24 to 48 postoperative hours so that they will receive adequate rest and comfort. Do not wait for the patients to ask, and make sure that they understand that if they are in pain they should ask for medication or assistance.

Increase Mobility

Position. Correct positioning of the hip joint is essential at all times because dislocation of the new joint can occur easily. (A dislocation is of even greater concern for a patient with a hemiarthroplasty, because the head of the prosthesis is larger and it must fit within the patient's acetabulum.) The involved leg should be kept in about 20 degrees of abduction and neutral rotation, and hip flexion should be less than 45 degrees for at least 2 weeks. There are a variety of methods used to help keep the involved leg in correct position. These are (1) a Thomas splint with a Pearson attachment, with or without traction, (2) a Hodgen splint, with or without traction, (3) a Kirschner wire inserted through the proximal tibia for traction and control of rotation, (4) a Hamilton-Russell traction, (5) a Buck's traction, (6) an Amsterdam sling, (7) abductor pillows (Figs. 6–17 A and B) or an abductor splint, (8) a short leg cast with attached spreader bar, and (9) regular pillows between the legs. A modified above-knee spica cast may be used for approximately 3 weeks if the hip was unstable at the completion of the operation.

Turning. Only turn the patient to the unaffected side, and use pillows or an abducter pillow between the patient's legs to keep the involved leg in abduction. If the patient is allowed to be turned to the affected side, the patient is generally turned no more than 45 degrees. If Buck's traction is used, disconnect the traction, turn the patient using pillows between the

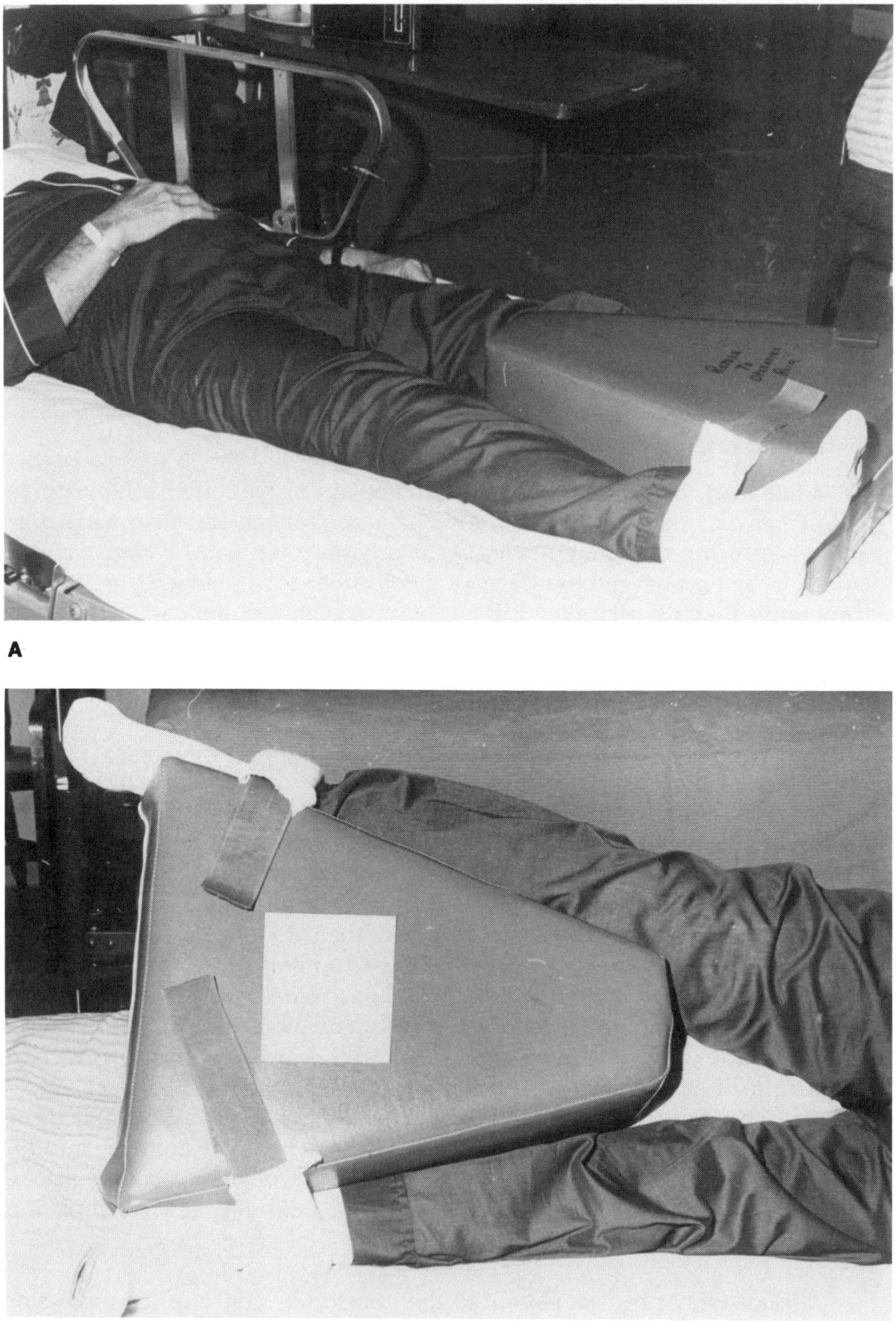

A

B

Figure 6–17. A. Abductor pillow. **B.** Abductor pillow (side lying). *(Courtesy of Carle Foundation Hospital and Clinic.)*

legs, reposition the traction on the other side of the bed, and reconnect the traction.

Exercises. Mild active and passive exercises are started the day of surgery and are carried out each hour while the patient is awake. On the second or third postoperative day, the patient may begin skateboard and knee flexion exercises for a total of 30 minutes twice a day. For skateboard and knee flexion exercises, several pieces of apparatus are needed (Fig. 6–18). One consists of a knee sling placed under the involved leg just above the knee and connected to a pulley on the overhead frame. A rope from the sling through the overhead pulley is attached to the center of a foot-long wooden roll held by the patient. The patient is then able to pull up on the sling, raise the leg, and flex the knee. The other apparatus utilizes a metal posterior splint. The splint goes beneath the patient's affected leg from the upper calf to the toes, and has three small wheels or rollers attached at its base, so that it can be thought of as a skate. The splint is lined with a towel for padding, and the leg is secured in the splint with an ace bandage. At the base of the splint, near the rollers, there are metal eyelets large enough to accommodate a rope. A wide board, with a pulley on each end, is placed flat across the foot of the patient's bed. A rope goes from the patient's right hand through the pulley attached to the right side of the board at the foot of the bed, through the eyelets at the base of the skate, through the pulley attached to the left side of the board, to the patient's left hand. The patient is then able to use the ropes and do a passive abduction and adduction (to the midline) exercise with the involved leg, pulling it back and forth over the board. The knee flexion and skateboard exercises are alternated during the 30-minute period. In the beginning the skateboard may be passive but as the patient gains more control over the muscles in the hip it becomes more of an active exercise. To prevent the involved leg from going past the midline, and to prevent a rope burn, the uninvolved leg is placed on a pillow that comes to the midline. Another exercise that patients may do later is riding a stationary bicycle (Fig. 6–19).

Ambulation. The patient usually comes to a standing position for the first time on the second or third postoperative day. The patient may get out of bed with assistance of the nurse or with the use of a tilt table, a Nelson bed, or a circolectric bed. In getting out of bed, it is usually much easier for the patient to keep the involved leg from crossing the midline and avoid flexing the affected hip more than 45 degrees, if it is done on the side of the uninvolved hip. For most patients, it is easier to keep the involved leg in abduction when returning to bed on the side of the affected hip. The patient usually begins walking using a walker with a four-point gait (Fig. 6–20) and then progresses to crutches and even canes by 6 weeks after surgery. Only partial weight bearing is allowed at first, but full weight is usually allowed by 6 weeks or longer.

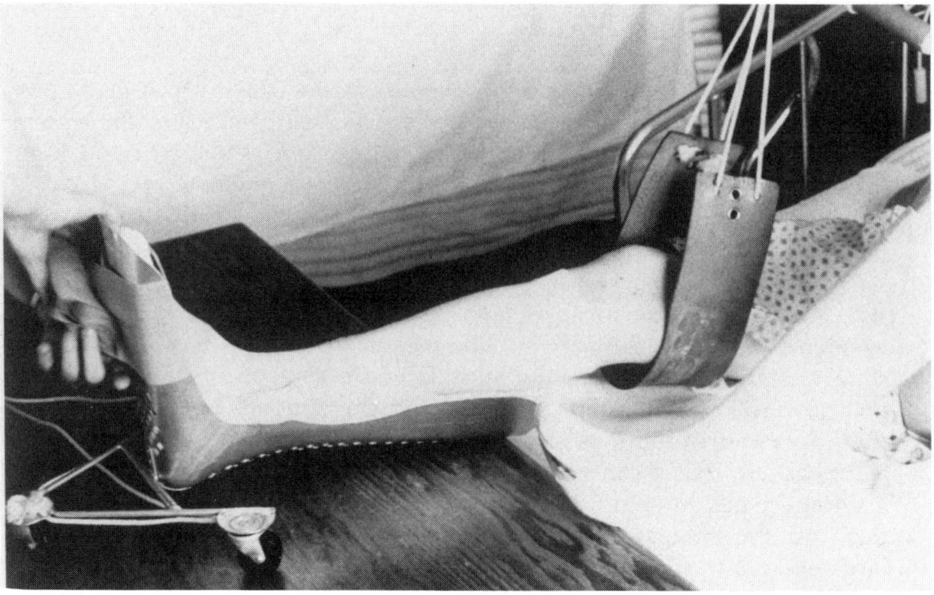

A

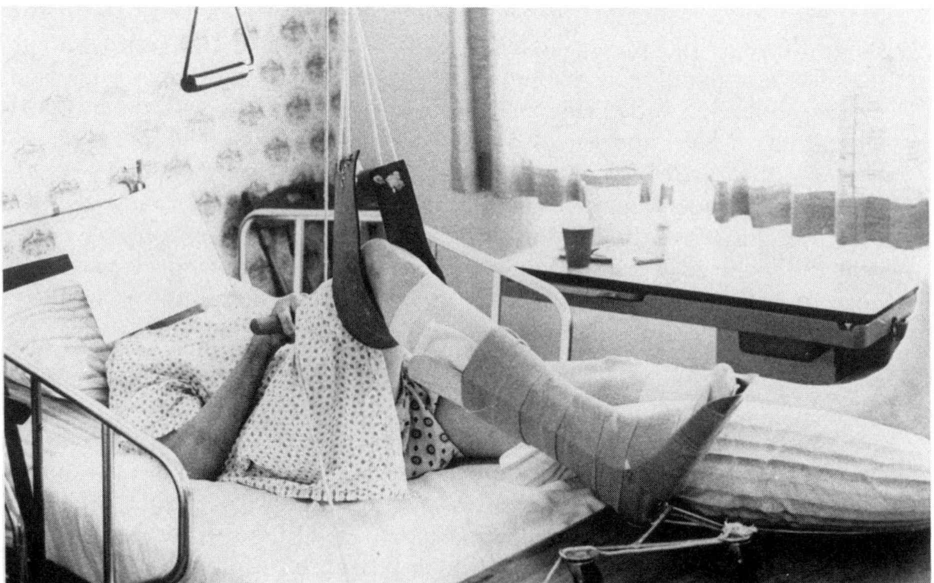

B

Figure 6–18. A. Application of skate. **B.** Skateboard and knee flexion exercise. *(Courtesy of Carle Foundation Hospital and Clinic.)*

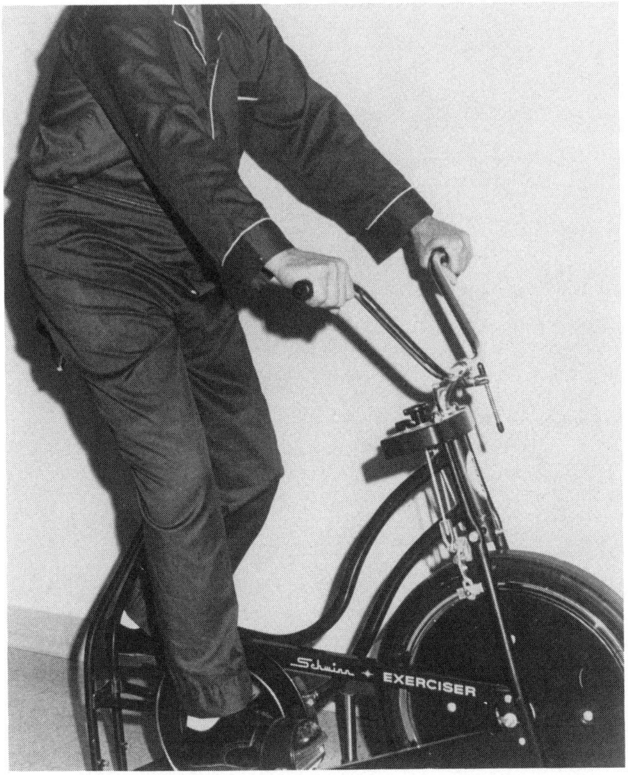

Figure 6–19. Stationary bicycle exercise. *(Courtesy of Carle Foundation Hospital and Clinic.)*

Sitting. Sitting in a chair may be started as early as the fourth postoperative day. The patient should be in a semierect position rather than a normal sitting position because the hip should not be flexed more than 45 degrees. That position can be achieved by placing pillows in the seat and the back of a chair with armrests, which prevents the patient from sitting at a right angle. Another way is to utilize the total hip chair (Fig. 6–21). Bathroom privileges, which allow the use of a stool with an elevated seat, may be started on the fifth postoperative day.

Patient Teaching. Spend time with the patient, the family, and significant others answering questions about the surgery, exercises, and planning for discharge. The usual hospital stay for a patient having a hip arthroplasty is 2 weeks or less; therefore, teaching and planning for discharge should start at admission and preoperative teaching. Points that are specific for recovery from hip arthroplasty and the prevention of dislocation, especially during the first 6 weeks, are (1) the importance of continuing with exercises so that hip flexion increases to 90 degrees and the patient can sit

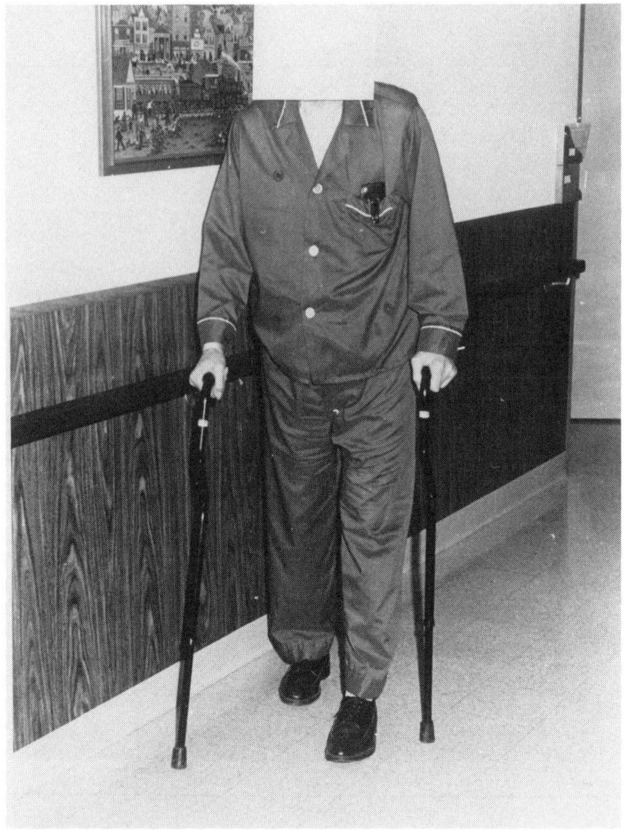

Figure 6–20. Four-point gait with canes. *(Courtesy of Carle Foundation Hospital and Clinic.)*

in a straight chair by 6 weeks postsurgery, (2) continuing to use the elevated toilet, (3) not crossing the legs when sitting, (4) using pillows between the legs at night to prevent the involved leg from crossing the midline, (5) taking showers and not tub baths, (6) continuing with crutches and partial weight bearing, (7) refraining from prolonged sitting or driving a car, (8) not bending over to pick anything up off the floor, tie a shoelace, or pull up linen in bed, (9) refraining from sexual intercourse until the 6-week check-up (some physicians do not impose that restriction, especially for women and for certain positions for men; discuss that point with the patient's physician), and (10) reporting any immediate signs of subluxation or dislocation of the hip, chest pain, excessive swelling in the leg, redness, tenderness, or swelling of the hip, bloody or purulent discharge from the incision, or urinary tract infection.

Prevent Complications. Potential complications following a total hip replacement are infection, dislocation, thrombophlebitis, pulmonary embo-

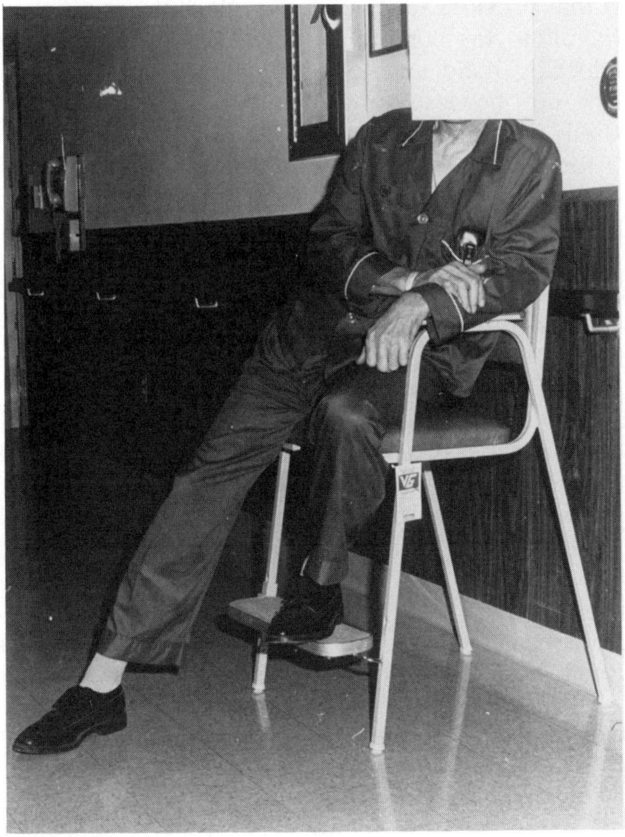

Figure 6–21. Total hip chair. *(Courtesy of Carle Foundation Hospital and Clinic.)*

lism, and fat embolism (especially for total hip arthroplasty and hemiarthroplasties). (See Table 6–2 and Chapter 3 for further discussion.)

Evaluation and Reassessment

The considerations discussed for the patient who has had an internal fixation apply here as well. Special emphasis should be given to evaluating the patient's compliance with the exercise regime to repair muscle tone and prevent a dislocation of the hip. Also check to be certain that the patient understands the extent of mobility restrictions that will apply after discharge from the hospital.

Noncemented Femoral Hip Arthroplasty

The most common complication of total hip arthroplasties is aseptic loosening of the femoral component. The bone cement interface is the area of failure in most instances, and it was felt that eliminating the need for cement would reduce loosening and give a longer lasting total hip arthroplasty. The alternative is to use a porous prosthesis that provides for bony ingrowth as the method of fixation. The porous material allows the bone to form within the pores of the prosthesis, causing an interlocking bond and long-lasting fixation. For such bony ingrowth to occur, there must be close contact between the bone and the porous surface of the prosthesis (Doheny, 1985).

The surgical procedure for a noncemented Austin-Moore femoral arthroplasty is much the same as for other total hip arthroplasties up to the point of femoral implantation. In the noncemented procedure, a bone cutter is used to cut pieces from the femoral head. The pieces are used to fill the fenestrations in the prosthetic stem, and they stimulate the formation of a bony bridge. The porous femoral prosthesis is then pounded down the femoral shaft. Prior to the final seating of the prosthetic collar, pulverized bone from the femoral head is packed into the proximal femur (Blake, 1985).

Postoperative care is the same as for other total hip arthroplasties except that the patients are kept on toe-touch weight bearing with crutches for at least 6 to 12 weeks (up to 6 months for some patients). That period of restricted weight bearing is necessary to insure proper tissue growth and avoid stress on the prosthesis, which could interfere with bony ingrowth and cause a loosening of the prosthesis.

Postoperative complications are the same as in other total hip arthroplasties. However, a small percentage of patients complain of a mild aching lateral midshaft pain. The pain usually resolves itself with time, but may be present for up to 1 1/2 years (Blake, 1985). Should replacement of the femoral component ever be necessary, this procedure would be simplified because only the proximal bony bridge would need to be broken for removal.

NEOPLASMS

All types of bone tumors may affect the hip. The most common benign tumors are osteochondroma, osteoid osteoma, and giant-cell tumors. The most frequent malignant tumors are myeloma, primary and secondary chondros osteogenic sarcoma, Ewing's tumor, fibrosarcoma, and chordoma. There is nothing that distinguishes primary bone tumors in the region of the hip from those elsewhere. Metastatic tumors are not uncommon in the hip, especially in the bone adjacent to the acetabulum and in the head and neck of the femur, as the blood supply there is relatively rich (Coventry, 1973, p. 391). (For a more in-depth discussion of pathology for these tumors, see Chap. 4.)

Each tumor, soft tissue or bony, is evaluated individually. The questions of benign or malignant, the possibility of local recurrence, the function of the hip, and the anatomical location are all considered in the treatment of neoplasms of the hip region. Excisional biopsy is preferable for such tumors as osteochondromas or osteo-chondrosarcomas to avoid any invasion of the tumor or any spilling of the malignant or potentially malignant cells. Similarly, tumors of the synovium are treated by complete excision of the synovium. In dealing with malignant tumors, the surgical approach is to avoid penetration of the tumor during the removal, whether it is to be by excision or amputation (Coventry, 1973, p. 402).

Surgical Procedure

Hip Disarticulation

Amputations through the proximal thigh and disarticulation at the hip joint are generally the result of trauma or neoplastic disease. Occasionally, amputations at this level may be necessitated by infection or the conversion of a severe congenital anomaly to fit a prosthesis (Coventry, 1973, p. 411). Amputations about the hip and the pelvis include those through the femur proximally from 5 cm distal to the lesser trochanter, disarticulations of the hip, and hemipelvectomy amputations (Edmondson & Crenshaw, 1980, p. 839). In the proper sense, amputation is a procedure that removes a part by cutting through one or more bones, while a disarticulation removes a part through a joint (Edmondson & Crenshaw, 1980, p. 822). Thus, a hip disarticulation is defined as the removal of a leg through the hip joint, and a hemipelvectomy is the removal of the lower extremity and a portion of the pelvis by cutting through one or more of the pelvic bones.

Hemipelvectomy

If an amputation is done for a malignant tumor in or about the hip, it is usually a hemipelvectomy amputation. The hemipelvectomy amputation, a radical and infrequently done procedure is known by many names, including interinnominoabdominal amputation, interabdominal amputation, interpelviabdominal amputation, iliabdominal amputation, transiliac amputation, transpelvic amputation, and hindquarter amputation (Edmondson & Crenshaw, 1980, p. 841). Because of the proximity of the hip joint to the upper part of the femur, a hip disarticulation is usually not appropriate. The hip disarticulation is a treatment for malignant tumors, but these tumors are usually lesions of the femoral shaft below the trochanter. A hemipelvectomy is not usually done for tumors of the lower grade malignancy, such as chondrosarcomas, occurring in areas where complete removal of the intact tumor is possible. Although a benign tumor, which is destroying function, can be removed from the head and neck of the femur and replaced by a prosthesis, or the acetabulum can be removed and replaced, these instances are rare. Complete replacement of most of the femur by homogenous bone has been reported occasionally in the literature. Occasionally special prostheses for the proximal end of the femur are made when the head and the neck must be removed.

In civilian life, a hip disarticulation is most often performed for bone and soft-tissue tumors of the thigh. The distal femur is a common site of osteogenic sarcoma. Amputation proximal to the bone in which the tumor occurs has resulted in statistically superior outcomes when compared to amputation through the same bone at a higher level. Thus a hip joint disarticulation is the level of choice for most malignant bone tumors of the thigh (Burgess & Zettl, 1973, p. 412).

The objective of postoperative medical management is to provide firm support to the operative site. In the past this was commonly accomplished by soft compression dressings. If soft tissue compression dressings alone are used, they should be adequately reinforced by pressure bandaging and kept under sufficient tension to control and hasten stump maturation. Today, it is common practice to utilize a rigid dressing and a postsurgical prosthetic fitting so that walking with progressive weight bearing can be started within a few days. The only absolute contradiction to immediate postsurgical prosthetic fitting is an actual or potential infection at the site of the amputation or an open amputation. The prosthetic fitting, usually applied by a prosthetist, consists of a rigid plaster of Paris dressing, a pylon going from the stump to the ankle with no hip or knee joints, and a foot–ankle assembly. The rigid dressing is applied to the hip in such a way that compression is firmly and evenly distributed over the end of the stump, both iliac crests, and the ischial tuberosity on the amputated side. The initial rolls of plaster are of elastic plaster of Paris, because it conforms to the contour of the stump better and permits easier control of tension. The outer rolls are of regular plaster of Paris, because the elastic plaster is not as strong as the conventional type. The prosthetic pylon and the foot–ankle assembly are aligned to allow a smooth gait that will not be fatiguing and will avoid excessive pressure on the stump. To make a swing-through gait easier, the length of the prosthetic fitting is 0.9 to 1.3 cm shorter than the length of the opposite leg. Some physicians have discontinued immediate postsurgical prosthetic fitting following hip disarticulation or hemipelvectomy amputations because available components do not allow the patient to sit comfortably and require ambulation on a pylon without a movable hip or knee joint. Furthermore, the hip disarticulation stump matures rapidly when treated by conventional methods, allowing early fitting with a properly articulated definitive prosthesis. After a minimum of 6 to 12 weeks following a hip disarticulation or hemipelvectomy, a Canadian hip disarticulation prosthesis or a modification of it, can be fitted (Edmondson & Crenshaw, 1980, pp. 845–846, 849, 857).

□ NURSING PROCESS (Table 6–7)

Assessment

Before surgery, the patient's general condition should be thoroughly evaluated. In all elective amputations, the prosthetist as well as the surgeon should evaluate the patient before surgery so that necessary measurements can be made, and a shoe for the prosthetic foot can be obtained if an immediate postsurgical prosthetic fitting is to be utilized. Psychological assessment of the patient preoperatively will greatly enhance postoperative nursing assessment and intervention. Even though the amputation may be elective, the operation may be a life-saving measure or a first step toward regaining function and decreasing pain. It is important that the patient understand the operation before it occurs so as to foster a positive attitude toward rehabilitation. Let the patient ask questions, and make the patient comfortable enough to express fears, anxieties, and negative feelings. Opportunities should also be given to the family and significant others to express their fears and anxieties. Observe interactions between the patient, the family, and significant others, specifically with regard to the topic of amputation. A visit by an amputee or an amputee's family may also be helpful.

Postoperatively, special assessment concerns focus on fluid and electrolyte balance, bleeding, and shock. Look for signs of bleeding along the incision line and posterior to it. Note the amount of drainage from the wound drains, assess for urinary output, and check the drying of the plaster cast if an immediate postsurgical prosthetic fitting was utilized. Note the location and intensity of pain. Observe the emotional responses to the surgery and attitudes toward the stump; most patients or family members will not look at the stump.

Nursing Diagnosis and Goal Formulation

The typical postsurgical nursing diagnoses are (1) alterations in comfort related to pain at the surgical site from the trauma to bone and soft tissue, (2) alterations in mobility related to the loss of a leg and the application of an immediate postsurgical fitting, (3) alterations in psychological well-being related to anxiety and knowledge deficit from the change in body image and concerns about future roles as husband/wife, employee, and member of society, and (4) potential complications related to surgical procedure.

Immediate goals are to have the patient experience (1) a decrease in the level of pain through repositioning and prescribed medications, (2) an increased potential for ambulation through bed exercises, getting out of bed as soon as possible, and an increased ability to sit by correct positioning in a chair, (3) a decreased anxiety about self-care, body image, and fears of future role performance by open discussions and increased knowledge, and (4) an absence of complications related to surgery. Long term goals are (1) to have the patient free of physical and emotional complications, (2) to maintain full functional capabilities of the rest of the body, and (3) to restore as much function as possible by the use of a prosthesis.

Planning and Intervention

Alleviate Pain. Routine nursing measures and prescribed medications may be utilized for pain relief. With the use of a rigid dressing, there is usually a decrease in the severity of pain after surgery. Strong opiates are often unnecessary or are only used for a few days. Phantom pain, i.e., pain in the amputated limb, is usually not relieved by medications. An immediate postsurgical prosthetic fitting usually decreases phantom pain, but having the patient describe the pain in detail may be the most beneficial. Although health personnel refer to such sensations as phantom pain, the sensation

TABLE 6–7. NURSING PROCESS FOR HIP DISARTICULATION AMPUTATION

Assessment	Nursing Diagnosis	Goal Formulation	Planning and Intervention	Evaluation and Reassessment
1. Assess the location, duration and severity of pain. Observe for verbal and nonverbal cues of pain. Check vital signs. Check for any areas of tightness from the rigid dressing.	1. Alteration in comfort: pain at the surgical site related to bone and soft tissue trauma.	1. Short-term goal: a decrease in the level of pain by repositioning, therapeutic communication, and prescribed medications. Long-term goal: free of pain.	1. Alleviate Pain Explain rationale for rigid dressing (if utilized). Utilize therapeutic communication to deal with real and phantom pain. Help with positioning. Administer pain medications as indicated.	1. Nursing measures, the rigid dressing and prescribed medications should keep the patient relatively comfortable.
2. Assess the level of strength in the upper extremity and uninvolved leg. Assess the patient's ability to do exercises. Assess the patient's ability to turn self. Assess the patient's ability to ambulate safely. Assess the patient's ability to sit.	2. Impaired physical mobility related to the loss of the leg.	2. Short-term goal: an increase in mobility through bed exercises and ambulation. Long-term goal: able to ambulate with assistive devices and to sit comfortably in a chair.	2. Increase Mobility *Position* Turn patient to either side (support leg on pillow when turned to involved side). Change position every 2 hours during the day and every 4 hours at night. Teach patient correct method of turning. Instruct on how to use trapeze. *Exercises* Instruct on exercises to increase strength in upper extremities and leg for crutch walking. Instruct on abdominal exercises.	2. The patient should be able to do exercises for ambulation without any problem, but may need further assistance with sitting exercises.

			Help with exercises that assist in sitting. *Ambulation* Demonstrate method of ambulation with and without pylon fitting and crutches.	
3. Assess for signs and symptoms of infection. Check vital signs. Assess duration, location, and severity of pain. Check for breaks in skin on the scrotum (males). Check anal area.	3. Potential for injury: infection related to breaks in skin integrity.	3. Short- and long-term goals: free of any complications.	3. Prevent Complications *Integumentary* Keep dressing clean and dry. Utilize preventive measures to keep from soiling dressing when patient eliminates. Do daily wound care. Encourage a well-balanced diet and plenty of fluids. *Potential Complications Due to Immobility* (See Chap. 3 and Table 6–2)	3. The patient should remain free of any complications.
4. Assess the patient's level of understanding about the rehabilitation process. Assess stage of adaptation to the disability. Assess concerns about future role as a husband/wife, employee, and member of society.	4. Potential knowledge deficit related to rehabilitation process and prognosis.	4. Short- and long-term goals: a decrease in anxiety through increased knowledge.	4. Patient Teaching Allow time for open discussion of feelings and about loss of limb. Spend time with family or significant other. Allow time to discuss future role performance and activity level. Discuss the purpose and rationale of the rigid dressing and potential for a prosthesis. Discuss potential complications and when to call the physician.	4. The patient should begin to adapt to the disability. The patient should be able to start talking about the amputation and looking at it. The patient should feel confident in continuing the rehabilitation process at home.

of pain is real to the patient, and might better be referred to as phantom sensations in discussions with the patient. Some physicians do not want phantom pain discussed with the patient before it occurs, believing that if it is not discussed it is less likely to occur. If phantom pain does occur in such instances, the patient may become frightened of what is happening and hesitant to mention it for fear that people will think their mental status is impaired. (For further discussion on phantom pain, see Chap. 2.)

Increase Mobility

Exercises. To increase the potential for ambulation and decrease complications, bed exercises, such as coughing, deep breathing, and the use of the trapeze, should be started as soon as the patient is awake after surgery. It will be easier for most patients to turn to the nonoperative side, but as the pylon is removed when they are in bed, they may turn to the operative side if the remaining leg is supported by pillows.

Ambulation. Early ambulation with limited weight bearing on the prosthetic fitting is very beneficial psychologically and lessens the emotional trauma from the loss of a limb. Most patients are up by at least 48 hours after surgery, even though the pylon fitting is often not applied until the drains are out, some 24 to 36 hours after surgery. Most younger patients will be able to stand in parallel bars or with crutches on the third or fourth postoperative day. Many are able to leave the hospital within 2 or 3 weeks, but will probably not be able to resume their occupation with the temporary prosthesis because of difficulties in sitting.

Sitting. Sitting with an immediate postsurgical prosthetic fitting following a hip disarticulation or a hemipelvectomy is difficult because the rigid dressing covers both iliac crests, the ischial tuberosity on the amputated side, and the stump area. Because there is no hip or knee joint, the patient is unable to bend from the iliac crest down on the affected side. Positions in which the patient could sit are those in which the patient is able to flex the uninvolved, but not the involved hip. In the hospital, a total hip chair may be available, and it will usually be easy for the patient to use. Continue to work with the patient on methods of using other chairs and what might be done at home. If a conventional soft dressing is used or if the prosthetic fitting is removed, the patient will have difficulty in learning to sit without support, because there is no femur on the involved side to help with balance. Special exercises and techniques need to be learned and practiced. The nurse needs to work closely with the patient and the physical therapist in those exercises.

Patient Teaching. Initially, it may be difficult for the patient to look at the stump, let alone handle the dressing or the prosthesis. It will take time, but the patient's acknowledgment is an important step in the rehabilitation process. The term stump may cause anxiety or feelings of degradation to the patient, so it is advisable to try to avoid the word, even though it seems to be the most descriptive term available.

Allow time for frank and open discussions about what the remaining portion of the hip looks like. Discuss the immediate prosthetic fitting, and note that although the pylon does not look like a leg, it does allow for ambulation and with pajamas it can be less noticeable in the hospital. Discussions with nurses, a rehabilitated amputee, and the prosthetist about what the prosthesis will look like (color, joints, and so on), and how it will function and what the patient will be able to do can be helpful.

Decrease fear about future role performance by health education and candid discussions of what to expect from the permanent prosthesis. Discuss the requirements of the patient's present job and how the patient's potential to return to it or to another related job. The social worker should work with the nurse, physical therapist, prosthetist, and physician to help the patient deal with those problems.

To increase the patient's self-esteem, provide opportunities for patients to be alone with their families. Encourage the patient to express concerns about any impairment in family roles. Treat the family as the unit of care, and enlist the family's support of the patient by supporting them in adjusting to the patient's surgery. Help them communicate with the physician, and keep them informed of the patient's daily progress. Utilize the patient's concern for the family to motivate the patient to actively participate in the rehabilitation process.

Prevent Complications. Of special concern with a hip disarticulation or hemipelvectomy are nursing measures to prevent problems with elimination and to maintain skin integrity. Preoperatively the patient was given enemas to cleanse the bowel. The patient with a hemipelvectomy may have the anus temporarily sutured closed or sealed off with oiled silk during surgery. Defecation is encouraged after the second day, aided by the use of neostigmine and a gentle enema on the fourth or fifth day, if needed. A Foley catheter is usually inserted preoperatively and removed about the fourth or fifth day postoperatively.

The skin is prepared preoperatively from the costal margins proximally to both knees distally. In surgery, the scrotum may be either stitched or strapped to the uninvolved thigh. Implement nursing measures to prevent skin infection. The incisional sutures are usually removed on the fourteenth day. If the patient has a postsurgical prosthetic fitting, the cast will be changed at that time. Casts may also be changed if they are too loose. (For patient education regarding cast care, see Appendix B.)

Evaluation and Reassessment

The considerations discussed for the patient who has had an internal fixation apply here as well, but the following points should be kept in mind. In evaluating pain, determine whether phantom pain is present. See how well the patient is able to ambulate and sit. Finally evaluate how well the patient and the patient's family are adjusting to the change in body image, and whether they have reached the stage of acceptance.

UPPER LEG (DISTAL TWO-THIRDS OF THE FEMUR)

Trauma

FRACTURES

Shaft of the Femur

A fracture of the femoral shaft is a relatively common injury in adults and children. The fracture is usually produced by trauma, and may be associated with multiple system injuries. Because the femur is the largest bone of the body and the principal weight-bearing bone in the leg, fractures may result in prolonged restrictions on mobility. With a fracture of the femoral shaft, the line of pull and the great strength of the muscles of the hip and thigh usually produce marked displacement of the bone fragments. The affected leg appears shortened and the thigh may present anterior and lateral angulation, with the lower portion of the leg lying in an abnormal rotation. The patient is unable to move the leg, and attempts to do so cause severe pain. The fracture is typically accompanied by extensive hemorrhage into the soft tissue of the thigh, sometimes severe enough to precipitate shock. Generally the fracture is closed rather than open, and damage to the sciatic nerve may occur.

Methods of Surgical Repair
Several methods are available for treatment of femoral shaft fractures. The type and the location of the fracture, the degree of comminution, the age of the patient, and the patient's social and economic demands are factors in determining the method of care. A femoral shaft fracture in an adult can rarely be reduced and held in plaster immobilization because a cast cannot prevent displacement and angulation from the large, powerful muscles of the thigh. Femoral fractures are often treated in skeletal traction initially, followed by the use of a hip spica (see pp. 281 and 284–285 and Appendix B) or an ambulatory cast brace. If the fracture is treated surgically, one option is open reduction with a compression plate fixation. A second option is open reduction with the use of an intramedullary nail introduced across the fracture fragments. A third surgical option is closed reduction aided by the use of an x-ray image intensifier. A fourth surgical option is the use of external fixation devices. The exter-

nal fixation device method is the only one that does not utilize a period of skeletal traction.

Traction

Most patients with traumatic fractures of the femur are placed in either skin or skeletal traction for several days or weeks. That is true even though the patient may be placed later in a cast brace or have an open or closed reduction with some form of internal fixation. Some patients have skeletal traction as their only method of treatment. Traction is utilized to prevent further damage to soft tissue, nerves, and blood vessels, relieve muscle spasms, reduce the fracture, and provide immobilization to maintain alignment. More specifically, for patients with a fracture of the femur, the objective of the traction is to maintain abduction and external rotation of the distal fragment of the fracture. If there is any inward or outward bowing, the physician should be notified as the apparatus must be adjusted with proper slings and weights to counteract and correct that tendency toward deformity (Larson & Gould, 1978, p. 218).

Russell's or suspension traction (Fig. 6–22), in combination with skin or

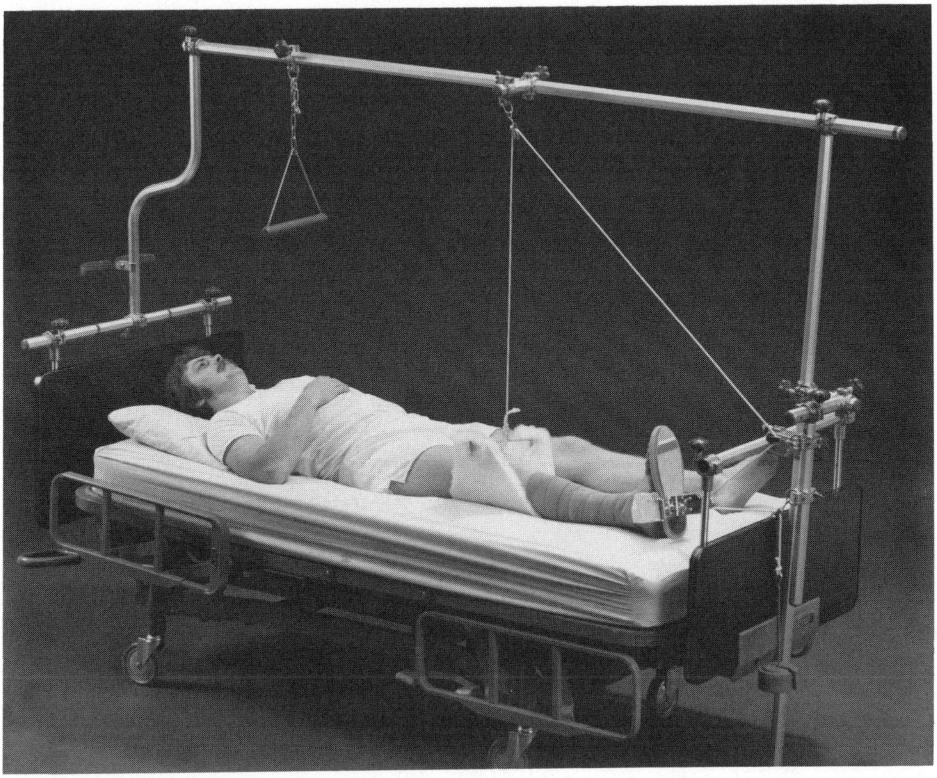

Figure 6–22. Russell's traction. *(Courtesy of Zimmer, Inc.)*

skeletal traction, may be utilized. If skeletal traction is used, a Steinmann pin or Kirschner wire is usually inserted through the tibia just below the tuberosity. Suspension is obtained by means of the Thomas splint and Pearson attachment, or with a Hodgen or Keller-Blake splint. The splint is usually elevated at a 45-degree angle to the bed. The Pearson attachment is fastened to the Thomas splint at the knee joint. The knee is flexed 45 dgrees, and the lower leg lies in the Pearson attachment, which is parallel to the bed (see Fig. 6–10). Balanced suspension traction is produced by a counterforce other than the patient's body weight. The extremity balances or floats in the traction apparatus. The line of traction on the extremity remains fairly constant, despite changes in the patient's position. The foot of the affected leg is prevented from developing footdrop by the use of a foot support that is clamped to the Pearson attachment. (For more information on traction, see Appendix A and pp. 278–279.)

Skeletal traction may be preferred to skin traction because of the length of time in traction and the considerable amount of weight that must be applied to overcome spasms of the thigh muscles. When reduction of the fracture has been accomplished, the amount of weight is usually reduced to prevent separation of the bone fragments. Traction must be continued until sufficient healing has taken place to permit crutch walking, or until sufficient callus has formed to permit the application of a hip spica or cast brace, or to have an open or closed reduction with internal fixation.

□ NURSING PROCESS (Table 6–8)

Assessment

The patient admitted with a fracture of the femoral shaft often has multiple injuries to other systems of the body, because femoral shaft fractures frequently result from "high energy" trauma. Because the femur is the longest bone and endures a tremendous amount of stress, it is the strongest bone in the body. The powerful muscles that surround the femur provide it with a plentiful blood supply. When fractures occur, even closed fractures, they are associated with significant blood loss, especially during the first 12 hours. Assess for signs of shock, and look for other injuries, especially internal or head injuries, that may have occurred at the time of the accident (Edmondson & Crenshaw, 1980, p. 594). For further details on assessment, see Chapter 2.

In the typical patient with a fractured femoral shaft, the leg tends to develop medial rotation of the lower fragment. The gluteus medius muscle has a tendency to pull the proximal fragment outward, and the strong pull of the adductor muscle group tends to cause outward bowing at the point of the fracture.

A neurovascular assessment is done to determine skin color, pulse, joint motion, and complaints of numbness, coldness, or swelling of the leg (Chap. 2). If there is an open fracture, note the amount and color of drainage.

TABLE 6–8. NURSING PROCESS FOR FRACTURED FEMUR TREATED WITH BALANCED SKELETAL TRACTION

Assessment	Nursing Diagnosis	Goal Formulation	Planning and Intervention	Evaluation and Reassessment
1. Assess the location, duration, and severity of pain. Check alignment of leg and traction. Assess the neurovascular status of the involved leg.	1. Alteration in comfort: pain in leg related to bone and soft tissue trauma.	1. Short-term goal: a decrease in pain through immobilization with traction. Long-term goal: free of pain.	1. Alleviate Pain Maintain traction. Keep from jarring traction. Teach relaxation techniques. Utilize distraction. Teach muscle setting exercises. Administer pain medications as indicated.	1. The traction should help to reduce pain. Relaxation techniques and muscle setting should help reduce muscle spasms. Medication should help to relieve pain not relieved by other methods.
2. Assess the patient's body alignment and the alignment of the involved leg. Check the traction for the correct amount of weight and the angle of pull. Assess the patient's ability to follow directions and do exercise regime. Assess the patient's ability to lift self with the use of the trapeze. Assess neurovascular status of in-	2. Impaired physical mobility: decreased leg function related to lack of bone stability.	2. Short-term goal: an increase in mobility through traction and exercises. Long-term goal: regain full function in the leg.	2. Increase Mobility *Position* Keep patient supine. Elevate head of bed as indicated for comfort. Teach patient how to use trapeze. *Exercises* Instruct on exercises for upper extremity and uninvolved leg. Instruct on muscle setting exercises (quadriceps and gluteal), plantar and dorsiflexion exercises and active range-of-motion exercises of the ankle.	2. The patient should understand the rationale for positioning and cooperation in maintaining the correct position. Exercises should be done by the patient on a regular basis. There should be no signs of hip flexion contractures, footdrop, or atrophy.

(continued)

TABLE 6–8. *(Continued)*

Assessment	Nursing Diagnosis	Goal Formulation	Planning and Intervention	Evaluation and Reassessment
volved leg and compare it with the uninvolved leg.			Teach exercises to increase upper extremity strength. *Traction* Maintain traction at all times. Keep leg in abduction. Keep traction apparatus off the bed. Keep correct amount of knee flexion. Keep the involved foot in correct alignment.	
3. Assess vital signs and observe the patient's color and temperature. Check skin turgor and mucus membranes texture. Assess fluid intake and output. Assess muscle tone and strength.	3. Potential fluid volume deficit related to decreased intake and volume loss secondary to surgery and trauma.	3. Short-term goal: fluid volume within normal limits. Long-term goal: free of circulatory problems.	3. Prevent Complications *Circulatory* Maintain hydration. Offer fluids patient likes on a regular basis. Change patient's position slowly. Apply elastic stockings to uninvolved leg. Teach exercise program.	3. The patient should remain well hydrated with good muscle tone and skin turgor.
Auscultate the chest for lung clearance. Check respiratory rate, depth, and rhythm. Assess patient's color.	Potential alteration in respiratory function: impaired gas exchange related to pulmonary and fat emboli.	Short- and long-term goals: free of any respiratory complications.	*Respiratory* Keep patient well hydrated. Administer anticoagulant drugs. Teach coughing and deep breathing exercises.	The patient should remain free of respiratory complications.

Check for any shortness of breath or chest pain. Check for any signs of petechiae.			Teach muscle setting exercises. *Occurrence of Emboli* Immobilize patient. Elevate head of bed. Start oxygen. Notify physician.	
Assess posterior bony prominences for signs of pressure. Assess the involved leg especially behind the knee and in the heel area where it rests on the sling. Check for pressure where ever the traction equipment makes contact with the patient's skin. Assess the pin site for any signs of infection.	Potential impairment in skin integrity: disruption of skin layers related to pressure. Potential for injury: infection at pin site related to skeletal traction.	Short- and long-term goals: free of any problem with skin integrity.	*Integumentary* Apply eggcrate, sheepskin, or other protection to patient's bed. Teach patient how to utilize trapeze to lift off bed and relieve pressure. Keep bed flat a portion of the day (to reduce skid). Keep pressure from traction equipment off patient's skin. Reposition involved leg to reduce any pressure at knee or heel. Keep dressing clean and dry.	The patient should remain free of any skin complications.
4. Assess the patient's level of understanding about the purposes and goals of the traction. Assess patient's understanding about injury and rehabilitation process.	4. Potential knowledge deficit related to traction and the rehabilitation process.	4. Short- and long-term goals: a decrease in anxiety through an increased knowledge.	4. Patient Teaching Discuss the rehabilitation process. Discuss the rationale for use of traction. Instruct in self-help. Include patient's family and significant other in teaching plan. Implement handicrafts or other activities for bed patients.	4. The patient, family, and significant other should understand the various steps in the rehabilitation process and why traction was used.

Observe the emotional reaction of the patient, the family, and significant others. Many times fractures of the femur occur to working-age adults during their leisure time activities, and the patient feels guilty about how the accident occurred and about missing work.

Nursing Diagnosis and Goal Formulation

Nursing diagnoses for a typical patient with a fractured femur are (1) alterations in comfort related to pain in the thigh from trauma to bone and soft tissue, (2) alterations in mobility related to lack of bone stability, (3) alterations in psychological well-being related to anxiety and knowledge deficit from loss of mobility and rehabilitation, and (4) potential complications related to trauma and immobility.

Short-term goals are to have the patient experience (1) a decrease in pain through the use of specific nursing measures, traction, and prescribed medications, (2) an increase in mobility through exercise, positioning, and maintaining traction, (3) a decrease in anxiety through increased knowledge about the injury and the process of rehabilitation, and (4) an absence of complications from surgery and immobility. Long-term goals are to have the patient free of pain and able to walk without a limp or an assistive device.

Planning and Intervention

Alleviate Pain. In the beginning, patients placed in balanced skeletal traction following a fractured femur have pain due to soft tissue and bone trauma. Medications are ordered to help relieve the pain temporarily, and being in traction helps greatly in the long run. The traction helps to align the bone fragment, to counteract the muscle spasms that pull the bone out of alignment, and to maintain immobilization. Pain usually increases if the traction is readjusted or if someone disturbs the traction equipment, or if the patient moves the affected leg out of alignment.

Increase Mobility

Position. The patient must be taught the correct body and leg positioning, and the importance of staying in the proper position and not readjusting any part of the apparatus. Patients need to know how much movement is allowed, the ways in which they can help themselves, and the importance of reporting any pain, pressure, or discomfort that develops. Most patients with a fractured femur in balanced skeletal traction lie supine. Some, depending on the level of the fracture and their general condition, may be able to tilt to the side, and most are able to move rather freely in bed. They may sit up with the use of the overhead trapeze or have the head of the bed elevated, generally at 30 degrees and at 45 degrees for meals. However, some patients may have restrictions on the amount of elevation allowed because it may reduce countertraction (i.e., the effective weight of the patient's body that balances the weights on the traction). To prevent hip flexion contractures, the head of the bed must be completely lowered several times daily. This provides for extension of the hip joints.

The position of the extremity in suspension traction is determined by the fracture, but usually the extremity is held in a neutral position or in a position of slight internal rotation. The amount of abduction may vary. The position the patient assumes in bed affects the amount of abduction maintained, and if the patient lies diagonally, abduction is lost. A short footboard or a small flexion pillow for the uninvolved foot helps the patient maintain the desired position. With suspension traction, the knee of the uninvolved leg should be at the same level as the fastening of the Pearson attachment onto the Thomas splint.

With the use of the suspension traction, the patient is able to pull on the trapeze, push down with the uninvolved leg and lift the buttocks off the bed. This greatly helps in getting the patient on the bedpan, changing linen, and giving skin care to the coccyx area. When the patient raises him- or herself in the suspension apparatus, the line of traction remains unchanged. The suspension thus allows freedom for the body as a whole while efficient traction on the leg is maintained.

Exercises. Exercise increases circulation and maintains muscle tone and must be part of the care for a patient in skeletal traction. Muscle weakness and contractures occur from disuse. No unnecessary stiffness or atrophy should be allowed to occur because of the immobilization of the injured leg. Exercises for the uninvolved portions of the body should include flexion and extension of the hip and knee of the unaffected leg; range of motion at the ankle; plantar and dorsiflexion of the foot; quadriceps, gluteal, and abdominal setting exercises; exercises to develop the extensors of the elbows and wrists (to facilitate future crutch walking); and breathing exercises. Encourage activities of self-care and the use of the trapeze if the patient's arms will allow.

Patients tend to guard joints near a fracture; therefore, explanations and encouragement are needed to promote the active and passive exercising of the foot and to prevent a contracture of the Achilles tendon of the affected leg. Quadriceps and plantar and dorsiflexion exercises are also part of the exercise program for the affected leg (see pp. 258–259). Quadriceps muscles begin to atrophy in about 1 week if not used.

Patient Teaching. The accident was an emotional as well as physical shock to the patient, and being placed in balanced skeletal traction can be a very fearful experience. Even though explanations were given when the traction was applied, most patients are unable to fully comprehend them. Once things have settled down, discuss the traction equipment and its purposes with the patient, the family, and significant others. Reinforcing what the different purposes of the traction are when you are working with it or asking the patient to participate will also increase the patient's understanding.

Know what the physician has told the patient and what the plan of treatment will be. Will the patient be in the traction for a few days before surgery, and if surgery, what method? Will the patient later be put in a cast brace, or is traction the only method of treatment? If traction is the only treatment, the patient may remain in traction 3 months or more. If traction is not to be the only method of treatment, patient education should be started concerning follow-up care. Of course the answers need to be given with the clarifier that plans can change based on the patient's response to traction. Do not forget to make time to discuss with the patient the emotional reaction to the accident, and what effect is has had on his or her life and the lives of others.

Prevent Complications. The patient in balanced skeletal traction is prone to all the complications of bedrest discussed previously, especially emotional boredom. In addition, the following problems are of particular concern.

Circulatory. When a bone is fractured, surrounding soft tissue, blood vessels, and nerves are also injured, and there may be enough blood loss to cause shock. Generally the patient is most vulnerable to shock during the first 12 hours.

Respiratory. The patient with a closed fractured femur is at risk of fat emboli and respiratory complications due to bedrest.

Integumentary. In administering care, make sure that there is no pressure on the popliteal space or on the lateral aspect of the leg over the head of the fibula. Reposition the patient and/or slings to relieve any pressure. Institutions differ over how to care for the pin tract sites. Some want the original dressing to go untouched unless infection is suspected. Others want the site treated daily with an anti-infective agent like betadine. However, the use of an iodine preparation for skin care around pins is questionable. Still others want the site left exposed. Whatever the method, teach the patient to recognize the signs and the symptoms of infection.

Evaluation and Reassessment

A patient in balanced skeletal traction should feel reasonably comfortable, that is, free of any severe pain. A neurovascular evaluation of the affected extremity should find good nerve and vascular function. In evaluating whether traction is being maintained, note the alignment of the body and the leg. Evaluate whether the patient is complying with exercise regime and rehabilitation program. The patient should be free of potential complications such as pressure areas, footdrop, hip flexion contractures, or other effects of immobility. If the goals have not been met, both the goals and the plan of care must be reassessed and the nursing process begun again.

Cast Brace

Fractures of the distal half of the shaft of the femur can be treated for 1 to 6 weeks with skeletal traction, after which the traction is removed and a femoral cast brace applied. By that time, the soft tissues have started to heal and swelling is reduced.

A cast brace (Fig. 6–23) is a combination of cast and brace made up of three components. First, there is a patellar weight-bearing cast on the lower leg, either as a short leg cast or a cylinder cast. Second, there is an ischial weight-bearing cast on the thigh, molded well around Scapra's triangle, the ischial seat, and the greater trochanter. The thigh component is applied snugly to increase the hydrodynamic compressive effect of the thigh muscles and to provide for immobilization of the fracture fragments. Third, there is an external polycentric knee hinge that connects the below the knee portion to the thigh portion and that allows 90 degrees of knee flexion. The cast brace allows

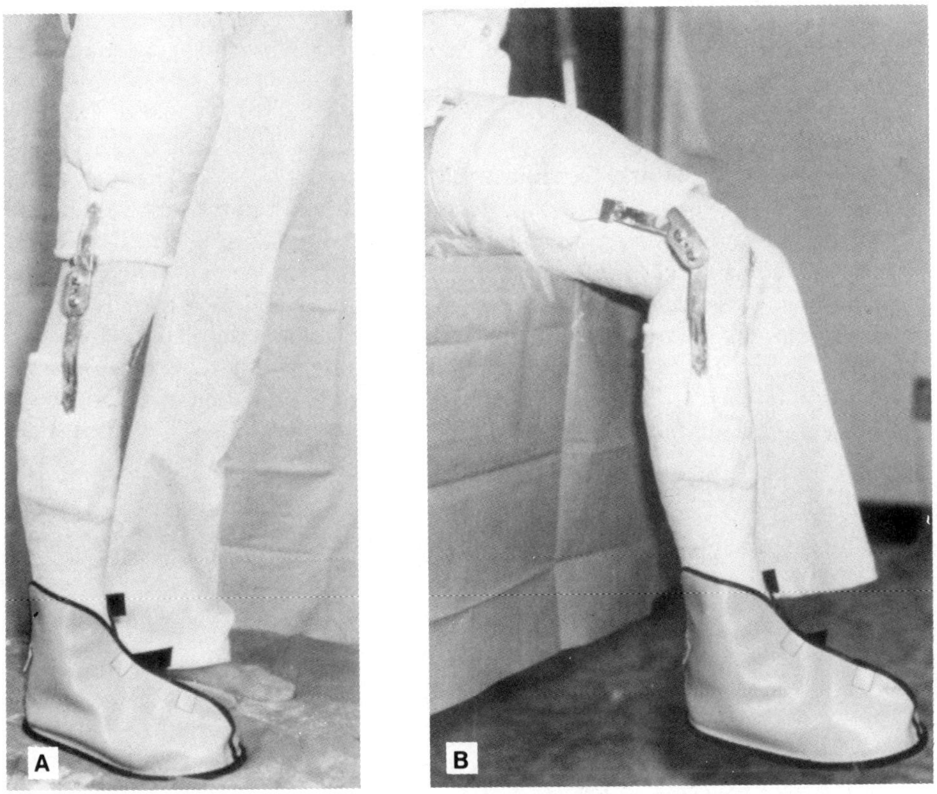

Figure 6–23. Cast brace. **A.** The patient standing with a cast shoe and the brace in full extension. **B.** The patient sitting with the knee bent to a comfortable angle. *(From Lewis, R. C.* Handbook of traction, casting and splinting techniques. *Philadelphia: Lippincott, 1977, p. 95, with permission.)*

for mobility of both hip and knee joints while allowing a fairly normal gait when ambulating.

Cast bracing is based on the concept that weight bearing is always a physiological activity and will promote the formation of bone. It allows early ambulation with partial weight bearing, which promotes healing by adding pressure to the fracture site, by improving circulation, by mobilizing muscles, and by lessening edema in the capsules and joint structures of the knee (Brunner & Suddarth, 1980, p. 1284).

□ NURSING PROCESS (Table 6–9)

Assessment

The overall condition of the patient has generally stabilized before the cast brace is applied, but the nurse needs to assess the involved leg after the cast brace is applied. Assess the amount, kind, and location of pain. Check the neurovascular status of the affected extremity. Check the skin around the edge of both casts, and note any complaints or discomfort at the proximal or distal ends. Ensure that the hinges of the cast brace are functioning. Do a general assessment of each cast as discussed in Appendix B.

Nursing Diagnosis and Goal Formulation

The nursing diagnoses and long-term goals for a patient in a cast brace remain the same as they were when the patient was in skeletal traction. The short-term goals are to have the patient experience (1) a decrease in pain through specific nursing measures and prescribed medications, (2) an increase in mobility through exercises and controlled ambulation, (3) a decrease in anxiety through increased knowledge about the purpose and function of the cast brace, its role in the process of rehabilitation, and how to do crutch walking, and (4) an absence of complications.

Planning and Intervention

Alleviate Pain. Measures to alleviate pain are the same as those for skeletal traction and a patient in a long leg cast.

Increase Mobility. Exercises and turning procedures for a patient with a cast brace are the same as those for a patient with a long leg cast (discussed in Appendix B).

Ambulation. Even though the patient may start ambulating as soon as the cast is dry, care should be taken the first time the patient gets up because he or she has been on bedrest for some time. The patient will be using crutches, allowing partial weight bearing on the affected leg. The hinges at the knee are unlocked before the patient starts to get out of bed, and are locked before the patient stands and begins to walk. When the patient

TABLE 6–9. NURSING PROCESS FOR FRACTURED FEMUR TREATED WITH A CAST BRACE

Assessment	Nursing Diagnosis	Goal Formulation	Planning and Intervention	Evaluation and Reassessment
1. Assess the duration, location, and severity of pain. Observe for verbal and nonverbal signs of pain. Assess the neurovascular status of the involved leg.	1. Alteration in comfort: pain in the leg related to soft tissue and bone trauma.	1. Short-term goal: a reduction in the amount of leg pain. Long-term goal: free of any pain.	1. Alleviate Pain Keep the involved leg elevated when sitting or lying. Teach muscle setting exercises. Utilize distraction and repositioning. Teach relaxation techniques. Administer prescribed medication.	1. The patient should remain relatively free of pain.
2. Assess the position of the leg. Check the neurovascular status. Check the strength in the upper extremities and uninvolved leg. Assess the patient's ability to do the exercise regime. Check that the hinges on the cast are in working condition.	2. Impaired physical mobility: decreased leg function related to lack of bone stability.	2. Short-term goal: an increase in mobility through exercises and immobilization with a cast brace. Long-term goal: regain full function in the involved leg.	2. Increase Mobility *Position* Place patient in a position of comfort. Keep the leg elevated. Make sure leg is positioned safely. *Exercises* Teach quadriceps and gluteal setting exercises. Teach active range-of-motion exercises for the ankle. Instruct on exercising all uninvolved joints. Instruct on exercises to increase upper extremity strength for crutch walking.	2. The patient should utilize correct positioning in bed and ambulate safely. The patient should be able to demonstrate ability to do exercises without supervision.

(continued)

TABLE 6–9. ***(Continued)***

Assessment	Nursing Diagnosis	Goal Formulation	Planning and Intervention	Evaluation and Reassessment
			Ambulation Instruct on 4-point crutch gait. Make sure patient knows how to go up and down stairs and how to get in and out of a chair. Teach patient to flex the knee while sitting and to do flexion and extension exercises.	
3. Assess for signs of swelling. Assess the neurovascular status. Assess the patient's ability to do exercises. Check the position of the leg when the patient is lying and sitting. Check for tightness of the cast.	3. Potential alteration in tissue perfusion: edema related to soft tissue and bone trauma.	3. Short-term goal: a decrease in the amount of swelling around the knee. Long-term goal: free of any circulatory problems.	3. Prevent Complications *Circulatory* Explain to the patient that swelling at the knee usually occurs. Encourage quadriceps setting and knee flexion and extension exercise. Elevate leg when sitting or lying.	3. The patient should remain free of any circulatory problems.

Assess skin at cast edges (especially the proximal edge along the groin and gluteal areas and the distal edge at the knee). Assess for location, duration, and severity of pain. Check tightness of cast.	Potential impairment of skin integrity: pressure areas or a break in skin integrity related to the cast.	Short- and long-term goals: free of any integumentary problems.	*Integumentary* Petal rough cast edges. Utilize a small amount of cornstarch to smooth the skin and reduce irritation. Check when placing patient on bedpan so as not to pinch the skin along proximal edge of cast. Reposition leg every 2 hours to ease pressure. Follow up any complaints of pain and discomfort. *Potential Complications Due to Immobility* (See Chap. 3 and Table 6–2)	The patient should remain free of any break in skin integrity.
4. Assess the patient's level of understanding about the rehabilitation process, cast care, and home care.	4. Potential knowledge deficit related to the rehabilitation process, cast care, and home care.	4. Short- and long-term goals: a decrease in anxiety through increased knowledge.	4. Patient Teaching Discuss the various steps in the rehabilitation process. Discuss cast care. Demonstrate methods of bathing and dressing with a cast brace on. Discuss techniques for getting into a car or utilizing public transportation. Include family and significant other in teaching plan.	4. The patient, family, and significant other should feel confident about the patient going home.

gets onto a commode or into a chair, the hinges are unlocked again. A priority for the nurse assisting with ambulation is to check the status of the hinges.

Exercises. The patient will continue to do the exercises started while the patient was in balanced skeletal traction. The patient can now do flexion and extension exercises while sitting, which is probably a more comfortable position than standing or lying supine.

Patient Teaching. First and foremost, the patient should understand the purpose of the cast brace and how it works, and why he or she should not try to adjust or alter it. Teach the patient, the family, and significant others about the general care of the cast brace and the involved leg, and discuss home care and safety precautions (Appendix B).

Prevent Complications

Circulatory. Nursing care for a patient with a cast brace is similar to that of the patient in a long leg cast with one major difference: patients with a cast brace frequently have swelling above the knee. After traction is removed and the cast brace is applied, the patient frequently has swelling about the knee and to some degree in the toes, especially after ambulation. The knee may swell up to twice the normal size and cause the cast to feel tight. Even though that is an expected outcome and will gradually subside over time, there are a number of measures that may facilitate the process. Explain to the patient why that phenomenom occurs, and that it is not a cause for alarm. Encourage quadriceps setting exercises, exercising the knee with flexion and extension, and elevating the complete leg when not weight bearing. Teach the patient to report any changes in neurovascularity, e.g., tingling, numbness, or coldness in the involved leg (Chap. 2) and how to elevate the casted leg.

Integumentary. Pressure areas are a potential problem with any cast, but with the cast brace this is especially true. The thigh component has a particular tendency to develop pressure areas, because the proximal edge extends well into the groin and gluteal areas, and the distal edge presses against the swelling at the knee. An activity that seems to present added skin problems is getting on and off the bedpan because it may pinch the skin along the proximal edge of the cast. Measures to help relieve the discomfort are to reposition the casted extremity to ease pressure on specific areas. Make sure there are no rough edges on the cast. Petal the cast edges as indicated. Sometimes a small amount of cornstarch will help to smooth the skin and reduce irritation. Follow up all complaints of pain or discomfort.

Evaluation and Reassessment

The considerations discussed for the patient who has had an internal fixation apply here as well. Special emphasis should be given to evaluating the patient's response to the cast brace and understanding of home care instructions and safety precautions.

Open Reduction with Plates and Screws

Plates and screws are commonly used for internal fixations of fractures involving the upper or lower thirds of the femur and for fractures unsuitable for intramedullary nailing. For fixation by plates and screws (Fig. 6–24), the AO plate or dynamic compression plate is used. The plates may be placed on two sides of the bone at right angles to each other. When plates and screws are used for internal fixation of femoral shaft fractures, weight bearing and unprotected ambulation are usually not allowed as early as they are when repair is an intramedullary nail. The plates are usually removed after 24 months provided that union is complete.

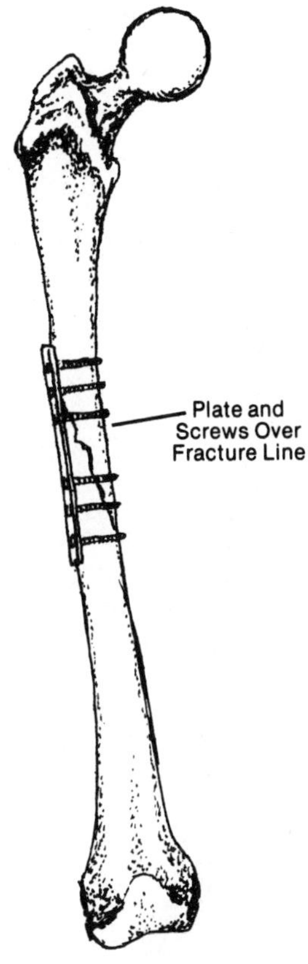

Figure 6–24. Open reduction and internal fixation, fractured femur. *(From Brantley, P., & Analla, M., 1980, p. 82. Courtesy of Howmedica.)*

Intramedullary Fixation

In adults with closed uncomminuted fractures through the narrow portion of the medullary canal, intramedullary fixation is the treatment of choice. A variety of intramedullary fixation devices exist (Fig 6–25), including the Rush rod, the cloverleaf Küntscher nail, the double I-Beam nail, Schneider's self-broaching nail, the AO femoral nail, and the Hanson-Street diamond-shaped nail. The nail must be of sufficient length and strength and of sufficient size to completely fill the medullary canal for fixation to be secure.

The two most serious complications are nonunion and infection. Nonunion is usually the result of failure to accomplish fixation because the nail is too small or the fracture is too far proximal or distal in the shaft; thus the nail cannot completely fill the medullary canal and control rotation. Fixation is also poor in fractures that are too comminuted. The development of infection after intramedullary fixation is serious as it greatly increases the likelihood of nonunion. Even if union does occur, it may take years. Amputation may be the ultimate result of an infection (Edmondson & Crenshaw, 1980, p. 607).

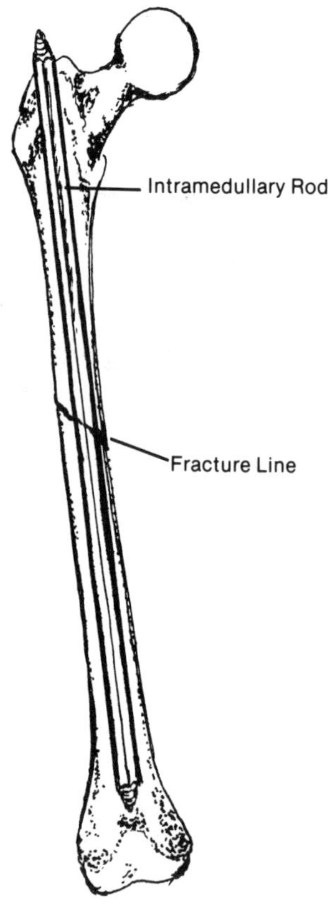

Figure 6–25. Reduction and internal fixation, fractured femur: intramedullary rod. *(From Brantley, P., & Analla, M., 1980, p. 81. Courtesy of Howmedica.)*

Open Method. Open intramedullary nailing of the femur involves inserting a nail after surgical exposure of the fracture. After reaming the proximal and distal canals, a guide wire is driven up the proximal segment until it exits from the superior neck at the base of the trochanter or through its medial margin. The intramedullary nail is introduced over the guide wire, driven down the medullary canal across the fracture site and into the distal fragment, usually to the level of the proximal pole of the patella, as reduction is accomplished.

Postoperative care consists of support, not immobilization, provided by a Thomas splint for 5 to 7 days. Quadriceps settings and plantar and dorsiflexion exercises are usually started as soon as the patient recovers from anesthesia. It is important to begin these exercises and to continue them, as they maintain muscle tone and strength that compress the fracture and probably stimulate local vascularity (Edmondson & Crenshaw, 1980, pp. 597–602).

Closed Method. Closed intramedullary nailing is a method to nail shaft fractures of long bones without exposing the fracture site. It was first advocated by Küntscher in 1940, but has become more widely used with the development of image intensifier television fluoroscopy. With the closed method an incision is made proximal to the greater trochanter, and a hole is made in the trochanter just medial to its tip. The nail is then driven down the medullary canal across the fracture site toward the condyles. The fracture site may be manipulated to get the nail across the fracture, but the fracture site is never opened (Edmondson & Crenshaw, 1980, pp. 603–607).

Postoperative care usually consists of balanced suspension with a Thomas splint for 3 to 4 days, and early active quadriceps and plantar and dorsiflexion exercises. As soon as muscle control of the leg is gained, ambulation on crutches is permitted with no weight bearing. Progressively increasing weight bearing is permitted as roentgenographs indicate progress and complete union. Often union is rapid, and unrestricted weight bearing may be permitted by 10 to 12 weeks. When the rigidity of fixation is not optimal because of comminution or other problems, alterations in the rehabilitation program and delay in weight bearing may be required (Edmondson & Crenshaw, 1980, pp. 603–607).

External Fixation

External fixation is often indicated for patients who have a lot of soft tissue damage as well as an open fracture, and are thus not candidates for open reduction and internal fixation or skeletal traction. Two heavy Steinmann pins are inserted proximal to the fracture and two are inserted below the fracture and immobilized by the use of external devices such as the Hoffman or Wagner devices. These devices are particularly applicable when there is a severe open fracture accompanied by extensive soft tissue injury. In those instances, the major complications are infection, tissue necrosis, misalignment, and fracture instability that can delay healing and endanger the extremity. In instances with less severe tissue damage, the four Steinmann pins may be incorporated into a plaster total contact thigh cast. (For more details on the care of a patient with an external fixation, see Chap. 7.)

Fractures of the Distal Third of the Femur

Fractures of the distal third of the femur can be classified into supracondylar fractures without joint involvement and condylar fractures with joint involvement.

Supracondylar fractures not involving the joint, which are undisplaced or impacted fractures, can usually be treated with a few days of traction followed by application of a cast brace. For severely displaced and comminuted fractures, the usual treatment is skeletal traction with a Kirschner wire near the tibial tuberosity. After reduction has been obtained and maintained for 2 to 3 weeks, the leg can usually be placed in a femoral cast brace and ambulation permitted (Edmondson & Crenshaw, 1980, p. 587).

For supracondylar fractures not involving the joint, open reduction and internal fixation is usually only done for fractures secondary to a pathological process or when the condition of the patient will not permit bed confinement for traction. Such internal fixations are usually repaired using Blount or Elliott blade plates, straight plates, Rush pins, and other devices. Complications that can occur are infection, nonunion, and restriction of motion (Edmondson & Crenshaw, 1980, p. 587).

Condylar fractures involving the joint may be unicondylar or bicondylar. A common method of treatment is skeletal traction with a pin through the tibia near the tuberosity, and if necessary an additional pin through the distal fragment of the femur, with light traction used to help with positioning. Open reduction may be necessary following a period of traction. Unicondylar displaced fractures may be treated with an open reduction and internal fixation using Knowles pins and cancellous screws. When the posterior part of the medial femoral condyle is sheared off, an open reduction and internal fixation with a lag screw may be used. For T condylar fractures, a method of fixing the fracture would be a plate, Knowles pins, and four screws (Edmondson & Crenshaw, 1980, p. 587–593).

Pathology

NEOPLASMS

Amputations

Above the knee (AK) amputations of the lower extremity may be the result of a number of disorders, including infections, neoplasms, and traumatic injuries. Most, however, are the result of peripheral arterial disease.

By far the most frequently encountered form of peripheral arterial disease is arteriosclerosis obliterans, or peripheral arterial insufficiency, an organic disease of the arteries of the legs. The disease causes the arteries to become narrowed and obstructed so that the legs and feet do not receive enough blood. The obtructions usually are permanent, and the disease is therefore chronic. Arteriosclerosis obliterans is a disease restricted almost exclusively to adults and is usually manifested at ages over 50. Diabetes mellitus appears to increase the prevalence and severity of the disease, as does cigarette smoking. Circulation to the legs can be improved by growing (or grafting) new blood vessels and by increasing the volume of blood carried by unblocked arteries. Femoral–popliteal bypass surgery is also used to relieve this condition. If these methods fail, however, an amputation may be necessary.

The nursing assessment of the patient before surgery emphasizes a circulatory assessment of the lower extremities. Probably the most important assessment is for arterial pulsation. The assessment proceeds from the dorsalis pedis, to the posterior tibial, the popliteal, and finally the femoral artery. Note how distally you were able to detect a pulse, bearing in mind that in the normal healthy population, 7 percent lack a dorsalis pedis pulse, and 3 percent lack a posterior tibial pulse (Brunner & Suddarth, 1980, p. 618). Use Doppler to help in the assessment of the pulse. Note any intermittent claudication, that is a pain, ache, cramp, or feeling of severe fatigue that affects the muscles distal to the occluded artery after exercise, and that is usually relieved by rest. Assess skin temperature, looking for alterations in the skin temperature of the patient's lower extremities by using the dorsum of your hand or the back of a finger. Compare one extremity to the other, unless both are involved. Note the skin color changes that occur in various positions. Abnormal postural color changes are pallor (which indicates a cessation of capillary flow), cyanosis (which indicates an obstruction to the outflow of blood), and rubor (which indicates an excessive flow of blood because of arterial and capillary dilation). Note any ulceration or gangrenous appearance, especially in the terminal segment of the toes or the heel.

Surgical Procedure

Amputation through the thigh (AK amputation) is the second most frequent kind of amputation, exceeded only by below-knee procedures. Because in the AK amputation the patient's knee joint is lost, it is extremely important that the stump provide a good fit for the prosthesis. The conventional constant-friction knee joint in most AK prosthesis extends 9 to 10 cm distal to the end of the prosthetic socket, so the femur must be amputated sufficiently proximal to the knee to allow room for the joint in the prosthesis. Thus, most AK amputations are performed anywhere from 10 cm above the knee joint to 10 cm below the hip joint.

In a closed AK amputation, the skin flaps are usually equal, hence the suture line divides the anterior and posterior portions of the stump. The femur is severed about 5 cm proximal to the muscles and skin, the blood vessels are ligated and cut, the sciatic nerve is ligated and cut approximately 5 to 7.5 cm proximal to the end of the bone. The muscles are either sutured over the distal end of the femur or holes are made in the distal end and the muscles are sutured to the bone (myoplasty). Penrose drains or plastic tubes for suction drainage are placed deep into the wound and the skin flaps are closed. An immediate postsurgical fitting is then applied to the femur, with one strap going around the waist and a second going over the shoulder. (See the section on hemipelvectomy and hip disarticulation for further details on immediate postsurgical prosthetic fittings.) For patients without an immediate postsurgical fitting, a pressure dressing is applied and a procedure for stump wrapping is instituted (Fig. 6–26).

When there is an infection or potential infection an alternative procedure known as a guillotine or open amputation is usually done. In a guillotine amputation the bone, skin, and muscle tissues are all resected at the same level. The blood vessels are ligated, but the skin is not sutured closed to allow for

---

Begin by explaining to the patient that the purpose of the procedure is to help reduce swelling and shape the stump for a prosthesis. Explain the procedure to the patient as you are doing the bandaging, as the patient must learn to do it by himself or herself.

Sew three 4-inch elastic bandages together end-to-end and roll them into one long bandage or use a special elastic bandage designed for stump wrapping. Make figure 8 turns with the bandage, wrapping the stump around the top of the patient's leg, downward under the stump, and back to the groin area. Keep the bandage roll away from the stump and avoid going straight around the stump, as that is apt to interfere with circulation.

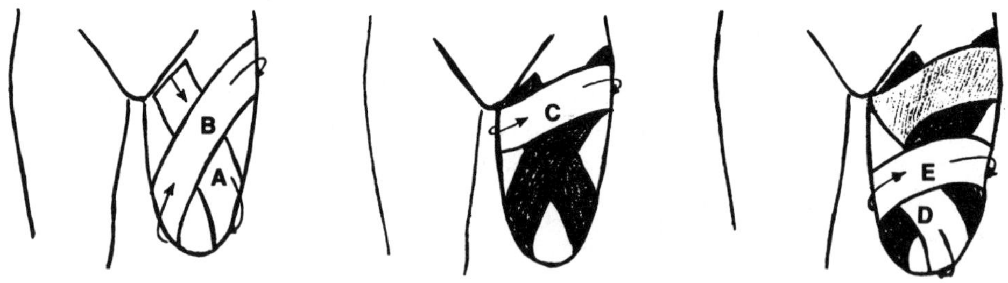

To begin, have the patient in a semi-Fowler's position or sitting on the side of the bed. Hold the end of the elastic bandage at the top medial anterior surface of the patient's leg or, even better if the patient is able, ask the patient to hold the bandage. Bring the bandage diagonally downward toward the distal end of the patient's stump and loop the bandage around the end of the stump *(A)*.

While applying even pressure, bring the bandage diagonally upward over the anterior of the stump up to the groin *(B)*, and bring the bandage around the back of the stump and across the front *(C)* to anchor the proximal ends of turns *(A)* and *(B)*. That completes the first figure 8 and it will no longer be necessary to hold the end of the bandage.

Continue around the back of the patient's stump once again and bring the bandage from high on the medial side down to the lateral aspect of the distal end of the stump *(D)*. Bring the bandage about halfway up the back toward the medial side of the stump, and continue across the front going slightly upward *(E)*.

Figure 6–26. Bandaging an above-knee amputation. *(Modified from Bandaging Instruction for Above-the-Knee Amputations, Department of Physical Medicine and Rehabilitation, University of Illinois at the Center Research and Educational Hospitals, Chicago, Illinois [undated].)*

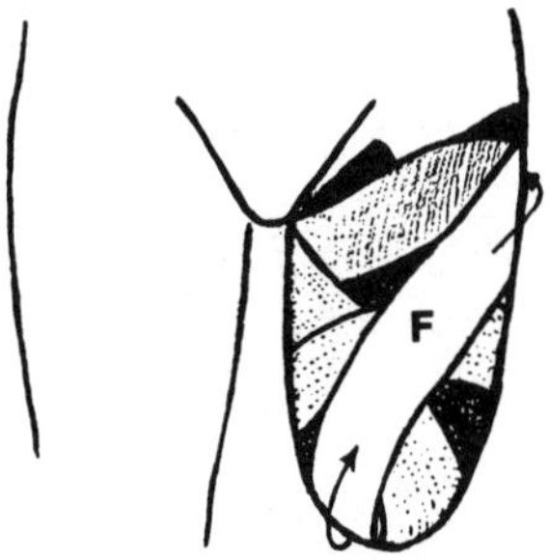

Then bring the bandage down the back to the end of the stump on the medial side, and up the front diagonally toward the hip on the lateral side *(F)*. (Turns *D, E,* and *F* make the second figure 8.)

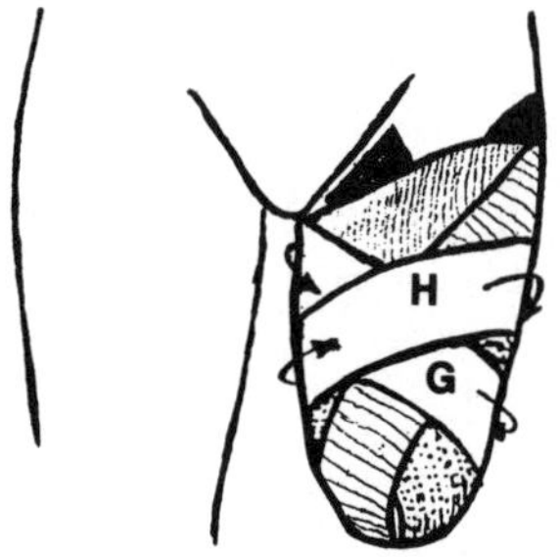

Continue around the back of the leg and up on the medial side, and then bring the bandage across the front, going slightly downward *(G)*. Next, bring the bandage around the back going slightly upward, and continue that upward motion across the front of the stump *(H)*.

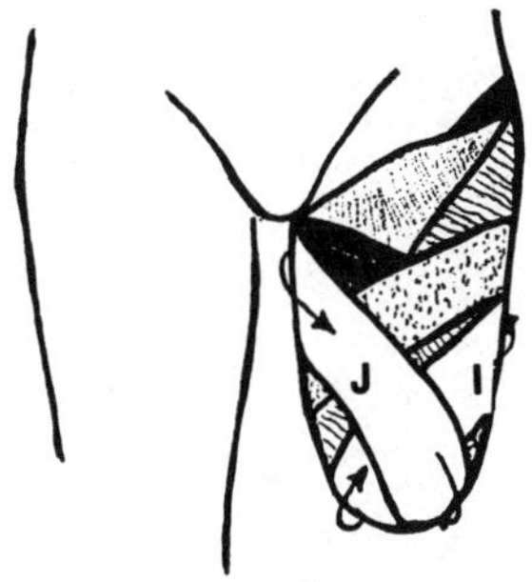

Bring the bandage downward across the back to the end of the stump on the medial side, and then bring it halfway up the front toward the lateral side *(I)*. Continue the upward motion around the back of the stump to the upper medial side, and then angle the bandage downward across the front to the end of the stump on the lateral side *(J)*. Repeat the figure 8 turns at least once more to the groin, to cover all of the fatty tissue high on the inside of the thigh.

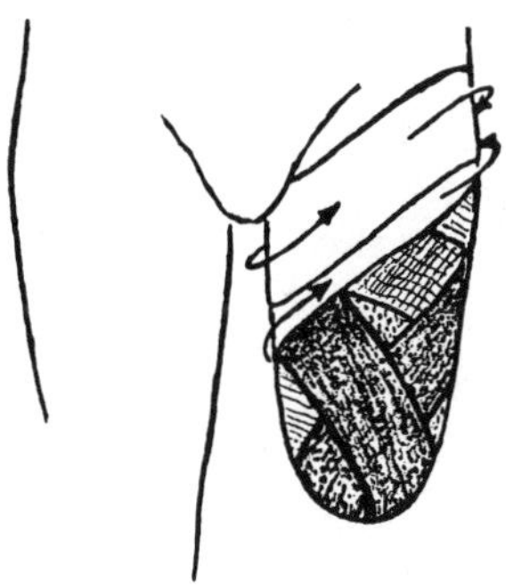

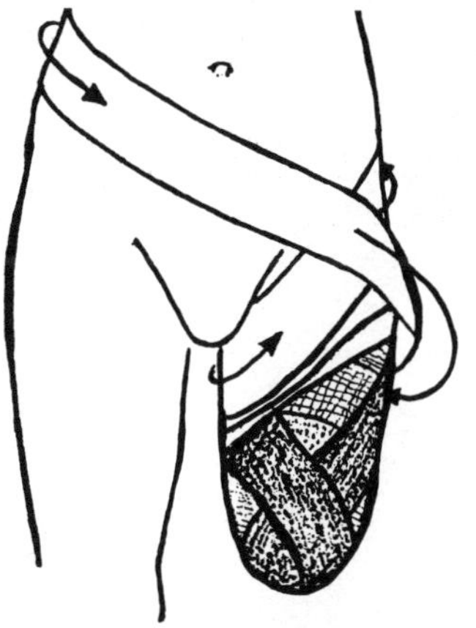

To prevent the bandage from slipping, bring it diagonally over the patient's buttocks to the opposite iliac crest, and then diagonally across the lower abdomen toward the lateral side of the stump, resuming figure 8s until the stump is completely covered and the elastic bandage is exhausted.

Finally, secure the bandage with clips, safety pins, or adhesive tape. If clips or safety pins are used, make sure they are on the anterior surface of the stump to prevent pressure areas from developing. Chart the procedure, the patient teaching, and the patient's response.

TABLE 6–10. NURSING PROCESS FOR ABOVE-KNEE AMPUTATION WITH A RIGID DRESSING

Assessment	Nursing Diagnosis	Goal Formulation	Planning and Intervention	Evaluation and Reassessment
1. Assess the location, duration, and severity of pain. Observe for verbal and nonverbal cues of pain. Assess for tightness of the cast. Assess for drainage.	1. Alteration in comfort: pain in the leg related to bone and soft tissue trauma secondary to amputation.	1. Short-term goal: a decrease in the amount of leg pain. Long-term goal: free of pain.	1. Alleviate Pain Keep the foot of the bed elevated the first 24 hours after surgery. Help reposition the leg. Utilize distraction and other noninvasive nursing measures. Teach relaxation techniques. Discuss phantom pain. Apply pressure to the end of the stump.	1. Nursing measures and medications should keep the patient fairly comfortable. Discussions and the utilization of pressure at the end of the stump should help reduce phantom pain.
2. Assess patient's ability to do exercises. Assess strength in upper extremity. Assess ability to utilize crutches.	2. Impaired physical mobility: decreased ability to move related to loss of leg.	2. Short-term goal: an increase in mobility through the use of a cast, temporary foot, and crutches. Long-term goal: able to walk safely with a prosthesis.	2. Increase Mobility *Position* Teach use of the trapeze. Place in a position of comfort while supine. Change position every 2 hours when awake and every 4 hours at night. Place sand bags or trochanter roll along lateral side of leg. Place the patient prone with no pillows under the abdomen for 30 mintues to 2 hours at least twice a day. (Gradually increase to 6 hours out of every 24 hours.) *Exercises* Encourage active range of motion of all uninvolved joints. Teach muscle setting exercises (quadriceps and gluteal setting). Teach hip extension, adduction,	2. The patient should be able to do exercises without supervision, but initially may need help in changing position. There should not be any internal rotation, abduction or flexion contractions. In using crutches and a temporary foot, the patient should be carrying most of the body weight on the hands rather than on the temporary foot.

			and abduction exercises. Teach exercises to increase strength in the upper extremities for crutch walking *Ambulation* Instruct on using a 3-point crutch gait (when the patient is not using a temporary foot). Instruct on partial weight bearing (usually only 35–40 pounds) for patients with a temporary foot. Assist with walking.	
3. Assess for signs of infection. Assess level of pain or discomfort. Check vital signs.	3. Potential for injury: infection related to incision.	3. Short- and long-term goals: free of any signs of infection.	3. Prevent Complications *Integumentary* Keep cast dry. Encourage a well-balanced diet and plenty of fluids. Encourage adequate rest. Teach exercises. Administer antibiotics as prescribed.	3. The patient should remain free of any signs of infection.
4. Assess the patient's level of understanding about the rehabilitation process and prognosis.	4. Potential knowledge deficit related to rehabilitation process and future ambulation.	4. Short- and long-term goals: a decrease in anxiety through increased knowledge.	4. Patient Teaching Allow time for discussion of feelings about loss of limb. Discuss changes in body image. Discuss future role performance and activity level. Discuss the potential affect on work and social and personal role performance. Spend time with family and significant other. Discuss the purpose and rationale of the rigid dressing. Discuss potential complications and when to notify physician.	4. The patient should begin to accept changes in body image. The patient should be able to verbalize the beginning stage of acceptance of the amputation. The patient, family, and significant other should be able to discuss the amputation and potential changes in lifestyle.

open drainage of any purulent exudate. The stump is then covered with a bulky compression dressing.

To prevent the skin and muscles from receding from the end of the bone, the extremity is put in skin traction with approximately 5 pounds of weight. There are a number of methods for applying the traction. One is to apply three or four strips of adhesive tape over the dressing and attach them to a piece of wood distal to the end of the stump, which is then connected by a rope and pulley to weights at the foot of the bed. Another is to put a stockinette over the dressing and tie a knot in the end of the stockinette, which is connected to the rope leading to the traction apparatus. After a period of antibiotic therapy and skin traction, the patient returns to surgery for a closed amputation.

□ NURSING PROCESS (Table 6–10)

Assessment

The assessment of a patient following an AK amputation is very similar to that for a patient with a hip disarticulation. If the patient has had an open amputation, check the position of the patient and the traction apparatus to make sure the pull is correct. Note the color and the amount of drainage. Assess the emotional status of the patient. If the patient has had a closed amputation because of a peripheral vascular disease, the patient will have had preoperative teaching. For patients with traumatic injuries, however, there is frequently little time to prepare them and their family.

Nursing Diagnosis and Goal Formulation

The nursing diagnosis for a typical patient with an AK amputation is the same as for a patient with a hip disarticulation. Immediate goals are the same, except the second short-term goal is to have increased ambulation by bed exercises (and traction, if an open amputation). The long-term goals are the same.

Planning and Intervention

Alleviate Pain. See pain relief measures discussed for patients with a hip disarticulation. The traction used in an open amputation, by applying a continuous pull, helps to prevent or reduce pain from muscle spasms.

Increase Mobility. To increase potential for mobility and to decrease complications, bed exercises, such as coughing and deep breathing, exercises for all uninvolved joints, and the use of the trapeze, should be started as soon as the patient recovers from anesthesia. The patient with an immediate postsurgical fitting can turn to either side. Put a pillow between the legs, keeping the stump in correct alignment when turning and resting on a side. Most patients will not want to turn and will need encouragement. Some may prefer lying on the uncasted extremity.

For patients with immediate postsurgical fitting, early ambulation with limited weight bearing on the prosthetic fitting is very beneficial psychologically, and lessens the emotional trauma from the loss of a limb. Most patients are up as soon as the drains are removed, 24 to 48 hours after surgery. Patients generally start ambulating early, although their pylon fitting does not have a knee joint and requires them to walk stiff-legged.

Even after ambulation has begun, patients need to remember proper positioning in bed and must continue to exercise. One recommended exercise is to squeeze a pillow between the legs. (Once the exercise is done remove the pillow to prevent abduction and place a trochanter roll or sandbag along the side of the leg to prevent abduction or external rotation.) Encourage the patient to have the bed flat several times a day and lie prone for a least 30 minutes twice a day. These two procedures help to prevent hip flexion contractures. The patient is encouraged to work on upper extremity exercises to assist with ambulation. Once patients have developed good balance when standing, they should stand, with proper support, and swing the affected extremity back and forth. This procedure helps with hip flexion and extension. Other exercises may be required by the patient's physician and the physical therapist.

For patients with an open amputation and skin traction, maintain the traction as though it were skeletal traction. Do not release the traction without a physician's order. (For more details on traction, see Appendix A.)

Patient Teaching. The areas covered in the care of a patient with a hip disarticulation apply here. An open amputation may be particularly traumatic, and it is important to spend time with the patient discussing the traction, how long it will be on, and the treatments that will follow.

Prevent Complications. Infection or potential infections are of special concern for a patient with an open amputation. If the amputation resulted from osteomyelitis, the patient may be in isolation.

Evaluation and Reassessment

The considerations discussed with regard to an internal fixation and a hip disarticulation apply here. Special attention should be given to evaluating how well the patient is able to ambulate and if the patient has accepted the change in body image. If the patient has an open amputation, check to see if the stump is infection-free.

REFERENCES

Amstutz, H. C. Total hip replacement. In R. G. Tronzo (Ed.), *Surgery of the hip joint.* Philadelphia: Lea & Febiger, 1973.

Armstrong, M. E., Dickason, E. J., Howe, J., et al., *McGraw-Hill handbook of clinical nursing.* New York: McGraw-Hill, 1979.

Blake, S. A. Noncemented femoral prosthesis: Intraoperative focus. *Orthopaedic Nursing,* 1985, *4* (1), 40–42.
Brunner, L. S., & Suddarth, D. S. *Medical–surgical nursing,* (4th ed.). Philadelphia: Lippincott, 1980.
Burgess, E. M., & Zettl, J. H. Amputations and prosthetic management of the hip. In R. G. Tronzo (Ed.), *Surgery of the hip joint.* Philadelphia: Lea & Febiger, 1973.
Compere, E. L. *Orthopaedic surgery.* Chicago: Year Book Med. Pub., 1974.
Coventry, M. B. Tumors in and about the hip. In R. G. Tronzo (Ed.), *Surgery of the hip joint.* Philadelphia: Lea & Febiger, 1973.
Doheny, M. O'B. Porous-coated femoral prosthesis: Concepts and care considerations. *Orthopaedic Nursing,* 1985, *4* (1), 43–45.
Donahoo, C. A., & Dimon, J. H. III. *Orthopedic nursing.* Boston: Little, Brown, 1977.
Edmondson, A. S., & Crenshaw, A. H. *Campbell's operative orthopaedics.* St. Louis: C. V. Mosby, 1980.
Gartland, J. R. *Fundamental of orthopaedics.* Philadelphia: W. B. Saunders, 1979.
Ghista, D. N., & Roaf, R. *Orthopaedic mechanics: Procedures and devices.* New York: Academic, 1978.
Larson, C. B., & Gould, M. *Orthopedic nursing* (9th ed.). St. Louis: C. V. Mosby, 1978.
Luckmann, J., & Sorenson, K. C. *Medical–surgical nursing: A psychophysiologic approach* (2nd ed.). Philadelphia: W. B. Saunders, 1980.
Roaf, R., & Hodkinson, L. J. *Textbook of orthopaedic nursing* (2nd ed.). London: Blackwell, 1975.
Tronzo, R. G. Fractures of the hip. In R. G. Tronzo (Ed.), *Surgery of the hip joint.* Philadelphia: Lea & Febiger, 1973.
Warwick, R., & Williams, P. L. *Gray's anatomy* (35th Brit. ed.). Philadelphia: W. B. Saunders, 1973.

BIBLIOGRAPHY

Aaron, R. K. Total joint orthroplasty. *Surgical Clinics of North America,* 1983, *63* (3), 697–714.
Beanland, D. An exercise program for total hip replacement. *Orthopedic Nurses' Association Journal,* 1978, *5* (2), 36.
Beeson, P. B., & McDermott, W. *Cecil-Loeb textbook of medicine.* Philadelphia: W. B. Saunders, 1971.
Blake, S. A. Noncemented femoral prosthesis: Intraoperative locus. *Orthopaedic Nursing,* 1985, *4* (1), 40–42.
Bosch, A. V., & Corzatt, R. D. Internal fixation of trochanteric fractures by the Ender method. *Orthopedic Nurses' Association Journal,* 1978, *5* (7), 22–25.
Brantley, P., & Analla, M. *The nurse and orthopedic surgery.* Rutherford, N.J.: The Orthopedic Nurses' Association, Inc. in cooperation with Howmedica, Inc., 1980.
Burgess E. M. Amputations. *Surgical Clinics of North America,* 1983, *63* (3), 749–770.
Butterfield, S., Quosous, S., & Reschaurer, R. Ender intramedullary nailing of pertrochanteric fractures. *Orthopedics,* 1979, *2* (5), 507–512.
Cailliet R. *Soft tissue pain and disability* (5th ed.). Philadelphia: F. A. Davis, 1981.
Canale, S. T., & Manugian, A. H. Irreducible traumatic dislocations of the hip. *Journal of Bone and Joint Surgery,* 1979, *61A* (1), 7–14.
Carini, G. K., & Birmingham, J. J. *Traction made manageable.* New York: McGraw-Hill, 1980.

Catchings, C. Fractures of the shaft of the femur. *Orthopedic Nurses' Association Journal,* 1978, *5* (1), 18–20.
Ceccio, C. M. Postoperative pain relief through relaxation in elderly patients with fractured hips. *Orthopaedic Nursing,* 1984, *3* (3), 11–19.
Christianson, F. Closed wound irrigation in orthopedics. *Orthopedic Nurses' Association Journal,* 1979, *6* (9), 359–366.
Clissold, G. *The body's response to trauma: Fractures.* New York: Springer, 1973.
Crowninshield, R. D., Brand, R. A., Johnston, R. C., & Milroy, J. C. An analysis of femoral component stem design in total hip orthroplasty. *Journal of Bone and Joint Surgery,* 1980, *62* (1), 68–78.
Czitrono, A. A., & Pritzker, K. P. Simple bone cyst causing collapse of the articular surface of the femoral head and incongruity of the hip joint. *Journal of Bone and Joint Surgery,* 1980, *62A* (5), 842–845.
Darst, B. I have a new hip. *American Journal of Nursing,* 1978, *9,* 1489–1490.
DeGowin, E. L., & DeGowin, R. L. *Bedside diagnostic examination* (3rd ed.). New York: Macmillan, 1976.
DeLee, J. C. Intra-asseous lipoma of the proximal part of the femur. *Journal of Bone and Joint Surgery,* 1979, *61A* (4), 601–603.
DeLee, J. C., Evans, J. A., & Thomas, J. Anterior dislocation of the hip and associated femoral-head fractures. *Journal of Bone and Joint Surgery,* 1980, *62A* (6), 960–964.
Doheny, M. O'B. Porous-coated femoral prosthesis: Concepts and care considerations. *Orthopaedic Nursing,* 1985, *4* (1), 43–45.
Dorr, L. D. Pulmonary emboli following total hip orthroplasty: Incidence study. *Journal of Bone and Joint Surgery,* 1979, *61A* (7), 1083–1087.
Duerksen, J. R. Hip fractures: Special considerations for the elderly patient. *Orthopaedic Nursing,* 1982, *1* (1), 11–19.
Dunnery, E. Fractured hip: How to move patients safely. *RN,* 1979, *42* (6), 44–57.
Fries, J. F. *Arthritis, A comprehensive guide.* Menlo Park, Calif.: Addison-Wesley, 1982.
Galante, J. O. Causes of fractures of the femoral component in total hip replacement. *Journal of Bone and Joint Surgery,* 1980, *62A* (4), 670–673.
Hamilton, A. Home instructions: Amputee with prosthesis. *Orthopedic Nurses' Association Journal,* 1979, *6* (2), 72–77.
Hoppenfeld, S. *Physical examination of the spine and extremities.* New York: Appleton-Century-Crofts, 1976.
Iverson, L. D., & Clawson, D. K. *Manual of acute orthopaedic therapeutics.* Boston: Little, Brown, 1977.
Kavanaugh, J. H. Multiple myeloma, amyloid orthropathy, and pathological fracture of the femur. *Journal of Bone and Joint Surgery,* 1978, *60A* (1), 135–137.
Lane, J. M., Sculco, T. P., & Zolan, S. Treatment of pathological fractures of the hip by endoprosthetic replacement. *Journal of Bone and Joint Surgery,* 1980, *62A* (6), 954–959.
Mallory, T. H. The evolution of the Buck-32 total hip prosthesis. *Clinical Orthopedics,* 1980, *147,* 148–153.
Marquart, E. T. Posterior dislocation of the hip and femoral head fracture: Consultation corner. *Orthopedics,* 1979, *2* (4), 424–428.
McBeath, A. A. Late complications of total hip replacement and their prevention. *Current Practice in Orthopaedic Surgery 1979,* 1979, *8,* 58–77.
McBryde, A. M. Jr. Benign (intracapsular) tumors of the hip. *Current Practice in Orthopaedic Surgery 1977,* 1977, *7,* 154–179.
Meador, R. Learning to live with a new leg. *American Journal of Nursing,* 1979, *79* (8), 1393–1395.

Mnaymney, W., & Temple, W. Modified hemipelvectomy utilizing a long vascular myocutaneous thigh flap. *Journal of Bone and Joint Surgery,* 1980, *62A* (6), 1013–1015.

Petty, W., & Goldsmith, S. Resection orthroplasty following infected total hip orthroplasty. *Journal of Bone and Joint Surgery,* 1980, *62A* (6), 889–896.

Rauscher, N. A. Pathological femur fracture due to bone cyst. *Orthopedic Nurses' Association Journal,* 1978, *5* (10), 12–15.

Seinsheimer, F. Subtrochanteric fractures of the femur. *Journal of Bone and Joint Surgery,* 1978, *60A* (3), 300–306.

Stevens, D. B. Method of operative treatment for intertrochanteric fractures of the femur. *Current Practice in Orthopaedic Surgery 1977,* 1977, *7,* 56–78.

Stillman, M. J., & de Tornyay, R. Nursing decisions: Series 3, No. 9, Experience in clinical problem solving. Mike J.: A young man with a fractured femur. Part 1: Traction. *RN,* 1978, *41* (7), 63–73.

Swinson, D. R., & Swinburn, W. R. *Rheumatology.* New York: Wiley, 1980.

Turek, S. L. *Orthopaedics, principles and their applications* (3rd ed.). Philadalphia: Lippincott, 1977.

VanAudekurcke, R., Martens, M., Mulier, J. C., & Stuyck, J. Experimental study on internal fixation of femoral neck fractures. *Clinical Orthopedics,* 1979, *141,* 203–212.

Wu, K. K., et al. The surgical technique for forequarter amputation: A clinical analysis of ten cases. *Orthopedics,* 1978, *1* (6), 457–461.

7

THE KNEE AND LOWER LEG

Chapter 7 focuses on the care of patients with traumatic pathological conditions affecting the knee and the lower leg. The chapter starts with a brief review of anatomy to help the nurse understand the rationale underlying nursing care. Next, discussions center on conditions affecting the knee from a minor sprain to amputations, with emphasis on the clinical assessment and the nursing care associated with surgical procedures. The final major section of the chapter focuses on traumatic and pathological conditions that affect the lower leg.

ANATOMY

BONES

The bones of the knee and lower leg are the femur (Chap. 6), the tibia, the fibula, and the patella (Fig. 7–1). The tibia and the fibula are the medial and lateral bones of the lower leg. The tibia is the stronger of the two, and except for the femur is the longest bone of the skeleton. Its lower end is smaller than the upper end, and on its medial side a stout process, the medial malleolus, projects downward beyond the rest of the bone. The upper end is expanded, providing a weight-bearing surface for the body weight transmitted through the lower end of the femur. The proximal end of the tibia is comprised of two prominent masses, the medial and lateral condyles, and a smaller projection, the tibial tuberosity. The fibula is much more slender than the tibia, and is not a weight-bearing bone. The lower end or lateral malleolus projects downward to a lower level than the tibia and lies on a more posterior plane (Warwick & Williams, 1973, p. 366).

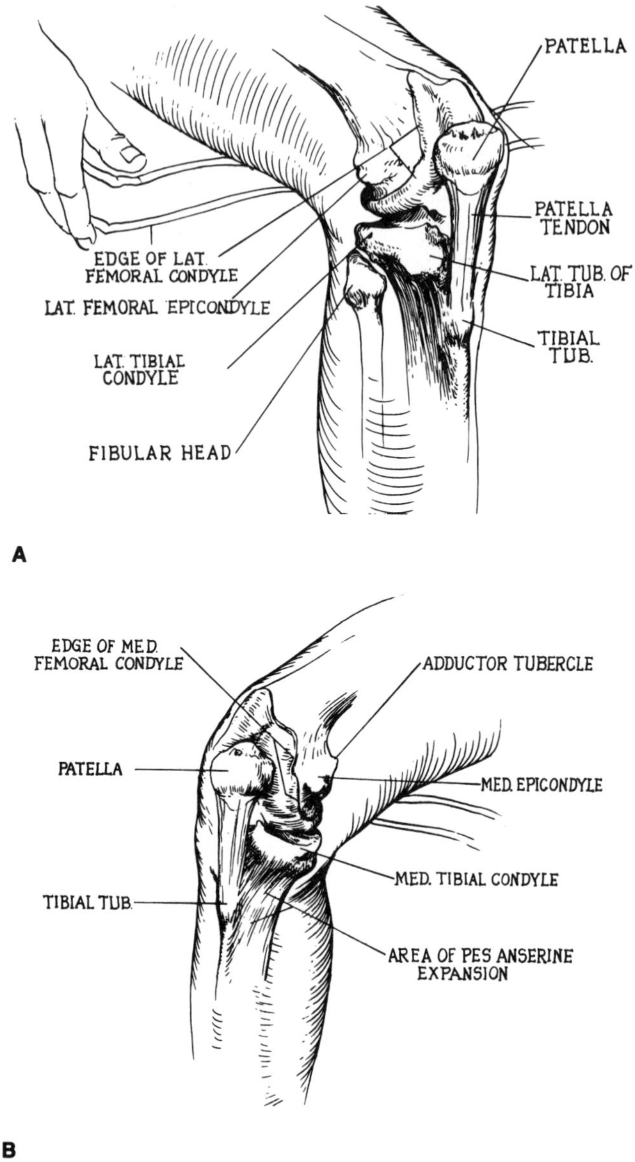

Figure 7–1. A. Anatomy of the knee joint, anterolateral aspect. **B.** Anatomy of the knee joint, anteromedial aspect. *(Figures 7–1, 7–2, 7–4 through 7–7, 7–10, and 7–11 are reproduced from Hoppenfeld, S., 1976, with permission.)*

Patella

The patella (see Fig. 7–1) is the largest sesamoid bone, that is, the largest bone that is embedded within a tendon. The anterior surface is convex, perforated by nutrient vessels, and marked by numerous rough, longitudinal striae. The patella is anterior to the knee joint and embedded within the substance of the quadriceps tendon. A thin layer of quadriceps tendon passes over the anterior surface of the patella to join the patellar tendon, which inserts distally into the tibial tubercle. When a person is standing, the lower limit of the patella lies more than 1 cm above the line of the knee joint. The patella is separated from the skin over the joint by a bursa as well as by the tendon of the quadriceps femoris (Warwick & Williams, 1973, p. 364).

The function of the patella, in addition to protecting the femoral condyles from injury, is to increase the mechanical advantage of the quadriceps tendon. Active knee extension is achieved by the quadriceps muscles. The muscle forces are transmitted to the patella through the quadriceps tendon, then to the patellar tendon, and finally to the tibia at the tibial tubercle. When the knee is extended, the force the quadriceps muscles must exert is influenced by the patella, because the patella causes an increase in the length of the moment arm through which the quadriceps muscles work. If the patella is removed, the moment arm is shortened and the muscular force required to extend the knee increases. The quadriceps muscles cannot provide this additional force, and hence the knee cannot be fully extended if the patella is absent.

MUSCLES

The knee is a modified hinge (or ginglymus) joint between the femur and the tibia. It is surrounded by a thick synovial membrane that secretes the synovial fluid that lubricates the joint. Because flexion and extension are its principal movements, with only a small amount of rotation of the tibia possible, two main groups of muscles are involved in movements of the knee. The flexor (hamstring and gastrocnemius) muscles bend the knee, and the extensor (quadriceps femoris) muscles cause the knee to straighten. A major function of both groups is to hold the knee in any desired position so that it is a stable and reliable supporting structure.

NERVES

The muscles of the knee joint are enervated by the femoral nerve on the anterior position of the thigh (supplying the quadriceps) and the sciatic nerve on the posterior surface (supplying the hamstring and the gastrocnemius). Division of either or both of these nerves therefore seriously impairs the action of the knee. The knee joint may also be deprived of its sensory nerve supply as a result of disease, and is then vulnerable to repeated trauma because no pain is felt (Roaf & Hodkinson, 1975, p. 352).

BURSA

The knee is supplied extensively with protective bursae (Fig. 7–2). These are sacs composed of a synovial membrane that contains synovial fluid, and they

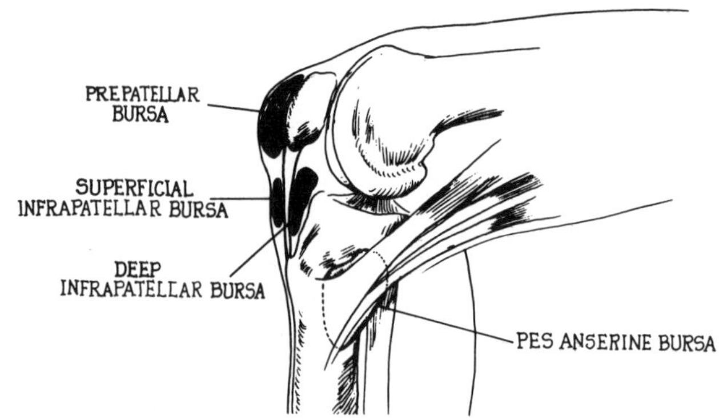

Figure 7–2. Clinically significant bursae of the knee.

are situated between two surfaces to minimize the friction between them. For example, one bursa extends up from about one-third of the length of the thigh behind the quadriceps, and another is on the anterior surface of the tibia. As a result of infection, surgery, or trauma, these bursae can become distended with the products of the lesion such as blood, pus, or increased synovial secretions (Roaf & Hodkinson, 1975, p. 353).

THE KNEE JOINT

The knee is the largest joint in the body, and plays a key role in human locomotion (Warwick & Williams, 1973, p. 450). At the same time it is one of the joints most frequently affected by trauma because of its anatomical structure, its exposure to external forces, and the functional demands placed upon it (Edmondson & Crenshaw, 1980, p. 884–885).

The bones of the knee joint are the femur, the patella, and the tibia (see Fig. 7–1). The joint surface of the distal femur has two condyles. Between the condyles anteriorly is the saddle-shaped femoral patellar surface, upon which the patella glides. Between the condyles inferiorly is the femoral tibial surface, which has a deep U-shaped notch, the intercondylar fossa. The joint surface of the proximal tibia, called the tibial plateau, has two articular indentations separated by the raised intercondylar eminence. All of the articular surfaces of the femoral condyles, the tibial condyles, and the dorsal aspect of the patella are covered by 3 to 4 mm of cartilage.

Meniscus

The hinge effect of the knee joint is produced by the rounded femoral condyles and the shallow depressions of the tibial plateaus. The tibial spine (or intercondylar fossa) is a twin-peaked projection that lies between and separates the tibial plateaus. Lying on top of the tibia are two incomplete rings or semilunar-shaped pieces of fibrocartilage known as the medial and lateral menisci (Fig. 7–3). The menisci cover one-half to two-thirds of the articular surfaces of each tibial plateau. The menisci move forward and backward with the tibia and promote a snug fit between the femur and the tibia when the joint is in extension.

The Fibrous Capsule

The ligaments of the joint comprise the fibrous capsule which surrounds and supports the joint. Those ligaments are the ligamentum patellae, the tibial (medial) and fibular (lateral) collaterals, the oblique and arcuate popliteal, the anterior and posterior cruciate (see Fig. 7–3), and the transverse ligaments. The fibrous capsule is augmented by the tendons of the muscles that surround the joint.

The fibrous capsule is blended above on each side with the origin of the corresponding head of the gastrocnemius, and centrally it is strengthened by the oblique popliteal ligament. On the medial side the fibers are attached to the medial surfaces of the femoral and tibial condyles beyond the articular surfaces. Thus, the fibrous capsule blends with the posterior part of the tibial

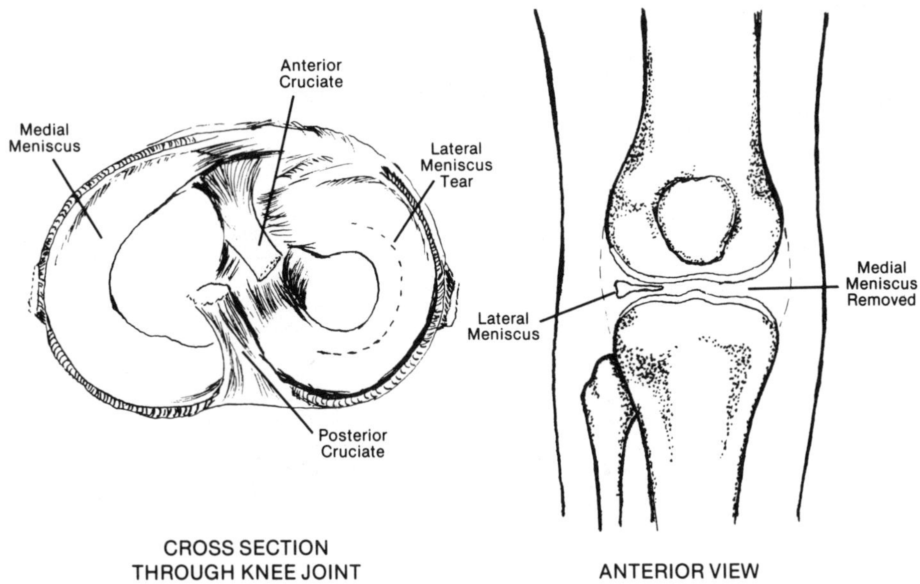

Figure 7–3. Anatomy of the knee. *(From Brantley, P., & Analla, M., 1980, p. 92. Courtesy of Howmedica.)*

collateral ligament of the joint. On the lateral side the fibers are attached to the femur above the origin of the popliteus and descend over the tendon to the lateral condyle of the tibia and the head of the fibula. Anteriorly, the fibrous capsule is entirely absent above the patella and the patellar area (Warwick & Williams, 1973, p. 451).

Within the joint are two strong ligaments known as the anterior and posterior cruciate ligaments, named because they run in a crisscross fashion from the femur to the tibia. The anterior cruciate ligament goes from the anterior surface of the tibia to the posterior aspect of the femur and acts to prevent forward displacement of the tibia on the femur. The posterior cruciate ligament goes from the posterior surface of the tibia to the anterior aspect of the femur and acts to prevent backward displacement of the tibia on the femur (Gartland, 1979, p. 405–406).

The extracapsular ligaments are strong bands that pass from the femur to the tibia. In particular, there are strong ligaments on the lateral and medial aspects known as the collateral ligaments. The medial stability of the knee joint is increased by the medial collateral ligament, which runs from the medial femoral condyle to the medial tibial condyle. The deeper layer of that ligament is attached to the outer border of the medial meniscus. The lateral stability of the knee joint is increased by the lateral collateral ligament, which runs from the lateral femoral condyle to the fibular head, but has no attachment to the lateral meniscus (Gartland, 1979, p. 405).

Blood Supply

The popliteal artery, a continuation of the femoral artery, has five branches in the area of the knee joint: the medial and lateral superior geniculars, the middle genicular, and the medial and lateral geniculars.

THE KNEE

Trauma

INTERNAL DERANGEMENTS OF THE KNEE JOINT

The term internal derangement is loosely applied to a variety of intra-articular and extra-articular disturbances of the knee joint, usually of traumatic origin, which interfere with the function and mechanics of the joint. The pathological changes that take place in the knee immediately after trauma depend on the nature and the severity of the injury (Edmondson & Crenshaw, 1980, p. 894).

Lesions of the Meniscus

Injuries to one or other meniscus are common and result from twisting strains applied to the knee when it is slightly flexed or when it is in full flexion. A twisting force applied to the knee joint may trap a meniscus between the femur and tibia to produce the familiar "torn cartilage" lesion. To produce a tear, the knee joint must be first rotated in a flexed position to trap the meniscus and then extended to produce the tearing force on the tissue. This combination of motions is frequently encountered in athletics. (A meniscus cannot be torn while the knee is in full extension.) The torn or detached portion of the meniscus may become displaced toward the joint and jammed between the articular surfaces of the femur and the tibia, arresting all movement and producing a "locked" knee.

Medial Meniscus

Medial meniscus tears are nine times more common than tears of the lateral meniscus. This is believed to occur because the medial meniscus has less mobility, being more securely attached to such neighboring structures as the deep layer of the medial collateral ligament, and is therefore less able to adapt to sudden changes of position. Furthermore, during rotation of the flexed or partially flexed joint, the medial meniscus moves through a greater interval than the lateral meniscus, and is therefore subject to more stress. At the same time, the medial fibers of the popliteus may prevent the lateral meniscus from being trapped between the articular surfaces (Edmondson & Crenshaw, 1980, p. 896).

Two types of medial meniscus tears occur most frequently. One, the "punch-press" effect of the femoral condyle on the trapped meniscus causes a splitting of the meniscus along its longitudinal axis, producing the so-called "bucket handle" tear. Here, the inner portion of the torn cartilage may get displaced into the joint and cause locking (Edmondson & Crenshaw, 1980, p. 898). The bucket handle tear is the lesion usually present in an athlete with a "trick knee." The joint may be unlocked by manipulation, but healing of the tear does not occur because the largely avascular meniscus has a limited capacity for regeneration, and a tear cannot be expected to heal unless it has occurred close to the capsule (Edmondson & Crenshaw, 1980, p. 897). Treatment is usually the surgical removal of the torn meniscus.

In the second type of medial meniscus tear, the meniscus is torn along the transverse axis. The tear usually does not cause locking of the joint. Pain is produced by momentary impingement of the irregular meniscus between the femur and the tibia when the knee is in motion. Symptoms of a transverse tear of the meniscus can frequently be relieved by the use of anti-inflammatory drugs, combined with putting the joint at rest for a period of time. If symptoms persist, operative excision of the meniscus is indicated.

Lateral Meniscus

Lateral meniscus lesions include tears and cystic degeneration. Tears similar to those of the medial meniscus may involve the lateral meniscus, though they are much less common. On the other hand, cystic degeneration is more common in the lateral meniscus than in the medial (Edmondson & Crenshaw, 1980, p. 898). In this condition, thought to be caused by repeated trauma, multiple cysts containing gelatinous material appear within the peripheral border of the meniscus. The cysts may cause pain and often can be seen and palpated along the lateral border of the knee joint. Treatment is surgical removal of the cysts.

Post-Trauma Assessment. The differential diagnosis of internal derangement of the knee is somewhat difficult but it can be made by taking a careful history and doing a thorough examination of the knee. It is often necessary for the examination to be supplemented by roentgenograms, arthrography, or arthroscopy (Chap. 2). When a meniscus has been injured, the capsular and ligamentous structures, and even the articular surfaces, may also have been injured.

A history of the injury is important to establish that the lesion is of traumatic origin and that the meniscus was previously sound. In tears of abnormal or degenerative menisci, a history of specific injury may not be obtained, for example in middle-aged persons who sustain a weight-bearing twist of the knee or have pain after squatting. These patients may recall symptoms of mild catching, snapping, or clicking, and occasional pain and mild swelling in the joint, but may not seek medical care until the tear increases and causes locking or lack of stability in the knee (Edmondson & Crenshaw, 1980, p. 898).

The symptoms of the more typical traumatic tears of a normal meniscus are as follows: (1) *Locking.* Even though locking is a classic symptom of a meniscal tear it must be emphasized that an intra-articular tumor, an osteocartilagenous loose body, and other conditions may also cause locking. A locked knee may not be recognized unless the extension of the affected knee is compared with that of the other knee. In "true" locking, there is something within the joint that prevents full extension. "False" locking is also possible, especially after an injury that causes hemorrhaging into the posterior part of the capsule or a spasm of the hamstring muscle (Edmondson & Crenshaw, 1980, p. 898). (2) *"Giving Way."* A sensation of "giving way" may be felt by the patient during a rotary movement of the knee. The sensation may result from a tear in the posterior part of the meniscus, but may also be produced by other conditions, especially loose bodies, chondromalacia of the patella, and instability of the joint resulting from injury to ligaments or weakness of the supporting musculature, especially of the quadriceps (Edmondson & Crenshaw, 1980, p. 898). (3) *Pain.* Probably the most important physical finding is localized tenderness over the medial and lateral joint line or over the periphery of the meniscus. Menisci are without nerve fibers, except at the periphery, but the pain may result in synovitis and traumatized capsular tissues. The pain is frequently aggravated by forced rotation of the foot and leg, and pain or a click may be produced by the McMurray test. To do the McMurray test (Fig. 7–4) for the medial meniscus, stand on the patient's affected side and have the patient lie supine. Take hold of the patient's heel and flex the leg fully. Then place your other hand on the affected knee with your fingers touching the medial joint

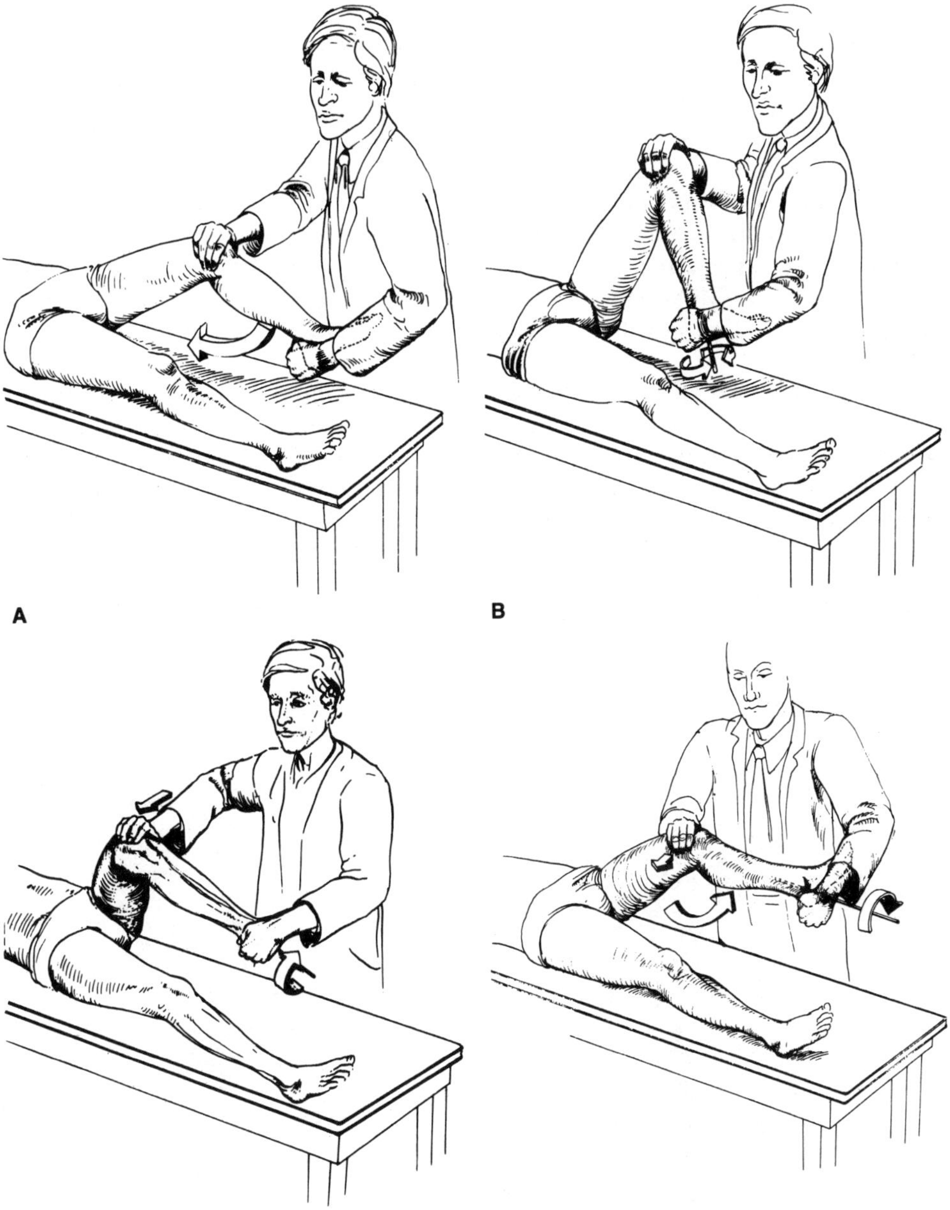

A B C D

Figure 7–4. A. The McMurray test for meniscal tears. Flex the knee. **B.** With the knee flexed, internally and externally rotate the tibia on the femur. **C.** With the leg externally rotated, place a valgus stress on the knee. **D.** With the leg externally rotated and in valgus, slowly extend the knee. If a click is palpable or audible, the test is considered positive for a torn medial meniscus, usually in the posterior position.

line. Keeping the knee completely flexed, rotate the leg externally as far as possible, and then slowly extend the knee. As the femur passes over a tear in the meniscus, a click may be heard or felt. To examine the lateral meniscus, palpate the posterolateral margin of the joint while internally rotating the leg as far as possible and slowly extending the knee, listening and feeling for a click. A click produced by the McMurray test usually occurs between complete flexion of the knee and 90 degrees, and indicates a posterior peripheral tear of the meniscus. Popping, which occurs at a greater degree of extension, suggests a tear of the middle and anterior positions of the meniscus. Thus the position of the knee when the click occurs helps to identify the location of the lesion. A negative McMurray test, however, does not rule out a tear (DeGowin & DeGowin, 1976, p. 741; Edmondson & Crenshaw, 1980, p. 899; Hoppenfeld, 1976, p. 191).

Another test to aid in the diagnosis of a torn meniscus is Apley's grinding test. Begin with the patient lying prone on the examining table, and flex the affected knee to 90 degrees. The affected leg is pulled upward to distract the joint, and then rotated to place rotational strain on the ligaments (Fig. 7–5). When ligaments are torn, that part of the test is usually painful, which indicates a lesion of the tibial collateral ligament. Next, with the knee in the same position, the foot and leg are pressed downward into the knee and rotated as the joint is slowly flexed and extended. When the medial meniscus is torn, popping

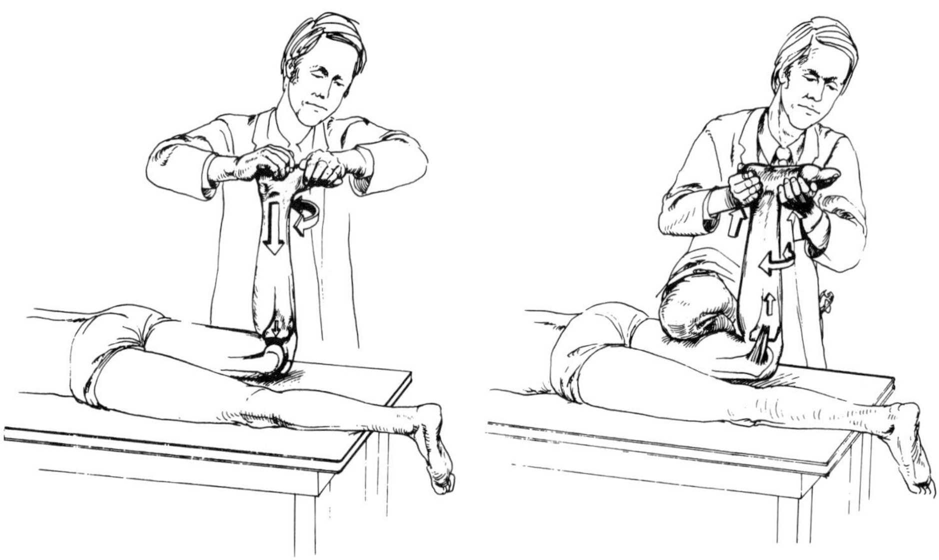

A B

Figure 7–5. A. Apley's compression test for meniscal tear. **B.** Apley's distraction test for ligamentous damage.

and pain localized to the joint line may be noted (DeGowin & DeGowin, 1976, p. 742; Edmondson & Crenshaw, 1980, p. 899; Hoppenfeld, 1976, p. 191). (4) *Effusion.* Effusion indicates an irritation to the synovium. Alone, effusion has limited diagnostic value, especially as tears that occur within the body of the meniscus or in a degenerative area may not produce an effusion. To help determine if there is a large amount of effusion in the knee, a test for ballotable (i.e., rebounding) patella can be done. To do the test, instruct the patient to relax the quadriceps muscles and then gently extend the knee until the leg is straight. Next, push the patella backward into the trochlear groove, quickly releasing it (Fig. 7–6). When the patella is forced into the trochlear groove the fluid under the patella is forced to the sides of the joint. When the patella is quickly released, the fluid flows back to its former position, forcing the patella to rebound (Hoppenfeld, 1976, p. 195). If only a minimal amount of effusion is in the knee joint, the ballotable patella test is not diagnostic. To test for minimal effusion (Fig. 7–7), have the patient's knee in extension, and then "milk" the fluid down from the suprapatellar pouch and over from the lateral side into the medial side of the knee. After the fluid is collected on the medial side of the knee joint, gently tap the medial side and observe how much fluid flows to the lateral side (Hoppenfeld, 1976, p. 196). (5) *Atrophy of the Musculature.* Atrophy of the musculature about the knee, especially of the vastus medialis component of the quadriceps muscle, suggests a recurring disability of the knee, but does not indicate its cause (Edmondson & Crenshaw, 1980, p. 898).

Surgical Repair. An immediate operation is not always necessary following a meniscus injury. Some injuries may recover if immobilization is accomplished and a walking leg cast is applied for 3 to 6 weeks. Unfortunately, most tears

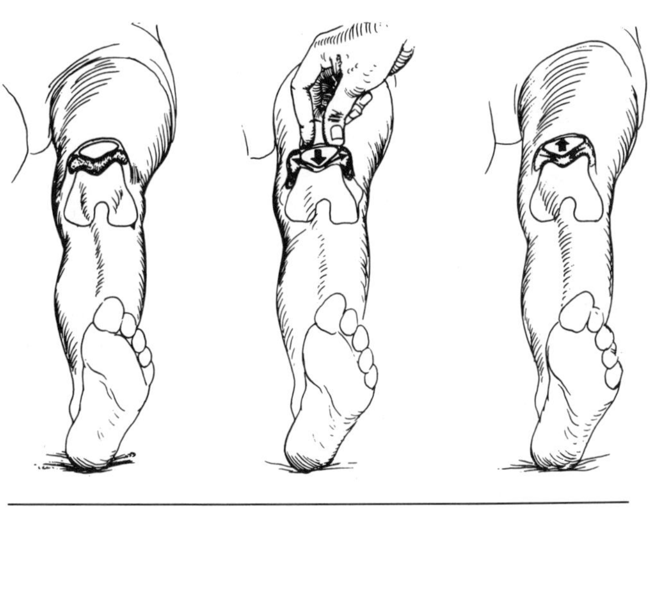

Figure 7–6. Test for major effusion; a ballotable patella.

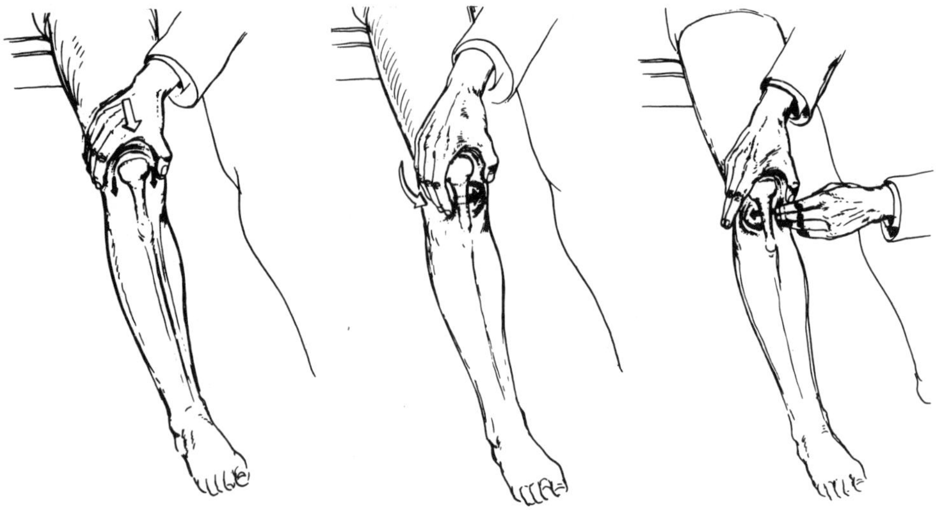

Figure 7–7. Test for minor effusion.

occur in areas where healing cannot be expected, and consequently it is rare that the symptoms are permanently relieved without surgery.

MENISECTOMY. A menisectomy or removal of a meniscus is indicated for a knee that locks or for a patient who experiences recurrent pain and limitation of motion from a torn cartilage. The surgery may be done in one of two ways. One is by making a surgical incision into the knee joint, with the knee in a flexed position, the meniscus is separated from its anterior tibial attachment, then from its middle and posterior peripheral attachments, and removed. After an examination of other structures in the knee for possible pathology, the incision is closed, and a compression dressing with a knee immobilizer, posterior splint, or cylinder cast applied.

ARTHROSCOPY. An alternative method of removing a torn meniscus is through an arthroscope (Fig. 7–8). This method is invasive because the scope is inserted into the joint through small puncture wound(s) that permit visual inspection, irrigation with a saline solution, and the introduction of cutting instruments. The torn meniscus is removed in very small pieces. If there is also damage to ligaments, that damage cannot be repaired through the scope, and a surgical incision is required.

Patients having arthroscopic surgery for the removal of a meniscus require basically the same nursing care as other patients with knee surgery. However, the patient having arthrosopic surgery usually does not have an immobilizing device, has only a small dressing, and usually does not have many complaints

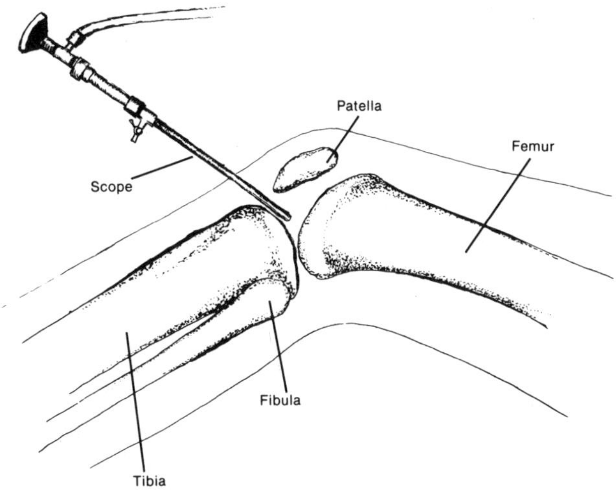

Figure 7–8. Arthroscopy of the knee. *(From Brantley, P., & Analla, M., 1980, p. 88. Courtesy of Howmedica.)*

of discomfort. Most patients want to ambulate soon after recovering from the anesthesia, but this usually is not allowed if the standard postoperative regime for knee surgery is followed (see the discussion following).

□ NURSING PROCESS (Table 7–1)

Assessment

The initial postsurgical assessment of a patient following a menisectomy is very similar to that of a patient following a total knee replacement (see pp. 375–376). The patient has a compression bandage of Webril or some other fluffy absorbent material, and the knee is immobilized in extension by a posterior splint, a "cotton" cast (e.g., an O'Donoghue), or a knee immobilizer (Fig. 7–9). Check for any tightness, pain, or circulatory impairment that could be related to pressure from the dressing or immobilizing device. A neurovascular assessment of the affected leg (pulse, temperature, color, capillary filling, edema, sensory and motor function) should be made (Chap. 2) and the position of the leg checked for proper alignment and elevation on pillows. Ice bags are placed along the incisional area. Check that they are not placed on top of a wet cast, as the weight of an ice bag can indent the cast.

Nursing Diagnosis and Goal Formulation

The nursing diagnoses for a typical patient following a menisectomy are (1) alterations in comfort related to knee pain from soft tissue trauma and surgery, (2) alterations in mobility related to lack of joint mobility from

TABLE 7–1. NURSING PROCESS FOR MENISECTOMY WITH KNEE SPLINT

Assessment	Nursing Diagnosis	Goal Formulation	Planning and Intervention	Evaluation and Reassessment
1. Assess for location, duration and severity of pain. Observe for verbal and nonverbal cues of pain. Check the position of the leg. Check for tightness of the dressing or knee splint. Assess neurovascular status.	1. Alterations in comfort: pain in the knee related to soft tissue trauma.	1. Short-term goal: a reduction of pain in the knee through immobilization and prescribed medications. Long-term goal: free of pain.	1. Alleviate Pain Keep the leg elevated. Place ice bags along the incisional area of the knee. Keep the leg in correct alignment. Utilize noninvasive nursing measures. Teach relaxation techniques. Administer prescribed medications.	1. The patient should remain relatively comfortable with correct positioning and prescribed pain medication.
2. Assess the tightness of the knee splint. Assess the neurovascular status. Check for correct positioning of the splint. Check for correct positioning and elevation of the leg. Assess the patient's ability to do exercises. Observe patient's ability to ambulate safely.	2. Impaired physical mobility: decreased knee function related to soft tissue trauma.	2. Short-term goal: an increase in mobility through immobilization and controlled exercises. Long-term goal: regain full function in the knee.	2. Increase Mobility *Position* Place the patient in position of comfort. Keep the leg elevated for 24–48 hours. Keep the leg elevated when sitting. Keep the leg in extension for 10–14 days. *Exercises* Start the patient on quadriceps and gluteal setting exercises the afternoon of surgery or first postoperative day.	2. The patient should be able to keep the leg elevated and do the required exercises. However, in the beginning they may need a lot of emotional encouragement and some physical help in doing the straight leg raises. The exercise regime should be done every hour with an initial goal of five repetitions of the straight leg raises.

			Encourage straight leg raises as soon as physically possible. Instruct on exercises to increase strength in the upper extremities for crutch walking. Start gentle flexion exercises when sutures are removed (usually 2 weeks after surgery).	
			Ambulation Demonstrate crutch walking (toe touch but no full weight bearing). Assist with early ambulation. Demonstrate how to go up and down stairs and how to get in and out of a chair.	The patient should be able to ambulate safely with crutches.
3. Assess the neurovascular status. Check the leg for tightness of the splint. Check for level of pain.	3. Potential for injury: neurovascular deficit related to soft tissue trauma and knee splint.	3. Short- and long-term goals: free of any neurovascular deficit.	3. Prevent Complications *Circulatory* Keep the leg elevated. Place ice bags along the incision line. Utilize nursing measures to prevent or reduce swelling. Keep knee splint straps secure but not too tight. *Potential Complications Due to Knee Surgery* (See Table 7–3, Total Knee Arthroplasty) *Potential Complications Due to Immobility* (See Chap. 3 and Table 6–2).	3. The patient should be free of any complications.

(continued)

TABLE 7–1. *(Continued)*

Assessment	Nursing Diagnosis	Goal Formulation	Planning and Intervention	Evaluation and Reassessment
4. Assess the patient's level of understanding about the rehabilitation process and home care.	4. Potential knowledge deficit related to rehabilitation process.	4. Short- and long-term goals: a decrease in anxiety through increased knowledge.	4. Patient Teaching Discuss the rehabilitation process. Discuss the importance of the exercise program and of no increase in weight bearing until allowed by physicians. Discuss home care and methods of dressing and bathing.	4. The patient should feel confident in continuing the exercise program (goal is 90 degrees of flexion and 50 repetitions of straight leg raises). Athletes may require 3 months of rehabilitation to regain mobility, strength, and agility for competitive sports.

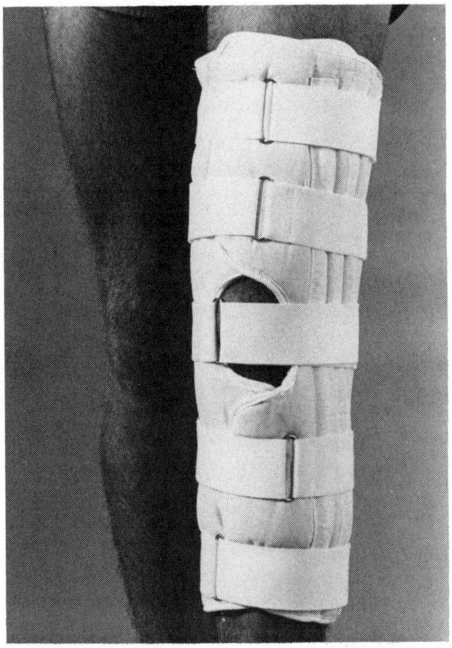

A

Figure 7–9. A. Knee immobilizer. *(Courtesy of Zimmer, Inc.)* B. Knee immobilizer (patient in bed). *(Courtesy of Carle Foundation Hospital and Clinic.)*

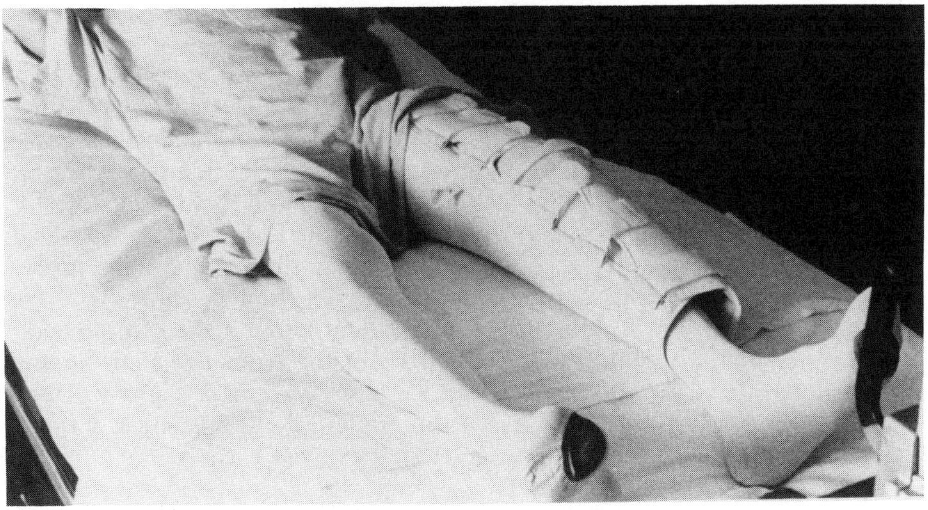

B

surgery and an immobilizing device, (3) alterations in psychological well-being related to anxiety and knowledge deficit about surgical procedure and future functional ability of the knee joint, and (4) potential complications related to surgical procedure and immobilizing device.

The short-term goals are to have the patient experience (1) a decrease in, if not relief of, all of the pain in the knee, (2) an increase in mobility through the use of exercises, (3) a decrease in anxiety through increased knowledge about surgical procedure and rehabilitation process, and (4) an absence of complications. Long-term goals are for the patient to be free of pain and able to return to normal activities.

Planning and Intervention

Alleviate Pain. Pain relief measures following a menisectomy involve keeping the leg elevated in extension for the first 24 to 48 hours postsurgery. Ice bags applied to the incisional area (but not directly over the incision) help to prevent pain by their local anesthetic effect and by reducing edema. Check ice bags for positioning and refill as needed. Muscle setting exercises help to increase circulation and decrease pain. Administer prescribed pain medications as necessary.

Increase Mobility

Position. The leg is usually kept in extension for 10 to 14 days, and elevated during the first 24 to 48 hours following surgery. The leg should also be elevated when sitting or lying.

Exercises. The patient begins a program of quadriceps (and gluteal) setting exercises (Chap. 6) either the afternoon of surgery or on the first postoperative day. It is better if the patient has learned the exercise program preoperatively, even if he or she needs to use the unaffected leg to practice. As soon as physically possible, the patient should begin straight leg raises. The patient may need a lot of emotional and physical support and encouragement with the straight leg raises. In the beginning the nurse or the physical therapist may have to lift the leg to a position of 60 or more degrees of hip flexion, and let the patient lower the leg to the bed. The nurse or the therapist still needs to assist the patient so that the leg does not drop to the bed. The quadriceps setting and straight leg lifts should be carried out every hour on the hour while the patient is awake. The goal is five repetitions of the leg raising exercise each time.

Ambulation. When the patient has developed good muscle control over the affected leg, he or she is allowed up with crutches. The patient is usually allowed to toe touch but not to have full weight bearing.

Patient Teaching. The patient is usually discharged from the hospital 3 to 5 days following surgery, when the patient is able to do leg lifts. When the sutures are removed (approximately 2 weeks postoperatively) the immobilized extension is discontinued and gentle flexion exercises of the knee are begun. The isometeric exercise program is continued until the patient is able to get 90 degrees of knee flexion. Some physicians encourage a home exercise program whereas others require that the patient come into the physical therapy department and work with a therapist. Active knee flexion without weight is continued until the patient has built up sufficient strength, usually 50 repetitions. The patient then goes on to weighted lifts.

The patient, the family, and significant others need to understand the importance of carefully following each step in the rehabilitation program. The premature use of heavy weights can produce pain and effusion and retard the healing process.

At discharge, ambulation with the use of crutches must be stressed. Even though the patient may not feel that crutches are required, they are needed until sufficient strength in the quadriceps has returned. The return function to the knee joint is directly proportional to the return of strength and muscle tone to the muscles of the knee and hip. Often several months are required for complete recovery. Athletes, even though their rehabilitation is often faster than others, may not regain sufficient mobility, strength, and agility to return to competitive sports for 3 months after a menisectomy.

Prevent Complications. The nursing measures discussed in the care of a patient following a total knee replacement apply here, although complications are much less frequent.

Evaluation and Reassessment

For a typical patient recovering from a menisectomy, the evaluation is similar to that of a patient following a total knee arthroplasty. Special emphasis should be given to evaluating the patient's compliance with the exercise regime and the patient's understanding of the mobility restrictions that will apply after discharge from the hospital.

Ligamentous Injuries of the Knee

The knee joint owes its stability to a strong and extensive capsule, formed by the collateral and cruciate ligaments, and surrounding muscles and tendons. Injury to any one of the ligaments affects locomotion and the stability of the knee. Knee ligaments are often injured in athletic activities and motor vehicle accidents. They may also occur in falls or when sudden severe stress or tension is placed on the ligament.

Classification of Ligamentous Injuries

In 1968 a Committee on the Medical Aspects of Sports of the American Medical Association published a handbook entitled *Standard Nomenclature of Athletic Injuries.* In that book a sprain is defined as an injury limited to ligaments (which attach bone to bone) and a strain as a stretching injury of a muscle or its tendinous attachment to bone.

Sprains of the knee are classified into categories depending on the degree of severity. A first-degree (mild) sprain of a ligament is defined as a tear of a minimum number of fibers of the ligament with localized tenderness but no instability of the knee. A second-degree (moderate) sprain has a disruption of more ligamentous fibers with more loss of function and more joint reaction but no instability of the knee. A third-degree (severe) sprain has a complete disruption of the ligament with resultant instability. Third-degree or severe sprains, which have instability of the knee, may be further classified as to the degree of instability demonstrated under stress testing of the joint. A one-plus instability indicates that the joint surfaces separate 5 mm or less; with a two-plus instability they separate between 5 and 10 mm; and with three-plus instability they separate 10 mm or more (Edmonson & Crenshaw, 1980, p. 918).

Treatment of a mild or first-degree sprain may be entirely symptomatic with the patient returning to normal activities within a few days. Usually rest, ice, and a compression bandage are all that is required. A moderate sprain usually requires some protection because a portion of a ligament has been torn, and although the remaining untorn portion may be able to stabilize the knee, the strength of the ligament has been significantly impaired. These patients are usually placed in a long leg cast with the knee flexed 30 to 45 degrees for 4 to 6 weeks. Recovery can usually be expected with no residual effects if a program of rehabilitative exercises is followed. Severe sprains often require surgical treatment and immobilization. By definition, the repair of a ligamentous injury of the knee involves surgical treatment of the acute injury. Optimally repair restores the anatomical integrity and tension in the torn ligament. After surgery for most ligament repairs, the leg is immobilized in a long leg cast with the knee flexed 45 to 60 degrees. The patient, the family, and significant others as well as the nurse should understand that ligament healing and return to normal function require 9 to 12 months. Repair is distinct from reconstruction, which refers to the surgical treatment of ligamentous laxity present 3, 4, or more months following injury (Edmondson & Crenshaw, 1980, p. 928).

Collateral Ligament Injuries

Medial (Tibial) Collateral Ligament

Medial stability of the knee is accomplished by the joint capsule and the medial (tibial) collateral ligament, which runs from the medial femoral condyle to the medial tibial condyle (DeGowin & DeGowin, 1976, pp. 742–743). Injuries of the tibial collateral ligament usually occur from forceful valgus bending of the knee joint. In such instances the femoral attachment is usually torn, though less frequently the tibial attachment is detached. The midportion of the medial collateral ligament is attached to the medial meniscus, so its injuries are properly associated with ruptures of the meniscus.

With an incomplete rupture of the tibial collateral ligament, pain is usually severe but function is not completely lost. The region around the ligament is tender and swollen. Lateral mobility of the joint is lacking. Individuals with a complete rupture of the ligament have pain and swelling at the site, and palpation may disclose a movable fragment of the bone where the ligament attaches to the bone. A slight lateral mobility indicates an accompanying rupture of the anterior cruciate ligament.

Lateral (Fibular) Collateral Ligament

Rupture of the fibular (lateral) collateral ligament is produced by a severe varus bending of the knee, and is rather uncommon. Usually the fibular attachment is torn, and the head of the fibula may be avulsed. Tenderness occurs on the lateral aspect of the bone between the lateral femoral epicondyle and the fibular head. If there is a complete severance of the lateral collateral ligament, the ends may be palpated. Crepitus may be elicited to indicate avulsion of the fibular head. A slight lateral mobility of the knee may be present. A frequent complication of a ruptured fibular ligament is damage to the common peroneal nerve, thus the patient's ability to move the anterior and lateral muscles of the leg and the short extensors of the toes should be noted (DeGowin & DeGowin, 1976, p. 744).

Post-Trauma Assessment for Collateral Ligament Stability. Besides the symptoms noted above, a more extensive assessment of the lateral and medial collateral ligament needs to be done. One way to test the medial collateral ligament is to secure the patient's ankle with one hand and place the other hand around the patient's knee so that the thumb is against the fibular head. Push medially against the knee and laterally against the ankle in an attempt to open the knee joint medially (valgus stress). Palpate the medial joint line for any gapping. If a gap is present, the medial collateral ligament is not supporting the knee properly. When the stress on the knee is released, you can feel the tibia and femur "clunk" together (Fig. 7–10). To test the lateral collateral ligament, reverse the procedure (Hoppenfeld, 1976, p. 185). Most ligament injuries around the knee occur on the medial side. To summarize, an abnormal opening of the medial aspect of the knee joint noted when the medial collateral ligament is stretched with the knee partially flexed indicates damage to the medial collateral ligament. When an opening is noted on the lateral aspect of the knee joint, the lateral collateral ligament has been damaged (Gartland, 1979, p. 408–409).

After the medial collateral ligament repair is complete, suction drainage tubes are inserted, the surgical wound is closed, and the leg is placed in a long leg cast, with the knee flexed approximately 60 degrees and the tibia internally rotated. The same is true for a lateral collateral ligament repair, except that the tibia is externally rotated.

□ NURSING PROCESS (Table 7–2)

Assessment

The initial assessment for a patient following a repair of a collateral ligament follows the format for the patient having a total knee replacement

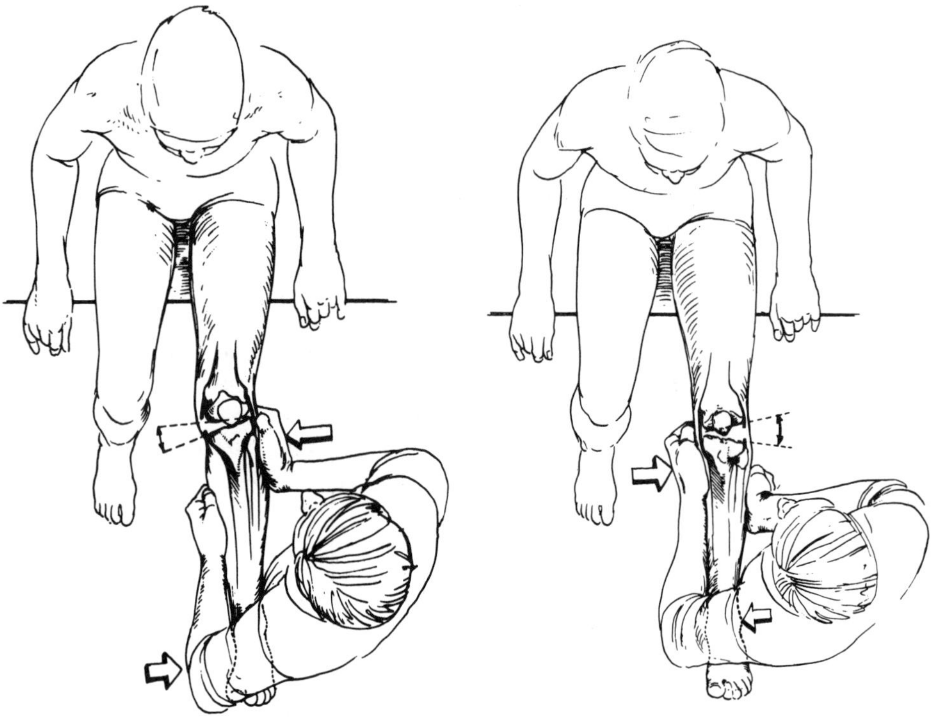

A B

Figure 7–10. A. To test the medial collateral ligament, apply valgus stress to open the knee joint on the medial side. **B.** To test the lateral knee for stability, apply varus stress to open the knee joint on the lateral side.

(see pp. 375–376). In the present case, however, the leg is in a long leg cast with the knee flexed 60 degrees and the tibia internally rotated (externally rotated for a lateral collateral ligament repair). The leg can be elevated either on several pillows or supported by a heavy canvas sling. Check to make sure that the canvas is sufficiently wide to distribute the weight and that it is not cutting into the wet cast. If the leg is on pillows, make sure that the pillows are positioned so that the leg is secure. Note the neurovascular status of the affected extremity and any complaints of discomfort.

Nursing Diagnosis and Goal Formulation

Nursing diagnoses and goal formulation are similar to those given for a patient following menisectomy (see pp. 349 and 354).

TABLE 7–2. NURSING PROCESS FOR REPAIR OF COLLATERAL LIGAMENT AND APPLICATION OF A LONG LEG CAST

Assessment	Nursing Diagnosis	Goal Formulation	Planning and Intervention	Evaluation and Reassessment
1. Check vital signs. Assess location, duration, and severity of pain. Check cast for pressure areas. Check position of leg.	1. Alteration in comfort: pain in the knee related to soft tissue trauma.	1. Short-term goal: a decrease in the level of pain through immobilization and prescribed medications. Long-term goal: free of pain.	1. Alleviate Pain Elevate the leg on pillows or with overhead slings. Place the leg in correct alignment; reposition as needed. Place ice bags along suture line. Teach relaxation techniques. Administer prescribed medications as indicated.	1. After the first 24 hours the patient should remain relatively comfortable with minimal amounts of medications.
2. Check the elevation of the leg. Check the cast for tightness. Assess the patient's strength in the upper extremities and uninvolved leg. Assess the patient's ability to do the exercises and to ambulate safely.	2. Impaired physical mobility: decreased knee function related to soft tissue trauma.	2. Short-term goal: an increase in mobility through controlled exercises. Long-term goal: regain full knee function.	2. Increase Mobility *Position* Keep the leg elevated without pressure on the heel. Turn patient to a position of comfort with leg elevated. *Exercises* Teach quadriceps and hamstring isometric exercises to be done every hour (starting day of surgery). Assist with leg lifts. Instruct on exercises to increase strength for crutch walking.	2. The patient should be able to keep the affected leg elevated, but will likely need help in turning. The patient should be able to do the isometric exercises without supervision, but will probably need help in doing leg lifts with the long leg cast in place.

(continued)

TABLE 7–2. *(Continued)*

Assessment	Nursing Diagnosis	Goal Formulation	Planning and Intervention	Evaluation and Reassessment
			Ambulation Ambulation begins when patient is able to lift the casted leg off the bed. Demonstrate crutch walking (no weightbearing on affected leg). Demonstrate how to get in and out of a chair and how to go up and down stairs using crutches.	The patient should be able to ambulate safely with crutches.
3. Assess the neurovascular status. Check the leg for any tightness of the cast or pressure areas. Check for level of pain.	3. Potential for injury: neurovascular deficit related to soft tissue trauma and cast application.	3. Short- and long-term goals: free of any neurovascular deficit.	3. Prevent Complications *Circulatory* Keep the leg elevated. Apply ice along incision line. Utilize nursing measures to prevent or reduce swelling. Bivalve cast as needed. Notify physician of any abnormal neurovascular response.	3. The patient should remain free of any complications.

Assess the skin along the edges of the cast. Assess for any pressure areas over bony prominences. Assess if something has been placed inside the cast.	Potential for injury: a break in skin integrity related to application of the cast.	Short- and long-term goals: free of any break in skin integrity.	*Integumentary* Keep the leg elevated. Utilize nursing measures to prevent or reduce swelling. Petal rough cast edges. Prevent the leg from lying on hard surfaces. *Potential Complications Due to Knee Surgery* (See Table 7–3, Total Knee Arthroplasty) *Potential Complications Due to Immobility* (See Chap. 3 and Table 6–2)	
4. Assess the patient's level of understanding about rehabilitation process and home care.	4. Potential knowledge deficit related to lack of knowledge about the rehabilitation process.	4. Short- and long-term goals: a decrease in anxiety through increased knowledge.	4. Patient Teaching Discuss the various stages in the rehabilitation process. Discuss cast care. Demonstrate methods of bathing, sleeping, and dressing with a long leg cast on. Discuss ways to reduce problems in traveling by car or public transportation. Include the family and significant other in teaching plan.	4. The patient should feel confident in going home and continuing the rehabilitation process.

Planning and Intervention

Alleviate Pain. Measures discussed to relieve pain for the patient following a total knee replacement apply here (see pp. 377 and 382).

Increase Mobility

Position. Insure that the position of the elevated leg does not lead to back discomfort or cause the proximal portion of the cast to irritate the soft tissue of the leg. Check to see that there is no pressure on the patient's heel and that the leg supports do not apply pressure.

Exercises. Encourage the patient to begin quadriceps and hamstring isometric exercises the first day postsurgery, and to continue with them every waking hour. Assist the patient with leg lifts to strengthen the hip flexors and abductors as soon as the patient is able. (For further discussion, see pp. 358–359 and 384.)

Ambulation. Ambulation is usually allowed as soon as the patient is able to lift the casted leg off the bed. Crutch walking is allowed with a three-point gait and no weight bearing on the affected leg.

Patient Teaching. The patient's length of stay in the hospital depends primarily on the rate of physical recovery. The emotional status of the patient, the family, and significant others affects how willing and able the patient is to do the exercises. As a whole, most patients are able to go home on crutches 4 to 10 days or sooner after surgery. The patient needs to understand the role of exercises is the rehabilitation of the knee and follow a home exercise program. The cast is usually changed about 2 weeks after surgery, and the new cast left on for another 6 to 8 weeks. (For discussion of home care with a long leg cast, see pp. 396 and 403 and Appendix B.) It usually takes about 12 months for maximum strength and function to be attained after ligament repair.

Prevent Complications. The nursing care to prevent complications following a collateral ligament repair is similar to that following a total knee replacement, except that the patient may develop problems related to a long leg cast. (For further nursing measures, see pp. 386–390 and 402–403.)

Evaluation and Reassessment

For a typical patient recovering from a collateral ligament repair, the evaluation is similar to that of a patient following a total knee arthroplasty. Special emphasis should be given to evaluating the patient's compliance with the exercise regime, understanding of the care required for the casted leg, and ability to ambulate.

Cruciate Ligament Injuries

The anterior and posterior cruciate ligaments are instrumental in preventing anterior and posterior dislocation of the tibia relative to the femur. These ligaments are intracapsular, originating on the tibia and inserting into the inner sides of the femoral condyles.

Violent injuries to the knee joint often rupture the anterior cruciate ligament. At the time of the injury, the patient has a great amount of pain, followed by hemarthrosis. The joint is usually in a slightly flexed position. In order to correctly determine the amount of injury, the swelling must subside or the blood must be aspirated from the knee joint. If not treated, the patient may later have symptoms of instability of the knee during activities such as walking down stairs (Hoppenfeld, 1976, p. 186).

An injury to the posterior cruciate ligament usually results from a direct blow on the head of the tibia while the knee is flexed. The signs are similar to those of an anterior cruciate ligament injury.

Post-Trauma Assessment for Cruciate Ligament Injuries

To test the integrity of the cruciate ligaments, the test for the draw sign is usually done. The patient must be lying supine with the affected knee flexed at 90 degrees and that foot flat on the table. Sit on the patient's foot to stabilize it. Cup your hands around the patient's knee, placing your fingers in the area of insertion of the medial and lateral hamstrings (in the popliteal fossa) and your thumbs along the lateral and medial line of the joint. To test the anterior cruciate ligament, pull the head of the tibia toward you so that it glides on the femoral condyles. If the tibia slides forward more than 1 cm, that is a positive anterior draw sign, and the anterior cruciate ligament may be torn (Fig. 7–11). However, always check the other knee for comparison, because a few degrees of anterior draw may be normal if an equal amount occurs in both knee joints (Hoppenfeld, 1976, p. 186).

To test the posterior cruciate ligament assume the same position, but push the head of the tibia away from you. If the tibia slides backward on the femoral condyles, that is a positive posterior draw sign, indicating that the posterior cruciate ligament is damaged. Again, check the other knee for comparison. An isolated tear of the posterior cruciate ligament is rare (DeGowin & DeGowin, 1976, p. 744; Hoppenfeld, 1976, p. 186).

Nursing Care Following Cruciate Ligament Repair

After an anterior cruciate ligament repair is completed (Fig. 7–12), suction drainage tubes are inserted, the surgical wound is closed, and the knee is immobilized in a long leg cast with 45 to 50 degrees of knee flexion and with the tibia slightly internally rotated. When the surgery has only been to repair a posterior cruciate ligament, the leg is immobilized in a long leg cast with 30 degrees of knee flexion. When a medial or lateral collateral ligament repair is performed along with the posterior cruciate ligament repair, however, the knee is kept in 45 to 50 degrees of flexion.

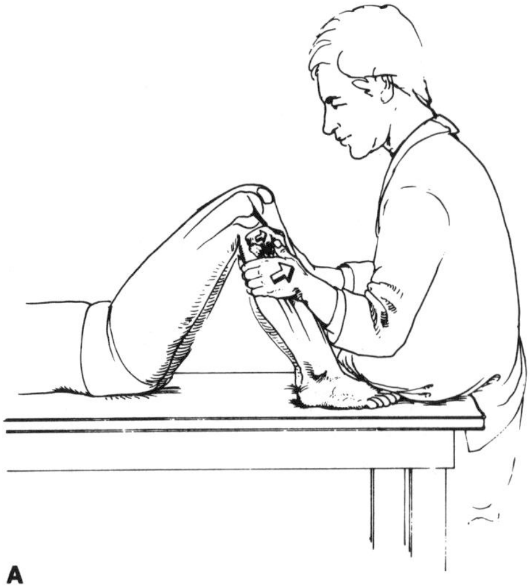

A

Figure 7–11. A. Position for eliciting the anterior draw sign. B. A positive anterior draw sign: torn anterior cruciate ligament. C. A positive posterior draw sign: torn posterior cruciate ligament.

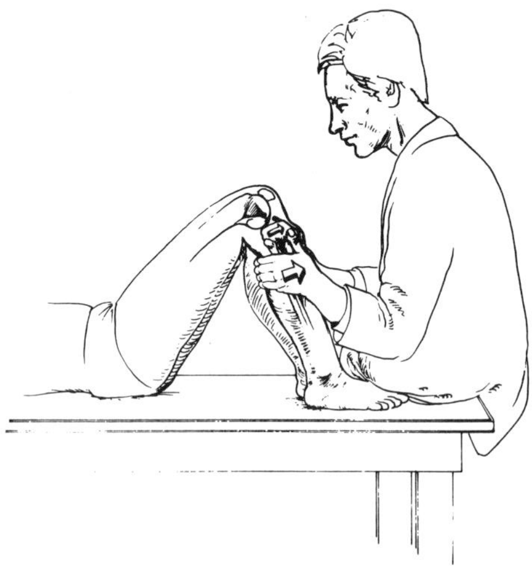

B

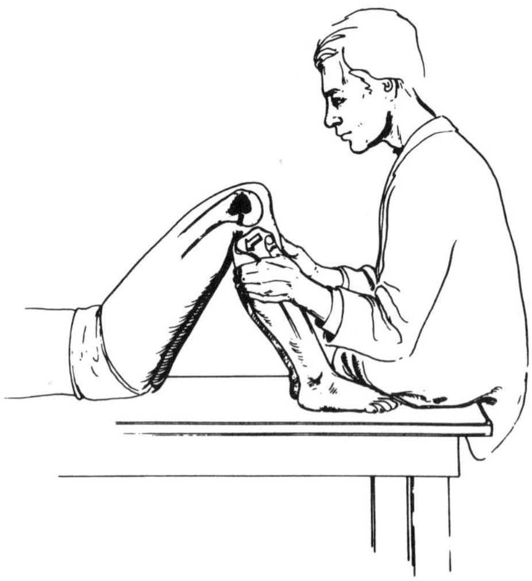

C

The nursing care for a patient following a repair of a cruciate ligament is similar to that following a collateral ligament repair. However, progressive quadriceps exercises are delayed until 6 to 8 weeks after cast removal, when hamstring strength is almost fully recovered. Such vigorous resistive exercises may disrupt or stretch the repaired cruciate ligament.

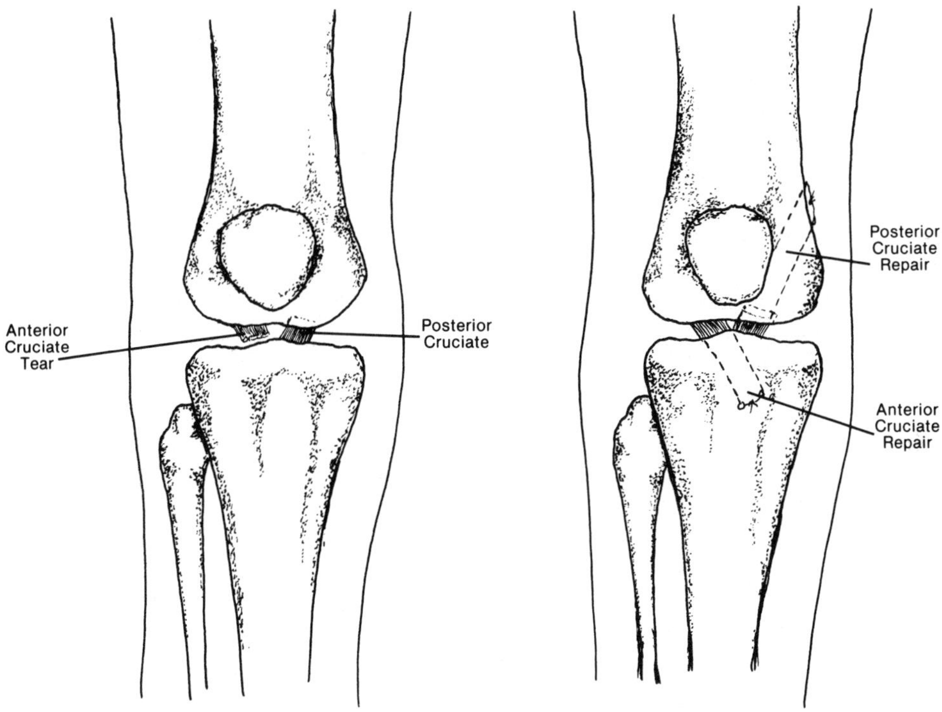

Figure 7–12. Repair of torn anterior or posterior cruciate ligaments. *(From Brantley, P., & Analla, M., 1980, p. 91. Courtesy of Howmedica.)*

INJURY TO THE QUADRICEPS EXTENSOR APPARATUS

The extensor apparatus of the knee begins with the quadriceps muscle, which blends into the quadriceps tendon. That tendon surrounds the patella, becoming the patellar tendon, which inserts into the tibial tubercle. When that apparatus is shortened, the knee extends. Any injury to the mechanism of the extensor apparatus, such as a rupture of the quadriceps tendon, a displaced fracture of the patella, a dislocation of the patella, a rupture of the patellar ligament, or an avulsion of the tibial tubercle, can result in an inability to adequately extend and stabilize the knee.

Disruption of the quadriceps extensor mechanism can occur due to direct or indirect trauma. Direct trauma usually results from a blow to the quadriceps muscle when it is contracted and the knee is slightly flexed. In an older person, a sudden violent contraction of the quadriceps muscle may also cause the extensor apparatus to rupture. The result is usually a separation of the tendon from the patella. The history given by aged, overweight, or poorly conditioned individuals frequently involves jumping from a chair or short height, which resulted in a severe pain in the anterior knee area, a felt or heard snapping of the knee, and a buckling of the knee joint. Examination of the leg reveals swelling and tenderness of the quadriceps tendon, and a sulcus (a furrow or depression) may be palpable. The patient is usually unable to extend the knee, although when the tear is incomplete, quadriceps function is present but diminished.

In a younger person, the injury is usually from athletic activities, and the avulsion is at the tendotubercle insertion. There is acute pain, tenderness, swelling, and impaired knee extension. A gap is usually palpable, and the patella is situated higher than normal. Such injuires can also occur from indirect trauma, such as when a running athlete is accelerating or decelerating (usually the latter).

PATELLAR FRACTURES

Patellar fractures occur frequently because of the patella's exposed position and the severe stresses that can be imposed upon it. The trauma can be either direct or indirect. The patient may give a history that includes a blow to the knee, a fall, or some other direct stress. In older, obese, or poorly conditioned individuals, indirect injury can occur from a jump, descending the stairs, or a forceful squat. An audible and painful snap frequently occurs, followed by a fall or loss of balance, and the individual is usually unable to extend the knee. Upon examination there is swelling about the patella, tenderness, and generally some effusion. The patella may reveal deformity, and occasionally fragments of the patella may be movable. Other fractures may require open reduction and internal fixation with the application of a long leg or cylinder cast (Fig. 7–13).

PATELLAR DISLOCATION

A dislocation in which the patella leaves the femoral groove can occur for various reasons, including severe falls, automobile accidents, and athletic injuries. The patient usually complains of the knee buckling, causing a fall, and pain in the anterior knee area. Effusion may occur but usually is not as severe as in an internal knee injury. There may be difficulty in extending the knee, but when the knee is extended the patella returns to its normal position. In chronic dislocations of the patella, examination reveals an excessive laxity of the extensor mechanism and excessive movement of the patella, generally in the lateral direction. The vastus medialis may be atrophic. Crepitation is felt and heard between the patella and its femoral groove. A recurrent dislocation of the pa-

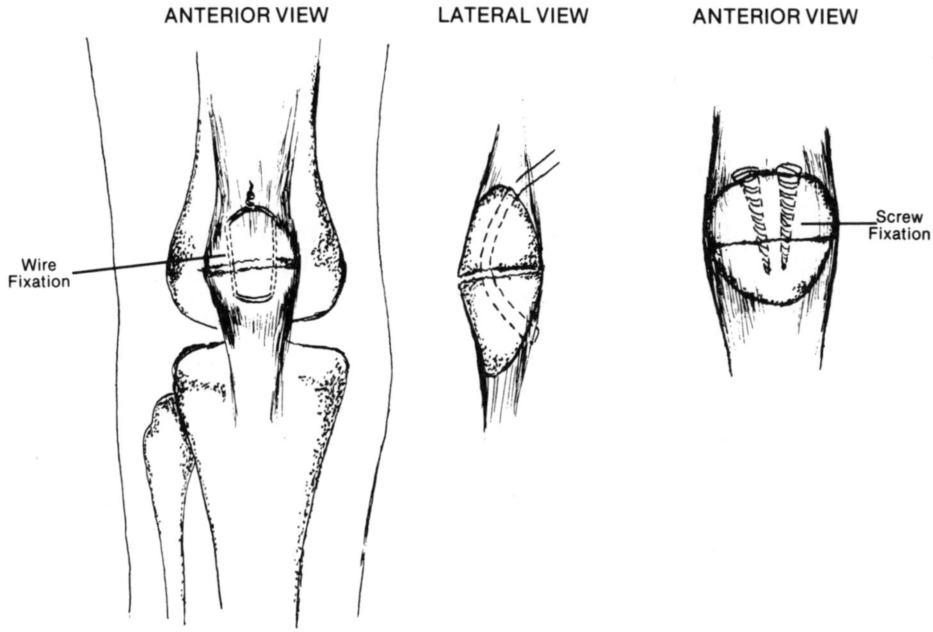

Figure 7–13. Open reduction and internal fixation, fractured patella. *(From Brantley, P., & Analla, M., 1980, p. 94. Courtesy of Howmedica.)*

tella is frequently associated with other knee pathology that impairs the extensor mechanism.

Treatment seeks to restore the continuity of the extensor mechanism and usually involves surgery. Ruptures of the quadriceps tendon and patellar ligament are usually repaired surgically, and the knee is protected in extension for at least 3 weeks. Early range-of-motion exercises are then begun to prevent knee stiffness. Surgical repair for a dislocation is aimed at changing the quadriceps pull, restoring the depth of the femoral sulcus, or decreasing the quadriceps laxity. The knee is protected for a period and then gentle exercises are started. For fractures of the patella, a conservative approach may be utilized, which first reduces joint effusion by aspiration and then application of a posterior mold splint to fully extend the knee. Ice is used until the swelling subsides, and then the posterior splint is changed to a cast for a period of 4 to 8 weeks. Surgical intervention for a fractured patella may involve replacement and fixation of the fragments, removal of the entire patella, removal of all fragments, or replacing the patella with a prosthesis.

OTHER TRAUMATIC INJURIES TO THE KNEE

Fractures of the Tibial Condyles

A fracture through one of the tibial condyles is one of the most common fractures involving the knee joint. This injury may be produced by direct compression, such as jumping down, or by a forceful abduction or adduction of the knee joint.

Fractures of the lateral tibial condyle occur more often than those of the medial tibial condyle because the lateral side of the knee is more exposed to trauma. A lateral force applied to the leg can cause both a fracture of the tibial condyle and a rupture of the medial collateral ligament.

Some tibial condyle fractures may be treated by closed reduction and the use of a long leg cast (see Appendix B). Others may be treated by skeletal traction (Chap. 6) or by open reduction with an internal fixation (e.g., a tibial bolt; Fig. 7–14) and a long leg cast applied for 6 to 8 weeks. The use of crutches without weight bearing on the affected leg is generally allowed in 3 to 5 days after surgery, but full weight bearing is not usually allowed for 10 to 12 weeks (Gartland, 1979, p. 426).

Dislocations of the Knee

A dislocation of the knee joint in an adult is usually produced by trauma, and can be either anterior, posterior, medial, or lateral, depending upon the position of the tibia in relation to the femur. Anterior dislocations are the most common. Most physicians accept closed reduction under general anesthesia and immobilization as the treatment of choice for most dislocations but some

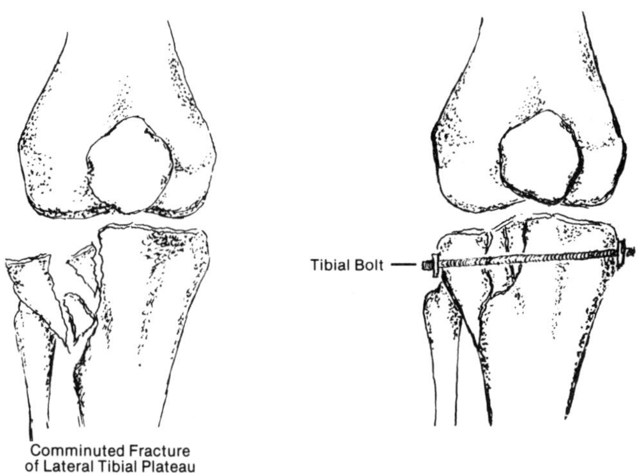

Figure 7–14. Open reduction and internal fixation, fractured tibial plateau. *(From Brantley, P., & Analla, M., 1980, p. 107. Courtesy of Howmedica.)*

physicians prefer open reduction to repair soft tissue damage. One serious potential complication is an injury to the popliteal artery, which may necessitate an amputation. Look for signs of vascular insufficiency or severe and increasing pain after reduction, which may indicate the possibility of vascular injury.

Traumatic Synovitis

A jarring or twisting injury to the knee may irritate the synovial membrane and cause an outpouring of normal appearing synovial fluid into the joint in the hours following the injury. Fluid distention of the joint and suprapatellar pouch may cause pain, limitation of motion, and a limping gait.

Traumatic synovitis may be suspected if injury to the joint surfaces, supporting ligaments, and menisci have been ruled out. Radiographic examination of the knee joint probably will be negative except for possible capsular swelling due to the accumulation of fluid (Gartland, 1979, pp. 410–411).

The treatment of traumatic synovitis usually consists of rest and support to the joint. Joint distension may be relieved by aspiration of the excess joint fluid.

Prepatellar Bursitis

The prepatellar bursa lies superficial to the distal end of the patella and the upper half of the patellar tendon. It may become acutely inflamed and swollen from local trauma or may be chronically irritated by repeated or prolonged kneeling. For that reason, the condition has been called "Housemaid's Knee" or "Nun's Knee." Clinically, a localized, well-circumscribed fluctuant mass may be palpated over the anterior aspect of the knee. The knee joint itself is not involved. Treatment usually consists of aspiration of the fluid, local injection of corticosteroids, and application of a pressure dressing. If the cause of the inflammatory response is infection, incision and drainage with proper antibiotic coverage are indicated. Occasionally, chronic recurrent enlargement justifies surgical excision of the bursal sac (Gartland, 1979, p. 164).

Pathology

ARTHRITIS AND INFECTIONS

Chondromalacia Patellae

Chondromalacia patellae or degenerative arthritis of the patellofemoral joint is as frequent and can be as painfully disabling as degenerative arthritis of the femorotibial joint (Cailliet, 1973, p. 248). Chondromalacia patellae frequently is a complication of other knee lesions, such as degenerative arthritis of the femorotibial joint or lesions of the cruciate or collateral ligaments. Its etiology is unclear, with possible causes including abnormal ridges on the femoral condyle, incongruity of the femoropatellar articulation, abnormal length of the infrapatella tendon, and malalignment of the patella. Signs of the chondromalacia include retropatellar aching, a feeling of crepitation, a feeling of the knee "giving way," and pain on descending stairs or rising from a chair. Upon examination of the knee, one finds a normal knee with tenderness over the medial aspect of the patella. When pressure is applied on the patella with simultaneous quadriceps contraction, crepitation and pain are elicited. Roentgenographic findings are negative until the condition is advanced.

Nonsurgical treatment usually consists of avoiding any irritating activity such as deep knee bends or squats. If pain persists brief immobilization in a cylindrical cast or retropatellar steroid injections may be used. Surgical intervention varies from arthrotomy and shaving the involved patella to a total patellectomy. One frequent approach is a combination of a patellar realignment and an excision of cartilage that modifies the Q angle (i.e., the lateral or medial patella deviation) (Cailliet, 1973, p. 248).

Degenerative Arthritis (Osteoarthritis)

Osteoarthritis involving the knee joint is a common and frequently progressive disorder seen mainly in middle-aged and older patients. It is characterized by deterioration of the articular cartilage, narrowing of the joint space, and overgrowth of the juxta-articular bone.

The knee joint, as a major weight-bearing joint, frequently becomes involved as part of a generalized disease process. Even though only one knee may be involved, it is not uncommon for osteoarthritis to affect both knees. Quite frequently, osteoarthritis affects one side of a knee joint more severely than the other, resulting in the development of an angular deformity at the knee. Narrowing of the medial side of the joint may cause genu varum deformity, whereas a genu valgum deformity may result from the narrowing of the lateral side of the joint. Long-standing or severe angular deformity may cause knee joint instability.

Osteoarthritis of the knee may also follow as a later complication of an intra-articular fracture of the joint or the removal of a torn meniscus.

Clinical Assessment

Osteoarthritis of the knee usually causes the patient to complain of pain, grating, and stiffness in the joint, and on occasion, of joint deformity with instability. Pain may be referred to the thigh and calf muscles. Synovial effusion in the knee is frequently present, and the patient may complain of a tightness in the back of the joint. The joint outlines may be distorted by the synovial effusion or by thickening of the synovial membrane. Some limitation of joint motion usually occurs, and a flexion contracture may develop. Roentgenographic examination of the knee joint may disclose narrowing of the joint space associated with sclerotic changes in the subchondral bone. Bone spurs may be seen along the joint margins and at the distal end of the patella. Changes may be more marked on one side of the joint than the other as discussed above. In advanced cases of osteoarthritis, the tibia may appear subluxed on the femur.

Medical Treatment

Symptoms produced by degenerative arthritis in the knee joint frequently may be relieved by the use of intra-articular hydrocortisone, following aspiration of any effusion present. Systemic use of anti-inflammatory drugs is helpful in relieving symptoms of pain and stiffness. Locally applied moist heat, mild support of the joint, and the occasional use of a cane to relieve stress to the joint may also be helpful in relieving symptoms.

Some patients require surgical treatment to relieve pain, correct deformity, or restore joint motion. The choice of surgical treatment depends on the specific findings of the history, the physical and roentgenographic examination, and the intended outcome. The surgical procedure may be a tibial osteotomy, a total knee arthroplasty, or an arthrodesis, and these procedures are described in a later section.

Rheumatoid Arthritis

Arthritis is discussed in detail in Chapter 4, but here we deal with rheumatoid arthritis (RA) as it relates to the knee joint. Rheumatoid arthritis is a systemic inflammatory disorder of connective tissue with primary involvement of the synovial membranes. Attention here is confined to the joints, tendons, and tendon sheaths, and the capsule of the knee.

Clinical Assessment

Usually RA has been clinically evident and diagnosed before the knee joints are involved. Synovial fluid drawn from the knee effusion is turbid with elevated specific gravity, slightly decreased sugar, and increased cellular inclusion. The disease process usually follows a sequence of events in which all of the tissues in and about the joint are involved sequentially. In the first phase there is usually only soft tissue involvement. This is primarily synovial hyperemia with joint effusion. The surrounding ligaments and capsule are stretched, swollen, and tender, and roentgenographic evidence reveals only soft tissue swelling with no articular changes. In the second phase there is pannus formation and evidence of nonarticular bone destruction, along with the continuation of synovitis. It is during this phase that the synovitis begins to invade the cartilage and the adjacent bone. Roentgenograms become diagnostic in this phase as there is now noticeable bone destruction (erosion) at the margins of the articular cartilage under the collateral ligaments and the appearance of decalcification. The knee joint space appears to remain intact on the roentgenogram, but by arthroscopic examination the presence of pannus and some erosion of cartilage is usually revealed. The third phase involves the beginning of the destruction of the cartilage and the erosion of subchondral bone. The joint space is now narrower, especially on the lateral aspect of the joint, and the knee joint is unstable. Soft tissue swelling usually lessens by the third phase, because by then the synovial tissue is more fibrotic and less inflamed. The periarticular swelling is firmer and feels thicker on examination. By the fourth phase there is joint destruction of varying degree with marked destruction of cartilage, which is apparent on the roentgenogram. There is marked joint laxity because of ligamentous involvement that causes subluxation and decreased joint function.

Medical Treatment

Treatment of a knee afflicted with RA consists of physical methods with prevention of deformity as the goal. Unlike other joints for which complete rest of prolonged duration is valuable, complete rest and immobilization is not appropriate in the knee because flexion contractures, quadriceps atrophy, fibrous adhesions with possible ankylosis, and subluxation are frequent and severe complications of immobility.

The position of flexion must be avoided during periods of exacerbation. Unfortunately, flexion is the position most comfortable to the patient, because it is promoted by both muscle spasm and joint capsule inflammation. Pillows under the knee during bedrest are not permitted. Posterior mold splints are sometimes used both to protect the extended knee and to help with comfort measures. The leg must be exercised periodically while in the splints. To do range-of-motion exercises to the knee, assist the patient in removing the leg from the splint and in doing gentle active and passive flexing and extending of the knee several times daily. This simple routine helps to prevent intra-articular fibrosis and capsular contractures. Heat or ice applications as tolerated by the patient can also be included in the exercise routine.

The quadriceps are to be exercised frequently. The exercises best tolerated during periods of exacerbation are the quadriceps setting and straight leg raises, either while in the cast or splint or during periods when the cast is removed. A gradual increase in quadriceps activity to active resistive exercises should be done as tolerated. Weight bearing is to be avoided except with the aid of crutches or a walker, and usually is not advisable if any flexion contracture exists. In general, the use of a brace to immobilize the extended knee is discouraged because it adds to further atrophy and dependence.

With the decrease of inflammation and associated spasm and painful joint motion, active exercises should be instituted. Once resistive exercises are initiated, they should be carefully supervised and done frequently during the day, with both the time and amount of exercise gradually increased. A patient's fear and low threshold of pain are strong factors that delay progress in rehabilitation efforts. Fear that pain means aggravation of the disease should be allayed, and realistic encouragement given. Some patients may require surgical treatment to relieve pain, correct deformity, or restore joint motion. The choice of surgical treatment depends upon the individual patient, the patient's physician, and the aims of the surgery. The surgical alternatives are a synovectomy, a total knee arthroplasty, or an arthrodesis.

Baker's (or Popliteal) Cyst

Baker's cyst is the name given to a firm, tense cystic mass occasionally found along the medial border of the popliteal space. The patient is usually a child, but popliteal cysts may also be seen in adults, particularly in patients with RA. Although the condition may represent herniation through the posterior capsule of the knee joint, most popliteal cysts are believed to be a fluid distention of the bursal sac associated with the gastrocnemius and semimembranosus muscles (Fig. 7–15).

No symptoms other than swelling may be noted, though the cyst may cause vague pain and discomfort associated with a sensation of weakness and "giving way." The cyst may be aspirated and injected with corticosteroids. Surgical excision may be required based on the intensity of the symptoms, or repeated aspiration and injection may be performed.

Loose Bodies

Loose bodies are fragments of cartilage, bone, or calcified tissue that lie free within a joint causing pain, joint irritation, and locking. Loose bodies have been

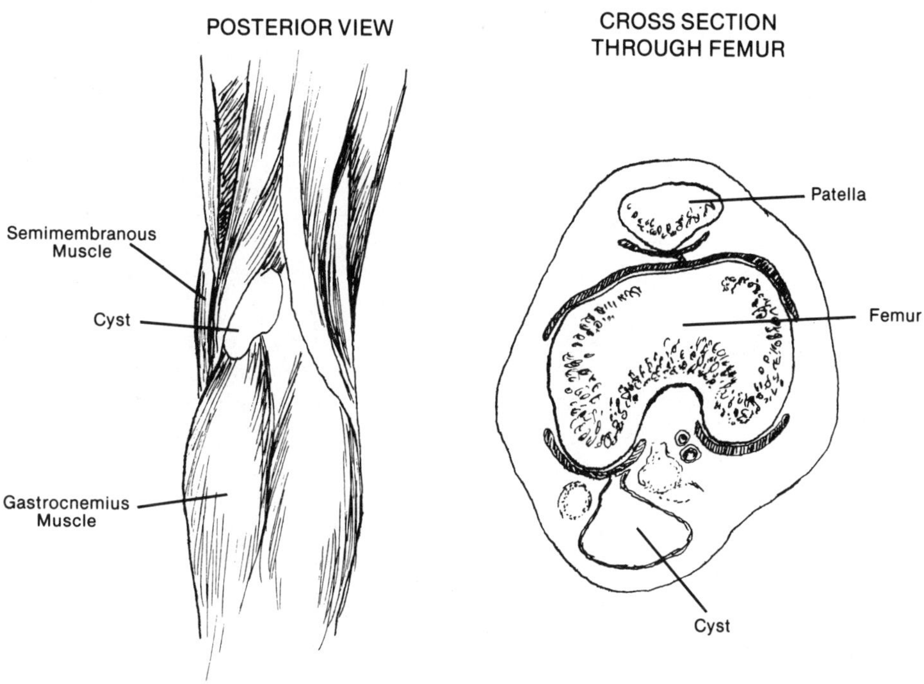

Figure 7–15. Baker's cyst. *(From Brantley, P., & Analla, M., 1980, p. 89. Courtesy of Howmedica.)*

discovered in practically every joint in the body, but occur most frequently in the knee. The fragments may be pieces of bone broken from the articular surface, such as a piece of tibial spine, a detached bone spur in an ostoarthritic knee joint, or a torn portion of a meniscus, or they may result from osteochondritis dissecans or osteochondromatosis. Locking occurs if a loose body becomes wedged between the bones, thereby forming a mechanical obstruction to complete extension.

Loose bodies containing bone or calcified cartilage are visible on roentgenographic examination. Loose bodies that are fragments of cartilage are not, but may be visualized by arthrography. They are removed from the joint by a surgical procedure known as an arthrotomy or arthroscopy. (See care of a patient following a menisectomy, pp. 349–355.)

Surgical Procedures

Synovectomy. A synovectomy is the surgical removal of the synovium. Persistent, unrelieved synovitis, usually related to RA, is the primary reason for a synovectomy, and the primary goal is to relieve pain. To be beneficial to the arthritic patient, the surgery must be done early in the course of the disease, prior to the onset of joint destruction. A late synovectomy may relieve pain, but it does not help restore functional effectiveness to the joint.

Nursing care following a synovectomy is similar to the care of a patient with a compression bandage and knee immobilizer. (See care following a menisectomy, pp. 349–355.) The leg is kept in extension with lateral rotation. The patient should do quadriceps setting exercises and ambulate with partial weight bearing, using crutches.

Proximal Tibial Osteotomy. A proximal tibial osteotomy is done to correct varus or valgus deformities of the knee. The procedure realigns the articular surfaces and thus distributes the weight more evenly on the joint, which relieves pain (Fig. 7–16). Healing is rapid because the surgery is performed through cancellous bone just proximal to the tibial tubercle.

The nursing care for a patient following an osteotomy is similar to that for a patient with an open reduction and a long leg cast. Because the affected leg will be slightly shorter after surgery, careful leg measurements need to be made so that the patient's shoes can be prepared with the proper amount of elevation.

Total Knee Replacement. A total knee replacement or total knee arthroplasty is surgery on an injured or diseased knee to reestablish a movable joint. The knee joint, like the hip joint, may be partially replaced (a hemiarthroplasty) or totally replaced. An arthroplasty consists of the replacement of the femoral condyles and the tibial plateau. The arthritic or diseased surfaces are removed and replaced by durable prosthetic components that are fixed firmly into place with methyl methacrylate bone cement. Some surgeons are now using porous-coated total knee prostheses that do not require any cement. There are two types of

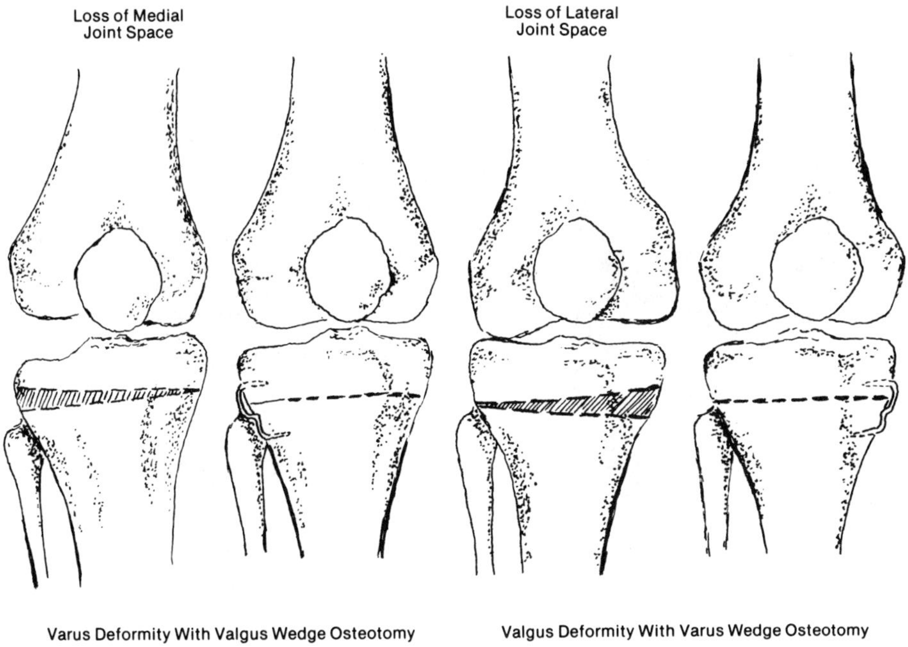

Figure 7–16. Proximal tibial osteotomy: varus or valgus closing wedge. *(From Brantley, P., & Analla, M., 1980, p. 105. Courtesy of Howmedica.)*

knee prostheses, the constrained (or hinged) and the nonconstrained (or unhinged). The nonconstrained type consists of two separate components, with the femoral component made of metal and the tibial component having a plastic articulating surface (Fig. 7–17). The stability of the unit or prosthesis is totally dependent upon good musculature and intact ligaments. The constrainted or hinged type is all metal (a cobalt–chrome alloy) and supplies its own stability (Fig. 7–18). The hinged type is indicated for unstable knees.

□ NURSING PROCESS (Table 7–3)

Assessment

The immediate postoperative assessment of a patient following a total knee replacement involves taking vital signs (pulse, respiration, and blood pressure), and observing the patient's general color and warmth. Usually, the patient's skin feels cool and the patient appears pale. The patient's level of consciousness and orientation should be determined. Have the patient cough and deep breathe and auscultate the chest for clearness of the lungs and any cardiac abnormalities. A neurovascular assessment of the affected

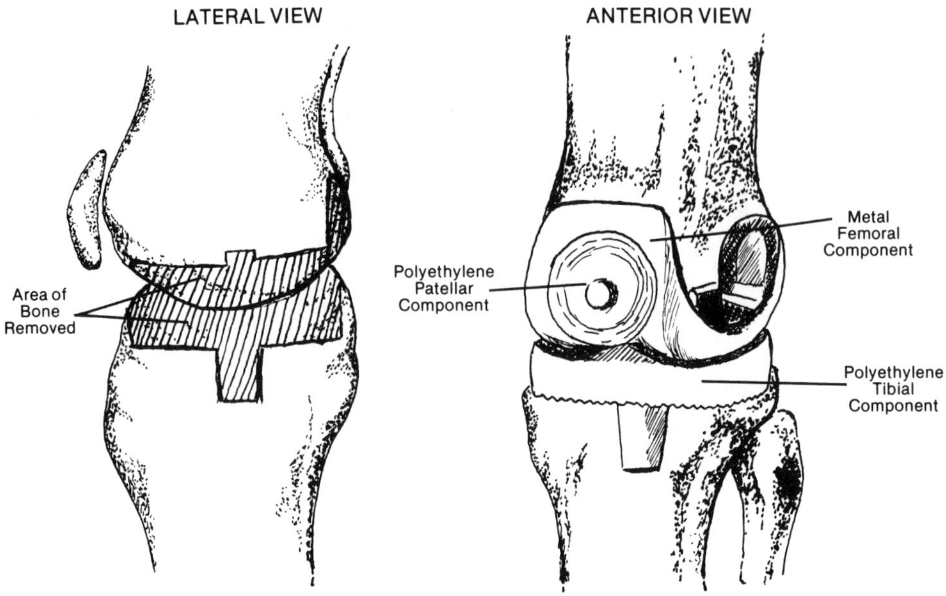

Figure 7–17. Total knee arthroplasty. *(From Brantley, P., & Analla, M., 1980, p. 98. Courtesy of Howmedica.)*

leg (pulse, temperature, color, capillar filling, edema, sensory and motor function) should be made (Chap. 2) and the position of the leg checked for proper alignment and elevation on pillows. The incisional dressing and the area posterior to the knee should be checked for drainage. The patient may have a compression dressing and the knee immobilized in extension with a knee immobilizer, a posterior plaster splint, or a cast. If the patient has wound catheters in place, note the color and amount of drainage, and whether the suction is working. Assess the type, severity, and location of pain and note whether the patient received pain medication in surgery or while in the postanesthesia room. Note the type of intravenous solution, the rate of flow, and the amount left in the bottle or bag. Obtain from the anesthesia and postanesthesia room records (or personnel) the amount of blood loss in surgery and the kind and amount of fluid replacement. Check the patient for bladder distention, urgency, or the need to void.

Nursing Diagnosis and Goal Formulation

The nursing diagnoses for a typical patient following a total knee replacement are (1) alterations in comfort related to knee pain from soft tissue trauma and surgery, (2) alterations in mobility related to lack of joint mobility from surgery and the immobilizing device, (3) alterations in psycho-

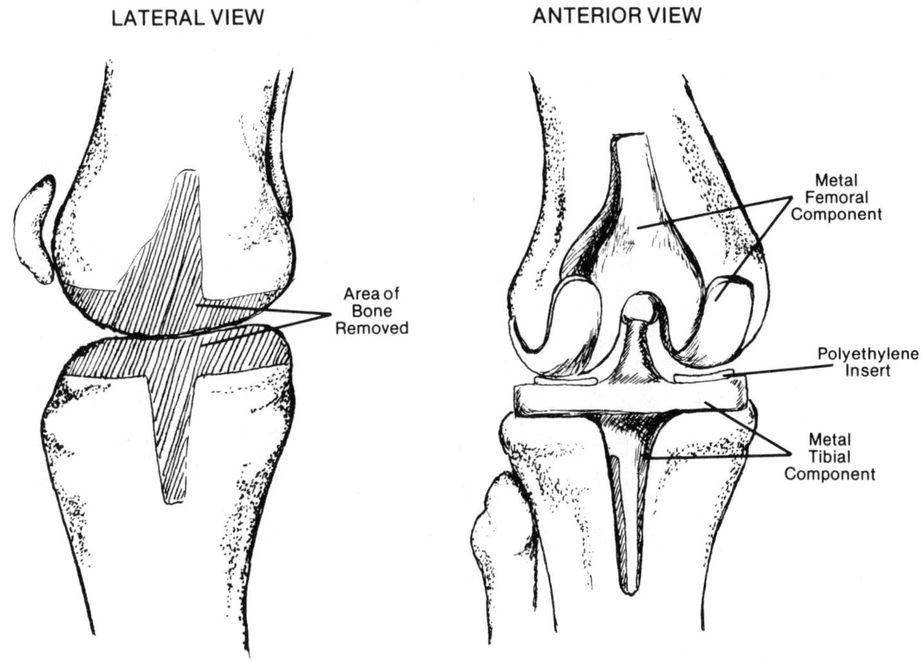

Figure 7–18. Hinged total knee arthroplasty. *(From Brantley, P., & Analla, M., 1980, p. 100. Courtesy of Howmedica.)*

logical well-being related to anxiety and knowledge deficit about the surgical procedure and the future functional ability of the knee joint, and (4) potential complications related to postoperative infection and decreased activity.

The short-term goals are to have the patient experience (1) a decrease in the amount, if not all, of the pain in the knee through nursing measures and prescribed medications, (2) an increase in mobility through the use of exercises and assistive devices, (3) a decrease in anxiety through increased knowledge about the procedure and the rehabilitation process, and (4) an absence of complications. Long-term goals are to have the patient free of pain and able to walk without discomfort, initially using a four-point gait and crutches, and without assistive devices by 6 months to a year.

Planning and Intervention

Alleviate Pain. Note the type, severity, and location of the pain to help determine the cause of the pain and thus the appropriate nursing measures. The patient who has had a total knee replacement will probably have more pain for a longer period of time than will a patient who has had a total hip

TABLE 7–3. NURSING PROCESS FOR TOTAL KNEE ARTHROPLASTY WITH KNEE SPLINT

Assessment	Nursing Diagnosis	Goal Formulation	Planning and Intervention	Evaluation and Reassessment
1. Assess the location, duration, and severity of pain. Observe for verbal and nonverbal cues of pain. Assess neurovascular status. Check the positioning of the leg.	1. Alteration in comfort: pain in the knee related to bone and soft tissue trauma.	1. Short-term goal: a decrease in the level of pain. Long-term goal: free of pain.	1. Alleviate Pain Elevate the leg on pillows. Keep the leg immobilized with knee splint. Reposition the leg by lifting gently. Apply ice bags along incision line. Utilize noninvasive nursing measures. Teach relaxation techniques. Administer medications as indicated.	1. The patient should need medication for the severe to moderate pain that occurs during the first 24–48 hours after surgery.
2. Check the positioning of the leg. Check for correct positioning of the splint. Assess the patient's ability to do the exercise regime. Assess strength in the upper extremities and uninvolved leg.	2. Impaired physical mobility: a decrease in knee function related to a lack of joint stability.	2. Short-term goal: an increase in mobility through immobilization and controlled exercises. Long-term goal: regain full knee function.	2. Increase Mobility *Position* Keep the leg immobilized with the knee splint. Keep the leg elevated. Elevate head of bed for comfort. *Turning* Turn to either side. Place pillows between legs to turn and provide support. *Exercises* Teach quadriceps and gluteal setting, plantar and dorsiflexion exercises and actual range of motion of the ankle (5 minutes every hour while awake). Demonstrate straight leg raising exercises.	2. The patient should be able to keep the leg elevated on pillows and in the correct alignment. Assistance should be available for turning and doing straight leg lifts. Exercise should be done without direct supervision because they were part of the preoperative teaching plan.

			Teach active range of motion to all uninvolved joints. Teach exercises to increase strength in the upper extremities. Teach patient to use a restorator when indicated.	
			Ambulation Demonstrate how to use the trapeze. Demonstrate walker use and crutch walking (partial-weight bearing).	Determine that the crutch walking gait has the correct amount of weight bearing.
3. Auscultate the chest for lung clearance. Assess the rate, depth and, rhythm of respirations. Assess for color. Check for shortness of breath or chest pain.	3. Potential alterations in respiratory function: ineffective airway clearance related to improper positioning and immobility.	3. Short- and long-term goals: free of any respiratory problems.	3. Prevent Complications *Respiratory* Instruct on turning, coughing, and deep breathing exercises. Elevate head of bed. Keep patient well hydrated. Utilize incentive respiratory device.	3. The patient's lungs should remain clear.
Check skin turgor and mucous membrane feature. Check neurovascular status. Assess for the "five Ps": (1) pain, (2) pain on passive motion, (3) paralysis, (4) paresthesia, and (5) pulselessness. Check vital signs.	Potential for injury: neurovascular deficit related to soft tissue swelling and knee splint. Potential fluid volume deficit related to decreased intake, lack of muscle tone, and volume loss in surgery.	Short- and long-term goals: free of any circulatory problem.	*Circulatory* Keep the patient well hydrated. Teach bed exercises. Apply elastic stockings. Encourage early ambulation. Administer anticoagulant drugs. Loosen any tight dressing or cast.	The patient should have good circulatory status with no problems.

(continued)

TABLE 7–3. *(Continued)*

Assessment	Nursing Diagnosis	Goal Formulation	Planning and Intervention	Evaluation and Reassessment
Assess intake and output. Auscultate for bowel sounds. Check for expulsion of flatus. Assess for nausea or anorexia. Assess abdomen for softness or distention.	Potential alteration in bowel elimination: constipation related to immobility and pain medications. Potential alteration in bowel elimination: ineffective bowel function related to immobility secondary to surgery.	Short- and long-term goals: normal peristalsis and regular elimination without pain or discomfort.	*Gastrointestinal* Administer parenteral fluid (first 24–48 hours after surgery). Keep the patient well hydrated. Start oral fluids when bowel sounds return.	The patient's nausea and vomiting should be self-limiting.
Check intake and output. Assess for any complaints of pain. Note frequency, amount, color, and odor of each voiding. Assess for bladder distention. Assess for possible sodium and potassium deficiency.	Potential alteration in urinary elimination: infection due to urinary stasis related to immobility.	Short- and long-term goals: void without pain or discomfort.	*Genitourinary* Utilize nursing measures to assist with voiding. Utilize nursing measures to help relax patient and relieve pain related to voiding. Start oral fluids when bowel sounds return.	The patient usually has difficulty in voiding immediately after surgery, but within 24–48 hours the patient usually diureses.

Assess how well the patient does the exercises. Check the number of degrees of knee flexion.	Potential alteration in mobility: stiff knee related to immobility.	Short- and long-term goals: move freely without any impediment of joint function.	*Musculoskeletal* Encourage the patient to continue exercises even though they may hurt. Encourage flexion to at least 90 degrees. Medicate before flexion exercises.	The patient should regain full range of knee function.
Assess incision for any signs of infection. Check vital signs. Assess area over bony prominences. Assess heel for any redness.	Potential for injury: infection related to surgical incision. Potential impairment of skin integrity: pressure areas related to immobility.	Short- and long-term goals: free of any pain or discomfort from pressure.	*Integumentary* Keep dressing clean and dry. Keep pressure off bony prominences. Keep knee splint secure but not too tight. Keep heel free of pressure.	The patient should not have any reddened areas or any signs of infection.
4. Assess the patient's level of understanding about the rehabilitation process and home care.	4. Potential knowledge deficit related to rehabilitation process and home care.	4. Short- and long-term goals: a decrease in anxiety through increased knowledge.	4. Patient Teaching Discuss the rehabilitation process. Encourage self-care. Discuss home resources for bathing, dressing, and ambulating. Discuss need to continue exercises. Include family and significant other in teaching plan.	4. The patient, family, and significant other should understand the rehabilitation regime and what the patient can and cannot do. There should be a decrease in the patient's anxiety level.

replacement. Following a total knee replacement, a typical patient will complain of severe to moderate pain for at least the first 24 to 48 hours, and some patients, even longer. Note the color and warmth of the toes, and check to see if the dressing, knee immobilizer, splint, or cast is too tight. Do a neurovascular assessment of the affected leg (Chap. 2). If circulatory impairment or swelling is noted, check the amount of elevation of the extremity. Elevate the leg (one pillow under the upper leg and two pillows under the lower portion) with the concept of "toes above the nose" but make sure that the elevation of the leg does not cause the patient low back discomfort. Adjusting the level of elevation of the leg, lowering the head of the bed, or turning the patient onto one side helps to relieve back pain. Check the ice bags that are along the incision site and refill as needed. They help to reduce swelling and thus prevent pain.

Sometimes the patient becomes anxious and tense, and tightens the muscles to prevent any movement. This increases the discomfort, but leads to even more tightening of the muscles. After reassuring the patient and getting the patient to relax the affected leg in your hands, use both hands and gently lift the leg and move it through its range of motion several times before repositioning it. Frequently the pain will go away or at least be reduced. In general, muscle setting exercises, which increase circulation, help to relieve pain and should be encouraged.

Patients having a total knee replacement may complain of pain in the back of the knee. If they had a knee flexion contracture before the surgery, it will be painful postoperatively because the contracted muscles are extended when the leg is held in extension. These patients may try to get out of the knee immobilizer or try to talk you into not putting the knee immobilizer back on, because they feel more comfortable when the knee is slightly flexed. It is important that they understand that keeping the knee flexed can impede their ambulation by causing a knee flexion contracture.

The nurse must be alert to any complaints of pain in the calf of the affected leg as that may not be a result of the surgery but an indication of thrombophlebitis. Patients may also complain of pain after each exercise session. This is to be expected, but can be prevented to some extent by giving the patient pain medications before the exercise. The pain needs to be relieved or it will interfere with the patient's program of rehabilitation, as he or she will not want to do the needed exercises.

Some patients ask for pain medications, others need to be encouraged to ask, and still others will not ask but will need to receive medication based on the nursing assessment. Following a total knee replacement, never let the patient go without pain medications just because he or she does not ask. For severe to moderate pain during the first 24 to 48 hours, most patients receive intramuscular injections of narcotics. For lesser pain, patients usually are on oral medications. Patients should know what medications are available, how often they are available, and that they are expected to ask for medications when they are needed. Some individuals are more willing to ask for medication if they know that it is not going to be a "shot."

Increase Mobility

Position. The patient having a total knee replacement will return from the postanesthesia room lying supine with the operated leg in an immobilizing device to keep it extended and elevated on pillows. The knee is usually kept in extension with a knee immobilizer, but some physicians may use posterior splints or cylinder casts. The knee immobilizer (various styles are available from different orthopaedic supply companies) holds the leg in extension and is usually more comfortable than a cast. Still, the knee immobilizer is not ideal for every patient. Even though immobilizers come in a variety of sizes, they do not fit the circumference and length of every leg, and some tend to slip when the patient gets out of bed. Some patients complain that the immobilizer is warm to wear, whereas still others find it very easy to take off when they are tired of it. In some instances, the nurse may need to use sheet wadding or Webril on the leg to improve fit, or even get another size after the compression dressing is off and the swelling is reduced. The knee immobilizer may be worn 24 hours a day (except during exercises) for 5 to 7 days, and then worn only at night.

If a cast has been applied, the general principles of cast care should be followed (Appendix B). Emphasis should be given to complaints of tightness or pressure at the operative site as the cast may need to be split and separated to relieve the pressure. Check the distal portion of the cast for pressure and irritation in the Achilles tendon area, and the proximal portion for irritation of the soft tissue of the groin.

The immobilized leg should be elevated in extension by the use of pillows, by elevating the foot of the bed, or by both, depending on the size of the patient. Elevation is used to help prevent and reduce edema, and the foot should normally be higher than the nose. If the patient is having increased swelling despite increases in the elevation of the leg, it may be necessary to lower the head of the bed. After 48 hours following surgery, the amount the leg is elevated may be decreased.

Turning. One of the first procedures is to turn the patient to the side. In most instances the patient has been supine since the night before surgery. With assistance, the patient can turn to either side but would probably prefer the unaffected side. With the nurse providing support along the entire length of the operated leg, the patient is able to turn, as discussed on pp. 258–259 and 383. The nurse must make sure that the head of the bed is lowered and that the leg does not twist as the patient turns. Once the patient has completed the turn, the operated leg is laid to rest on one to three pillows (depending upon the patient's size) to keep the leg in correct alignment.

Patients are usually able to assist in changing their own position while supine with the use of a trapeze and side rails. That helps to make the patient feel more independent and less uncomfortable, and assists the nurse in providing personal care.

Exercises. Exercises for the patient who has had a total knee replacement may begin from the day of surgery to several days postoperatively. If the patient has had preoperative teaching about the exercises and has practiced them, the patient will be able to do the exercises in the postanesthesia room. However, some physicians may not want exercises to begin that quickly.

Most patients will be doing quadriceps and gluteal setting exercises, range-of-motion exercises for the ankle, and plantar and dorsiflexion exercises of the affected leg, as discussed on pp. 258–259. Normally the patient will be asked to exercise 5 minutes out of every waking hour.

An additional exercise, which the patient may be required to do, is straight leg raises. The patient may find that hard to do in the beginning and thus the help of a nurse or a physical therapist, or the use of a sling, may be needed before the patient is able to do it without assistance. Some physicians will also have patients with total knee replacements do side-lying straight leg exercises, or lie prone and do knee flexion exercises. Other patients use a knee sling and do knee flexion exercises by the second or third postoperative day (after the wound catheters and the initial dressing have been removed). The knee flexion exercise is discussed on p. 295. Some patients with total knee replacement receive a whirlpool treatment before doing knee flexion exercises. The warm circulating water in the whirlpool increases the blood supply to the knee area and helps to relax the muscles in and around the knee joint. These patients probably still need oral pain medications before exercising.

Another exercise to increase flexion for the patient with a total knee replacement is the use of a restorator. A restorator is a set of bicycle-like pedals at the end of a pair of rods that attach to and extend forward from a chair. In a restorator exercise, the patient sits in the chair to which the restorator is attached, and the patient's feet are strapped onto the pedals. In the beginning the patient is able to sit and pedal with a minimum of knee flexion. As the patient's rehabilitation progresses, the pedals are moved closer to the chair, thus forcing the knee to flex more. The restorator exercise may be done for 30 minutes twice a day.

CONTINUOUS PASSIVE MOTION. Continuous passive motion (CPM) was first employed in the early 1960s. The involved extremity is placed in an electrically driven apparatus that continuously moves the involved joint through flexion and extension (Fig. 7–19). Since first described, the principle of continuous passive motion has been applied to several joints, including the knee, in situations where the healing of articular surfaces in joints is necessary, such as after the draining of a septic arthritic joint, postsynovectomy in a patient with RA, postarthroplasty in a patient with osteoarthritis, and after a loss of flexion caused by adhesions.

Passive motion, particularly if used continuously, reduces adhesions and stimulates healing, resulting in a stronger fixation. Continuous passive

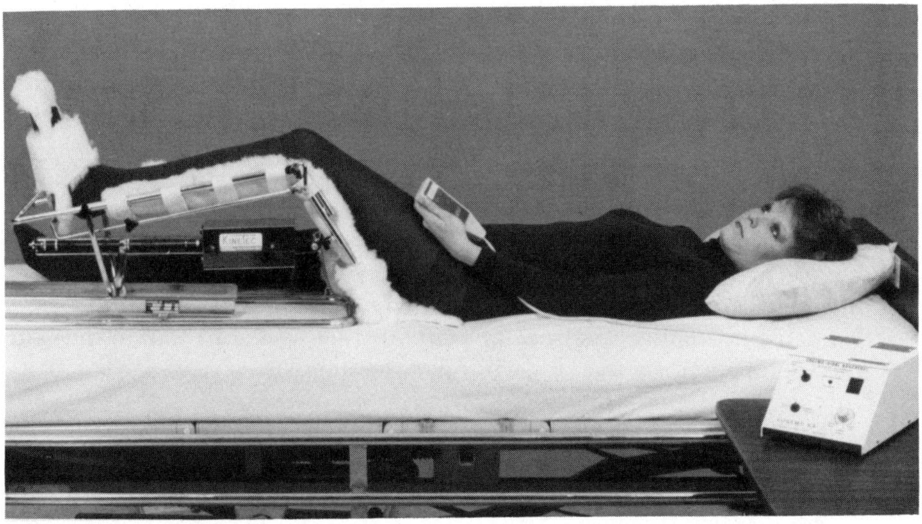

Figure 7–19. Continuous passive motion knee exerciser. *(Courtesy of Richards Medical Company. KINETIC is a registered trademark of COGEMO, an affiliate of Richards Medical Company.)*

motion following a knee arthrotomy or arthroplasty accelerates healing, increases range of motion, and maintains a higher level of muscle strength. Postoperative patients who experience CPM progress more rapidly, use fewer analgesics, and are discharged earlier with greater function than those patients whose joint is kept immobilized postoperatively (Strange & Johns, 1984).

To gain the most advantage from passive motion, it should be as continuous as possible, preferably 20 or more hours a day. Some physicians, however, may have the patient utilize CPM 4 hours once a day or 2 hours twice a day. The head of the bed can be elevated for comfort, but the patient must remain supine. The patient is prone to develop pressure areas, circulatory stasis, pulmonary stasis, and all the other sequelae of limited mobility.

Exercises like the ones discussed, or variations of them, may be incorporated into a home exercise program. The key to success is to restore the knee to at least 90 degrees of flexion, but the rehabilitation program for each patient should be individualized in terms of the patient's tolerance and rate of progression. Exercises for the rest of the body are also important to prevent the effects of immobility, and are discussed in Chapter 2.

Ambulation. The patient with a total knee replacement may start ambulating as soon as the wound catheters are discontinued and the initial dressing is removed. The patient is assisted out of bed with the knee immobilizer or cast still in place. In the beginning, walking may be done only with the assistance of health personnel or the use of a walker. The patient usually uses a four-point gait as it is a safe, slow gait and allows for partial weight bearing on the affected leg. (For a discussion of ambulation with a walker or crutches using a four-point gait, see Appendix C.) It makes no real difference which side of bed the patient gets out on, but the patient may find it easier to get out on the unaffected side and return on the affected side. By getting out on the unaffected side, the patient can use the overhead trapeze to support the upper body and slip the foot of the unaffected leg under the ankle of the operated leg to assist it to the floor. The same procedure can be done when getting back into bed on the other side. The patient should be encouraged to ambulate several times a day.

Sitting. Sitting is not usually a problem for the patient following a total knee replacement, but sometimes getting into and out of a chair, or on and off the toilet is a problem. A patient using crutches should be taught to back up until the back of the unaffected leg touches the seat, and then grip both crutches in the hand on the unaffected side. The patient should next bend at the waist and place the hand on the affected side onto the seat, and then move the affected leg forward and lower gradually onto the seat. To rise from the seat, the patient should reverse the procedure, pushing off against the seat with the hand on the affected side, and pulling the body upward with the other hand, which is holding both crutches.

Prevent Complications. Postoperative care for patient having a total knee replacement should recognize that most of these patients are not only weak from surgery but are elderly and have arthritis involving other joints in their body. In administering care and preventing complications, therefore, both orthopaedic and gerontological nursing concepts should be considered.

A total knee replacement is a major reconstructive procedure and therefore subject to the same local and systemic postoperative complications as other major surgical procedures. The likelihood of local complications is increased by the implantation of a large amount of foreign material on the joint surfaces and by the poor tissue tolerance to injury and stress common to these patients. The more commonly occuring complications are discussed here, along with prophylactic measures to prevent them.

Respiratory. Recumbency, the drugs used for pain relief that depress respiration, a decrease in the body's need for oxygen due to inactivity, and the resistance of the bed against the chest wall with bedrest are some of the factors that can lead to respiratory complications such as pneumonia and pulmonary embolism. Nursing measures should stress the prevention and quick observation of abnormalities. The patient is asked to do turning, coughing, and deep breathing exercises on a regular basis, and may also be asked to use an incentive respiratory device or other devices to facilitate respiratory hygiene. (For further discussion, see Chapter 2.)

Circulatory. Circulatory complications include such problems as dehydration from blood and fluid loss, circulatory overload, venous stasis, and orthostatic hypotension. The most common complications are probably pulmonary embolism and thrombophlebitis, because of the age of the patient, the immobility following surgery, and the use of a tourniquet during the operation.

Measures that help prevent these complications are bed exercises, especially the leg exercises discussed under mobility, and changing the position of the patient. The patient should be kept as active as possible with exercises and with ambulation, as tolerated. An elastic stocking, which extends from toes to groin, is usually applied to the unoperated leg before the patient returns to the unit, and to the operated leg after the initial compression dressing is removed. The stockings should be checked for any creases, wrinkles, or pressure areas, and should be removed for 1/2 hour twice a day. At that time inspect the legs and the feet, especially the heels, for any redness. Patients are frequently given anticoagulant medications, such as aspirin. (For further information, see Chap. 2.)

COMPARTMENTAL SYNDROME. One circulatory complication of special concern is known as compartmental syndrome, a condition in which progressive pressure within a confined space compromises the circulation and the function of tissues within that space. A compartment is enveloped by tough inelastic fascial tissue, and when swelling of the muscles occurs the fascia does not expand. In the lower leg that can occur in the anterior, lateral, superficial posterior, or deep posterior compartments. Such an ischemic condition can occur after unaccustomed strenuous activities, fractures (especially of the proximal tibia), or knee surgery. The onset of the symptoms can vary from as little as 2 hours to as much as 6 days after the trauma or surgery. If the pressure is not relieved within approximately 12 hours of the onset of the syndrome (i.e., from the onset of excessive intracompartmental pressure), irreversible nerve and tissue damage is likely to result, which can render the extremity useless because of contractures, paralysis, and loss of sensation, and in some cases, lead to amputation.

The orthopaedic nurse plays an absolutely vital role in detecting compartmental syndrome. In assessing for compartmental syndrome, remember the so-called "five P's." They are:

1. *Pain,* specifically progressive intense pain, a "red flag" is burning pain.
2. *Pain on passive motion,* as severe pain on passive motion of a distal

extremity is likely due to muscle ischemia. Two particularly significant signs are pain referred to the anterior compartment on passive plantar flexion of the toes, and acute calf pain on passive dorsiflexion of the foot (a positive Homan's sign).

3. *Paralysis,* as a decrease of the blood supply to the muscles leads to progressive paralysis of active voluntary function. To assess whether a motor nerve has been rendered ischemic, check the voluntary ability of the patient to flex and extend the toes.
4. *Paresthesias,* because as the sensory component of the peripheral nerve becomes progressively ischemic, the patient will notice numbness and tingling in the nerve that tranverses the involved compartment. The anterior compartment contains the deep peroneal branch, and its sensory area is the web space between the first and second toes. The posterior tibial nerve transverses the posterior compartment and supplies the plantar surface of the foot and toes.
5. *Pulselessness,* though it is the least important and least reliable of the signs. Peripheral pulses may remain intact in the presence of complete ischemia of a compartment. Capillary filling, pallor, and skin temperature are similarly of almost no help in making a timely diagnosis of compartmental syndrome. The physician may check the compartmental pressure by a variety of techniques.

Effective treatment depends upon early observation. Loosen any tight dressing or cast material that may be adding to the problem. There is disagreement about whether elevating the leg reduces swelling or further impedes circulation. If the intracompartmental pressure does not subside, the patient is returned to surgery for a fasciotomy. The incision in the fascia allows the muscles freedom to expand, relieving the pressure. The fascia is not sutured closed until all signs of swelling have subsided. The patient returns from surgery with an open lesion covered by dressings. Further surgery, and in some cases skin grafts, is needed to close the wound. To prevent disability the fasciotomy must be performed before the pressure damages the tissues.

Gastrointestinal. Immediately after surgery, the most common gastrointestinal problems are nausea and vomiting. They occur frequently, but are usually self-limiting. Parenteral fluids are usually administered for 36 to 48 hours following surgery, primarily to administer antibiotics, but those parenteral fluids can be used to help combat dehydration if nausea or vomiting persists.

Following a total knee replacement, the patient usually is able to tolerate fluids immediately after recovering from anesthesia, and a regular diet is tolerated quickly thereafter. Measures needed to assist with good nutrition should be stressed, with additional fluids and fibers in the diet as needed to combat the constipation that can occur as a result of immobility, medication for pain, and the patient's age. Note if any of the patient's oral medications, especially aspirin, are causing any digestive disorders. Other measures that help combat constipation are exercises and ambulation.

Genitourinary. Because of the anesthesia and the severe pain experienced immediately after surgery, some patients, especially elderly ones, may have difficulty voiding at first. Nursing measures should be directed toward relieving pain and relaxing the patient. It is helpful to get the patient in as near a normal voiding position as possible. A Foley catheter is usually not necessary following a total knee replacement.

In the first 24 to 48 hours following surgery some patients may have diuresis as a result of the intravenous fluids administered during surgery in order to maintain circulating volume. As a result, the patient may develop an electrolyte deficiency of sodium and potassium, and those electrolytes must be replaced.

Musculoskeletal. Nursing measures for patients following a total knee replacement should include measures to increase knee flexion. The goal is to have the patient regain as much active flexion in the knee as possible. Some patients will do the knee flexion exercises, but stop flexing when it begins to hurt. The patient should be encouraged to gradually increase the amount of flexion so that the ability to regain the desired 90 degrees of flexion will not be lost. If, despite such efforts, the patient is unable to regain 90 degrees of flexion, the physician may order a roentgenogram to determine if there is anything wrong with the prosthesis or the joint. If the roentgenogram is negative, the patient may be taken to surgery and the knee flexed 90 or more degrees under anesthesia. Immediately after that procedure, the patient will probably have pain and swelling in the knee, and the postoperative care for a patient following a total knee replacement should be reinstituted.

Integumentary. Following a total knee replacement, a patient is susceptible to pressure sores in the usual areas, and is particularly vulnerable on the heel because of the weight of the immobilized leg. Make sure that the patient's heel is "floating," i.e., that the leg is given sufficient support to reduce the weight on the heel. That can be done by keeping the leg elevated on a pillow, a folded bath blanket, or 2 to 3 inches of foam.

To enhance wound healing and avoid or control infection, physicians use wound catheters connected to continuous suction to remove blood from between layers of muscle and thus prevent any subcutaneous pooling of blood or fluid. Catheters are usually removed 36 to 48 hours postoperatively, after having removed an average of 300 to 500 cc of fluid. Because an effusion in the knee may occur, firm pressure on the bursae should be maintained. For that reason, a Jones pressure bandage, which extends from mid-calf to mid-thigh, hence well below and well above the bursae, may be applied (Roaf & Hodkinson, 1975, p. 353).

Once the catheters and initial dressing are removed, the incision line requires special care. It may just be left open to the air, but that is rare because the line is usually covered by a knee immobilizer. Most patients will have a small dressing over the suture line, with the incision cleaned daily with betadine, alcohol, or a similar solution. Observe the incision and the stab wounds left by the catheters for signs of infection, e.g., heat, swelling, redness, drainage, and hardness.

Problems, such as marginal wound necrosis, skin sloughs, hematoma formation, or wound dehiscence, can usually be detected easily. If the wound appears to be healing but the patient complains of unrelieved pain, there is a possibility of a local deep infection in the joint. This is a devastating complication that can lead to an arthrodesis or even an above-the-knee amputation. Such infections may not be observed for several weeks or even years postoperatively, and appear to be more frequent in patients with hinged prostheses.

Patient Teaching. Postoperative patient teaching for a patient having a total knee replacement emphasizes the exercise rehabilitation program. An exercise program is developed with the physical therapist before the patient leaves the hospital. The exercises will gradually increase in the level of exertion required, as weights will be added and the number of repetitions increased. It is a good idea for the patient to set aside specific times for exercise. One of the best times to exercise is after showering.

The patient should be encouraged to return to nearly full activity after discharge, as restrictions are few. The patient should avoid twisting the knee, walking on rough terrain, sitting for long periods, or bending the affected knee, and applying weight to it, such as in scrubbing floors or kneeling in prayer.

Immediately after discharge, the patient will need assistance at home because he or she is walking on crutches and tends to tire easily. Until the patient is quite ambulatory, elastic stockings have to be worn on both legs, and the patient usually needs help in getting them on, at least in the beginning. Crutch safety should be stressed. Pets or loose rugs could cause the patient to fall. It may be advisable to practice walking up and down stairs before discharge. No special chairs are necessary, but the patient should practice getting in and out of chairs. The patient should be encouraged to take showers instead of baths as he or she will find it too difficult and even painful to get into and out of a tub. The patient can use a stool in the shower for safety. If the patient has to step into a tub to shower, assistance may be needed initially to prevent falling. The patient, the family, and significant others must be taught the signs of infection discussed under potential complications of the integumentary system.

Evaluation and Reassessment

In evaluating the goal of alleviating pain in the knee, determine whether the individual is having any pain by verbal responses and by the patient's outward appearance, including facial grimacing during activities, the position assumed, and restlessness or sleeplessness. If pain still exists, determine the location, duration, and intensity of the pain, what aggravates and intensifies it, and what measures have been able to relieve it.

When evaluating care to increase mobility, determine the patient's compliance with the exercise routine and utilization of assistive devices such as trapeze, knee immobilizer, and walker or crutches. Evaluate the degree to which the patient has regained flexion in the affected knee, and the steadiness of the partial weight-bearing gait. Determine whether or not the patient, the family, and significant others have been able to follow the rehabilitation regime, how useful the discharge plan appears to be, and how well they understand what the patient can and cannot do. Regarding complications, look for the absence of contractures, pressure areas, decubiti, an elevated temperature, and other problem signs. If the goals have not been met, both the goals and the plan of care must be reassessed and the nursing process begun again.

Arthrodesis

An arthrodesis of the knee is a surgical fusion of the joint. It is indicated in infected knee joints or when the articular surfaces are so severely damaged that satisfactory function cannot be expected. Total knee arthroplasties are not effective for such patients. Arthrodesis also remains the salvage procedure of choice for failed reconstructive joint surgery. The goals of a knee arthrodesis are to decrease pain and allow mobility. However, the patient is left with a stiff knee. For that reason, the surgery is generally performed only if a single knee is involved.

A U incision is usually made on the anterior portion of the knee, and the articular cartilage is excised. A thin layer of subcortical bone is removed from the tibia and the femur to produce two flat surfaces, and the two bones are joined. (For an adult, 10 degrees of flexion and 10 degrees of external rotation of the tibia on the femur is considered the most useful position for walking or sitting.) Some form of fixation is then used to stabilize the joint for bone fusion. The preferred form of internal fixation is to use Steinmann pins with Charnley compression clamps (Fig. 7–20). If the compression method is not used, Knowles pins, a graft, or other methods of internal fixation are used because the position of the bone for fusion is difficult to maintain with external casting alone (Edmondson & Crenshaw, 1980, p. 1108).

□ NURSING PROCESS (Table 7–4)

Assessment

The nursing assessment is similar to that of a patient following a total knee replacement. However, the patient with an arthrodesis will have a long leg cast (groin to toe) and probably have external Charnley clamps laterally and medially that extend above and below the knee. (For further information, see pp. 375–376).

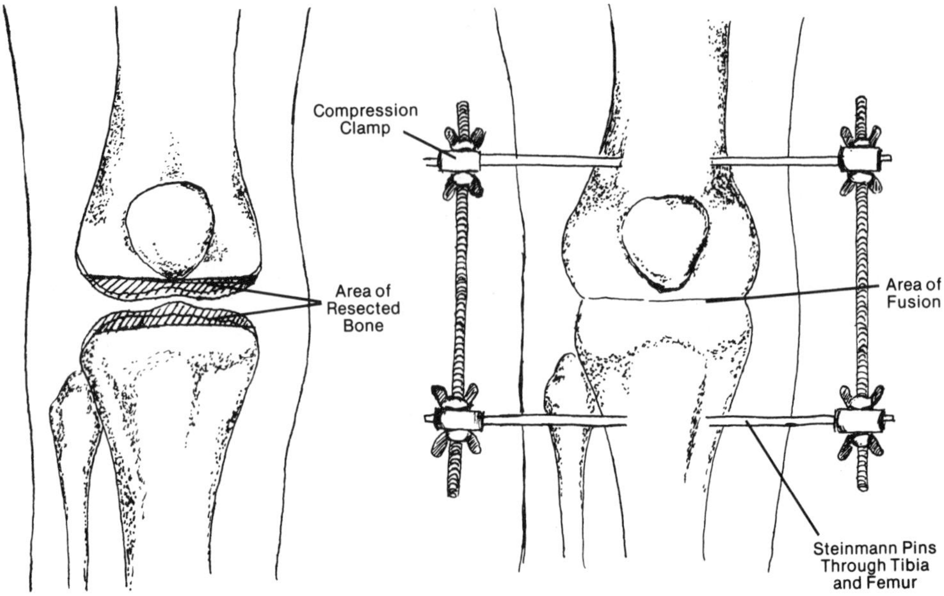

Figure 7–20. Arthrodesis of the knee. *(From Brantley, P., & Analla, M., 1980, p. 87. Courtesy of Howmedica.)*

Nursing Diagnoses and Goal Formulation

Nursing diagnoses and goal formulation are the same as those for a total knee replacement, except that the patient will ambulate with a stiff knee.

Planning and Intervention

Planning and implementation follow those for a patient with a total knee replacement, with a few modifications. For positioning, the leg is elevated and helped in extension with a cast that goes from the groin to the toes.

The exercises to be stressed are quadriceps and gluteal setting exercises, plantar and dorsiflexion exercises, and straight leg raises. There will be no flexion exercises. Initially, ambulation with crutches uses a three-point gait because no weight bearing is allowed on the affected leg for 2 to 4 weeks. After that time, the patient is usually allowed partial weight bearing, using a walking heel on the cast.

The patient needs some assistance in learning how to sit. The procedure for sitting follows that of a patient with a long leg cast or a knee immobilizer.

Patient Teaching. The patient, the family, and significant others need to understand that a period of immobilization after surgery is necessary for the knee joint to fuse. The patient will be in a cast, from the toes to the

TABLE 7–4. NURSING PROCESS FOR KNEE ARTHRODESIS WITH CHARNLEY CLAMPS AND A LONG LEG CAST

Assessment	Nursing Diagnosis	Goal Formulation	Planning and Intervention	Evaluation and Reassessment
1. Assess the location, duration, and severity of pain. Observe for verbal and nonverbal signs of pain. Check vital signs. Check cast for tightness. Assess the neurovascular status.	1. Alteration in comfort: pain in the knee related to bone and soft tissue trauma	1. Short-term goal: a decrease in pain through immobilization and prescribed medications. Long-term goal: free of pain.	1. Alleviate Pain Elevate the leg. Apply ice bags along both sides of the knee. Keep the leg immobilized. Utilize noninvasive nursing measures. Teach relaxation techniques. Administer prescribed medications.	1. Prescribed medication should relieve the pain and allow the patient to be fairly comfortable. However, the patient having an arthrodesis usually has more pain than one having an arthroplasty.
2. Check the position of the involved leg. Assess for correct body alignment. Check cast for tightness. Check position of clamps through the cast into the knee. Assess upper extremity strength for crutch walking.	2. Impaired physical mobility: a decrease in leg function related to lack of knee joint stability.	2. Short-term goal: an increase in mobility through controlled exercises and an assistive device. Long-term goal: gain optimal leg function with a fused knee.	2. Increase Mobility *Position* Keep the involved leg elevated. Place patient in a position of comfort (usually supine because of the clamps).	2. The patient should be able to keep body in correct alignment and keep the involved leg elevated.

(continued)

TABLE 7–4. *(Continued)*

Assessment	Nursing Diagnosis	Goal Formulation	Planning and Intervention	Evaluation and Reassessment
Assess the patient's ability to do required exercises.			*Exercises* Teach quadriceps and gluteal setting (5 minutes every hour while awake). Assist with straight leg exercises. Teach exercises to increase strength in upper extremities for crutch walking.	Even though there was preoperative instruction many patients need reinforcement of the importance of the exercises.
			Ambulation Demonstrate a nonweight-bearing crutch gait (for first 2–4 weeks) and partial weight bearing (after 4 weeks) with walking heel on the cast. Assist with getting out of bed. Demonstrate how to sit with a long leg cast.	The patient should be able to ambulate safely.
3. Assess for pain. Check for drainage or bleeding into the cast. Check vital signs. Assess neurovascular status. Reassess skin at the cast edges.	3. Potential for injury: Infection of soft tissue and bone related to surgical procedure.	3. Short- and long-term goals: free of any signs of infection.	3. Prevent Complications *Integumentary* Teach the signs and symptoms of infection. Encourage a well-balanced diet with plenty of fluids. Administer antibiotics as prescribed.	3. The patient should remain free of infection.

			Keep cast dry. Petal rough cast edges. *Potential Complications Due to Surgery and Immobility* (See Table 7–3, Total Knee Arthroplasty, and Chap. 3)	
4. Assess the patient's level of understanding of the rehabilitation process and future ability to walk. Assess level of adaptation to future restriction in knee flexion.	4. Potential knowledge deficit related to rehabilitation process and future mobility.	4. Short- and long-term goals: a decrease in anxiety through increased knowledge.	4. Patient Teaching Discuss the various stages in the long rehabilitation process. Discuss future ambulation. Discuss possible effect of fused knee on social, personal, and work life. Demonstrate cast care. Demonstrate methods of bathing and dressing with a long leg cast. Discuss ways to solve potential transportation problems. Include family and significant other in teaching plan. Allow time for open discussion of feelings.	4. The patient should have a decrease in anxiety and feel confident in going home. The patient should be in at least the beginning stages of adjusting to a change in body image. The patient should be able to verbalize an understanding of the long rehabilitation process.

groin with a window over the knee, for 2 to 3 weeks postsurgery, until the tendency for swelling subsides. The cast is then changed and left in place for another 10 to 12 weeks, or until substantial fusion has taken place. After the cast is removed, the leg is encased in a molded brace of suitable plaster or stiff leather with metal reinforcements, that extends from groin to ankle. This brace is worn by the patient night and day, until the fusion is solid, approximately 6 months.

Even after support is removed from the leg, the patient needs to take special care of the leg when walking. The affected leg should be carried through normally, rather than swung out to the side. When going up steps, the good leg should always lead, because the knee with the arthrodesis does not bend. The patient would otherwise have to tilt to the unaffected side and swing the affected leg out. When going down steps, similar considerations make it best for the patient to lead with the affected leg. When the surgical procedure entails the removal of a larger than normal amount of bone, the affected leg may be significantly shorter than the other leg; therefore an elevated shoe is needed on the affected side.

Evaluation and Reassessment

For a typical patient recovering from an arthrodesis of the knee, the evaluation is similar to that discussed for a patient following a total knee replacement. Special emphasis should be given to evaluating the patient's response to long-term immobilization of the knee in the initial stage, and the ability to walk in the later stage. Check that the patient understands the extent of ambulation possible, and how to care for the casted leg. Determine the patient's compliance with the exercise regime and understanding of the rehabilitation program.

Knee Disarticulation

A disarticulation of the knee or a knee bearing (KB) amputation is relatively rare. Physicians are reluctant to amputate the leg at that level because of difficulties in fitting a functional prostheses to half a joint. With advances in prosthetic devices those difficulties are being reduced, and knee disarticulations may in the future replace some above-knee amputation (Edmondson & Crenshaw, 1980, p. 836). Nursing care is similar to the care of a patient with an above-knee amputation (see pp. 330–334).

THE LOWER LEG

Trauma

FRACTURES OF THE TIBIA AND FIBULA

Trauma to the shin area is often sufficient to simultaneously fracture both bones of the lower leg. A direct blow to the anterior lower leg may cause a transverse fracture through the proximal, midshaft, or distal portions of the tibia and the fibula. The fractures are frequently comminuted, but torsional injuries to the leg occur causing a spiral or long oblique fracture.

Because the fibula is a nonweight-bearing bone, fractures of the fibula alone are rare. A fracture of the fibula alone usually remains in good alignment and requires no reduction, but the leg is immobilized in a cast.

The tibia is exposed to frequent injury, and because one-third of its surface is just below the skin, open fractures are more common in the tibia than in any other major bone. The blood supply of the tibia is also relatively vulnerable because its blood vessels are not enclosed in heavy muscles.

There are three methods for repairing fractures of the tibia: (1) closed reduction and cast, (2) internal fixation, and (3) use of an external fixation device. The choice of method depends primarily on the type and the location of the fracture.

Closed Reduction with Cast

Tibial fractures may be repaired using a closed method of reduction followed by the application of a leg cast in two ways. One is to use a long leg cast until the bone calcifies, i.e., for approximately 8 to 10 weeks. The second method is to apply a long leg cast for 2 to 4 weeks, and then change to a below-knee patellar-tendon-bearing cast until calcification is complete. In instances of delayed union, calcification may take 4 months or longer.

□ NURSING PROCESS (Table 7–5)

Assessment

Assessment of a patient following the application of a long leg cast for a fracture of the tibia includes a general assessment of the patient postanesthesia, as well as an assessment of the affected extremity. Listen to the patient's complaints, as trauma or surgery affecting an extremity produces swelling from bleeding and edema. Check for unrelieved pain and increasing pain or swelling. Ask the patient to localize the exact site of the pain. Check for tingling, coldness, numbness, and the patient's ability to move

TABLE 7–5. NURSING PROCESS FOR FRACTURED TIBIA TREATED BY CLOSED REDUCTION AND LONG LEG CAST

Assessment	Nursing Diagnosis	Goal Formulation	Planning and Intervention	Evaluation and Reassessment
1. Assess the location, and severity of pain. Observe for verbal and nonverbal signs of pain. Check vital signs. Check for tightness of cast. Assess neurovascular status.	1. Alteration in comfort: pain in the leg related to bone and soft tissue trauma.	1. Short-term goal: a decrease in pain through immobilization. Long-term goal: free of pain.	1. Alleviate Pain Elevate the leg on pillows or with overhead sling. Apply ice at fracture site. Utilize positioning and other noninvasive nursing measures. Teach relaxation techniques. Administer prescribed medications as indicated.	1. During the first 3–7 days after injury there is usually severe to moderate pain that requires medication. The pain is usually worse at night and when the foot is lowered for ambulation.
2. Check position of leg. Check for correct body alignment. Assess strength in upper extremities. Assess the patient's ability to do exercises. Assess ability to walk safely with crutches.	2. Impaired physical mobility: a decrease in leg function related to lack of bone stability.	2. Short-term goal: an increase in mobility through immobilization and crutches. Long-term goal: regain full function in the leg.	2. Increase Mobility *Position* Keep the leg elevated when lying or sitting. Keep patient supine or on uninvolved side using pillows to support casted leg. Teach patient how to use trapeze. *Exercises* Teach isometric leg exercises. Teach straight leg raises. Demonstrate exercises to increase upper extremity strength. *Ambulation* Assist the patient into chair or wheelchair. Demonstrate no weight-bearing crutch gait (three-point).	2. In the beginning assistance is usually needed for the patient to turn or change position. The patient should maintain strength and mobility, and be aple to ambulate safely with crutches.
3. Assess the neurovascular status. Check for any signs of swelling.	3. Potential for injury: neurovascular deficit related to soft tissue swelling and cast.	3. Short- and long-term goals: no circulation problems.	3. Prevent Complications *Circulatory* Keep the leg elevated when lying or sitting.	3. The patient should remain free of any neurovascular deficit.

Check for tightness of cast.			Apply ice at fracture site. Teach muscle setting exercises. Notify physician of any abnormal neurovascular response.	
Assess skin at the cast edges. Assess for potential pressure over bony prominences. Check for signs of edema.	Potential for injury: a break in skin integrity related to pressure areas or rough cast edges.	Short- and long-term goals: free of any skin problems.	*Integumentary* Petal rough cast edges. Keep cast off hard surfaces. Keep pressure off heel or any bony prominence. Utilize nursing measures to prevent or reduce edema. *Potential Complications Due to Knee Surgery* (See Table 7–3, Total Knee Arthroplasty) *Potential Complications Due to Immobility* (See Chap. 3 and Table 6–2)	The patient should be free of any break in skin integrity.
4. Assess for the patient's level of understanding about the rehabilitation process and self care.	4. Potential knowledge deficit related to rehabilitation process and self-care.	4. Short- and long-term goals: a decrease in anxiety through increased knowledge.	4. Patient Teaching Discuss the various steps in the rehabilitation process. Discuss the rationale for exercising and elevating the involved leg when sitting or lying. Discuss cast care. Demonstrate how to petal the cast. Demonstrate methods of bathing that are safe and keep the cast dry. Demonstrate methods of dressing with a long leg cast on. Discuss methods of sleeping (alone or with a partner). Include family or significant other in teaching plan.	4. The patient should feel confident in doing activities of daily living safely. The patient should demonstrate, through verbal responses, an understanding of the rehabilitation process and the role of exercise.

the toes. Note any discoloration of the toes; the color should be pink. Paleness and cold toes suggest an arterial obstruction, whereas blueness suggests a venous obstruction. Pinch the nail beds to assess capillary filling in the involved leg; a rapid return of color should appear when the pressure is released (Chap. 2). As the patient is in a long leg cast, only the femoral pulse is usually obtainable, and that is nondiagnostic as it is proximal to the injury. Always compare the uninjured leg with the injured leg.

The assessment of the cast depends on the type of material used for casting. Here the emphasis is on the assessment of a patient with a long leg cast made of plaster of Paris. (For more information on other types of casts, e.g., fabric tapes impregnated with resins, see Appendix B.) Observe the color of a freshly applied cast. A white shiny cast is one that is dry, whereas a moist cast has a dull gray look and a dull sound when tapped. Assess the complete cast, turning the patient to the unaffected side to check the back. At the edges of the cast, check for tightness or any skin irritation. At the distal end of the cast, check to make sure that the little toe is able to move freely. The linen should be off the cast, exposing it to the air to dry; that also serves to keep the linen dry. The complete leg is elevated by raising the foot of the bed, or by putting the leg in slings or on pillows. After several days, a postoperative assessment includes smelling both ends of the cast for signs of an infection under the cast.

Nursing Diagnosis and Goal Formulation

The nursing diagnoses for a typical patient with a fractured tibia and a long leg cast are (1) alterations in comfort related to pain in and below the joint from trauma to bone and soft tissue or surgery, (2) alterations in mobility related to lack of bone stability, (3) alterations in psychological well-being related to anxiety and knowledge deficit about loss of mobility, and (4) potential complications related to trauma and immobilization in a cast.

Short-term goals are to have the patient experience (1) a decrease in pain through nursing measures, cast immobilization, and prescribed medications, (2) an increase in mobility by positioning, exercise, and controlled ambulation, (3) a decrease in anxiety through increased knowledge about the purpose and function of the cast and the process of rehabilitation, and (4) an absence of complications. Long-term goals are to have the patient free of pain and able to walk without an assistive device.

Planning and Intervention

Alleviate Pain. Pain following a fractured tibia is usually severe for 3 to 7 days, but that varies depending on the type of fracture and the individual. Elevating the affected leg helps to reduce pain, but make sure that the patient is able to relax the leg in that position. Apply ice bags along the fracture site and refill as needed. Offer analgesics on schedule. Take the time to sit with the patient, the patient's family, and significant others for therapeutic communication.

Increase Mobility

Position. The patient with a fractured tibia and a long leg cast needs to be in bed with the involved leg elevated until the cast is dry, usually 24 hours but sometimes longer, depending on the cast. Make sure that there is no pressure on the soft tissue at the proximal end of the cast or on the patient's low back area.

Turning. Most patients are lying supine when they return to the unit, and would probably prefer to stay that way because they fear that moving will cause them pain. They must turn to their side, however, to promote homeostasis, to relieve pressure on the coccyx, and to allow the posterior side of the cast to dry. The procedure for helping a patient turn is the same as the one discussed for a patient following a fractured hip (see pp. 257–258). In most cases the patient is able to use the overhead trapeze and side rails to move all of the body except the affected leg. In the beginning, someone will need to lift and support the leg during the turn and then reposition the leg on pillows once the turn is completed. The patient may turn to either side, but would probably prefer the unaffected side.

Exercises. Patients in a long leg cast need exercise if they are to maintain strength and prevent the complications of immobility. General body exercises and self-care (as discussed for a patient following a fractured hip, pp. 258–260) as well as more specific exercises for the leg are involved. Joints above and below the cast need to be exercised to prevent stiffness. Encourage flexion and extension movements of the toes and as much range of motion of the hip as possible.

Muscle setting or isometric exercises are taught using the uninvolved leg so they can be done on the fractured leg while it is in the cast. Check with the physician on the specific exercises, when to start the exercises, and how much exercising should be done. The most frequently used exercises are quadriceps setting and straight leg raises. (For a discussion of these and of other possible exercises, see the care of a patient following a total knee replacement, p. 384.)

Ambulation. After the cast is dry, the patient is usually allowed up in a chair or a wheelchair. Discuss every step in the procedure with the patient. Alert the patient to the likelihood of increased pain when the affected leg is lowered, explain that the patient should arise slowly to prevent orthostatic hypotension, and tell the patient whether weight bearing is allowed. Initially, two nurses are needed to get the patient out of bed following the procedure discussed on p. 260 for pivoting a patient from a bed into a chair. One nurse is needed to support the casted leg and ease it to the floor while the second assists the patient. Once the patient is comfortably positioned in the chair, the casted leg is elevated.

If the patient is to be seated in a wheelchair, check that the wheelchair is locked and has a foot extension that can be elevated before beginning the procedure. Use the foot extension to elevate the leg, placing a pillow between the leg and the foot extension so that the casted leg will be more comfortable. The casted leg should be secured to the foot extension using a strap with a buckle, a towel and safety pins, or (preferably) wide adhesive tape. The tape holds the cast securely without damaging it, is easily removed, and can be used at home. A thin patient with a heavy long leg cast may be able to tip the wheelchair forward if he or she leans toward the foot. Discuss the problem with the patient, and consider adding sandbags to the back of the wheelchair. Because the foot extension does not elevate the leg relative to the body to the same degree as when the patient was in bed, the patient may experience some pain and swelling.

When patients are allowed to ambulate without weight bearing, they will use crutches with a three-point gait (Appendix C). Exercises to prepare a patient's upper extremities for crutch walking should be started as soon as the patient is physically able (see p. 259), but the patient may still tire easily at first. Patients who are allowed weight bearing will have a long leg cast with a walking heel. These patients may be advised to wear an elevated shoe on the unaffected side to equalize leg lengths so that they can walk with a more normal gait. (For further information on long leg casts, walking heels, crutch measurement, and ambulation with crutches, see Appendices B and C.)

Prevent Complications. Nursing measures to prevent the complications of bedrest are discussed in Chapter 3, and nursing measures to prevent complications that apply specifically to knee surgery on pp. 386–390. Only nursing concerns specific to a patient with a fractured tibia and a long leg cast are covered here.

Circulatory. Patients with fractures of the proximal tibia and those in long leg casts may develop compartmental syndrome. (see pp. 387–388).

Gastrointestinal/Genitourinary. Some patients have problems with the first voiding after surgery and most patients find it difficult to use a bedpan with their leg elevated in a long leg cast. The casted leg should remain elevated, however, to prevent increased blood flow and pain. If the cast is extra long, take care in removing the bedpan and urinal after use to prevent soilage. Because using the bedpan is awkward, some patients are reluctant to eat or drink. Note how much the patient is eating and drinking and encourage good nutrition with adequate fluid intake. Get the patient up to a bedside commode or to the bathroom as soon as possible.

Integumentary. Attention should be given to the positioning and turning of a patient with a long leg cast. The bed is normally equipped with an overhead trapeze, and the patient should be encouraged to lift and change positions frequently. Use pillows under the casted leg to prevent flat spots, especially on the heel and the posterior portion of the cast. Indentations in the cast can also occur when a flat hand is not used to handle a wet cast. Assess for pressure behind the knee in the popliteal area, at the proximal end of the fibula (on the lateral side of the leg where the peroneal nerve transverses), at the Achilles tendon, and on the heel, and reposition the patient as indicated.

Patient Teaching. Some patients find that lying supine is the most comfortable position for their leg. Others find it difficult to sleep at night lying supine. Sleepless patients tend to be a bother to other patients, and to worry excessively about their injury or other problems. The pain in the leg may also appear to become worse at night. Try therapeutic communication, back rubs, smoothing of the bedding, fluffing and repositioning pillows, and warm milk. Giving a second sedative or another pain medication should be done only after other methods fail. Patients who have difficulty sleeping at night frequently want to sleep late in the morning. They must understand that difficulties in sleeping should not be allowed to interfere with their rehabilitation program.

Patients with a fractured tibia and a long leg cast need emotional support from the staff, the family, and significant others. They may remember seeing people on the street with a long leg cast, and wonder why they are still in the hospital. Patients need to understand the location of the fracture, how it was reduced, why the exercises are necessary, and the need for their continued hospitalization.

Before discharge, the patient, the family, and significant others need to know about cast care, personal hygiene with a long leg cast, and ambulatory activities (Appendices B and C). If the hospital has a movie on cast care, make sure these patients have an opportunity to see it. Personal hygiene can present difficulties for the patient. Bathroom facilities should be convenient and allow the patient room to sit on the stool with the casted leg extended. Showering twice a week should be encouraged. Tub baths are difficult, inconvenient, and risk getting the cast wet, although patients often feel that sponge baths are inadequate. To protect the cast in the shower, it can be enclosed in a large plastic bag that is taped to the skin at the top (or commercial plastic cast cover). Initially, the patient needs assistance in getting the bag over the cast, and in getting into and out of the shower.

At home, it is essential that the patient realize the importance of elevating the leg when sitting, and continuing with the exercise regime. In bed, if the casted leg is elevated on pillows, a chair may be placed next to the bed to prevent the casted leg from falling to the floor. Patients who share their bed with another should realize that the cast can scratch and irritate, and is best placed on the side away from their bed partner. Patients in a long leg cast need not abstain from sexual activities, though they may have to adjust their positioning and wrap the casted leg with a sheet to prevent abrasions.

Evaluation and Reassessment

For a typical patient recovering from a closed reduction of a fractured tibia with a long leg cast applied, the evaluation is essentially the same as described for a patient who has had a total knee arthroplasty. Special emphasis should be given to evaluating the patient's compliance with the exercise regime and understanding of the care of the affected leg.

Internal Fixation

A second method of treatment for fractures of the shaft of the tibia is internal fixation. With closed internal fixation an intramedullary nail (e.g., a Lottes nail [Fig. 7–21], a Küntscher nail, or an AO slotted nail) is driven down the medullary canal of the tibia. The patient is usually placed in a long leg cast, with weight bearing, for 4 to 6 weeks. Three complications can commonly occur: (1) infection, (2) nonunion of the fracture site, and (3) migration of the nail. The nursing care is similar to that for a patient with a fractured tibia who has a long leg cast (see pp. 397–404).

In an open internal fixation, plates and screws (Fig. 7–22) are used, and the leg is usually placed in a long leg cast for 4 to 6 weeks with partial or full weight bearing. Complications following this procedure include infection, nonunion, breakage of the plate or screws, and loss of fixation. The nursing care is similar to that for a patient with a fractured tibia who has a long leg cast (see pp. 397–404).

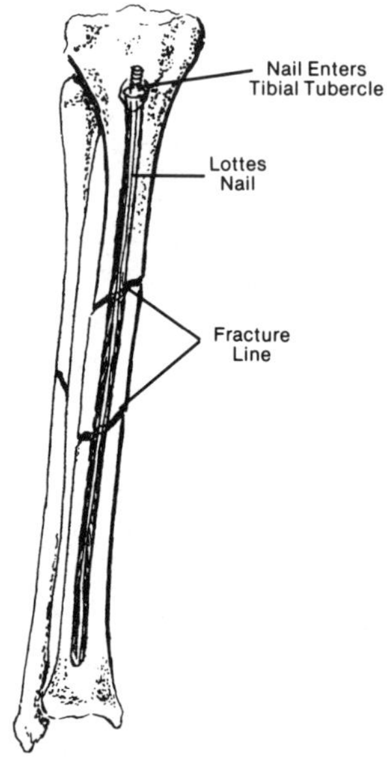

Figure 7–21. Open reduction and intramedullary fixation, fractured tibia: Lottes nail. *(From Brantley, P., & Analla, M., 1980, p. 108. Courtesy of Howmedica.)*

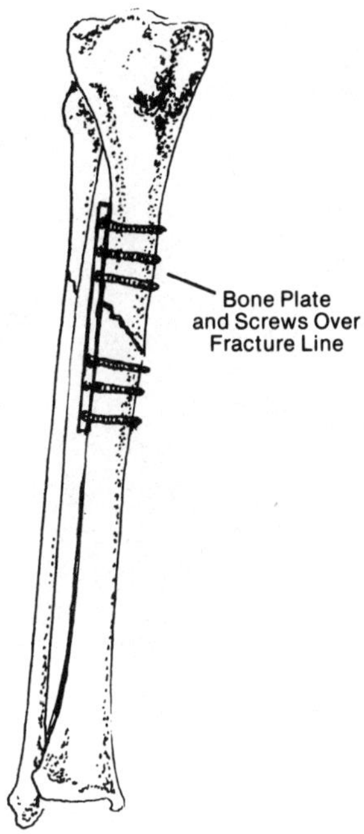

Figure 7–22. Open reduction and internal fixation fractured tibia: plate and screws. *(From Brantley, P., & Analla, M., 1980, p. 109. Courtesy of Howmedica.)*

External Fixation

External Fixation with Device

External fixation can be used for many fractures, and is widely used for open fractures of the tibia and the fibula where there is also marked soft tissue damage and skin loss. Normally, two or more heavy Steinmann pins are inserted proximal to the fracture and two distal to the fracture, and they are held in place by external devices such as Hoffman or Wagner devices (Fig. 7–23). With the use of a single or double frame mounting and universal joint clamps, segmental fracture fragments can be aligned. In open fractures needing that type of repair, instability, malalignment, and soft tissue complications with skin necrosis and deep infection are common. In many instances these patients may return many times for skin grafts.

□ NURSING PROCESS (Table 7–6)

Assessment

Patients treated with an external fixation device often have multiple injuries to other systems of the body. Assess for signs of shock and look for

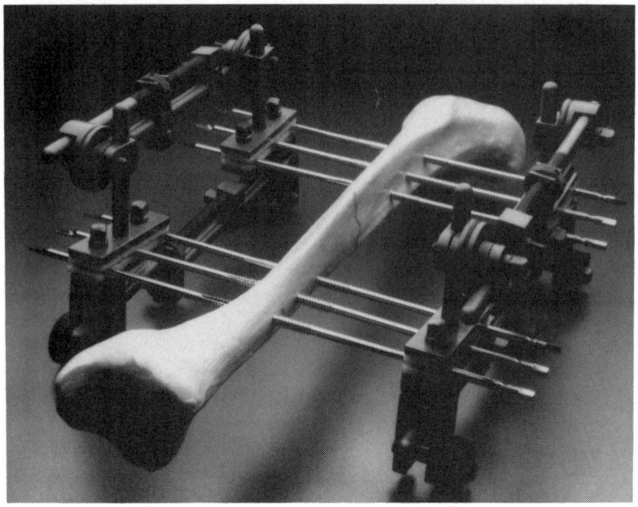

Figure 7–23. Zimmer Hoffmann-type external fixation system. *(Courtesy of Zimmer, Inc.)*

other injuries, especially internal or head injuries, which may have occurred at the time of the accident. A neurovascular assessment is done to determine skin color, joint motion, and complaints of numbness, coldness, or swelling of the leg (Chap. 2). Check for a pulse in the affected leg, starting at the most distal pulse. Assess any open skin area for obvious bleeding. Observe the emotional reactions of the patient, the family, and significant others to the open fracture site and the external fixation device. The injured leg and the apparatus can be disturbing to many.

Nursing Diagnosis and Goal Formulation

Nursing diagnoses for a typical patient with a fractured tibia and an external fixation device are (1) alterations in comfort related to pain in thelower leg from trauma to the bone and soft tissue, (2) alterations in mobility related to lack of bone stability, (3) alterations in psychological well-being related to anxiety and knowledge deficit from loss of mobility, and (4) potential complications related to trauma and an open wound.

Short-term goals are to have the patient experience (1) a decrease in pain through nursing measures and prescribed medications, (2) an increase in mobility through exercise, positioning, and the use of immobilizing devices, (3) a decreased anxiety through increased knowledge about the injury and the process of rehabilitation, and (4) an absence of complications. Long-term goals are to have the patient free of pain and able to walk without an assistive device.

TABLE 7–6. NURSING PROCESS FOR FRACTURED TIBIA TREATED WITH AN EXTERNAL FIXATION DEVICE

Assessment	Nursing Diagnosis	Goal Formulation	Planning and Intervention	Evaluation and Reassessment
1. Assess the location, duration and severity of pain. Assess neurovascular status. Check the position of the affected leg.	1. Alteration in comfort: pain in leg related to bone and soft tissue trauma.	1. Short-term goal: a decrease in pain through immobilization and prescribed medication. Long-term goal: free of pain.	1. Alleviate Pain Elevate the extremity. Make sure the leg is safely and securely positioned. Utilize therapeutic communication. Discuss treatment method. Teach relaxation techniques. Administer prescribed pain medications as indicated.	1. Medications and nursing intervention should relieve moderate to severe pain.
2. Check the position of the affected leg. Assess the neurovascular status of the affected leg. Assess the patient's ability to do exercises. Assess the patient's upper extremity strength. Assess the stability of the external fixation device.	2. Impaired physical mobility: decreased leg function related to lack of bone stability.	2. Short-term goal: an increase in mobility through the use of an external fixation device and crutches. Long-term goal: regain full mobility.	2. Increase Mobility *Position* Keep the leg elevated by securing ropes to the external fixation device and attaching them to the overhead frame. Reposition the leg by taking hold of the device on each side. Teach the patient how to use the trapeze to change position. Keep the patient supine.	2. The patient should keep the leg elevated until there is no longer concern about swelling.

(continued)

TABLE 7–6. NURSING PROCESS FOR FRACTURED TIBIA TREATED WITH AN EXTERNAL FIXATION DEVICE *(Continued)*

Assessment	Nursing Diagnosis	Goal Formulation	Planning and Intervention	Evaluation and Reassessment
			Exercises Teach quadriceps and gluteal setting exercises, plantar and dorsiflexion exercises and leg raises for the uninvolved leg. Teach range-of-motion exercises for both ankles. Start leg exercises on involved leg when condition allows. Teach exercises to increase strength in the upper extremities. *Ambulation* Demonstrate a nonweight-bearing gait for crutch walking.	The patient should be able to do the exercises on the uninvolved leg. The patient should be able to do crutch walking safely but may need a lot of encouragement because of the external device.
3. Assess for any drainage or odor from wound. Assess for skin tautness around the pins. Assess for pain. Check vital signs.	3. Potential for injury: infection related to an open wound and internal pins.	3. Short- and long-term goals: free of any signs of infection.	3. Prevent Complications *Integumentary* Do wound irrigations for the open contaminated wound. Do pin site care. Encourage a well-balanced diet with plenty of fluids. Administer prescribed antibiotics.	3. The patient should be free of any signs of infection.

			Potential Complications Due to Immobility and Trauma (See Table 7–3 and Chap. 3)	
4. Assess the patient's level of understanding about the method of treatment and the rehabilitation process. Check whether a social worker is needed.	4. Potential knowledge deficit related to treatment method and rehabilitation process.	4. Short- and long-term goals: a decrease in anxiety through increased knowledge.	4. Patient Teaching Allow time for open discussion about the injury, the external fixation device, and the long rehabilitation process. Teach the patient how to lift and move the leg utilizing the external fixation device. Teach the patient how to do pin care. Demonstrate methods of bathing and dressing with an external fixation device on the leg. Include family and significant other in the teaching plan. Teach the signs and symptoms of infection. Utilize a social worker to help with problems of hospital costs.	4. The patient should be able to discuss the injury and have a knowledge of the treatment method. The patient should be able to verbalize an understanding of the long rehabilitation process. The patient, family, and significant other should feel confident in moving the leg and doing pin care.

Planning and Intervention

Alleviate Pain. The patient requiring an external fixation for the treatment of a fracture is likely to have multiple problems, hence the complaints of discomfort may not be all bone related. Elevate the extremity to help prevent swelling and pain, and make sure the leg is safely and securely positioned. With an open lesion, the patient is likely to have had the external fixation device applied with very little explanation. Take time to have therapeutic communication with the patient, the family, and significant others. It promotes relaxation and can be very effective in reducing pain.

Increase Mobility

Position. Immediately after surgery the leg with the external fixation device is elevated. The general rule is that the leg should be higher than the heart; therefore, the patient may be asked not to have the head of the bed elevated more than a few degrees. The leg can be elevated using pillows, balanced suspension traction, or by securing ropes to the fixation device. Elevation is usually required until there is no longer concern about swelling.

The best way to reposition the affected leg is to lift it by taking hold of the device, and the patient, the family, and significant others need to know how to lift the leg using the device. The patient should be using the overhead trapeze to assist with body position changes.

Exercises. Active and passive range-of-motion exercises for all unaffected extremities should be stressed. For the affected leg, quadriceps and gluteal setting exercises, plantar and dorsiflexion exercises, leg raises, and range-of-motion exercises for the ankle should be done, though they may not be allowed immediately. Teach the patient these exercises using the unaffected leg.

Ambulation. Crutch walking without weight bearing while the external device is attached to the leg is not really difficult, but requires a psychological adjustment on the part of the patient. Reassure patients that they will succeed with time and practice. (For further discussion on crutch walking, see Appendix C.)

Prevent Complications. General nursing measures to prevent complications of immobility are discussed in Chapter 3. Only concerns specific to patients with an external fixation device are dealt with here.

Integumentary. Preventing infection of bone and soft tissue is a real concern. The patient is receiving antibiotics but special care should be given to the open wound, the specific method of treatment, and the amount of soft tissue damage.

For an open contaminated wound many physicians prescribe wound irrigation, a sterile procedure. Care should be taken to keep the upper leg and trunk dry, and disposable pads can be a great help. Care is also needed to prevent infection at the pin sites, and physicians have their own preferences for pin care. One method, for patients without an open lesion, is to regularly cleanse around the pins with an antiseptic solution and to apply a small amount of antibacterial ointment such as Neosporin.

Sometimes the skin around the pin sites is taut and causes discomfort. If no nursing measure relieves it, the physician may treat the problem by incising the skin around the pin.

Patient Teaching. Emotional support is needed to help the patient accept what has happened, the method of treatment, and the likelihood of a long hospital stay. Educate the patient about the location and type of fracture and the method of repair. The patient should realize that the external fixation device stabilizes the fracture, allowing time for the bone and the soft tissue to heal, and enabling the leg to be moved freely without injury. Allow time for an open discussion of the prognosis with the physician and the patient. A social worker may be of help if the patient is concerned about the costs of hospitalization and problems in returning to work.

Patients without open lesions may go home with the external fixation device; therefore, the patient, the family, or significant others will need to be instructed on how to do pin site care and how to cleanse the skin under the device. The patient must also know how to detect a possible infection, i.e., to look for redness, pain, heat, tenderness, hardness, or drainage. An easy plan for the patient is to write out the steps of care and the signs and symptoms of infection for the patient to take home and use as a reference.

Hygiene and dressing at home are similar to those of a patient with a cast (Appendix B). If slacks are desired, the side seams can be split and velcro straps attached to partially close the openings.

Evaluation and Reassessment

For a typical patient recovering from an open fracture of the tibia with soft tissue damage and an external fixation device, the evaluation is essentially the same as that described for a patient who has had a total knee replacement. Be sure to check the patient's compliance with the exercises and rehabilitation regimes. Special emphasis must be given to determine the patient's responses to the injury and the method of treatment. Continue to evaluate the responses of the patient, the family, and significant others to long-term immobilization of the involved leg (usually months and even longer with skin grafts) and the possibility of future hospitalization and surgery, bearing in mind the stages of adjustment discussed in Chapter 1. Regarding complications, look for the absence of pressure areas and decubiti, an elevated temperature, increasing pain, and other problem signs.

External Fixation with Plaster

Another external fixation technique has been used in the treatment of closed tibial shaft fractures, and in open fractures without extensive soft tissue damage or skin loss. Two pins are inserted in the tibia proximal and one distal to the fracture, and the pins are then incorporated in a plaster cast.

The initial cast is worn for 3 to 6 weeks. In stable transverse fractures with good opposition, the pins can be removed after 3 to 4 weeks, and in comminuted and oblique fractures, after approximately 6 weeks. A long leg walking cast is then applied, and weight bearing on crutches is allowed. Eight to ten weeks after surgery, the cast may be changed to a below-knee patellar tendon bearing cast until calcification is complete. The nursing care is similar to that for a patient with a fractured tibia and a long leg cast (see pp. 397–404 and Appendix B).

AMPUTATIONS

Amputations of the Lower Leg

Amputations of the lower leg may be the result of a number of disorders, including infections, neoplasms, (see Chap. 4), and traumatic injuries. Most, however, are the result of peripheral arterial disease.

The most common type of amputation today is the below-knee (BK) amputation, where the remaining tibia is 12.5 to 17.5 cm long, depending on the patient's height. (Usually 2.5 cm of bone length remains for each 30 cm of body height). Most physicians agree that the ideal level for a prosthetic fitting is about 15 cm.

The procedure is similar to the open or closed method of above-knee amputation discussed on pp. 326–327 and 330, except that there are two bones involved. The myoplasty attaches the muscles to the tibia because it is the weight-bearing bone. The fibula is usually severed proximal to where the tibia is severed so that the prosthesis will fit better.

Following a closed method of amputation the physician may use a compression dressing with ace bandages (Fig. 7–24). Although the patient may not wear a prosthesis, most physicians will have an immediate postsurgical prosthetic fitting applied that will extend from the stump to mid-thigh. The straps will go along the sides of the cast portion of the fitting and attach to the strap that goes around the patient's waist. No shoulder strap is necessary.

□ NURSING PROCESS (Table 7–7)

Assessment

The assessment of a patient following a BK amputation is similar to that for a patient with an above-knee amputation (see p. 332). If the patient has had a closed amputation because of a peripheral vascular disease, he or she would have had preoperative teaching. However, there is frequently little time to prepare patients with traumatic injuries. In such instances, assess the nature of the emotional reactions. Be alert to the possibility that there may be other physical injuries.

Nursing Diagnosis and Goal Formulation

The typical postsurgical nursing diagnoses for a patient with a BK amputation are (1) alterations in comfort related to pain at the surgical site from trauma to the bone and the soft tissue, (2) alterations in mobility related to loss of the lower leg and the application of an immediate postsurgical fitting, (3) alterations in psychological well-being related to anxiety and knowledge deficit about a change in body image and concerns about future ability to function, and (4) potential complications related to surgery and prosthesis.

Short-term goals are to have the patient experience (1) a decrease in the level of pain through repositioning, therapeutic communication, and prescribed medications, (2) an increase in mobility through bed exercises and early ambulation, (3) a decrease in anxiety by increased knowledge through open discussions, and (4) an absence of complications. Long-term goals are (1) to have the patient free of physical and emotional complications, (2) to maintain the full functional capabilities of the rest of the body, and (3) to restore as much leg function as possible by the use of a prosthesis.

Planning and Intervention

Alleviate Pain. Standard nursing measures for pain relief are utilized for the care of patients following a BK amputation (see pp. 303, 306, and 331). With the use of a rigid dressing, strong opiates are often unnecessary.

Increase Mobility. Immediately after surgery the patient's affected leg will be elevated for the first 24 hours. The patient should be encouraged to use the trapeze to change position in bed, and, initially with assistance, can turn to either side. When turning, the patient will probably prefer turning to the unaffected side, with pillows between the legs for comfort.

The patient should be encouraged to do quadriceps and gluteal setting exercises and to do leg raises with the affected extremity as soon as possible. Early ambulation with limited weight bearing on the prosthetic fitting is beneficial psychologically as it helps to lessen emotional trauma from the loss of the limb. Most patients are up within 48 hours after surgery with assistance. A patient with a BK amputation and an immediate postsurgical dressing will walk like a patient with an above-knee amputation, because the cast covers the knee, limiting mobility. Once the cast is removed and the prosthesis is applied, the patient regains the use of the knee and the prosthesis will supply a hinge joint for the ankle. (For further discussion on ambulating a patient with an immediate postsurgical fitting, see pp. 302, 327, and 330.)

Begin by explaining to the patient that the purpose of the procedure is to help reduce swelling and shape the stump for a prosthesis. Explain the procedure to the patient as you are doing the bandaging, as the patient must learn to do it by himself or herself.

Sew two 4-inch elastic bandages together end-to-end and roll them into one long bandage, or use a special elastic bandage designed for stump wrapping. Make figure 8 turns with the bandage, wrapping the stump around the upper portion of the patient's leg downward under the stump, and back to the upper portion. Keep the bandage roll away from the stump and avoid going straight around the stump, as that is apt to interfere with circulation. There should be more pressure at the end of the stump than at the top to insure proper venous blood return, but firm pressure should be used throughout.

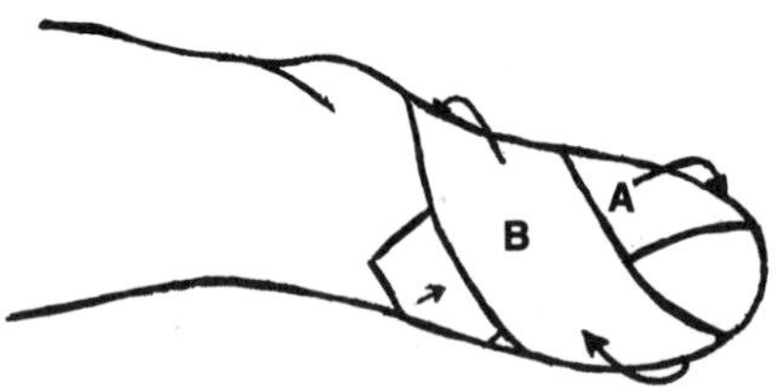

To begin, place the patient in semi-Fowler's position or have the patient sit on the side of the bed. With one hand, hold the end of the bandage on the medial side of the leg, just below the knee. With the other hand, bring the bandage across the front and downward to the distal end of the stump *(A)*. Bring the bandage across the back to the medial side, and then bring it up and across the front of the patient's leg *(B)*.

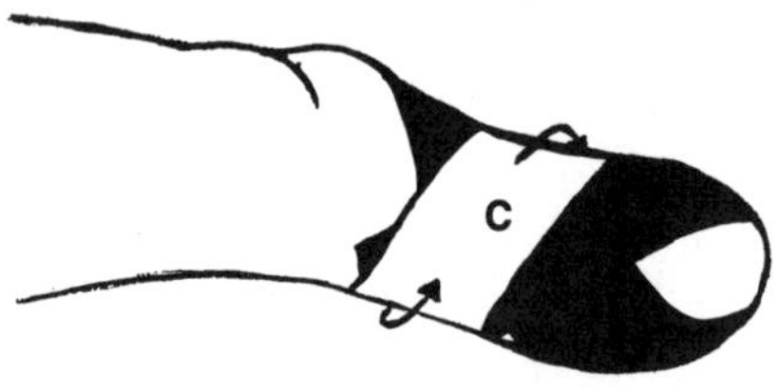

Bring the bandage across the back to the medial side and then bring it down and across the front of the stump *(C)* to anchor turns *(A)* and *(B)*. That completes the first figure 8 and it will no longer be necessary to hold the end of the bandage.

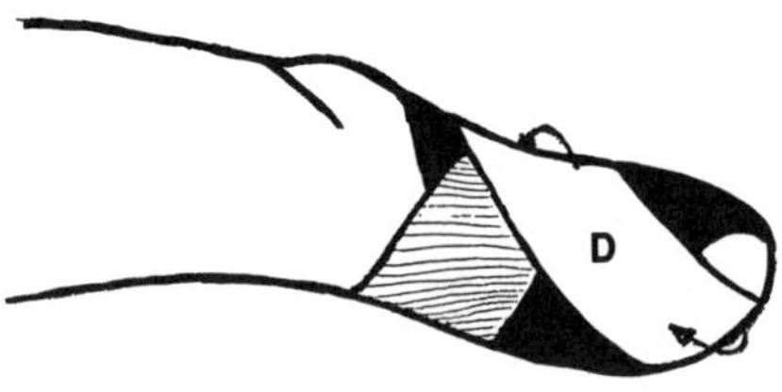

Continue around the stump, down the back to the medial end, and then up the front to the lateral side *(D)*.

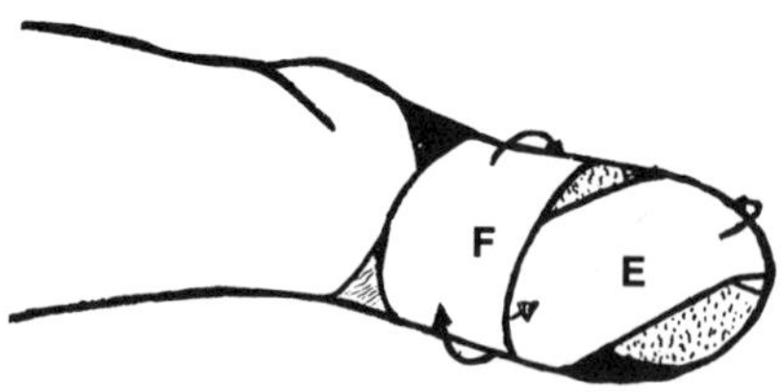

Continue diagonally up the back toward the medial side of the knee and then diagonally downward across the front of the leg to the lateral end of the stump *(E)*. Bring the bandage up the back, across the front just below the knee *(F)*.

Figure 7–24. Bandaging a below-knee amputation. *(Modified from Bandaging Instruction for Below-the-Knee Amputations, Department of Physical Medicine and Rehabilitation, University of Illinois at the Center Research and Educational Hospitals, Chicago, Illinois* [*undated*].*)*

Patient Teaching. Before a patient can accept a change in body image, he or she must first understand what has happened and what the prognosis is. For most patients following a BK amputation, the chances of returning to near normal activities are very good. Many are able to ambulate to a gait that is about indistinguishable from normal.

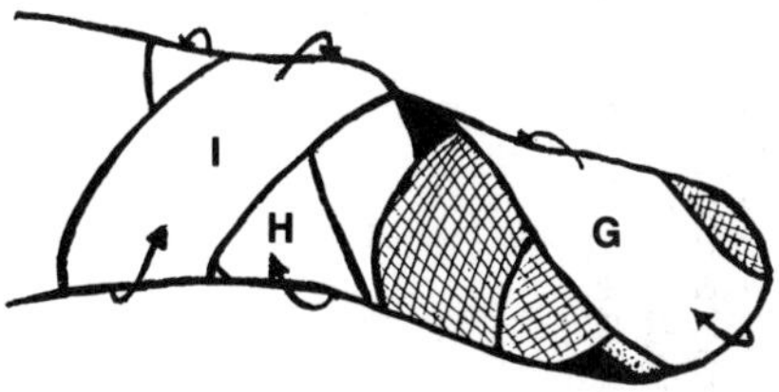

Continue around the leg and down the back to the medial end of the stump, and then go up the front to the lateral side of the knee *(G)*. Continue across the back of the leg and upward to above the knee cap *(H)*. Bring the bandage across the back again, and then cross the front of the leg in a downward fashion *(I)*.

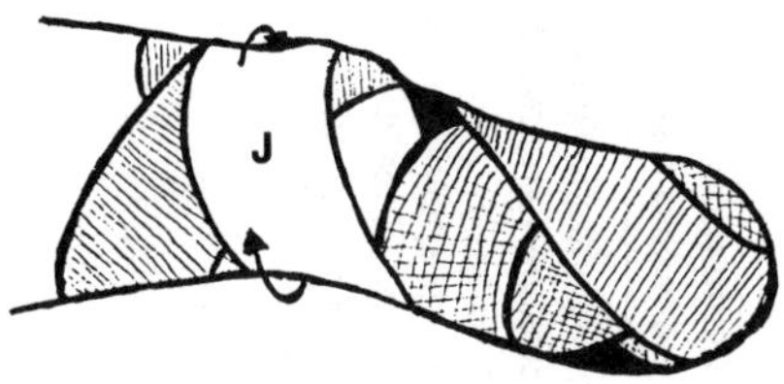

Bring the bandage across the back and then upwards across the front to the lateral side just above the knee *(J)*.

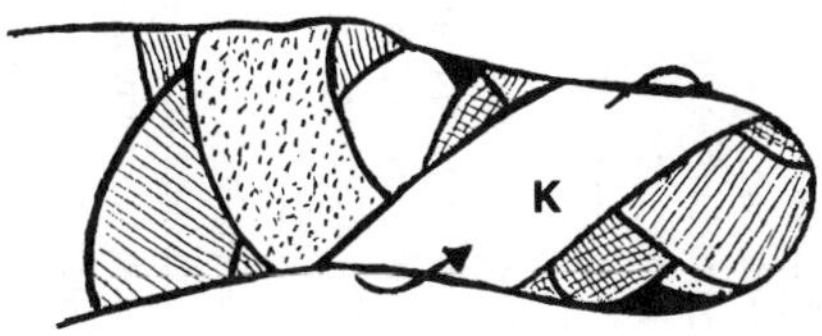

Bring the bandage down the back of the knee and then down the front of the stump *(K)*. Continue with figure 8 turns (*D, E, F,* and G) as long as the bandage permits.

Anchor with clips, safety pins, or adhesive tape. Chart the procedure, the patient teaching, and the patient's response.

Figure 7–24. *(continued)*

The patient, the family, and significant others need time to adjust to the amputation. The stages of adjustment to a disability, discussed in Chapter 1, come more easily to some patients than to others. The age of patients and the reasons for the amputation influence the adjustment process. (For more detailed discussion of adjusting to an amputation, see pp. 306–307.)

The teaching for cast care is the same as that for a patient with a long leg cast. Crutch walking will initially use a four-point gait, and the patient should know how to go up and down stairs before leaving the hospital.

Prevent Complications. Infection or potential infections are of special concern for a patient with a BK amputation, especially if the reason for the amputation was trauma or osteomyelitis. The patient with osteomyelitis may even be put in isolation. Complications from surgery and bedrest should be minimized by early ambulation, but the customary preventive measures need to be employed.

Evaluation and Reassessment

For a typical patient following a BK amputation, the considerations discussed for a patient who has had a total knee arthroplasty apply, but the

TABLE 7–7. NURSING PROCESS FOR BELOW-KNEE AMPUTATION WITH A RIGID DRESSING

Assessment	Nursing Diagnosis	Goal Formulation	Planning and Intervention	Evaluation and Reassessment
1. Assess the location, duration, and severity of pain. Observe for verbal and nonverbal cues of pain. Check for tightness of the rigid dressing.	1. Alteration in comfort: pain in the leg related to bone and soft tissue trauma.	1. Short-term goal: a reduction in leg pain. Long-term goal: free of any pain.	1. Alleviate Pain Elevate the foot of the bed. Keep the leg in correct alignment. Allow time for discussion of feelings. Teach relaxation techniques. Apply pressure to the end of the cast. Administer prescribed medications as indicated.	1. The patient should require medication to relieve the pain. Pressure applied to the distal end of the cast should help to reduce phantom pain.
2. Check the position of the leg. Assess for strength in the upper extremities. Assess for ability to do exercises. Check for tightness of the rigid dressing. Check for correct tightness of cast straps.	2. Impaired physical mobility: a decrease in leg function related to loss of a portion of the leg.	2. Short-term goal: an increase in mobility through exercises and crutch walking. Long-term goal: regain leg function through use of a prosthesis.	2. Increase Mobility *Position* Teach the patient how to use the trapeze. Place patient in a position of comfort while supine. Change position every 2 hours while awake and every 4 hours at night. Place the patient prone with no pillow under the abdomen for 30 minutes to 2 hours at least twice a day (gradually increase the time). *Exercises* Encourage active range of motion of all uninvolved joints. Teach quadriceps and gluteal setting exercises and leg raises.	2. The patient should be able to do the required exercises without supervision. After instruction and a demonstration, the patient should be able to ambulate safely with crutches.

			Teach hip extension, adduction and abduction exercises. Teach exercises to increase upper extremity strength. *Ambulation* Demonstrate a partial weight-bearing crutch gait.	
3. Assess for signs and symptoms of infection. Check vital signs. Assess for level of pain. Check for any bleeding or drainage in cast. Check for odor.	3. Potential for injury: infection related to surgical incision.	3. Short- and long-term goals: free of any signs of infection.	3. Prevent Complications *Integumentary* Encourage a well-balanced diet with plenty of fluids. Keep rigid dressing dry. Administer antibiotics as prescribed. Teach patient signs and symptoms of infection. *Potential Complications Due to Surgery and Immobility* (See Table 7–3 and Chap. 3)	3. The patient should remain free of any sign of infection.
4. Assess for the patient's level of understanding about the rehabilitation process and future ambulation. Assess the patient's stage of adaptation to the disability.	4. Potential knowledge deficit related to rehabilitation process and future ambulation.	4. Short- and long-term goals: a decrease in anxiety through increased knowledge.	4. Patient Teaching Allow time for open discussions of feelings about changes in body image and potential changes in work, social, and personal life. Discuss the various stages in the rehabilitation process. Teach the patient how to care for the cast. Discuss methods of bathing, dressing, and sleeping with a cast.	4. The patient should be able to verbalize an understanding of the rehabilitation process. The patient should be able to talk about the amputation and to view the leg. The patient should be able to start to discuss feelings about the loss of the leg. The patient, family, and significant other should feel confident in caring for the patient at home.

following points merit special attention. In evaluating pain, determine whether phantom pain is present. See how well the patient is able to ambulate and sit with the immediate postsurgical fitting. Evaluate how well the patient, the family, and significant others are adjusting to the change in body image, and whether they have reached the stage of acceptance.

Rupture of the Achilles Tendon

Traumatic rupture of the Achilles tendon is not uncommon, particularly among middle-aged men. Sudden contraction of the calf muscle with the foot fixed to the floor may cause the Achilles tendon to be pulled apart. The tendon rupture usually occurs within the sheath, leaving the sheath intact. The patient immediately notes sharp pain in the area and an inability to plantar flex the foot. On examination, a gap continuity of the tendon can be palpated.

An immediate surgical repair of the Achilles tendon is usually done. The major complication is skin necrosis during the healing process.

It is possible to treat this injury by the application of a walking cast with the foot held in marked plantar flexion. This position allows the ruptured tendon fragments to come together and reunite within the cast. This process usually takes between 6 and 8 weeks, but recurrence of the rupture following cast removal is not uncommon (Gartland, 1979, pp. 430–431).

Rupture of the Plantaris Tendon

The plantaris is a long, thin muscle in the calf that lies between gastrocnemius and soleus muscles. Rupture may occur with vigorous use of the legs, causing the patient to experience a sharp, stinging pain in the calf. Plantar flexion is unaffected and surgical treatment is not required. Rest, support to the calf, and the use of a heel lift are the only supportive measures needed (Gartland, 1979, p. 431).

REFERENCES

Cailliet, R. *Knee pain and disability*. Philadelphia: F. A. Davis, 1973.

DeGowin, E. L., & DeGowin, R. L. *Bedside diagnostic examination* (3rd ed.). New York: Macmillan, 1976.

Edmondson, A. S., & Crenshaw, A. H. (Eds.). *Campbell's operative orthopaedics* (6th ed.). St. Louis: C. V. Mosby, 1980.

Gartland, J. J. *Fundamental of orthopaedics* (3rd ed.). Philadelphia: W. B. Saunders, 1979.

Hoppenfeld, S. *Physical examination of the spine and extremities*. New York: Appleton-Century-Crofts, 1976.

Roaf, R., & Hodkinson, L. J. *Textbook of orthopaedic nursing* (2nd ed.). Oxford: Blackwell Scientific, 1975.

Strange, E., & Johns, J. Nursing care of the patient treated with continuous passive motion following knee arthroplasty. *Orthopaedic Nursing*, 1984, *3* (6), 27–32.

Warwick R., & Williams, P. R. *Gray's anatomy* (35th Brit. ed.). Philadelphia: W. B. Saunders, 1973.

BIBLIOGRAPHY

Aaron, R. K. Total joint arthroplast. *Surgical Clinics of North America,* 1983, *63* (3), 697–714.

Accardo, N. J., et al. Nailes total knee replacement procedure. *Orthopedics,* 1979, *2* (1), 37–45.

Ahstrom, J. P. Reliability of history and physical examination in diagnosis of meniscus pathology. *Current Practice in Orthopaedic Surgery, 1977,* 1977, *7,* 203–223.

Ahstrom, J. P. Rehabilitation of the knee. *Current Practice in Orthopaedic Surgery 1979,* 1979, *8,* 77–86.

Alms, M. Compartmental syndrome as a complication of the Hauser procedure. *Journal of Bone and Joint Surgery.* 1980, *62A* (2), 313.

Beeson, P. B., & McDermott, W. *Cecil-Loeb textbook of medicine.* Philadelphia: W. B. Saunders, 1971.

Berson, B. L., & Hermann, G. Torn discoid menisci of the knee in adults. *Journal of Bone and Joint Surgery,* 1979, *61A* (2), 303–304.

Bik, P. A. A patient undergoing a local, outpatient arthroscopy of the knee. *Orthopedic Nurses' Association Journal,* 1978, *5* (6), 22–24.

Brantley, P., & Analla, M. *The nurse and orthopedic surgery.* Rutherford, N. J.: The Orthopedic Nurses' Association, Inc. in cooperation with Howmedica, Inc., 1980.

Brodersen, M. P., Fitzgerald, R. H. Jr., Peterson, L. F. A., et al. Arthrodesis of the knee following failed total knee arthroplasty. *Journal of Bone and Joint Surgery,* 1979, *61A* (2), 181–185.

Burgess, E. M. Amputations. *Surgical Clinics of North America,* 1983, *63* (3), 749–770.

Cathings, C. Fractures of the shaft of the femur. *Orthopedic Nurses' Association Journal,* 1978, *5* (1), 18–20.

Chick, R. R., & Jackson, D. W. Tears of the anterior cruciate ligament in young athletes. *Journal of Bone and Joint Surgery,* 1978, *60A* (7), 970–973.

Clayton, M. L., & Kagan, A. II. The rheumatoid knee. *Current Practice in Orthopaedic Surgery 1979,* 1979, *8,* 121–133.

Clissold, G. *The body's response to trauma: Fractures.* New York: Springer, 1973.

Cochran, G. Van B. *A primer of orthopaedic biomechanics.* New York: Churchill Livingstone, 1982.

Compere, C. L., Hill, J. A., Lewinick, G. E., & Thomson, R. G. A new method of patellectomy for patellofemoral arthritis. *Journal of Bone and Joint Surgery,* 1979, *61A* (5), 714–719.

Compere, E. L. *Orthopaedic surgery: A handbook of orthoperative surgery.* Chicago: Year Book Medical, 1975.

Convery, F. R., Minteer-Convery, M., & Malcon, L. L. The spherocentric knee: A re-evaluation and modification. *Journal of Bone and Joint Surgery,* 1980, *62A* (3), 320–327.

Crossland, S., & Deyerle, W. Compartmental syndrome. *Nursing 80,* 1980, *10* (11), 51–53.

Crotwell, W. A. The thigh-locer: ambulatory non-operative treatment of femoral shaft fractures. *Journal of Bone and Joint Surgery,* 1978, *60A* (1), 112–117.

Croushare, T. M. Battered body: A teenage amputee taught us four tips for better long-term care. *Nursing 78,* 1978, *8* (1), 36–41.

Croushare, T. M. Dealing with emergency amputations. *Nursing 80,* 1980, *10* (4), 82–83.

Dahlman, V., et al. The use of the Vidal-Adrey external fixators for open fractures and non-unions. *Orthopedic Nurses' Association Journal,* 1978, *5* (8), 33–37.

Das, A. K., & Mukherhee, D. R. Giant osteochondral base body of the knee joint. *Journal of Bone and Joint Surgery,* 1978, *60A* (4), 559–560.
Del Pizzo, W., Fox, J. M., Blazina, M. E., et al. Operative arthroscopy for the treatment of problems of the medial compartment of the knee. *Orthopedics,* 1980, *3,* 984–986.
Drennan, D. B., Lacher, F. B., & Maylahn, D. J. Fractures of the tibial plateau. *Journal of Bone and Joint Surgery,* 1979, *61A* (7), 989–995.
Fernley, H. T. Nursing care study: A patient with severe femoral shaft fracture. *Nursing Times,* 1978, *74* (24), 994–995.
Flarek, F. F. Method of skin closure following fasciotomy for anterior tibial compartment syndrome. *Orthopedics,* 1980, *3,* 223–224.
Flynn, L. M. The Nailes hinge knee prosthesis with axial rotation. *Orthopedics,* 1979, *2* (6), 602–605.
Folcik, C., & Dumas, K. Identifying a standard for pin care using the quality assurance approach. *Orthopaedic Nursing,* 1984, *3* (3), 17–34.
Fries, J. F. *Arthritis, a comprehensive guide.* Menlo Park, Calif.: Addison-Wesley, 1982.
Ghista, D. N., & Roaf, R. *Orthopaedic mechanics: Procedures and devices.* San Francisco: Academic, 1978.
Grana, W. A. Chronic instability of the knee. *Orthopedic Nurses' Association Journal,* 1979, *6* (8), 320–324.
Greenfield, G. R. Proximal tibial epiphysial fracture. *Orthopedics,* 1980, *3,* 747–750.
Harvie, K. W. A major advance in the central of post-operative knee pain. *Orthopedics,* 1979, *2* (1), 26–27.
Hernandez, V., & O'Connor, M. Case study: Arthroscopy for internal knee derangement. *Orthopedic Nurses' Association Journal,* 1978, *5* (4), 110–112.
Hui, F. C., & Fitzgerald, R. H. Hinged total knee arthroplasty. *Journal of Bone and Joint Surgery,* 1980, *62A* (4), 513–519.
Insall, J., Scott, W. N., & Ranawat, C. S. The total condylar knee prosthesis. *Journal of Bone and Joint Surgery,* 1979, *61A* (2), 173–180.
Iverson, L. D., & Clawson, D. K. *Manual of acute orthopaedic therapeutics.* Boston: Little, Brown, 1977.
Ivey, F. M., Blazina, M E., Faro, J. M., & Del Pizzo, W. Reoperation following patellectomy for chondromalacia. *Orthopedics,* 1979, *2* (2), 136–137.
Kleinman, R., Oda, M., & Horowitz, B. Supracondylar fracture of the femur as a complication of the patillar tendon bearing cast: A case report. *Orthopedics,* 1980, *3,* 1203–1205.
Kamisarz, J. M. Chondromalacia patella. *Orthopaedic Nursing,* 1984, *3* (3), 24–28.
Kryschyshen, P. L., & Fischer, D. A. External fixation for complicated fractures. *American Journal of Nursing,* 1980, *80* (2) 256–259.
Larson C. B., & Gould, M. *Orthopedic nursing* (9th ed.). St. Louis: C. V. Mosby, 1978.
Lowe, E. B. Jr. Diagnostic and operative arthroscopy. *Surgical Clinics of North America,* 1983, *63* (3), 599–606.
Lubinus, H. H. Patella glide bearing total replacement. *Orthopedics,* 1979, *2* (2), 119–127.
Lupin, A. E. Head off compartment syndrome before "it's too late." *RN,* 1980, *43* (12), 38–41.
Matsen, F. A., Winquist, R. A., & Krugmire, R. B. Jr. Diagnosis and management of compartmental syndromes. *Journal of Bone and Joint Surgery,* 1980, *62A* (2), 286–291.
McPoil, T. G., Burgtholdt, H. T., & Hunt, G. C. Modification of temporary below-knee sockets for amputees with absent or diminished sensation. *Physical Therapy,* 1980, *60* (4), 437–438.

Meador, R. Learning to live with a new leg. *American Journal of Nursing,* 1979, *79* (8), 1393–1395.

Mira, A. J. A critical analysis of quadriceps function after femoral shaft fracture in adults. *Journal of Bone and Joint Surgery,* 1980, *62A* (1), 61–67.

Mubarak, S. J., Owen, C. A., Hargens, A. R., et al. Acute compartment syndrome: Diagnosis and treatment with the aid of the Wick catheter. *Journal of Bone and Joint Surgery,* 1978, *60A* (8), 1091–1095.

Omer, G. E. Management of the painful extremity. *Current Practice in Orthopaedic Surgery 1979,* 1979, *8,* 86–99.

Peterson, H. A. Operative correction of post-fracture arrest of the epiphyseal plate. *Journal of Bone and Joint Surgery,* 1980, *62A* (6), 1018–1020.

Powell, M. *Orthopedic Nursing.* New York: Churchill Livingstone, 1976.

Rauscher, N. A. Pathological femur fracture due to bone cyst. *Orthopedic Nurses' Association Journal,* 1978, *5* (10), 12–15.

Reid, B. C. Ambulation aid for a bent knee spica. *Physical Therapy,* 1978, *58* (4), 448.

Riley, L. N., & Hungerfard, D. S. Geometric total knee replacement for treatment of the rheumatoid knee. *Journal of Bone and Joint Surgery,* 1978, *60A* (4), 523–527.

Sim, F. H., & Chao, E. Y. S. Prosthetic replacement of the knee and a large segment of the femur or tibia. *Journal of Bone and Joint Surgery,* 1979, *61A* (6), 887–892.

Strange, E., & Johns, J. Nursing care of the patient treated with continuous passive motion following knee arthroplasty. *Orthopaedic Nursing,* 1984, *3* (6), 27–32.

Spickler, L. Soft tissue injuries of the knee. *Orthopedic Nurses' Association Journal,* 1979, *6* (10), 409–414.

Sprales, K. J. Nursing care of skeletal pins: A closer look. *Orthopaedic Nursing,* 1985, *4* (1), 11–19.

Swinson, D. R., & Swinburn, W. R. *Rheumatology.* New York: Wiley, 1980.

Tjörnstrand, B., Hagstedt, B., & Person, B. M. Results of surgical treatment for non-union after high tibial osteotomy in osteoarthritis of the knee. *Journal of Bone and Joint Surgery,* 1978, *60A* (7), 973–977.

Tremblay, G. R., Laurin, C. A., & Drovin, G. The challenge of prosthetic cruciate ligament replacement. *Clinical Orthopedics,* 1980, *147,* 88–92.

Turek, S. R. *Orthopaedic Principles and their applications* (3rd ed.). Philadelphia: Lippincott, 1977.

Van Der Linden, W., & Larsson, K. Plate fixation versus conservative treatment of tibial shaft fractures. *Journal of Bone and Joint Surgery,* 1979, *61A* (6), 873–878.

Votz, R. G. A method of skeletal traction to protect a reattached patillar tendon following total knee replacement. *Journal of Bone and Joint Surgery,* 1979, *61A* (7), 1109–1110.

Wall, J. J. Compartment syndrome as a complication of the Hauser procedure. *Journal of Bone and Joint Surgery,* 1979, *61A* (2), 185–191.

Walsh, C. R., & Wirth, C. R. Total knee arthroplasty: Biomechanical and nursing considerations. *Orthopaedic Nursing,* 1985, *4* (1), 29–34.

Wilber, M. C., & Evans, E. B. Fractures of the femoral shaft treated surgically. *Journal of Bone and Joint Surgery,* 1978, *60A* (4), 489–491.

Whipple, T. L., & Bassett, F. N. Arthroscopic examination of the knee. *Journal of Bone and Joint Surgery,* 1978, *60A* (4), 444–453.

Wilde, A. H. Management of complications after knee replacement. *Current Practice in Orthopaedic Surgery 1979,* 1979, *8,* 121–133.

Wilson, F. C., Fajgenbaum, D. M., & Venters, G. C. Results of knee replacement with the Walldius and geometric prosthesis. *Journal of Bone and Joint Surgery,* 1980, *62A* (4), 497–503.

Winquist, R. A., & Hanse, S. T. Segmental fractures of the femur treated by closed intramedullary nailing. *Journal of Bone and Joint Surgery,* 1978, *60A* (7), 934–939.

Wolfgang, G. L. Unicompartmental modular total knee arthroplasty. *Orthopedics,* 1980, *3,* 313–318.

Zimmer. *The traction handbook.* Warsaw, Ind.: Zimmer, USA, 1980.

8

THE ANKLE AND FOOT

Chapter 8 focuses on the treatment and associated care of traumatic and pathological conditions of the ankle and the foot. Conditions ranging from common ankle and foot problems, such as corns, calluses, sprains, and fractures, to fusion and reconstructive surgical procedures are discussed. The chapter begins with a review of the anatomy of the ankle and the foot.

ANATOMY

BONES

The talocrural or ankle joint is a uniaxial joint. It is formed by the talus, the tibia, and the fibula and is stable because of its mechanical configuration and ligamentous supports. The lower end of the tibia and its medial malleolus, the lateral malleolus of the fibula, and the inferior transverse tibiofibular ligament together form a deep recess in which the body of the talus is embraced. The ankle bones are connected by a fibrous capsule, and by several ligaments (Fig. 8–1), specifically the deltoid, anterior, and posterior talofibular, and calcaneofibular ligaments (Warwick & Williams, 1973, p. 460).

The skeleton of the foot (Fig. 8–2) has three parts: the tarsus (or hindfoot), the metatarsus (or midfoot), and the phalanges (or forefoot). The seven tarsal bones make up the skeleton of the posterior half of the foot. The tarsal bones are arranged in proximal and distal rows with an additional bone interposed between the two rows on the medial side. The proximal row is comprised of the talus and the calcaneus. The distal row, from medial to lateral, is composed of the medial cuneiform, intermediate cuneiform, lateral cuneiform, and cuboid bones. On the medial side the navicular bone is interposed between the

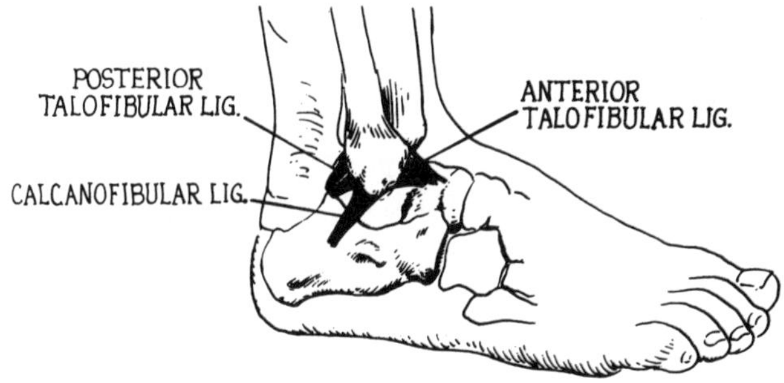

Figure 8–1. Three important ligaments of the lateral aspect of the ankle. *(Figures 8–1, 8–3 through 8–6, 8–13, 8–16 through 8–19, and 8–21 through 8–24 are reproduced from Hoppenfeld, S., 1976, with permission.)*

head of the talus and the cuneiforms. Laterally, the calcaneus articulates directly with the cuboid.

The five metatarsal bones are situated in the distal part of the foot, connecting the tarsus to the phalanges. They are numbered one through five from the medial side. The metatarsals are miniature long bones possessing a shaft, a base or proximal end, and a head or distal end. The bases articulate with the distal row of the tarsus and with one another. The heads articulate with the proximal phalanges of their respective digits.

The 14 phalanges correspond in number and general arrangement to the phalanges of the hand. There are two phalanx bones in the big toe, and three is each of the other toes. The terminal phalanx of the big toe normally shows a small degree of valgus (lateral) deviation; such deviation may also be seen in the proximal phalanx even in persons who have never worn shoes (Warwick & Williams, 1973, p. 392).

ANKLE MOVEMENT

When the foot is dorsiflexed, the talus is forced between the two malleoli and no lateral rotation is possible, but when the foot is plantar flexed, some lateral motion is allowed. The neutral or plantar flexed positions are thus more vulnerable to possible injury. The lateral and medial collateral ligaments stabilize the ankle yet permit plantar and dorsiflexion. The medial ligaments are taut in the neutral position, but the posterior strands relax in plantar flexion and the anterior fibers relax in dorsiflexion. The lateral collateral ligaments have a central axis and remain taut in all ranges of plantar and dorsiflexion. The ligaments run from the malleoli to the talus, calcaneus, and navicular bones. They are supplied with sensory nerves that, when stretched, evoke a reflex muscle spasm that protects the joint from further motion (Cailliet, 1981, p. 3–15).

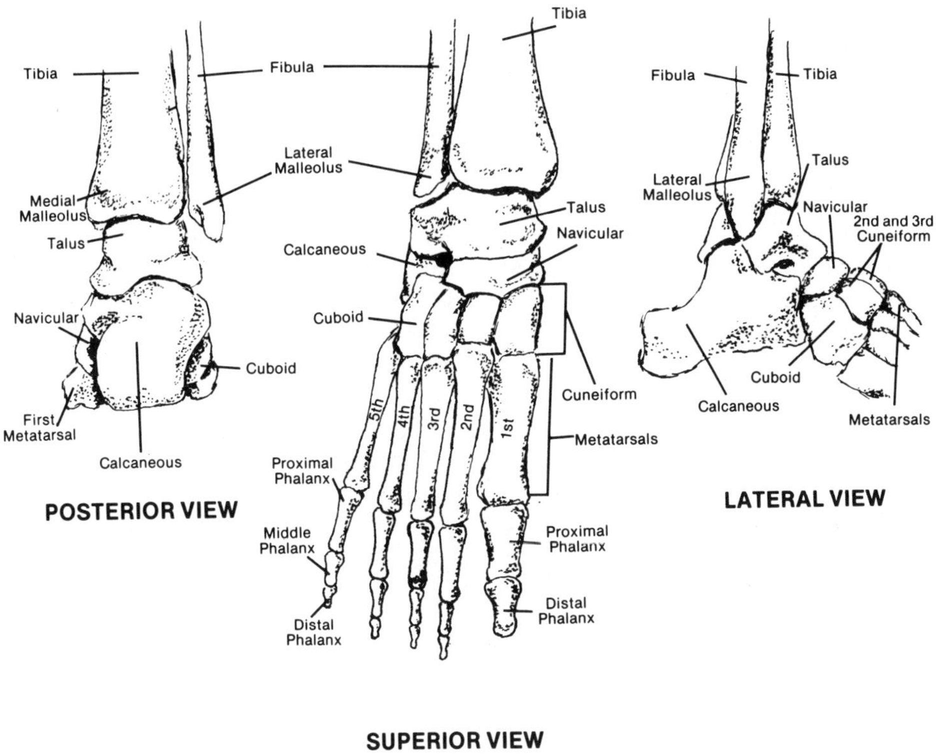

Figure 8–2. Skeletal anatomy of the foot and ankle. *(From Brantley, P., & Analla, M., 1980, p. 112. Courtesy of Howmedica.)*

THE FIBROUS CAPSULE

A fibrous capsule surrounds the ankle joint. It is thin in front and in back and attaches to the borders of the articular surfaces of the tibia and the malleoli, and below, to the talus close to the margins of the trochlear surface (except in front, where it is attached to the dorsum of the neck of the talus). The fibrous capsule is supported on each side by strong collateral ligaments.

A synovial membrane lines the capsule, and the joint cavity ascends for a short distance between the tibia and the fibula.

LIGAMENTS OF THE ANKLE

Stabilizing the medial side of the ankle both anteriorly and posteriorly is the strong, flat, triangular deltoid ligament, which consists of five components. The deep component attaches to the undersurface of the medial malleolus and the body of the talus. The four superficial components are the tibionavicular and anterior talotibial components anteriorly, the calcaneotibial component centrally, and the posterior talotibial component posteriorly.

Laterally there are three ligaments that help to stabilize the ankle. The anterior talofibular ligament, which is 2 to 2.5 mm thick, attaches anteriorly to the border of the lateral malleolus and anteriorly to the neck of the talus. The calcaneofibular ligament, which is stronger than the anterior talofibular ligament, attaches superiorly to the tip of the lateral malleolus and inferiorly to the lateral surface of the calcaneus. It is the only lateral ligament that is extracapsular. The posterior talofibular ligament, which is the strongest lateral ligament, attaches anteriorly to the digital fossa of the fibula and posteriorly to the lateral tubercle on the posterior aspect of the talus. A fourth ligament, the lateral talocalcaneal ligament, supports the subtalar joint and lies between the anterior talofibular ligament and the calcaneofibular ligament, blending with both.

The ligaments that bind the distal tibia and the fibula together are (1) the anterior and posterior inferior tibiofibular ligaments, which attach superiorly and medially to the tibia and inferiorly and laterally to the fibula, (2) the inferior transverse ligament, which attaches laterally to the lateral malleolus and medially to the posterior border of the distal articular surface of the tibia, and (3) the interosseous ligament, the strongest bond between the bones, which attaches to the contiguous rough surfaces of the tibia and the fibula.

TENDONS, VESSELS, AND NERVES

Starting from the medial side, the tendons, vessels, and nerves of the ankle are, in front, the tibialis anterior tendon, the extensor hallucis longus tendon, the anterior tibial vessels, deep peroneal nerve, the extensor digitorum longus tendon, and the peroneus tertius tendon. From behind, there are the tibialis posterior tendon, the flexor digitorum longus tendon, the posterior tibial vessels, the tibial nerve, and the flexor hallucis longus tendon. In the groove behind the fibular malleolus, there are the peroneus longus and peroneus brevis tendons.

Arteries supplying the joint are derived from the malleolar branches of the anterior tibial artery and from the peroneal arteries. The nerves are derived from the deep peroneal and tibial nerves.

MUSCLES OF THE ANKLE JOINT

When the body is in an erect position the foot is at right angles to the leg. The active movements of the ankle joint are those of dorsiflexion and plantar flexion. In dorsiflexion the angle between the front of the leg and the dorsum of the foot is diminished, whereas in plantar flexion that angle is increased. Slight amounts of side-to-side gliding movement, and rotation, abduction, and adduction are permitted when the foot is in plantar flexion. To obtain dorsiflexion, the muscles used are the tibialis anterior muscle, assisted by the extensor digitorum longus, extensor hallucis longus, and peroneus tertius muscles. For plantar flexion, the muscles used are the gastrocnemius and soleus, assisted to a lesser degree by the plantaris, tibialis posterior, flexor hallucis longus, and flexor digitorum longus muscles.

THE ANKLE

Trauma

A force applied to the ankle joint may cause a strain, a sprain, a ligamentous rupture, a dislocation, a fracture, or a combination of injuries, depending on the nature and the amount of force applied (Gartland, 1979, p. 443). The most severe injury to the ankle is the fracture–dislocation, the least severe is the strain, and the most common is the sprain.

STRAIN

A strain to the ankle is an overstretching of the ligaments without disrupting the integrity of their fibers or avulsing them from their bony attachments. The strained ankle retains normal joint stability, and a strain is usually considered a minor injury that heals within a few weeks with minimal care.

SPRAIN

A sprain of the ankle joint is a stretching injury of the joint capsule and supporting ligaments by a twisting force (Gartland, 1979, p. 433). It occurs most frequently when a stress is applied to an ankle in an unstable position. The ankle is most unstable when plantar flexed, and it is in that position that forceful inversion or eversion will stretch the ligaments. This action can occur when running, walking over uneven ground, or even from unaccustomed walking in high heel shoes (Cailliet, 1981, p. 117).

Sprains may be classified according to the amount of soft tissue injury. Type I sprains involve trauma with minor ligamentous injuries, type II sprains involve incomplete ligamentous injuries, and type III sprains involve complete disruption of the ligament (Edmondson & Crenshaw, 1980, p. 873). Doctor Watson-Jones once said, "It is worse to sprain an ankle than to break it," because a fracture will receive treatment whereas a sprain may be neglected or receive inappropriate care. (For further discussion on sprains, see Chap. 7.)

Eversion and abduction of the foot may result in disruption of the deltoid ligament, whereas inversion stress may cause ligamentous disruption on the lateral side of the ankle. Diagnosis and treatment are dependent on an understanding of the ligamentous structure about the ankle. The most common sprain occurs from inversion stress while the foot is slightly plantar flexed, and results in stretching the lateral collateral ligaments (Cailliet, 1981, p. 118). The anterior talofibular ligament is the most commonly affected. If the inversion stress occurs with the ankle at a right angle, the calcaneofibular ligament receives the stretch force.

Post-Trauma Assessment

When assessing a patient who has an ankle injury with a possible sprain of the ankle joint, obtain information on how the injury occurred, what position the foot was in, what the person heard or felt, and how long ago the injury occurred. With a sprain, you would expect to find that there was a forced inversion with the foot plantar-flexed, and that a short time after injury there was a great amount of swelling, tenderness, and stiffness of the joint. The tenderness is localized mostly along the stretched ligament (e.g., to the tissues immediately below the lateral malleolus). When walking there is instability of the ankle and severe discomfort. Within a few days an area of ecchymosis develops, caused by blood seeping beneath the deep fascia. The discoloration may even go as far as the toes.

Roentgenograms are usually negative, and arthrograms for ligamentous injuries of the ankle are of limited value. Upon physical examination of a possible sprained ankle, look for evidence of ligamentous injury and test the ankle for instability. Because the anterior talofibular ligament (Fig. 8–3) is the ligament most often involved in ankle sprains, tenderness elicited along its course may indicate such damage. To test that ligament (Fig. 8–4), do an inversion stress test by turning the patient's foot into plantar flexion and inversion. If inversion stress increases the pain, there is a distinct possibility that the ligament is sprained or torn. The inversion stress test indicates the condition of the talofibular ligament but does not give evidence of joint stability. Usually, a tear in that ligament allows the talus to slide forward on the tibia because the anterior talofibular ligament is the only structure preventing subluxation of the talus. Therefore, test for anterior instability between the tibia and the talus using the anterior draw sign (Fig. 8–5). In performing the anterior draw sign test, the patient sits on the edge of the table or bed with the legs dangling and the feet in a few degrees of plantar flexion. Place one hand on the anterior aspect of the lower tibia and grip the calcaneus in the palm of your other hand. Then, draw (pull) the calcaneus and talus anteriorly, while pushing the tibia posteriorly (see Fig. 8–5). Normally, the anterior talofibular ligament is tight in all positions of the ankle joint, and there should be no forward movement of the talus on the tibia. Under abnormal conditions the talus slides anteriorly from under the cover of the ankle joint (positive draw sign); you may even feel a "clunk" as it moves (Hoppenfeld, 1976, p. 321).

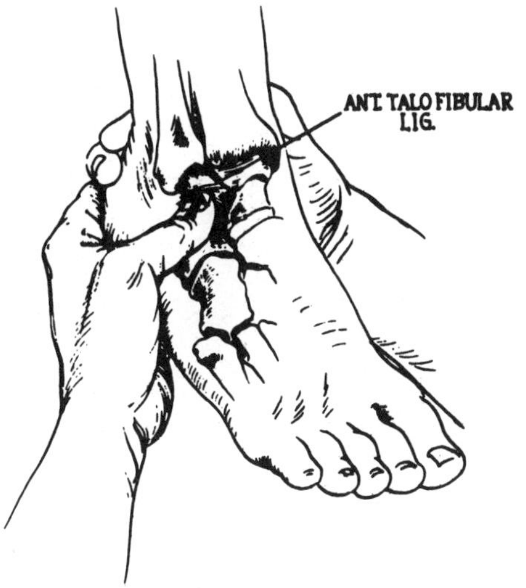

Figure 8–3. Palpation of the sinus tarsi.

To test the stability of the deltoid ligament on the medial side, stabilize the patient's leg around the tibia and the calcaneus and evert the foot (Fig. 8–6). If the deltoid ligament is torn, you may feel a gross gapping at the joint. The posterior talofibular ligament can be torn only in conjunction with the other lateral ligaments. It takes a massive trauma to the ankle joint, such as a dislocation, to damage the posterior talofibular ligament (Hoppenfeld, 1976, p. 222).

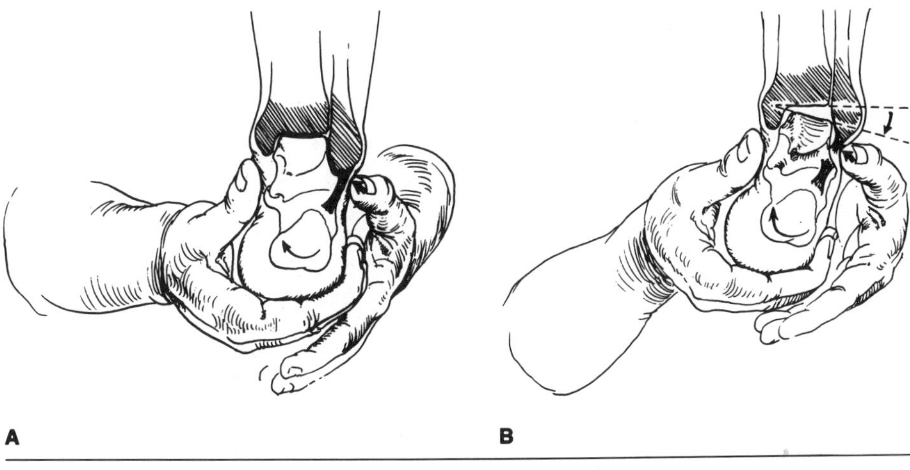

A B

Figure 8–4. A. A test to evaluate the stability of the anterior talofibular and the calcaneofibular ligaments. **B.** The ankle is unstable if the anterior talofibular and calcaneofibular ligaments are torn.

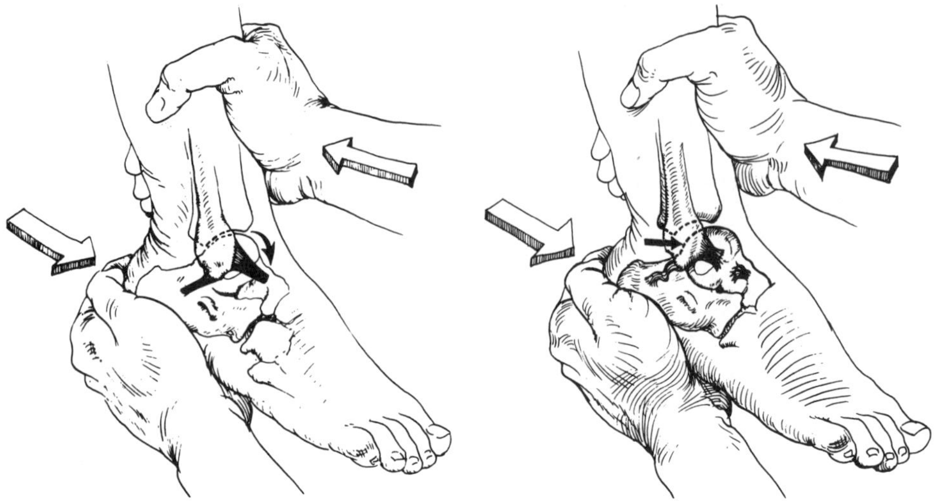

A B

Figure 8–5. A. The anterior draw sign test to evaluate the intactness of the anterior talofibular ligament. **B.** A positive anterior draw sign.

After the tests are completed on the involved foot, test the normal one as a means of comparison to determine the extent of abnormal gapping. Stress roentgenograms are usually the best way to confirm the physical findings described above.

Medical Treatment

The majority of type I or II sprains or ligamentous injuries can usually be treated by rest and support with excellent prognoses for return of normal function. In a type III sprain, where a complete dissolution of fibers has occurred, immobilization is essential. Usually the acute symptoms subside over a

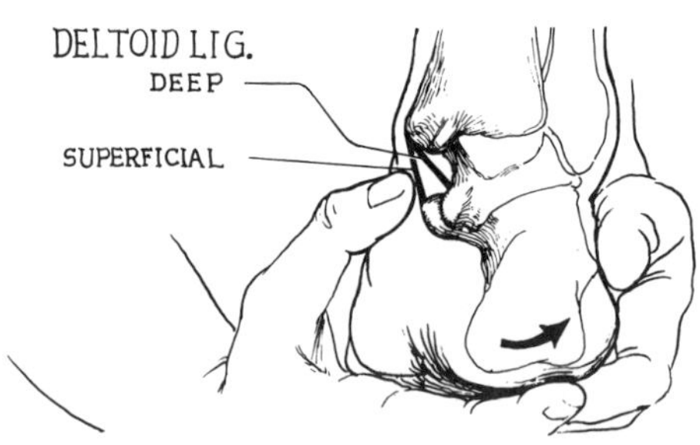

Figure 8–6. Pain elicited upon eversion may be due to a sprain of the deltoid ligament.

period of weeks, but some tenderness and swelling may persist about the lateral aspect of the ankle.

□ NURSING PROCESS (Table 8–1)

Assessment

For patients with a cast or elastic wrap on the foot, it is necessary to check the neurovascular status of the toes. Determine the circulation by noting any swelling, the temperature and color of the skin of the toes and the foot, and the circulation as evidenced by the blanching test (after the toenails are gently compressed between the thumb and the fingers and then released, the color of the toenail beds should quickly change from white to pink). There may very well be discoloration and swelling of the foot or toes due to the trauma of injury. To help determine the temperature of the affected foot, check the temperature of the uninvolved foot. Determine the motor function by evaluating the patient's ability to wiggle or move the toes. Check to make sure the swelling, cast, or dressing is not impeding the movement. Determine the sensory response as indicated by any complaints of numbness, tingling, or lack of feeling in any of the toes when tested by sharp or dull touch. Determine the amount, kind, and location of pain. Check the positioning of the affected foot. It should be elevated and safely secured in that position, with no pressure on the heel, support for the complete leg, and support for both sides of the leg to prevent rotation.

Nursing Diagnosis and Goal Formulation

Nursing diagnoses for a typical patient with a sprained ankle are (1) alterations in comfort related to pain from trauma to the ligaments that stabilize the ankle, (2) alterations in mobility related to lack of stability in the affected ankle, (3) potential complications related to trauma to the supporting ligaments in the ankle, and (4) alterations in psychological well-being related to anxiety and knowledge deficit about the injury and the method of treatment.

Short-term goals for a typical patient with a sprained ankle are to experience (1) a decrease in the amount of pain by immobilization or prescribed medications, (2) an increase in mobility within a few days through the use of assistive devices, (3) an absence of complications from the decreased activity of the ankle, and (4) a decrease in anxiety through patient understanding of the injury, the method of treatment, and the preventative measures. Long-term goals are to have the patient free of pain and swelling and to have return of normal function with no residual effects.

Planning and Intervention

Alleviate Pain. Nursing measures to help alleviate ankle pain immediately following a sprain are to immobilize the ankle, elevate the foot and the

TABLE 8–1. NURSING PROCESS FOR SPRAINED ANKLE TREATED WITH AN ELASTIC BANDAGE WRAP

Assessment	Nursing Diagnosis	Goal Formulation	Planning and Intervention	Evaluation and Reassessment
1. Assess for the location, duration, and severity of pain. Assess the neurovascular status. Check the tightness of the elastic bandage.	1. Alteration in comfort: pain in the ankle related to soft tissue trauma.	1. Short-term goal: a reduction in ankle pain through immobilization. Long-term goal: free of any ankle pain.	1. Alleviate Pain Elevate the foot. Keep pressure off the heel. Immobilize the ankle with an elastic bandage. Apply ice bags to the ankle. Teach relaxation techniques. Administer pain medication as indicated.	1. The patient should remain relatively free of pain with the use of pain medication.
2. Check for any swelling in the foot and the ankle. Assess the neurovascular status. Check the positioning of the foot. Check for elevation of the foot.	2. Impaired physical mobility: decrease in ankle motion related to soft tissue swelling and lack of joint stability.	2. Short-term goal: an increase in joint mobility through immobilization and controlled exercise. Long-term goal: regain full function in the ankle.	2. Increase Mobility Immobilize the ankle with an elastic bandage. Keep the leg elevated when lying or sitting. Start ambulation on the first day. Demonstrate crutch walking. Teach range-of-motion exercises of the ankle.	2. Determine that the patient is able to crutch walk and perform other activities of daily living effectively.

3. Assess the tightness of elastic bandage. Assess the patient's ability to do the exercises.	3. Potential for impaired mobility related to lack of ankle joint stability.	3. Short- and long-term goal: regain ankle joint stability.	3. Prevent Complications Teach isometric peroneal muscle exercises. Discuss applying 1/4-inch laterally based heel wedge to the shoe worn on the involved foot.	3. The patient should remain free of any complications.
4. Assess knowledge level in relation to the cause of the injury and rehabilitation process.	4. Potential knowledge deficit related to rehabilitation process.	4. Short- and long-term goal: a decrease in anxiety through an increase in knowledge.	4. Patient Teaching Discuss the mechanism of injury and the healing process. Demonstrate how to wrap an elastic bandage around the ankle. Demonstrate methods of soaking the ankle. Discuss scheduling of activities. Discuss the need for ambulation and ankle exercises. Demonstrate crutch walking.	4. The patient should verbalize understanding of the injury and that the healing process takes from 4 1/2–26 weeks or more, depending on the severity of the sprain. The patient should demonstrate how to wrap an ankle and crutch walk safely.

ankle, and use ice packs and medications as prescribed. Immobilization helps to relieve the pain by preventing movement and thus reducing stress to the affected ligaments. Pain is intensified by the immediate swelling that occurs after the injury. Swelling can be reduced by the elevation of the affected foot on two or three firm pillows, a commercial cast elevator, or slings. Reposition pillows as necessary, being sure to keep the patient's heel (or toes, when the patient is prone) off the pillows. Place pillows on both sides of the patient's thigh to help prevent hip rotation. Elevation of the extremity must be maintained even while the patient is up in a chair. When the patient is in a wheelchair, the affected leg is placed on the legrest on a pillow so that the leg does not rest on a hard surface. Then, elevate the leg on the legrest and secure the leg to the legrest with a belt or other support. If a cast is on the leg, use a 2-inch strap of tape, or several if the patient is in a long leg cast. If the patient is sitting in a regular chair, the foot can be elevated on a stool or the seat of another chair on which a pillow has been placed. If the foot is allowed to hang distal to the major portion of the body, swelling will increase. Ice packs along the lateral side of the ankle help to control the immediate swelling. Once the bleeding into the tissues has subsided, the patient without a cast can have the foot and the ankle soaked in hot water to relieve residual edema and tenderness.

Increase Mobility. When a patient has injured the ligaments that stabilize the ankle, rest and support for the ankle are needed so that healing can occur and function return. Rest and support for the ankle can be maintained by wrapping the ankle in an elastic bandage, by strapping the joint with tape, or in severe cases by supporting the ankle in a plaster splint or cast for 3 to 6 weeks. The immobilization allows the stretched and attenuated ligaments to be in anatomical position during the healing process. Even though immobilization helps to relieve pain and is beneficial in helping to reduce swelling, early ambulation seems to produce results superior to immobilization alone. Protection of the ankle followed by early mobilization and range-of-motion exercises are sometimes seen as the best approach. A cane or crutches are often needed to assist in the initial ambulation. Make sure the patient has a safe steady gait with the correct amount of weight bearing.

Prevent Complications. The most common long-term complication of ankle sprain is lateral talar instability. The patient may complain of recurring sprains or frequent giving way of the ankle. Some measures that have helped are isometric peroneal muscle exercises that improve stability for the lateral side of the ankle. The patient needs to understand the exercises, how to do them, why they are important, and to set aside time for doing them. A 1/4-inch laterally based heel wedge is also helpful for mild instability. If these measures are ineffective, a surgical repair of the peroneus brevis tendon may be needed.

Patient Teaching. Patient education is vital to reduce patient anxiety, to gain patient cooperation in administering care, and to have the patient accept the responsibility of self-care. Explain to the patient how the injury occurred, and if appropriate the need for proper footwear. Help the patient understand that the injury involves ligaments and not bones, but specific care is needed for healing to occur.

If the patient has an elastic wrap, demonstrate to the patient and the family how to rewrap the ankle. Allow them time to practice wrapping using the unaffected ankle. (If the patient has a cast, see Appendix B for a discussion on cast care.) Discuss a method of soaking the foot at least twice a day. The water should be warm, not hot, and the ankle should be soaked for at least 20 minutes at a time. Discuss the scheduling of the soaks with the patient so time is allotted and not forgotten, and discuss possible activities the patient can do while soaking the foot (i.e., reading, watching television, and doing handiwork, crafts, or other hobbies).

Help the patient understand the importance of ambulation and range-of-motion exercises, even though there may be some pain. If the ankle has been immobilized in a cast for 3 to 6 weeks there will be a need for peroneal stretching exercises to gradually return the ankle joint to full function. Demonstrate crutch walking and allow time for a return demonstration, especially of the patient's ability to go up and down the stairs and to get in and out of a chair. (For futher discussion of crutch walking, see Appendix C.)

Evaluation and Reassessment

Evaluate the amount of pain. Has the pain been reduced or has it increased over time? Is the pain on ambulation increasing? Determine if the patient is able to crutch walk and perform other activities of daily life effectively. The average duration of discomfort has been reported to be anywhere from 4 1/2 to 26 weeks, or even longer, depending on the severity of the sprain.

DISLOCATION

Dislocation of the ankle without fracture of either the medial or lateral malleolus or of the anterior or posterior lip of the distal articular surface of the tibia is extremely rare. Usually any ankle dislocations that do occur are easily reduced by closed methods, but posterior dislocation of the fibula behind the tibia can contribute to difficulty with closed reduction and thus may require open reduction (Edmondson & Crenshaw, 1980, p. 421).

FRACTURES

Besides ligamentous and soft tissue injuries, trauma to the ankle joint can cause bone injuries. Ankle fractures may be classified along anatomical lines, such as monomalleolar, bimalleolar (Pott's), or trimalleolar (Cotton) fractures, or by the mechanism of injury. An explosion fracture of the ankle, i.e., a malleolar fracture with a comminuted fracture of the distal tibial articular surface and the distal third of the tibia, is usually produced by a fall from a height. Sometimes an immediate open reduction may be extremely difficult or impractical. In such cases, a closed reduction of the fracture may be possible using traction through a transverse calcaneal pin or manipulation with a tibial pin proximal to the fracture in addition to the calcaneal pin. Both require a plaster cast with pins incorporated. If there are difficulties in reduction or healing, an arthrodesis of the ankle joint may be required later (Edmondson & Crenshaw, 1980, pp. 559–560).

Monomalleolar Fractures

Most monomalleolar fractures fall into one of three categories. First, there are supination–eversion fractures, where eversion is defined as an external or lateral rotation. The supination–eversion fracture is a spiral oblique fracture of the distal fibula associated with a rupture of the deltoid ligament or a fracture of the medial malleolus. Second, there are pronation–abduction fractures, which produce a transverse fracture of the medial malleolus associated with an oblique fracture of the tibia. Third, there are pronation–eversion fractures, which are characterized by a deltoid tear or a fracture of the medial malleolus associated with a spiral oblique fracture of the tibia (Edmondson & Crenshaw, 1980, pp. 552–553). In all cases, closed reduction with short leg cast is usually the treatment of choice (for nursing care for a patient with a short leg cast, see pp. 447 and 450).

Trimalleolar or Cotton Fractures

Trimalleolar fractures usually require open reduction. In addition to fractures of the medial malleolus and fibula, the posterior lip of the articular surface of the tibia is fractured and displaced, allowing posterior and lateral displacement and external rotation with supination of the foot (Edmondson & Crenshaw, 1980, p. 577). Each fracture is repaired by first reducing the fracture to anatomical position and then fixating it with mechanical devices such as screws or pins. Care following skin closure is similar to that given to patients with an internal fixation of a bimalleolar fracture (see pp. 437–442).

Bimalleolar or Pott's Fractures

Bimalleolar fractures can be reduced by either the open or closed methods. Closed reduction frequently can be accomplished once the swelling has been reduced, but often the anatomical position of the ankle is not maintained. In up to 20 percent of the bimalleolar fractures, intra-articular injuries to the talus and tibia are present and are untreated when closed reduction is utilized (Edmondson & Crenshaw, 1980, p 553). For most displaced bimalleolar fractures, treatment by open reduction and internal fixation of both malleoli is essential to restore the ankle joint (Fig. 8–7). To repair the joint various methods are used, such as oblique pins, screws, Kirschner wires, or even a small plate.

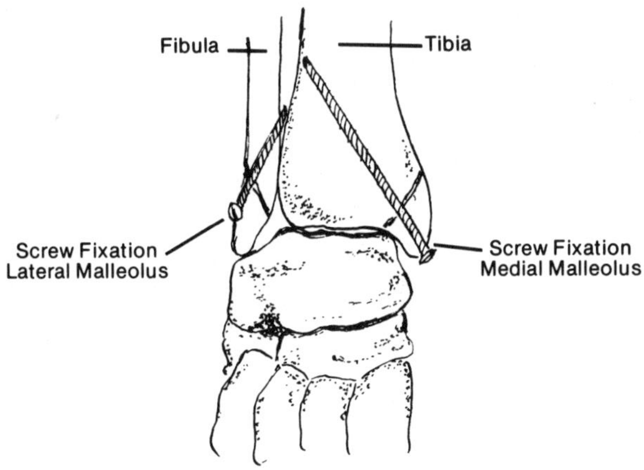

Figure 8–7. Open reduction and internal fixation, fractured medial or lateral malleolus or both. *(From Brantley, P., & Analla, M., 1980, p. 125. Courtesy of Howmedica.)*

☐ NURSING PROCESS (Table 8–2)

Assessment

Patients with a cast on the ankle, in foot traction, or with a bulky dressing need to have the neurovascular status of the foot checked (Chap. 2). There may be swelling due to the trauma or the surgery. In addition to possible discoloration of the skin from bleeding, there may be some discoloration from Betadine or other solutions used as preoperative preparation if an open reduction was done or if pins were inserted for traction. Determine the amount of pain, and whether the pain is due to nerve pressure or circulatory impairment.

For patients with an open reduction, determine the amount of bleeding. Note the size of any bloody area that appears on the cast or dressing. Be sure to check beneath the leg, especially on the lateral or medial sides of the ankle. Check frequently during the first 24 hours for any increase in the size of the bloody area. Bloody areas in the plaster cast retain their bright red color. Remember, bleeding into a wet plaster cast disperses the blood through the plaster, sometimes giving the impression that a lot more bleeding has occurred than actually has.

Nursing Diagnosis and Goal Formulation

For a typical patient with a Pott's fracture, the nursing diagnoses are (1) alterations in comfort related to pain from trauma and surgery, (2) alterations in mobility related to lack of bone stability in the ankle, (3) potential complications related to the fracture and the surgical procedure, and (4) alterations in psychological well-being related to anxiety and knowledge deficit about the injury and the prognosis.

Short-term goals for a typical patient with a Pott's fracture are to ex-

TABLE 8–2. NURSING PROCESS FOR FRACTURED ANKLE TREATED WITH AN OPEN REDUCTION, INTERNAL FIXATION, AND CAST

Assessment	Nursing Diagnosis	Goal Formulation	Planning and Intervention	Evaluation and Reassessment
1. Assess for the location, duration, and severity of pain. Check the tightness of the cast. Assess neurovascular status. Check for any swelling.	1. Alteration in comfort: pain in the ankle related to soft tissue and bone trauma.	1. Short-term goal: a decrease in pain through immobilization. Long-term goal: free of pain.	1. Alleviate Pain Securely elevate the foot. Keep pressure off the heel. Place ice bags along both sides of the ankle. Teach relaxation techniques. Administer pain medications.	1. Medications should keep the patient comfortable. Pain or throbbing in the foot when it is first lowered to the floor should be expected.
2. Assess neurovascular status. Assess strength in the upper extremities. Check elevation of the foot. Check for correct alignment.	2. Impaired physical mobility: a decrease in ankle function related to bone instability.	2. Short-term goal: an increase in mobility through immobilization. Long-term goals: regain full function in the ankle.	2. Increase Mobility *Position* Teach how to use the trapeze. Keep foot elevated on pillows. Turn patient to any position of comfort. *Exercise* Teach active dorsiflexion exercises (if front of cast has been removed). Teach isometric and straight leg raising exercises. Teach exercises to build up muscles for crutch walking. *Ambulation* Ambulate with nonweight bearing on affected leg. Demonstrate crutch walking (three-point gait).	2. The foot should be kept elevated except during ambulation. The patient should be able to ambulate safely using crutches and a three-point gait.

3. Assess the neurovascular status. Check for areas of swelling. Check for tightness of the cast.	3. Potential for injury: neurovascular deficit related to soft tissue swelling.	3. Short- and long-term goal: free of any neurovascular deficit.	3. Prevent Complications *Circulatory* Keep foot elevated. Utilize nursing measures to reduce any swelling. After surgery, do neurovascular checks every 15 minutes for the first 2 hours, every 30 minutes for the next 2 hours, every 60 minutes for the next 2 hours, every 2 hours for the next 18 hours, then at least at the beginning of every shift. Report any neurovascular abnormalities. Split cast as indicated.	3. The patient should remain free of any circulatory or integumentary problems.
Assess skin along cast edges for irritation. Assess for any pressure over bony prominences. Check cast for any drainage.	Potential impairment of skin integrity related to cast. Potential for injury: infection related to surgical incision and pressure areas.	Short- and long-term goal: free of any break in skin integrity or infection.	*Integumentary* Trim and petal cast edges. Replace window in cast securely. Elevate leg. Instruct on well-balanced diet.	
4. Assess knowledge of rehabilitation process. Assess ability to walk with crutches.	4. Potential knowledge deficit related to rehabilitation process.	4. Short- and long-term goal: a decrease in anxiety through an increase in knowledge.	4. Patient Teaching Discuss the rehabilitation process. Include family and significant other in teaching plan. Instruct on cast care. Teach how to do neurovascular checks. Go over methods of bathing and dressing.	4. Determine that the patient has been provided with sufficient data to feel confident about going home with a cast and ambulating on crutches.

perience (1) a decrease in the amount of pain in the ankle by immobilization and medications; (2) an increase in mobility by the use of a cast and crutches; (3) an absence of complications; and (4) a decrease in anxiety through the patient's understanding of the injury and the treatment method. The long-term goals are to have the patient free of pain and to have return of function to the ankle in approximately 12 weeks with no residual complications.

Planning and Intervention

Alleviate Pain. The foot should be elevated on pillows with the "toes above the nose." The heel should be off the pillows, to reduce pressure on the heel while the elevation is helping to prevent or reduce swelling. If the elevation of the foot of the bed is sufficient, make sure the heel is off the end of the bed. To help prevent discomfort caused by swelling, ice bags may be placed along both sides of the ankle, but not at the site of the swollen toes. These bags should not be filled heavily with ice, and air should be eliminated before the bags are closed. The pressure of heavy ice bags on a swollen and painful ankle has been known to cause great discomfort to the patient and considerable interference with circulation. Medicate the patient as needed for pain after first assessing the complaints of pain to make sure it is from the surgery or trauma and not from nerve pressure or circulatory impairment.

Increase Mobility. If both malleoli have been securely fixed, the ankle is usually immobilized in a short leg cast from the toes to the tibial tuberosity to prevent rotation. In many instances the distal portion of the front of the cast is removed as early as the third day so daily active dorsiflexion of the ankle may be carried out. The cast is then put back together and secured. That routine may be continued for 4 to 6 weeks, or until there is evidence of union. At that time, the cast is completely removed, and active range-of-motion exercises and protected weight bearing using crutches are begun. Those measures are continued until union is complete. If the lateral malleolus has not been securely fixed, the patient may be placed in a long leg cast (midthigh to toes with the knee flexed at 45 degrees and the foot in mild plantar flexion and internal rotation). If the long leg cast is utilized, it is used for only 4 to 6 weeks and then a short leg cast is worn until union is achieved. As a rule, malleolar fractures require 10 to 12 weeks to unite.

Depending on the amount of swelling, patients with a Pott's fracture may be able to ambulate on crutches shortly after surgery. Until there are signs of union, the patient is not allowed weight bearing; therefore, the patient will need to utilize a three-point crutch gait (Appendix C). Teach the patient exercises to help build up strength in the arms. Before getting the patient out of bed to walk with crutches, explain that there will be pain or throbbing in the affected foot when it is lowered to the floor, and that the foot may become discolored. When the patient sits in a chair or returns to bed, the foot should once more be elevated, and the normal color will return.

If the patient needs a bedpan, keep the leg elevated on pillows while placing a fracture bedpan under the patient's buttocks from the side of the body opposite the cast. If the patient is able to assist, have him or her use the trapeze to lift the buttocks off the mattress while you slide the bedpan under them. Another approach is for the patient to use the trapeze to lift while at the same time pushing against the bed with the uninvolved leg. (For care of a patient following repair of a fractured hip, see Chap. 6.)

Prevent Complications. The complications most common with Pott's fractures are incomplete reduction, nonunion, and infection at the fracture site. Although they are not necessarily problems that can be prevented by nursing measures, the alert nurse should be able to detect symptoms of such conditions so that appropriate action can be taken.

Skin complications can easily occur. Patients who have plaster of Paris casts following an open reduction do not have a stockinette under the plaster. Thus, edges of the cast are rough and need to be petaled when the cast is dry to protect the skin. (For discussion on how to petal a cast and the care of a cast, see Appendix B). When a window is made in the cast to change a dressing or to remove sutures, make sure the cast window is replaced and secured with tape so there will not be swelling at the site of the window.

Patient Teaching. The patient needs answers to questions concerning the postoperative course of treatment, the length of time before weight bearing, and the length of time of immobilization. The amount of time off from work depends on the patient's condition, the type of work, and the health and safety policies of the patient's employer.

Once the patient is allowed to return home, make sure the patient, the family, and significant others understand cast care, how to detect complications related to the cast, and how to perform personal hygiene with a cast (Appendix B). One thing some patients want to do is drive their car. Driving may not be feasible unless the patient's right leg is unaffected and the patient has a car with an automatic transmission.

A patient going home immediately after have a cast applied (following a closed reduction) must be even more knowledgeable about the cast. Teach the patient how to assess for neurovascular deficiencies. Have the patient contact the physician if any of the following occur: (1) increasing pain, (2) pain unrelieved by prescribed medication, (3) swelling unrelieved by elevating the leg for at least an hour, (4) a change of sensation in the toes (e.g., numbness, tingling, or burning), (5) decreased movement or loss of movement in the toes, (6) a change in skin color above or below the cast, (7) a bad smell coming from inside the cast, (8) a warm area or fresh stain on the cast, (9) a foreign object dropped into or stuck in the cast, and (10) a weakened, cracked, loose, or tight cast.

Instruct the patient to keep the plaster cast elevated on two pillows and uncovered for at least 48 hours (or as ordered by the physician) as the cast dries. In addition, instruct the patient to use the palms and not the fingertips to frequently change the position of the casted leg on the pillows. Remind the patient that all these measures promote even cast drying and help reduce swelling. Warn the patient that the wet cast will feel heavy, but reassure that as the cast dries it will get lighter. Caution the patient against walking on the cast before weight bearing is allowed.

Discuss the observations necessary to ensure comfort and prevent complications. For example, show the patient how to move the toes to assess motion. Because the leg will be in the cast for some time, explain the importance of exercise in preventing complications. Also, demonstrate how to perform any special exercises ordered. Emphasize cast care as discussed in Appendix B. Give the patient a copy of home care instructions.

Evaluation and Reassessment

Determine whether the patient has been provided with sufficient data to feel confident about going home with a cast and ambulating on crutches. If not, ask specific questions to determine what the patient does not understand, and explain it again. Postoperative pain should have been reduced by nursing measures and medication. If not, observe for signs and symptoms of complications or consider the possibility of requesting a change in pain medications.

Pathology

ARTHRITIS AND INFECTIOUS DISEASES

Rheumatoid Arthritis

The ankle is a joint with sizable synovium that can become inflamed. With rheumatoid arthritis, the synovitis may also injure the adjacent ligaments so that the ankle joint slips, or subluxes, the ligaments are strained, and pain and instability result (Fries, 1982, p. 180). Walking on an unstable ankle increases trauma to the joint, but if the ankle is stabilized, walking is to be encouraged to prevent stiffness. Unless the ankle is carefully supported by splints during the acute stage of rheumatoid arthritis of the ankle, an equinus deformity can develop and rapidly become fixed. An equinus deformity of long duration is corrected by lengthening the tendo calcaneus and dividing the posterior capsule. If the joint is ankylosed, an osteotomy is made to realign the foot, the tendo calcaneus is lengthened if necessary, and the ankle is then fused (Edmondson & Crenshaw, 1980, p. 1171).

The development of a stiff flat foot and a valgus heel deformity produce symptoms in patients with rheumatoid arthritis. A painful rheumatoid arthritis of the ankle can be relieved by a period of nonweight bearing and local steroid injections. A painful ankle may also be helped by wearing supportive ankle boots or ankle braces rather than regular shoes. Crutches or a cane are often a help during a period of exacerbation, as they take weight off a painful ankle (Swinson & Swinburn, 1980, pp. 56–57).

Ankle fusion for severe rheumatoid arthritis has been a satisfactory procedure. However, careful evaluation of the ipsilateral subtalar and knee joints should be done before the ankle is fused. When the subtalar joint is involved, fusing the ankle joint can concentrate the stresses on that joint and cause considerable pain. In such a situation, a total ankle arthroplasty may be indicated. For rheumatoid arthritis of the subtalar joint for which surgical treatment is necessary, a triple arthrodesis (see pp. 460–461) is usually the procedure of choice, but the functional status of the ankle joint influences the decision.

Rheumatoid tenosynovitis about the ankle and the subtalar joint may be symptomatic and disabling. Excision of diseased sheaths or of an exostosis associated with the tibialis posterior or peroneal tendons can often relieve symptoms sufficiently to avoid an ankle fusion (Edmondson & Crenshaw, 1980, p. 1173).

Osteoarthritis

Osteoarthritis, a degenerative process of the articular cartilage, rarely becomes as advanced in the ankle as it does in the hip or the knee unless intensified by an underlying disease process or trauma. Consequently, when advanced osteoarthritic changes develop in the ankle joint, contributory factors are sought in determining an appropriate corrective regime. The main underlying factors could be idiopathic, trauma, infection, other forms of arthritis, neoplasia, deformity, or blood dyscrasia (Turek, 1977, p. 266).

Most patients with osteoarthritis of the ankle give a history of sustaining a fracture, fracture–dislocation, or infection of the ankle joint some years previously. Gradually, symptoms typical of osteoarthritis appear, namely pain and stiffness pronounced at rest and relieved by activity, heat, and salicylates. Swelling in the joints may be due to increased joint fluid (which can be confirmed by aspiration) or may be caused by thickening of the capsular tissues. There is usually moderate generalized tenderness, and joint motion is often restricted. The gait is typically antalgic, short and halting, with a painful dorsiflexion just before the toe is lifted off.

Roentgenography demonstrates that the joint space becomes gradually narrowed as the subchondral cortex becomes dense and irregular. Beneath the subchrondral cortices, cysts may develop. Marginal bony outgrowths appear, particularly at the anterior tibial border. There may be evidence of an old malunited fracture, a deformed, dense astragalus suggesting an old avascular necrosis, a punched out gouty lesion, or severe demineralization and erosive defects that suggest an infectious or rheumatoid process (Turek, 1977, p.

1267). Locally, arthrography may demonstrate intra-articular soft tissue pathology.

Osteoarthritis of the ankle joint is not necessarily painful and disabling. Intermittent episodes can often be controlled by conservative means, such as rest, no weight bearing, application of heat, and salicylates, but these means are only temporarily effective in most cases. The ankle can be immobilized in a bivalved cast or plaster support, or placed in a brace that limits the motion of the ankle. Injections of corticosteroids into the joint space can provide temporary symptomatic relief. Persistence of symptoms, particularly pain severe enought to constitute a continuous disability, is an indication for surgical intervention. The surgery may be: (1) debridement and synovectomy, to maintain joint motion by removing loose bodies and part of the synovium; (2) denervation of the ankle joint, particularly the distal branches of the posterior tibial nerve and the lateral terminal division of the deep peroneal nerve to relieve pain; (3) arthrodesis or fusion of the ankle joint to eliminate motion and relieve pain; and (4) total ankle replacement (Turek, 1977, p. 1268).

Tuberculosis of the Ankle and the Foot

As tuberculosis spreads through the blood from a primary source, usually in the lungs, it often lodges simultaneously at various sites throughout the foot. Both the ankle and the foot are almost always simultaneously involved, as the disease moves through intercommunicating synovial channels or along soft tissue planes. The first and most common manifestation of infection is a synovitis of the ankle or tarsal joints. Subsequent manifestations can follow two different patterns. In one, there is a disease of the synovium or extrasynovial soft tissues that spreads to involve several joints and causes pain, tenderness, local heat, and diffused swelling. In the other, there is a localized bone lesion that at first produces low-grade symptoms, such as a chronic, dull aching, with inflammatory signs developing much later.

Certain bones appear more predisposed to tuberculosis. In infants, they are the metatarsals; in children, the tarsal bones; and in adults, the ankle bones. In older adults, the talus is the bone must often involved, with simultaneous infection of the subtalar and sometimes the talonavicular joint.

The onset of the disease is insidious, and may appear as a synovitis of the ankle joint causing effusion, periarticular soft tissue swelling, limitation of ankle motion, pain, limp, local warmth, and tenderness. Characteristically, the soft tissue swelling is doughy, only slightly tender, and barely warm. It tends to subside at rest and reappears with walking. Eventually, the swelling becomes persistent, pain increases in intensity, and ankle motion becomes progressively restricted. As the subastragalar joint becomes increasingly involved, pain occurs with each step at heel-strike. The pain is situated in the hindfoot and the peroneal areas and can be reproduced by passive side-to-side movement of the heel. The swelling extends about the dorsolateral aspect of the tarsal area, and as the infection extends toward the tarsometatarsal joint. One can reproduce the pain and demonstrate involvement of the distal joint by torsion (i.e., twisting the forefoot while the heel is held immobilized). More often the presence of tuberculosis is discovered on roentgenograms.

Medical Treatment

Antituberculosis drug regime is instituted, even if surgery is indicated, and may be started several months before surgery. To immobilize the ankle, a cast is applied from the upper thigh to the toes with the ankle at 10 degrees of equinus so that a functional position is attained in the event that fusion takes place as healing occurs. When drug therapy and immobilization are instituted early, these nonoperative treatments produce an apparent "cure" in 90 percent of the patients, and many will regain normal function (Turek, 1977, p. 1269).

The objectives of surgery for tuberculosis of the ankle area are to remove grossly diseased tissue, to improve the effectiveness of antituberculosis drugs, and, if possible, to prevent involvement of the adjacent joints, thereby preserving motion. A highly variable degree of involvement and distribution of infective foci requires a wide variety of applicable procedures, including (1) arthrotomy for synovial biopsy, partial synovectomy, and debridement and curettage of surface lesions, (2) excision of an isolated large bone lesion, with or without bone grafts, (3) total ostectomy of one or several bones (e.g., astragalectomy, metatarsectomy), (4) arthrodesis, and (5) amputation (e.g., of an infected toe) (Turek, 1977, p. 1269).

Arthrodesis

An ankle arthrodesis (fusion) (Fig. 8–8) is an operation to induce bony ankylosis in the ankle joint (1) to relieve pain, (2) to halt disease, or (3) to provide stability. The operative technique for fusion may be (1) intra-articular, (2) intra-articular and extra-articular, or (3) extra-articular. The choice of technique

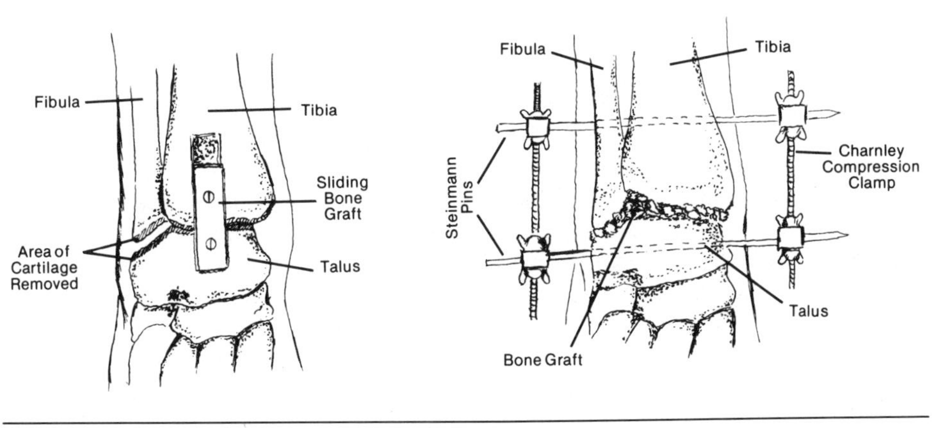

Figure 8–8. Anterior view, ankle fusion. *(From Brantley, P., & Analla, M., 1980, p. 127. Courtesy of Howmedica.)*

for any given patient depends on the patient's age, the pathological process involving the joint, and the presence or absence of a gross deformity in the joint.

With the intra-articular method, the articular surfaces are denuded to permit the approximation of cancellous bony surfaces and to allow for a more satisfactory correction of any deformity. Grafts of autogenous cancellous bone help to achieve more rapid and certain fusion. This method is used if there is a need to remove diseased tissue, as is often the case in tuberculosis.

A combination of intra-articular and extra-articular techniques is useful in many different circumstances, including tubercular, infected, and arthritic joints. The joint capsule is incised, as much of the synovium as possible is excised, the articular surfaces are denuded, and bone grafts are placed across the joint.

An extra-articular arthrodesis is a method of obtaining a union between normal bony surfaces entirely outside the joint capsule. Many of the extra-articular techniques devised for tubercular joints are now used in conjuction with intra-articular techniques.

SURGICAL PROCEDURE. Indications for an arthrodesis are pain and disability due to rheumatoid, traumatic, or degenerative arthritis, or to a malunited fracture of the ankle. In a typical ankle fusion procedure (see Fig. 8–8), the first step is to denude the surfaces of the talus, the tibia, and both malleoli and correct any deviations from correct alignment. A bone graft (e.g., a sliding graft from the anterior distal tibia, the proximal tibia, or the iliac crest) is then placed across the joint line of the anterior distal tibia and the talus. Steinmann pins can then be placed across the talus and the tibia where Charnley compression clamps are applied to them. Additional bone chips may then be added to fill in any space between the malleoli and the talus. The procedure may also be done utilizing bone grafts alone or utilizing Steinmann pins and Charnley clamps without a sliding bone graft. The patient is then placed in a short leg cast.

☐ NURSING PROCESS (Table 8–3)

Assessment

After a general assessment for a postoperative patient, special emphasis should be given to the fused ankle. The patient will be in a short leg cast with or without Steinmann pins and Charnley compression clamps. Check the neurovascular status of the involved foot (Chap. 2). Note any bleeding into the cast. The foot, elevated on pillows, should be free of any pressure areas, especially around the heel. The Steinmann pins and Charnley compression clamps should be free of any entanglement with the linen and in most instances sterile corks or other protective devices are placed over the sharp ends of the pins. Check the cast for pressure areas and for dryness if a plaster of Paris cast is used. Assess the patient for pain due to surgery. Correct the positioning of the involved leg and make certain that the total body is in correct alignment.

With an ankle fusion, most surgical procedures involve a bone graft. The most common donor site is the iliac crest. Check the dressing for any bleeding and pain at the donor site.

Nursing Diagnosis and Goal Formulation

The nursing diagnoses for the typical patient after an ankle fusion are (1) alterations in comfort related to pain from surgery, (2) alterations in mobility related to surgical fusion of the ankle joint, (3) potential complications related to surgical procedure and decreased activity, and (4) alterations in psychological well-being related to anxiety and knowledge deficit about injury, surgical procedure, and prognosis.

Short-term goals are (1) an absence of pain in the ankle, (2) a return of mobility with ankle immobilized in a cast and the use of assistive devices, (3) an absence of complications from surgery and decreased activity, and (4) a decrease in anxiety through an understanding of the surgical treatment and the prognosis. Long-term goals are to have the ankle free of pain and to have a stable ankle joint that permits walking with a safe gait.

Planning and Intervention

Alleviate Pain. Nursing measures that focus on pain relief are elevating the leg to prevent or reduce swelling, using ice bags, and placing the leg in correct anatomical alignment. The patient can help keep the affected leg in alignment and should be advised to look down along the leg periodically to see that it is properly positioned. Normally a line from the anterior superior spine to the second toe should pass over the mid-patella. If the position is incorrect, pain is likely to result. To allow for swelling, a rectangular window is sometimes cut in the cast over the dorsum of the foot and ankle. The window is then held loosely in place with bandages.

Increase Mobility. To increase mobility the focus of nursing care is to help the patient develop arm strength for crutch walking. Many of these patients may have been on crutches previously, but with a different gait. In every case, it is necessary to check the correctness and safety of gait. Because of the short leg cast, first ambulation on crutches is with a three-point nonweight-bearing gait.

The period of immobilization depends on the type of fusion and the results of roentgenograms. For postsurgical patients with a short leg cast and Steinmann pins, the cast is worn for 4 to 6 weeks with nonweight bearing. The pins are then removed and a walking boot cast is applied and worn for another 4 to 6 weeks until the fusion is solid. Other patients may receive a boot or walking cast 4 weeks after surgery, and partial weight bearing may be cautiously resumed. Full weight bearing is usually delayed for 8 to 12 weeks after the operation. Cast immobilization is continued

TABLE 8–3. NURSING PROCESS FOR ANKLE FUSION WITH CAST APPLICATION

Assessment	Nursing Diagnosis	Goal Formulation	Planning and Intervention	Evaluation and Reassessment
1. Assess the location, duration, and severity of pain. Assess the tightness of the cast. Check for areas of swelling.	1. Alteration in comfort: pain in the ankle related to bone and soft tissue trauma.	1. Short-term goal: a reduction in ankle pain. Long-term goal: free of any pain.	1. Alleviate Pain Elevate the involved foot. Keep pressure off of the heel. Apply ice bags along the sides of the ankle. Administer pain medications. Utilize noninvasive nursing measures.	1. The patient should remain relatively free of pain in the ankle and donor site with medication.
2. Check the positioning of the foot and total body. Check that the foot is securely elevated. Assess the patient's ability to ambulate safely with crutches.	2. Impaired physical mobility: a decrease in ankle function related to joint instability.	2. Short-term goal: an increase in mobility through immobilization. Long-term goal: regain optimal function with a fused ankle.	2. Increase Mobility *Position* Keep the foot elevated with no pressure on the heel. Turn to any position of comfort. Teach how to use trapeze. *Exercises* Teach isometric, straight leg and upper extremity exercises for crutch walking and active range-of-motion exercises for all unaffected joints. *Ambulation* Demonstrate crutch walking using a three-point gait.	2. The foot should be kept elevated except during ambulation. Exercises should be done without supervision. Ambulation should be done safely with no weight bearing for the first 6 weeks, partial weight bearing for the next 4 weeks, and then full weight bearing at 8 (to 12) weeks. Some patients should wear a cast for 2–3 months after surgery.

3. Assess the neurovascular status. Check for any areas of swelling. Check position of the leg.	3. Potential for injury: neurovascular deficit related to soft tissue swelling.	3. Short- and long-term goal: free of any neurovascular deficit.	3. Prevent Complications *Circulatory* Keep the foot elevated. Utilize nursing measures to reduce any swelling. After surgery, do neurovascular checks every 15 minutes for the first 2 hours, every 30 minutes for the next 2 hours, every 60 minutes for the next 2 hours, every 2 hours for the next 18 hours, and then at least at the beginning of every shift. Report any neurovascular abnormalities.	3. The patient should be free of any circulatory or integumentary complications.
Note any drainage. Check for any signs of infection. Note any complaints of pressure areas over bony prominences.	Potential for injury related to surgical incision. Potential impairment of skin integrity: pressure area related to the cast.	Short- and long-term goal: free of any integumentary complications.	*Integumentary* Discuss a well-balanced diet. Trim and petal cast edges. Report any signs of pressure. *Potential Complications* Complications of immobility (see Chap. 3).	
4. Assess knowledge level about the rehabilitation process and self-care.	4. Potential knowledge deficit related to rehabilitation process and self-care.	4. Short- and long-term goal: a decrease in anxiety through an increase in knowledge.	4. Patient Teaching Discuss the various steps of the rehabilitation process. Discuss cast care. Include family and significant other in the teaching plan. Discuss methods of bathing and dressing.	4. Determine if the family and significant other have been provided with data to cope with the long-term rehabilitation and the potential permanent changes in gait.

until the ankle joint is solidly fused. Some patients have cast walking delayed for 2 or 3 months after surgery and then after an additional 3 to 4 months go into a short leg brace with a rigid ankle joint. The short leg brace is worn until roentgenograms show a solid fusion.

Prevent Complications. Following an ankle arthrodesis, the most common potential complications are infection, nonunion, and malunion. To prevent complications from decreased activity, the nurse needs to focus on the total patient. Exercises for all uninvolved joints, to be done at least twice a day, should be encouraged. In the absence of other pathology, the patient is able to do most of the activities of daily living. Work with the patient and occupational therapist in developing activities to help stimulate both the patient's mind and body.

Patient Teaching. Patient teaching plays a vital role in helping the patient and the family adjust to the long rehabilitation period. Make sure the patient has a clear understanding of crutch walking, cast care, personal hygiene, and dressing with a short leg cast on. Teach the patient how to walk with a safe gait and without ankle motion. In doing so, remember that the position of the fused ankle and the condition of the other joints of the foot influence how well the patient is able to walk.

Evaluation and Reassessment

Evaluation and reassessment of the nursing care of a patient following an ankle arthrodesis concentrates on the type and the amount of pain and the effective measures taken to relieve the pain. If the pain has increased, is the neurovascular status good, is the cast too tight, or are there signs of an infection?

Determine if the patient, the family, and significant others have been provided with data to cope with the long rehabilitation and the potential of a permanent change in gait. If not, review the content area that is unclear. Support persons, such as clergy, psychiatric nurses, or support services personnel, may be useful in helping the patient adjust to the change in body image.

Total Ankle Arthroplasty

Total ankle arthroplasty is used for patients with severe traumatic, degenerative, and rheumatoid arthritis, avascular necrosis or absence of the talus, and failure of ankle fusion. There are numerous total ankle arthroplasty designs available, consisting primarily of polyethylene and stainless steel components (Fig. 8–9). These are classified as constrained or semiconstrained (i.e., restricted motion) joints and nonconstrained (i.e., unrestricted motion) joints. The total ankle surgical procedure involves osteotomies of portions of the distal tibia and the proximal talus. A proximal metallic tibial component and its poly-

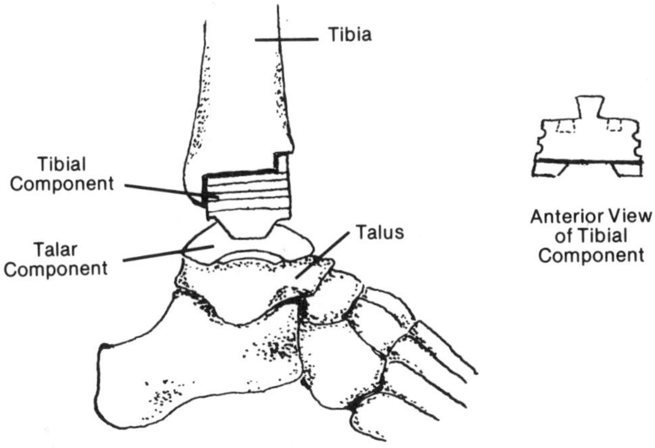

Figure 8–9. Total ankle arthroplasty, lateral view. *(From Brantley, P., & Analla, M., 1980, p. 113. Courtesy of Howmedica.)*

ethylene talar dome component are then cemented into place with methyl methacryalate. Suction drainage tubes are brought out through a puncture wound proximal to the incision. The wound is closed and a bulky pressure dressing and posterior plaster splint (to decrease edema after surgery) are applied (Edmondson & Crenshaw, 1980, p. 2157).

□ NURSING PROCESS (Table 8–4)

Assessment

After a general assessment for a surgical patient, special emphasis should be given to the reconstructed ankle. The patient will return to the unit with a large dressing, and in most instances a posterior splint to keep the ankle in correct alignment. Assess the extremity for nerve and circulatory function (Chap. 2). Assess for the type, amount, and kind of pain. Check that the leg is elevated and secure. (For further discussion on the assessment, see assessment of the patient with a sprained ankle, p. 431.)

Nursing Diagnosis and Goal Formulation

Nursing diagnoses for a typical patient following a total ankle arthroplasty are (1) alterations in comfort related to pain from the surgical procedure, (2) alterations in mobility related to lack of ankle joint stability, (3) potential complications related to surgical procedure and decreased activity, and (4) alterations in psychological well-being related to anxiety and knowledge deficit about the injury, the surgical procedure, and the prognosis.

Short-term goals are (1) a reduction of soft tissue swelling to decrease pain, (2) an increase in ankle mobility through controlled exercises, (3) an

TABLE 8–4. NURSING PROCESS FOR TOTAL ANKLE ARTHROPLASTY WITH POSTERIOR SPLINT

Assessment	Nursing Diagnosis	Goal Formulation	Planning and Intervention	Evaluation and Reassessment
1. Assess for location, duration, and severity of pain. Check for areas of swelling.	1. Alteration in comfort: pain in the ankle related to bone and soft tissue swelling.	1. Short-term goal: a relative state of comfort. Long-term goal: free of pain.	1. Alleviate Pain Elevate the foot. Apply ice along the sides of the ankle. Teach relaxation techniques. Administer pain medications.	1. Pain should be relieved with nursing measures and prescribed medications.
2. Assess neurovascular status. Check for correct alignment of the foot. Assess the ability to do exercises and to ambulate with crutches. Assess strength in the upper extremities for crutch walking.	2. Impaired physical mobility: decreased ankle function related to lack of joint stability.	2. Short-term goal: an increase in joint function through controlled exercises. Long-term goal: regain optimal ankle function.	2. Increase Mobility *Position* Keep the foot elevated on pillows. Turn to any position of comfort. Instruct on how to use trapeze. *Exercises* Teach gentle active range-of-motion exercises for the foot and active range of motion for all other joints. Instruct on exercises to the upper extremities for crutch walking. Teach quadriceps and gluteal setting exercises. *Ambulation* Demonstrate crutch walking. Ambulate on the second postoperative day with no weight-bearing on the involved foot.	2. The foot should be kept elevated and range-of-motion exercises done without supervision. Ambulation with no weightbearing on the involved foot and with the use of crutches should be accomplished safely.

3. Assess the neurovascular status. Check for areas of swelling and tightness of splint or dressing. Check that the foot is elevated.	3. Potential for injury: neurovascular deficit related to soft tissue swelling.	3. Short- and long-term goal: free of any neurovascular complications.	3. Prevent Complications *Circulatory* After surgery, do neurovascular status checks every 15 minutes for the first 2 hours, every 30 minutes for the next 2 hours, every 60 minutes for the next 2 hours, every 2 hours for the next 18 hours, and then at least at the beginning of every shift. Encourage gentle range-of-motion exercises. Keep foot elevated.	3. The patient should remain free of any neurovascular deficit.
Check for tightness of the splint. Assess the skin along the edges of the splint. Note any drainage.	Potential for injury: infection related to surgical incision or a break in skin integrity.	Short- and long-term goal: free of any break in skin integrity or infection.	*Integumentary* Pad the edges of the splint. Keep dressing clean and dry. Utilize measures to reduce swelling.	There should be no signs of a break in skin integrity or infection.
4. Assess knowledge of rehabilitation process and self-care.	4. Potential for knowledge deficit related to the rehabilitation process and self-care.	4. Short- and long-term goal: a decrease in anxiety through an increase in knowledge.	4. Patient Teaching Discuss the various steps in the rehabilitation process. Include family and significant other in the teaching plan. Clarify any questions. Discuss methods of bathing and dressing.	4. Determine that the patient feels confident in ambulating and in giving self-care. The patient should understand the exercise regime and the rehabilitation process.

absence of complications from the surgical procedure and decreased activity, and (4) patient understanding of the surgical procedure and the prognosis for ankle function. Long-term goals are to have the ankle free of pain and with restored function.

Planning and Intervention

Alleviate Pain. Nursing measures to help reduce and relieve pain are similar to those discussed for a patient with a fractured ankle (see p. 440).

Increase Mobility. The leg is elevated as much as possible until soft tissues have healed. When wound suction drainage tubes are removed, approximately 24 to 48 hours after surgery, the patient is allowed up with no weight bearing. The bulky dressing and the posterior splint are removed on about the fifth postoperative day, and may be replaced with a short leg cast. Short periods of weight bearing are then begun when tolerated by the patient, but elevation of the leg should be encouraged for at least 2 weeks following surgery. Approximately 2 weeks after application, the cast is removed and a range-of-motion exercise program emphasizing dorsiflexion should be instituted (Edmondson & Crenshaw, 1980, p. 2157).

Prevent Complications. Complications following a total ankle arthroplasty are similar to the major complications following a total knee arthroplasty (Chap. 7). Special attention should be given to the prevention of infection.

Patient Teaching. Explain the purposes and importance of elevating the foot and avoiding weight bearing until soft tissue healing has occurred. Work with the physical therapist, the patient, and the patient's family in implementing the exercise regime. Help the patient work out a time schedule so adequate time is allowed to do the exercises without being rushed.

Discuss with the patient and the patient's family the rehabilitation process, so that they will have realistic expectations about the surgery and the likelihood of the patient's regaining function of the ankle and the ability to walk. It should be stressed that to obtain maximal return of function, the patient must conscientiously follow the prescribed exercise regime.

Evaluation and Reassessment

The patient should have minimal pain and stiffness, which are usually relieved by medication and exercise. If swelling does occur, elevate the foot and continue with the exercises. If the swelling continues to increase and pain is not relieved by medication, notify the physician.

Determine how confident the patient feels in ambulating and in giving self-care. Check that the patient understands the exercise regime and the rehabilitation process. It may be beneficial for the patient to again talk with someone who has had a total ankle arthroplasty so that the patient's expectations will be realistic.

AMPUTATIONS

Amputations near the ankle are relatively infrequent, but may be done for severe trauma and infection. The most common such amputation, the Syme amputation (Fig. 8–10), is done at the level of the distal tibia and the fibula 0.6 cm proximal to the ankle joint, and the durable skin of the heel flap is used to provide the weight-bearing skin (Edmondson & Crenshaw, 1980, p 831). The amputation must leave a weight-bearing stump and enough space between the end of the stump and the ground so that a prosthesis with a functioning ankle joint can be worn.

The prosthesis, which must accommodate the distal tibial metaphysis, is rather large and bulky. For that reason, a below-knee amputation is often recommended for women. The prosthesis is a molded plastic socket with a removable medial window to allow passage of the bulbous end of the stump through its narrow shank, and a solid-ankle-cushion-heel (SACH) foot.

Most patients following a Syme amputation have a cast. Sutures are usually removed after 2 weeks. Weight bearing is not allowed for at least 8 weeks (others may have weight bearing much sooner). A walking cast is then applied and left on until arthrodesis is complete. The focus of nursing care is in helping the patient and significant other to adjust to the change in body image and in learning to walk with or without a prosthesis. (For further discussion of nursing care, see the amputation discussions in Chaps. 6 and 7.) The two most common causes of an unsatisfactory Syme amputation are the posterior migration of the heel pad and skin slough.

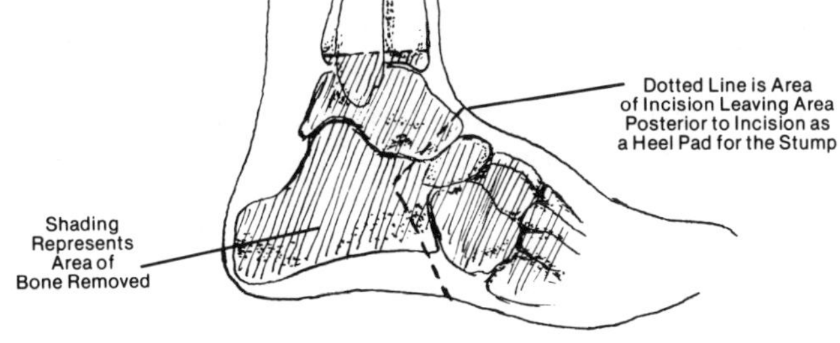

Figure 8–10. Syme's amputation. *(From Brantley, P., & Analla, M., 1980, p. 114. Courtesy of Howmedica.)*

THE FOOT

Trauma

FRACTURES

Heel Fractures

A fracture is suspected when a patient has pain in the heel following trauma. The calcaneus is the most frequently fractured of the tarsal bones. Fractures may be caused by a powerful contraction of the gastrocnemius and soleus muscles or by direct trauma to the heel (e.g., when a falling person lands on the feet). As a rule, two general types of fractures occur, avulsion fractures through the posterior portion of the bone, and comminuted or crush fractures involving the talocalcaneal joint (Gartland, 1979, p. 451). A fracture of the calcaneus may also be accompanied by a compression fracture of a vertebra or an avulsion of the Achilles tendon from its insertion.

Characteristic signs of a fractured calcaneus bone are that the heel is broadened, and the hollows beneath the malleoli are obliterated because of exudate. Later ecchymosis appears around the heel. All movements of the calcaneus are painful and markedly restricted. Roentgenograms help to confirm the presence, site, and extent of the fracture (Cailliet, 1981, p. 115).

Medical treatment is focused on restoring the contour of the bone, particularly the plantar surface and the talocalcaneal joint, while maintaining joint motion. Many of the fractures are treated with no attempted reduction, but by compression dressings, nonweight bearing, and early joint motion. Fractures with substantial widening of the calcaneus, however, are usually reduced by manual compression and are immobilized using a short leg cast. (For nursing care of a patient with a short leg cast, see pp. 437–442.) Some fractures may require surgical intervention. Depending on the location of the fracture and the degree of comminution, the fracture may be repaired by skeletal traction, pin fixation, or open reduction with bone graft.

Fractures of the calcaneus may result in prolonged incapacity and in some cases permanent disability and pain. The major complication is the development of traumatic arthritis at the talocalcaneal joint. If this occurs, the patient will have pain on weight bearing, particularly with motions requiring eversion and inversion of the foot. If the patient persists despite nonoperative methods, a triple arthrodesis may be done.

Metatarsal Fractures

Fractures of the metatarsal bones are common, and may be caused by twisting injuries of the forefoot or by heavy objects dropping on the foot. A fracture through the neck of the metatarsal may allow the metatarsal head to displace toward the sole of the foot. Repairs are directed at restoring and maintaining the normal alignment of the longitudinal arch and preventing the subsequent development of a painful plantar callus (Gartland, 1979, p. 450).

Many displaced metatarsal fractures can be treated by closed reduction and immobilization in a short leg cast. If that is unsuccessful, skeletal traction, percutaneous pinning, or open reduction with internal metallic fixation (using Kirschner wires) may be done (Fig. 8–11). If an open reduction with internal fixation is done, a short leg cast is usually applied. After 3 weeks, the Kirschner wires are removed and a walking boot cast is applied for another 3 to 5 weeks, until the fracture is well healed (Brantley & Analla, 1980, p. 124).

March Fractures

A march fracture is a stress fracture of a metatarsal shaft, often involving minimal or no trauma. Such fractures can occur during a long march, hence the name. Roentgenograms may be negative initially because the fracture is hairline with no displacment of fragments. Later, as callus forms around the fracture, roentgenography reveals that a fracture existed. Clinically, there is a tenderness at the middle of the involved metatarsal shaft, flexion or extension of the toes may be painful. Treatment usually consists of avoidance of weight bearing or walking, depending upon the severity of the symptoms. When

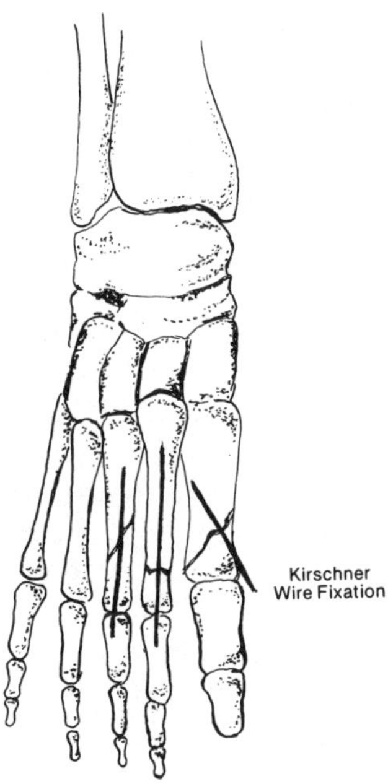

Figure 8–11. Open reduction of fractured metatarsal. *(From Brantley, P., & Analla, M., 1980, p. 124. Courtesy of Howmedica.)*

symptoms are severe, a walking cast may be applied for 3 to 4 weeks (Cailliet, 1981, p. 280).

Fractures of Toes

A toe fracture is usually caused by trauma, such as by a weight falling on a toe or by stubbing a toe while barefoot. As a rule, these are painful but not serious injuries. The objective of treatment is to maintain the alignment of the toes so that overlapping or hammertoe does not occur. Frequently this can be accomplished by strapping the broken toe to its neighbor or simply by wearing a sock. If multiple toe fractures are present, a walking cast may be applied for immobilization (Gartland, 1979, p. 450). (For nursing care of a patient with a short leg cast, see pp. 437–442.)

Pathology

ARTHRITIS AND INFECTIOUS DISEASES

Rheumatoid Arthritis

Rheumatoid arthritis frequently affects the forefoot, and leads to the development of stiff painful feet. With rheumatoid arthritis, there is inflammation and subluxation of the metatarsophalangeal (MTP) joints. Typically, the forefoot broadens and the metatarsal heads are depressed into the sole of the foot. The subluxation is upward producing a clawing of the toes (Garland, 1979, p. 144; Swinson & Swinburn, 1980, pp. 44–45). The skin under the subluxed joints becomes thickened to form calluses, producing a sensation that has been compared to walking on marbles. The arthritis may also affect the ankle joint, producing pain and decreased movement, especially when walking. The subtalar and tarsal joints may become involved, causing a stiff flat foot with a valgus heel deformity.

The problem of MTP subluxation and callus formation can be dealt with in a number of ways. Simple paring of the callus can reduce discomfort, but that has to be repeated. Wearing pads that lie just behind the MTP heads takes some of the weight off the MTP joint. Attaching a transverse metatarsal bar to the patient's shoe can serve the same purpose. Another nonsurgical approach is to provide surgical shoes, which are designed to fit the sole of the patient's foot so that body weight is well distributed and every part of the foot is well supported.

In many patients, Fowler's operation, where the painful MTP joints (or the metatarsal heads) are excised (Fig. 8–12), may be necessary to allow the toes to drop down into a more functional position (Gartland, 1979, p. 114; Swinson & Swinburn, 1980, p. 56).

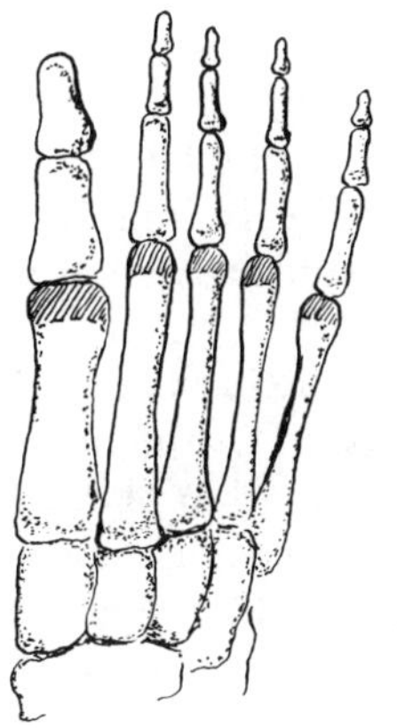

Figure 8–12. Excision of metatarsal head. *(From Brantley, P., & Analla, M., 1980, p. 121. Courtesy of Howmedica.)*

Osteoarthritis

The joint in the foot that most frequently develops osteoarthritis is the big toe joint (i.e., the first MTP joint). The condition, which is more common in men, is characterized by spurring (osteophytosis) around the MTP joint, producing a stiff and painful toe known as hallux rigidus. Treatment is by adapting shoes to prevent the bending of the first MTP joint during walking. If that is ineffective, fusion of the joint or Keller's operation may be indicated.

Hallux valgus is associated with the development of osteoarthritis of the first MTP joint together with bunion formation. This deformity is more common in women, and is aggravated by wearing shoes with high heels or shoes that do not provide proper support to the forefoot. Pain is common and is usually due to an inflammation of the associated bunion. (For further discussion of hallux valgus, see pp. 468–471.)

Traumatic Arthritis

Arthritis of the subtalar joint frequently follows trauma, such as a fracture of the calcaneus. Pain that is felt within the heel may be referred from an arthritic subtalar joint. Movement of the subtalar joint is painful, and roentgenograms usually reveal an irregularity of the bones between the talus and the calcaneus. Crepitation may be elicited by joint motion, and tenderness can be caused by pressure over the sinus tarsi in front of the lateral malleolus. Muscle spasm, especially of the peroneal group, may occur, producing a "splinting" of the subtalar joint. Weight bearing is painful, but rest gives relief. Conservative treatment is usually unsatisfactory, and surgical fusion may be necessary if symptoms persist (Cailliet, 1981, p. 114).

Posterior Calcaneal Bursitis

Pain and tenderness of the posterior aspect of the heel may be due to a postcalcaneal bursitis, an inflammation of the bursa located between the Achilles tendon and the skin (Fig 8–13). The condition is usually caused by friction from ill-fitting shoes, and is common in women who wear high heels. The bursa is usually visibly inflamed and often distended with fluid. Chronic irritation thickens the walls of the bursa and the overlying skin.

Examination reveals an inflamed and thickened area at the back of the heel, produced by the rubbing of the upper margin of the shoe. Treatment begins with properly fitted shoes that have moderately low heels. Moleskin placed over the thickened skin prevents further friction, or the back of the shoe may be cut out or the heel of the foot raised inside the shoe to prevent further aggravation of the bursa. Surgical excision of the bursa is never indicated. Drainage of the swollen bursa may be accomplished by needle aspiration followed by the insertion of hydrocortisone into the bursal sac (Cailliet, 1981, p. 112).

Tuberculosis

Tuberculosis of the bones of the foot, particularly the calcaneus and the talus, may occur at any age. When several bones of the foot are involved, amputation has been the procedure of choice for adults, because the extensive excisions required usually leave a deformed and worthless extremity. Alternative surgical procedures, which may be used for less extensive infections, are curettage and bone excisions (Edmondson & Crenshaw, 1980, p. 1082). (For further discussion on tuberculosis of the foot and ankle, see p. 444.)

Arthrodesis

An arthrodesis of the foot may be done by a number of procedures. One is the Dunn arthrodesis, where the navicular is removed and the foot is displaced

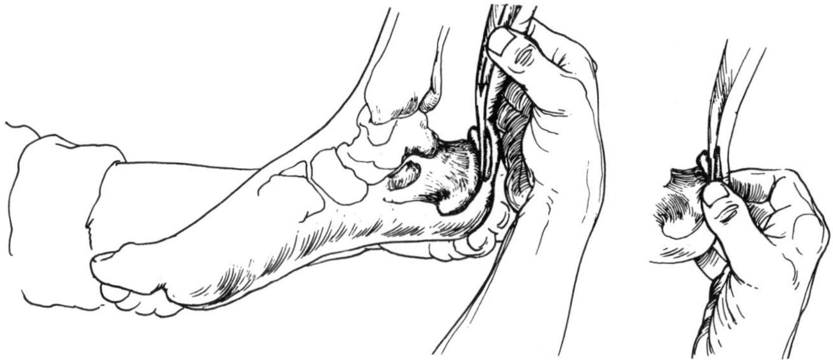

Figure 8–13. The Achilles tendon, or calcaneal, bursa.

posteriorly and fused. Another is the Hoke arthrodesis where the talar head and neck are removed, reduced in size by resection of the bone, replaced, and fused. This procedure permits backward displacement of the foot, but jeopardizes the blood supply to the talus. A third is the triple arthrodesis, which fuses the subastragalar, the astragaloscaphoid, and the calcaneocuboid joints to correct instability of the foot due to muscle imbalance (Fig 8–14). A triple arthrodesis is usually indicated when there is a deformity of the foot, with or without instability. After the surgery, the foot is placed in a long leg cast.

□ NURSING PROCESS (Table 8–5)

Assessment

The assessment of a typical patient with a triple arthrodesis is first a general assessment for a surgical patient. Specific emphasis should then be given to the foot that has been fused, as discussed in the assessment of a patient with a fractured ankle (see p. 437). The patient with a triple arthrodesis is likely to have more problems with postoperative bleeding, swelling, and especially pain, than a patient with a fractured ankle, because of the large amount of bone resection. Do not forget to assess the donor site if one was utilized.

Nursing Diagnosis and Goal Formulation

Nursing diagnoses for a typical patient following a triple arthrodesis are (1) alterations in comfort related to pain in the foot from pathology and

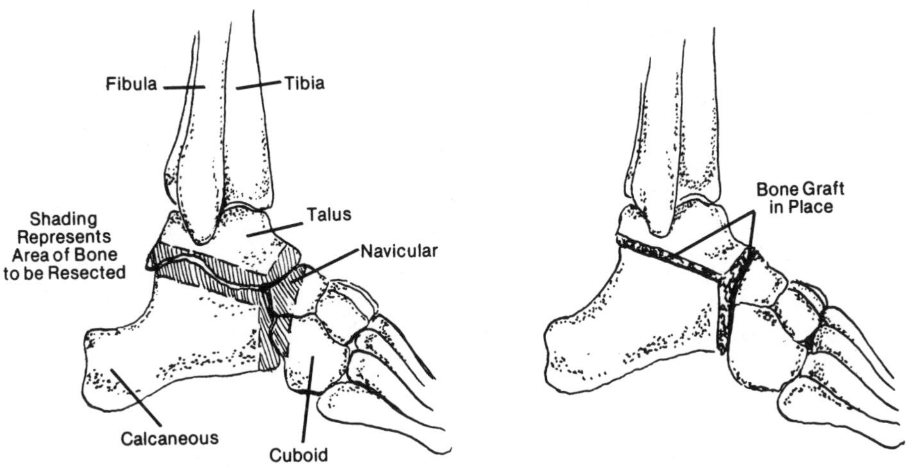

Figure 8–14. Triple arthrodesis, lateral view. *(From Brantley, P., & Analla, M., 1980, p. 126. Courtesy of Howmedica.)*

TABLE 8–5. NURSING PROCESS FOR TRIPLE ARTHRODESIS OF THE FOOT WITH EXTERNAL FIXATION AND CAST

Assessment	Nursing Diagnosis	Goal Formulation	Planning and Intervention	Evaluation and Reassessment
1. Assess the location, duration, and severity of pain. Check for elevation of the foot.	1. Alteration in comfort: pain in the foot related to bone trauma.	1. Short-term goal: a decrease in the level of pain through immobilization and prescribed medications. Long-term goal: free of pain.	1. Alleviate Pain Securely elevate the foot. Place ice bags along the sides of the ankle. Teach relaxation exercises. Utilize distraction. Administer prescribed medications.	1. Medications should relieve the pain from the large amount of bone resection.
2. Check the position of the foot. Assess the neurovascular status. Assess the ability to do exercises and walk with crutches.	2. Impaired physical mobility: decrease in foot rotation related to instability of joints.	2. Short-term goal: an increase in function through immobilization. Long-term goal: regain foot stability for walking.	2. Increase Mobility *Position* Keep the leg elevated (with pillows or overhead slings). Teach how to use the trapeze. Turn to any position of comfort. *Exercises* Teach active exercises for all unaffected joints. Instruct on exercises to build muscles in the upper extremities for crutch walking. *Ambulation* Demonstrate crutch walking.	2. The foot should be elevated until swelling subsides. Increase pain usually occurs when swinging the leg through in a three-point gait.
3. Assess the neurovascular status. Assess the amount of bleeding. Check for areas of swelling.	3. Potential for injury: neurovascular deficit related to soft tissue swelling.	3. Short- and long-term goal: free of any neurovascular complications.	3. Prevent Complications *Circulatory* After surgery, do neurovascular checks every 15 minutes for the first 2 hours, every 30 minutes for the next 2 hours, every 60 minutes for the next 2 hours,	3. Following a fusion of the foot there is more bleeding and swelling than following a fracture.

Check for any tightness of the cast.			every 2 hours for the next 18 hours, and then at least at the beginning of every shift. Report any neurovascular abnormalities. Keep the foot elevated.	The neurovascular status should remain deficit free.
Check for any signs of infection. Check the skin along the cast edges for irritation. Note the amount and color of drainage.	Potential for injury: infection related to surgical incisions and a break in skin integrity. Potential impairment of skin integrity: pressure areas related to cast.	Short- and long-term goal: free of any break in skin integrity or infection.	*Integumentary* Keep the foot elevated. Utilize nursing measures to reduce swelling. Trim and petal cast edges. Report any signs and symptoms of infection. Report any signs of pressure. *Other Potential Complications* (See text discussion.)	No signs of skin impairment or infection should occur.
4. Assess knowledge level of rehabilitation process and self-care.	4. Potential knowledge deficit related to rehabilitation process and self-care.	4. Short- and long-term goal: a decrease in anxiety through increased knowledge.	4. Patient Teaching Discuss the various steps in the rehabilitation process. Discuss cast care. Clarify any questions on exercises and ambulation. Include family in teaching plan. Discuss dressing and bathing.	4. The patient should have sufficient data to feel confident about going home in a cast with an external fixation device. The patient, family, and significant other should accept that walking with a fused foot involves a stiff "peg leg" gait.

surgical procedure, (2) alterations in mobility related to lack of joint stability in the affected foot, (3) potential complications related to surgical procedure and decreased activity, and (4) alterations in psychological well-being related to anxiety and knowledge deficit.

Short-term goals are (1) a decrease in pain in the foot, (2) an increase in mobility due to stabilized joints in the foot and the use of assistive devices, (3) an absence of complications from surgery or decreased activity, and (4) a decrease in anxiety due to knowledge of the surgical procedure and the prognosis. Long-term goals are to have the patient free of pain and able to walk without discomfort.

Planning and Intervention

Alleviate Pain. Nursing measures to relieve pain in the foot for a typical patient following a triple arthrodesis are principally the same as those for a patient with a fractured ankle. If signs of circulatory impairment occur, a large window over the anterior surface of the foot and the leg may be cut out of the cast.

Increase Mobility. To help regain and improve mobility, the casted leg is elevated immediately after surgery. The casted leg may be suspended from an overhead frame by two slings or a commercially available leg elevator until all swelling has subsided. After 10 to 14 days the long leg cast is removed and roentgenography done. If necessary, manipulation to correct alignment is made and a boot cast applied. Once the boot cast is in place, the patient is usually allowed up on crutches as tolerated. Approximately 6 weeks after surgery a walking cast is applied and controlled weight bearing begun. The cast is worn until solid bony union is demonstrated both clinically and roentgenographically, which is usually about 12 weeks after surgery.

After the cast is removed, the patient must learn to walk with a fused foot. Fusion of the calcaneus usually results in a stiff "peg leg" gait, with a lack of push off. Too much equinus produces a halting gait where the affected foot is kept in front of the body while walking. Thus the patient takes short steps with the arthrodesed foot being pushed ahead of the body, and larger steps when the other foot is brought up from the rear.

Prevent Complications. Nursing measures to prevent complications following a triple arthrodesis focus on infection prevention. Other possible complications are pseudoarthritis, malunion (especially if the cast was applied with the foot in an improper position), nonunion (particularly if the cast was removed too soon), and avascular necrosis of the body of the talus.

Patient Teaching. Help the patient develop a safe gait for ambulation, first with crutches, then with a walking cast, and finally with a fused foot. Help the patient and significant others adjust to the change in body image and the fact that the patient will always walk with a distinctive gait. (For patient teaching on cast care and ambulation, see Appendix B and Appendix C.)

Evaluation and Reassessment

Determine whether nursing measures and pain medications have relieved the pain. Sometimes the most distressing pain is at the donor site of the bone graft. The patient may complain of increased pain when swinging the leg through a three-point (nonweight bearing) gait. Pain that develops when the foot is lowered for crutch walking will usually subside after a period of elevation. If not, pain medications should be utilized.

Make sure the patient receives sufficient data to have a feeling of confidence about going home in a cast with an external fixation device and walking with crutches. Have the patient, the family, and significant others accepted that walking with a fused foot involves a stiff "peg leg" gait? More time with the patient may be needed in a stress-free environment to allow for free and open discussion about the patient's changed body image.

Arthrodesis of First Metatarsophalangeal Joint

Arthrodesis of the MTP joint of the great toe is done to salvage the foot after failure of other operations for hallux valgus and rheumatoid arthritis. It is especially useful for active young people who have a painful hallux rigidus. The procedure not only corrects the deformity of the MTP joint, but also reduces the varus deformity of the first metatarsal.

The procedure involves the excision of the bursa, trimming down the distal end of the metatarsal, and reaming out a hole at the proximal base of the phalanx. The bones are then correctly positioned for fusion. The amount of toe extension for men is usually 15 to 20 degrees. For women who wear medium heels it is 15 to 25 degrees, but for women who wear high heels at all times, 35 to 40 degrees of extension are usually needed. Some physicians recommend 15 degrees of extension for both, and thus limit their patients to a heel height of 3.8 cm. Once the toe is in the desired position, a long screw is inserted that extends almost the entire length of the metatarsal.

After surgery an elastic spica dressing is applied. Sometimes a cast is applied after surgery, and on the third or fourth postoperative day weight bearing is permitted using a shoe that has been cut away over the toe. For 6 weeks, the patient is not allowed to push off with the end of the toe while walking. Sometimes, during surgery, the bones are fixed with a Charnley compression clamp. The clamp is removed after 3 weeks, and a walking boot cast is worn for 3 more weeks.

Silastic Great Toe Implant (Swanson Design)

Patients with rheumatoid arthritis, hallux valgus, hallux rigidus, or a painful or unstable joint following a bunionectomy may be candidates for Silastic implants. The goal of a great toe Silastic implant is to relieve pain and provide stability. The procedure involves resection of the proximal third of the first proximal phalanx (Fig 8–15). Any exostosis (bony growth) of the metatarsal head is removed, providing a smooth articular surface. The medullary canal of the proximal phalanx is then reamed to accept the stem of the implant. The implant is then put in place (Brantley & Analla, 1980, p. 116).

After surgery a bulky dressing is applied for 3 to 5 days. A dynamic splint is then applied to maintain alignment while allowing motion. The splint is worn constantly for 3 to 4 weeks, and then only at night for 4 to 6 weeks more. Guarded weight bearing is started at 3 weeks in a wooden-soled postoperative boot. Potential complications following the surgery are infection, dislocation, or breakage of the implant.

DISORDERS OF THE ARCH

Flatfoot or Pes Planus

The Latin term *pes planus* and its English equivalent, flatfoot, are generally used to designate any deformity of the foot in which the longitudinal arch is depressed. Clinically, different types of pes planus are distinguished based on whether the arch is relatively too flexible or too rigid and whether the peroneal muscles are spastic or normal. The three principal types are (1) the flexible type with normal peroneals (pronation); (2) the rigid type with normal peroneals (structural flatfoot); and (3) the rigid type with spastic peroneals (spastic flatfoot) (Edmondson & Crenshaw, 1980, p. 1715; Turek, 1977, p. 1285).

The most common type of flatfoot in the adult is pronation (Fig. 8–16).

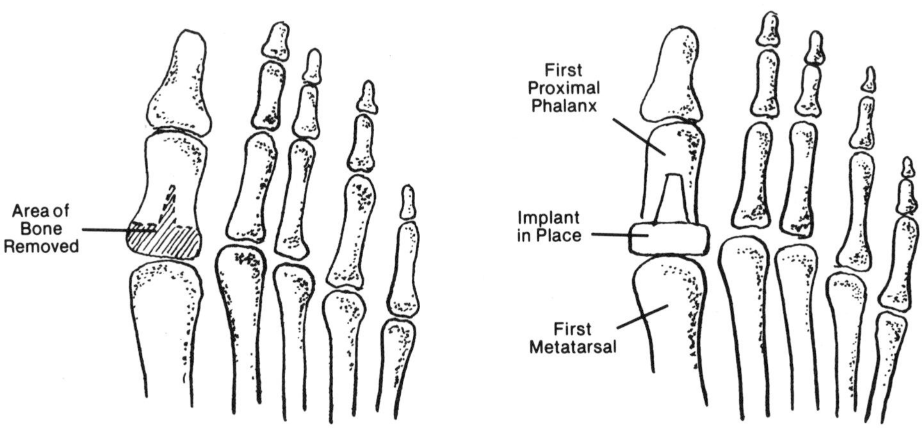

Figure 8–15. Silastic great toe implant: Swanson design. *(From Brantley, P., & Analla, M., 1980, p. 116. Courtesy of Howmedica.)*

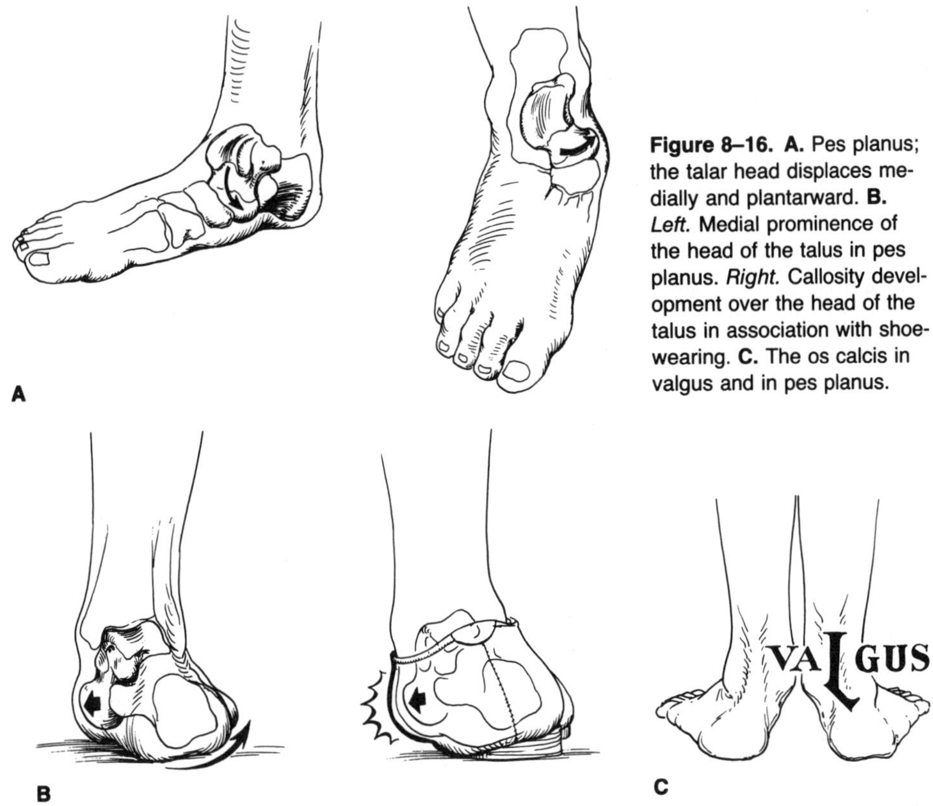

Figure 8–16. A. Pes planus; the talar head displaces medially and plantarward. **B.** *Left.* Medial prominence of the head of the talus in pes planus. *Right.* Callosity development over the head of the talus in association with shoe-wearing. **C.** The os calcis in valgus and in pes planus.

Some patients give a history of wearing shoe corrections in childhood. Others may ignore having problems with their feet until the onset of foot pain. In these instances, arch breakdown is usually brought about by occupational demands of prolonged standing or walking, by obesity, by poor muscle tone, or by the use of shoes that do not give adequate support. In other instances, severe pronation in the adult may be associated with severe sweating of the feet, edema about the foot and ankle, and varicose veins. The symptoms produced by pronation of the longitudinal arch in adults can usually be relieved by the use of resilient longitudinal arch supports. Exercises can be helpful. One is to have the patient stand with the feet and toes inverted (rotated inward along the longitudinal axes) so that the weight is borne on the outer border of the feet. The exercise should be repeated 30 times. Another exercise for the longitudinal arch is done by rising on the balls of the feet, raising the heels, and everting the ankles. The exercise is usually repeated 20 to 30 times. Painful feet in the adult caused by structural or spastic flatfeet may require operative fusion of the subtalar joints (a triple arthrodesis) for pain relief (Gartland, 1979, p. 443).

Metatarsalgia

If the bones forming the metatarsal arch bear a disproportionate amount of weight, thick calluses may form on the ball of the foot and the patient may experience a painful burning sensation in that area with weight bearing. That condition is known as metatarsalgia. Metatarsalgia occurs primarily in adults and is more common in women. It may occur alone, but it is frequently seen in association with pronation. In addition to callus formation and burning pain in the front of the foot, tenderness to palpation is usually noted *between* the metatarsal heads on the dorsum of the foot. Severe cases may be associated with clawing of the toes.

Symptoms can usually be relieved by the use of metatarsal arch supports. These come in various sizes and are placed in the shoe to lie just behind the metatarsal heads. Another method of treatment is to provide sufficient room for the muscles that support the metatarsal arch. Therefore, adequate shoe width in the metatarsal region is necessary. Many of these patients need shoes with an EE or EEE width, which can be difficult to obtain.

Exercises that help to relieve symptoms are those that strengthen the muscles of the arch. One exercise is the "towel" exercise. A towel is placed on the floor, and the feet are placed parallel to each other about an inch apart, with the heels just over the back edge of the towel. The toes of each foot are then contracted in succession so that the towel is gradually accumulated under the arch. Another exercise is the "marble" exercise. Ten to twelve marbles are placed on the floor, and are picked up, moved, and released using the toes and the flexor tendons. Pencils may be used instead of marbles, or the toes may be contracted rhythmically over the edge of a step or a large book upon which the patient is standing (Gartland, 1979, pp. 444–445).

DEFORMITIES OF THE TOES

Hallux Valgus (Bunion)

Hallux valgus is a deformity of the foot characterized by (1) a valgus deformity of the great toe at the MTP joint so that the base of the proximal phalanx is subluxed laterally; (2) a medial prominence of the first metatarsal head (the bunion); and (3) a varus deformity of the first metatarsal (Fig. 8–17). Hallux valgus may occur with rheumatoid arthritis and osteoarthritis, and may be bilateral or unilateral (Cailliet, 1981, p. 293; Edmondson & Crenshaw, 1980, p. 1715).

As hallux valgus develops, the increase in the varus of the first metatarsal decreases the power of the great toe to push off in walking. Thus the load carried by the second and third metatarsal heads increases, callosities develop beneath them, and the area becomes painful. Corns, calluses, hammertoes, subluxations of joints, and other afflictions of the foot are therefore often associated with hallux valgus of long duration, and all must be treated if discomfort in the foot is to be relieved.

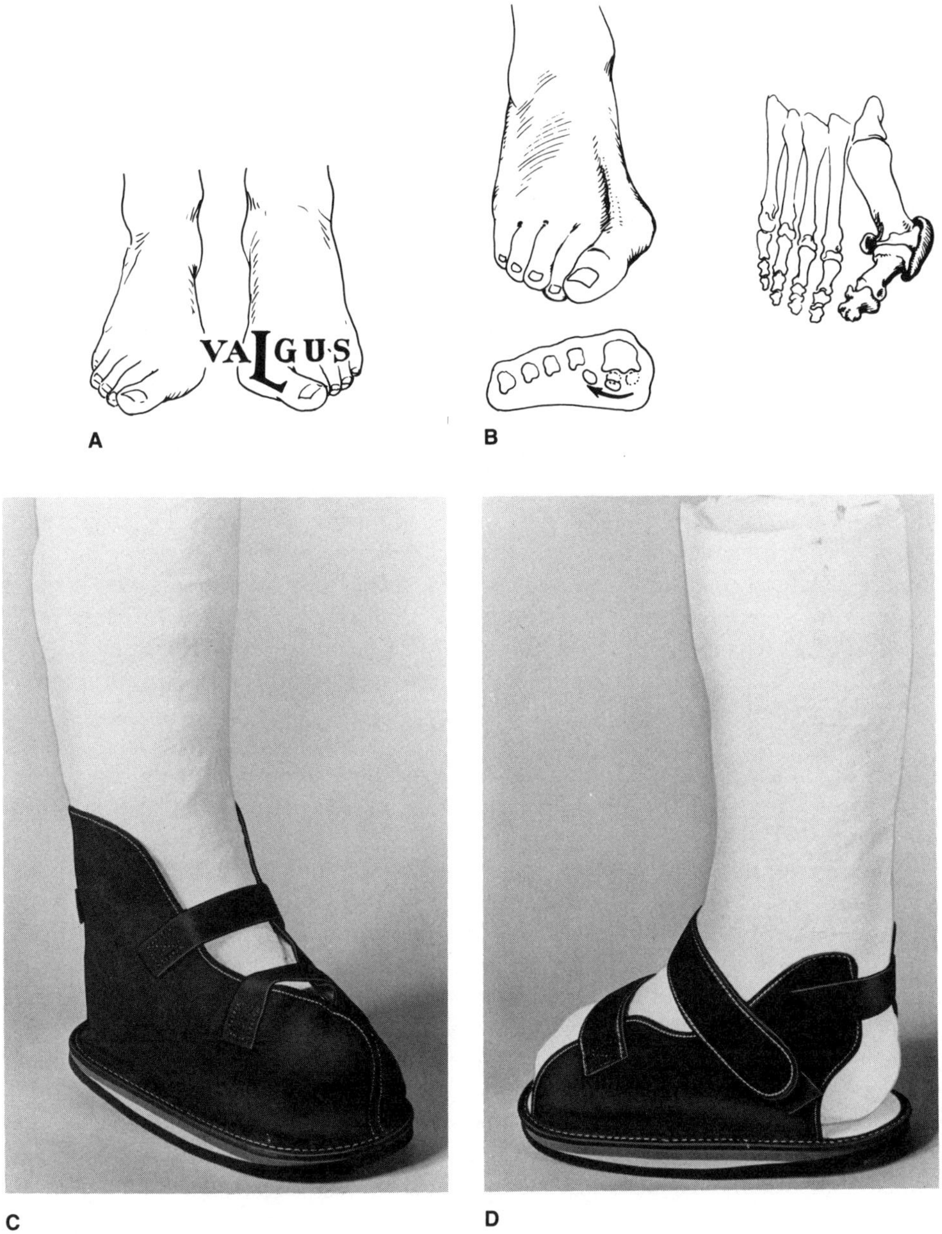

Figure 8–17. A. Hallux valgus. The "L" in valgus refers to the lateral deviation of the phalanx. **B.** Hallux valgus with bunion formation. **C.** Cast boot. **D.** Cast shoe. *(Figs. 8–17C and D courtesy of Zimmer, Inc.)*

Surgical Treatment of Hallux Valgus (Bunionectomy)

Surgery is indicated in hallux valgus primarily to relieve pain. The surgical procedure should (1) correct the valgus deformity of the proximal phalanx, (2) remove any exostotic bone from medial and dorsal aspects of the first metatarsal head, and remove the bursa when necessary, (3) correct the varus deformity of the first metatarsal, (4) correct any excessive tightness of the extensors of the great toe, and (5) correct any associated deformities of the forefoot, such as corns, hammertoes, and subluxations of joints (Edmondson & Crenshaw, 1980, p. 1716).

Six different operations have been devised to correct hallux valgus. The McBride operation frees the adductor hallucis tendon from the proximal phalanx and attaches it to the first metatarsal so the proximal phalanx no longer is pulled into valgus position, which helps correct the varus deformity of the first metatarsal. That procedure is used in younger and middle-aged patients when the deformity is only moderate, as it only involves a revision of soft tissue.

The Keller operation resects the proximal half of the proximal phalanx of the great toe, which shortens the toe and relaxes the conjoined adductor tendon and the contracted lateral part of the joint capsule, correcting the deformity. A Kirschner wire is inserted longitudinally through the great toe and into the first metatarsal. The Keller procedure is used for most patients who require excision of bone, especially for those with hallux rigidus and with lesser degrees of degenerative arthritis of the first MTP joint. Patients should be advised that for several months after surgery the toe will be floppy and plump, that it will be permanently shortened, and that active control of it will be slightly impaired.

The Stone operation consists of an incomplete resection of the first metatarsal head. It is used, though not frequently, in the treatment of hallux rigidus and hallux valgus.

The Lapidus operation is designed to narrow the angle at the base of the first and second metatarsals, remove any exostotic bone from the head of the first metatarsal, and release the pull of the adductor hallucis. The first metatarsocuneiform joint and the adjacent bases of the first and second metatarsal are arthrodesed to hold the first metatarsal shaft in alignment. Weight bearing after surgery is delayed until fusion takes place, which requires some 2 to 3 weeks. The procedure is used in patients with hallux valgus where the primary deformity is congenital varus angulation of the first metatarsal, and the associated valgus angulation of the great toe is secondary.

The Mitchell operation involves an osteotomy made through the first metatarsal, which displaces the metatarsal head laterally and slightly plantarward. Because the time required for healing after osteotomy is longer than for most other surgeries for hallux valgus, the Mitchell operation is usually more suitable for young and middle-aged patients who can calcify bone more rapidly and are better able to ambulate without weight bearing than are the elderly. Significant arthritic changes or limitations of motion in the MTP joint may make the Mitchell operation unsuitable.

The Joplin operation was devised not only to correct hallux valgus but also to reduce splaying of the foot and varus deformities of the first metatarsal. The procedure is rarely used today.

□ NURSING PROCESS (Table 8–6)

Assessment

After a general assessment of the total patient, the focus is on the affected foot. On the patient's return from surgery after a bunionectomy, check the neurovascular status of the toes at least every 2 hours for the first 24 hours, and then every 8 hours, even if the patient has no complaints. Note the temperature and skin color of the toes, and if there is any swelling or drainage. To help determine the temperature of the affected foot, check the temperature of the other foot. There may be some discoloration of the toes from solutions used in the surgical preparation of the foot. Checking the circulation of the toes by blanching may also be impaired or incomplete because of the surgical procedure performed. For example, following a Keller procedure, which included a correction of a hammer toe, pins, protective splints, or casts may extend over the end of the foot. Temperature may thus be the most important measure for assessing circulatory status. Bloody drainage is usually not present on the external dressing or cast. Determine the motor function of the foot by evaluating the patient's ability to wiggle or move toes. Check to make sure the swelling, cast, splints, or dressing are not impeding movement. Determine the sensory response as indicated by any complaints of numbness, tingling, or lack of feeling in any of the toes when tested by a sharp or dull touch. Postoperative pain in the foot may make it difficult for the patient to distinguish between pain from the operation and pain due to nerve pressure or circulatory impairment. Determine the amount, kind, and location of pain. Note the amount of elevation of the foot and whether it is safely secured in that position with no pressure on the heel. There should be support under the full length of the leg, and support along both sides of the leg to prevent rotation. No linen should be in contact with the elevated foot, and ice bags should be placed alongside the foot for the first 24 to 48 hours.

Nursing Diagnosis and Goal Formulation

Nursing diagnoses for a typical patient following a bunionectomy are (1) alterations in comfort related to pain in the bones and the MTP joint of the great toe from surgery, (2) alterations in mobility related to lack of stability in the joints of the great and second toe, (3) potential complications related to surgical procedure, and (4) alterations in psychological well-being related to anxiety and knowledge deficit about the surgical procedure and the rehabilitation process.

The short-term goals for a typical patient following a bunionectomy are (1) an absence of pain in the foot and toes by elevation, immobilization, and medications; (2) an increase in mobility by the use of a cast, splints,

TABLE 8–6. NURSING PROCESS FOR BUNIONECTOMY

Assessment	Nursing Diagnosis	Goal Formulation	Planning and Intervention	Evaluation and Reassessment
1. Assess for location, duration, and severity of pain. Check neurovascular status. Check for any areas of swelling.	1. Alteration in comfort: pain in the toes related to bone and soft tissue trauma.	1. Short-term goal: a decrease in pain through elevation and medication. Long-term goal: free of pain.	1. Alleviate Pain Elevate the foot. Place ice bags along the medial side of the foot. Keep linen off the toes. Utilize distraction techniques. Teach relaxation techniques. Administer pain medications.	1. During the first 24–48 hours, medication should be administered every 3–4 hours, even with nursing measures.
2. Check that the foot is elevated securely. Check that the foot is in correct alignment. Assess ability to ambulate without assistance. Check neurovascular status.	2. Impaired physical mobility: decrease in foot function related to instability of the great and second toes.	2. Short-term goal: an increase in mobility through immobilization. Long-term goal: regain optimal function in the foot.	2. Increase Mobility *Position* Keep the foot elevated. Place the bed in semi-Fowler's position. Teach patient how to use the trapeze. Turn to any position of comfort. *Exercises* Active range of motion of all unaffected joints. Encourage quadriceps setting, plantar and dorsiflexion exercises for 5 minutes every hour.	2. Pain or throbbing usually occurs when the foot is lowered during ambulation. The patient should ambulate safely using an assistive device.

			Instruct on exercises to build up strength in the upper extremities for crutch walking. *Ambulation* Demonstrate how to use a walker or do crutch walking (see text for specific ambulation technique based on surgical procedure). Instruct patient to use cast boot or wooden shoe in ambulating.	
3. Assess for signs and symptoms of infection. Note any drainage. Assess for any areas of swelling.	3. Potential for injury: infection related to break in skin integrity.	3. Short- and long-term goal: free of any signs of infection.	3. Prevent Complications *Integumentary* Keep dressing clean and dry. Report any signs and symptoms of infection. Keep linen off the toes. *Other Complications* (see text)	3. The patient should remain free of any signs of infection.
4. Assess the patient's knowledge level of the rehabilitation process for the surgical procedure used.	4. Potential knowledge deficit related to the rehabilitation process.	4. Short- and long-term goal: a decrease in anxiety through an increase in knowledge.	4. Patient Teaching Discuss the rehabilitation process for the procedure used (see text). Discuss method of bathing. Instruct patient to discard old shoes. Clarify any questions concerning ambulation.	4. The patient should have the knowledge to feel confident in going home and caring for self.

special shoes, and crutches, (3) an absence of complications, and (4) a decrease in anxiety through knowledge of the surgery and the rehabilitation. Long-term goals are to have the patient free of pain and to have return of toe and foot function with no residual complications.

Planning and Intervention

Alleviate Pain. The foot is usually elevated higher than the heart for the first 72 hours to prevent or reduce swelling. With the foot elevated, the heel must be free of pressure. To promote comfort and prevent swelling after surgery, ice bags are placed along the side of the foot at the incision site. Ice bags should not be placed directly on swollen toes as that will only increase pain. The source of the swelling is in the area of the incision, thus the ice is needed there. A surgical glove, a small plastic glove, or a small plastic bag filled with ice may be sufficient, and it can be secured alongside the foot by a roll of gauze or adhesive tape (if the patient has a cast).

The linen needs to be kept off the foot to reduce pressure. This can be accomplished by a bed cradle, a footboard at the end of the bed, or rods attached to the bed frame that support the linen and thus prevent it from touching the foot. Such precautions are especially important for patients with a Kirschner wire, as the linen can catch on the wire and cause an increase in pain, bright red drainage, and may even dislodge the wire.

During the first 24 to 48 hours the patient may need pain medication every 3 hours, even with the above nursing measures. Once the patient starts to ambulate there may be throbbing pain in the foot. The source of pain must be determined. It could be from the surgical procedure, the cast, or from a distorted or unnatural gait.

Increase Mobility. For the first 48 to 72 hours the patient is usually on bedrest. Active range-of-motion exercises to all unaffected joints are usually started immediately after surgery. Encourage quadriceps setting exercises and, if the foot is not in a cast, plantar and dorsiflexion exercises of the ankle for 5 minutes every hour the patient is awake. Exercises to build up strength in the upper extremities are started if the patient will be using crutches.

The patient is encouraged to turn and change position in bed while still keeping the foot elevated. In the beginning it is usually necessary to assist the patient in turning by holding and turning the affected foot, repositioning the pillows, and replacing the foot on the pillows. The patient can lie prone, but it is difficult to do so and still keep the foot elevated, the toes free of pressure, and the ice bags in place.

Different surgical procedures allow ambulation, with or without weight bearing, at different times. Following a McBride procedure, the patient is usually allowed up in a chair or wheelchair after 72 hours, and guarded weight bearing is started 12 to 14 days postsurgery. An elastoplast dressing is usually worn until the wound is healed and the sutures removed. An adhesive strapping to hold the toes in slight varus is then worn for 2 to 3 weeks before the patient is allowed to gradually resume activities. With a Keller procedure, the patient will have a Kirschner wire protruding from the end of the great toe, which may or may not be covered by a small cork. The Kirschner wire and dressing are usually removed at approximately 12 to 14 days after surgery, and walking is then begun. After a Mitchell procedure, the great toe is splinted in 5 degrees of flexion and in slight varus position, usually by means of tongue blades applied to the dorsal, medial, and plantar aspects of the foot and the toe. The splint is removed after 10 days, and a walking boot cast is applied and worn until the osteotomy heals (approximately 4 to 8 weeks). Following a Stone procedure, full weight bearing is allowed as soon as the patient is comfortable, usually 2 or 3 days postsurgery. The dressing and sutures are usually removed 8 to 10 days after surgery, and a felt pad is placed between the great and second toes. The pad is usually worn for 2 to 3 weeks and then replaced with a smaller pad that is worn for 4 to 5 months. At about 4 weeks postoperatively, a normal, large, soft shoe can be worn by the patient.

Pain or throbbing in the foot may be experienced when the patient begins to ambulate, with or without crutches. Patients are usually very apprehensive about bumping their toes. They tend to distort their normal gait to avoid pressure on the toes and the forefoot, and thus tend to walk on their heels, which usually causes pain in the ankles or calves.

Prevent Complications. The major complication following a bunionectomy is infection. Other complications from the procedure include (1) recurrence of the deformity, (2) a hallux varus deformity, (3) clawing of the great toe, (4) necrosis of the edges of the wound, (5) numbness of the great toe, (6) limitation of motion of the MTP joint, and (7) contractures of the web between the first and second toes.

Patient Teaching. Efforts should focus on the specific type of surgical procedure and the rehabilitation process. If the patient is to ambulate on crutches, reinforce the instructions given by the therapist. Patients need encouragement and understanding to overcome their hesitancy to walk on the affected foot. In the beginning, patients will not want to walk on the foot at all. Then they tend to walk on the heel, before developing a flat-footed gait with no push off that can be used until healing is complete. Patients may need to be reminded that correct posture helps avoid fatigue. They should also be instructed as to the importance of frequent rest periods, with the foot elevated, during the convalescent period.

Patients need to understand that it is necessary for them to discard their old shoes, because they are shaped to their foot before surgery and therefore apply stress to the corrected foot. Following a Keller procedure, however, patients may use an old pair of shoes cut out over the great toes until the wire is removed. Following a McBride procedure, some patients may need properly placed metatarsal pads in their shoes for several months.

For patients who are discharged with a cast, information on cast care needs to be given (see Appendix B). All patients should be instructed on the signs and symptoms of an infection and what to do if an infection develops.

Evaluation and Reassessment

Determine whether postoperative pain in the foot has been relieved by nursing measures and pain medication. Evaluate the circulation and neurological status of the foot. Check that the dressing or the cast is not too tight and that there is no swelling of the toes. The leg should be correctly aligned and elevated on pillows. When walking with crutches, the patient should have a safe, steady gait. If not, more instruction and work with the therapist may be needed. Determine whether the patient feels confident about going home with a dressing and pins or a cast. If not, ask questions to determine what the patient does not understand, and explain it again.

Bunionette (Tailor's Bunion)

Bunionette, or tailor's bunion, is a varus angulation of the fifth toe at the MTP joint that tends to develop in splayed (or flat) feet. Pressure from poorly fitted shoes may then cause chronic inflammation of the bursa on the lateral aspect of the fifth metatarsal head and a hard corn on the dorsolateral aspect of the proximal interphalangeal joint of the fifth toe (Fig. 8–18). When surgery is indicated by chronic pain, one of two procedures is generally done. In the first

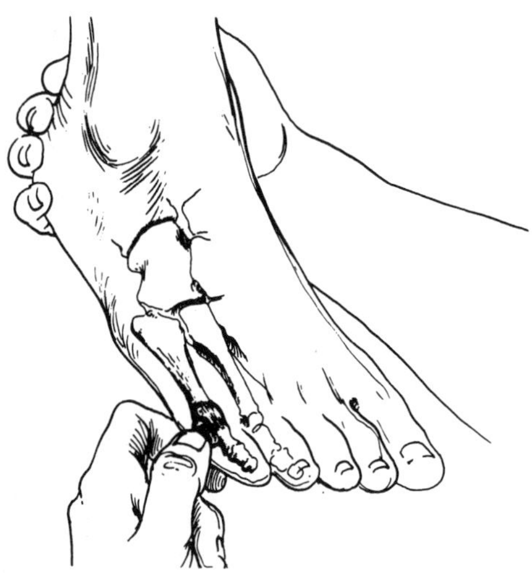

Figure 8–18. Tailor's bunion.

procedure, the lateral third of the fifth metatarsal head is resected, and in the second, the entire head of the fifth metatarsal is removed. The procedures shorten and realign the fifth toe, relieving pressure on any hard corn that may be present.

After surgery a compression dressing is applied. Weight bearing is resumed approximately 10 days after surgery, using shoes with the part over the fifth metatarsal head removed to prevent pressure. Wide shoes with medium or low heels should be worn for several months after surgery. A circular elastic metatarsal support that holds the metatarsal heads in close alignment during weight bearing is useful during the first few weeks after surgery to help prevent recurrence of the deformity.

Hammertoes

With a hammertoe deformity, the proximal interphalangeal joint is flexed and the distal interphalangeal joint is either flexed or extended. The metatarsal head is depressed and prominent on the plantar surface of the foot, causing a painful callosity to develop (Fig. 8–19). Irritation from shoes may cause corns to develop on the dorsum of the flexed proximal interphalangeal joint and on the end of the toe. The deformity may affect one or more toes and may either be congenital or acquired. When acquired, it is usually caused by wearing poorly fitted shoes, and is often associated with hallux valgus. The second toe is most often affected.

A more common surgical procedure to correct the deformity (Fig 8–20) is the resection of bone from the middle phalanx and the head of the proximal phalanx to allow the toe to be straightened and the remaining osseous surfaces to be opposed. The bones are then fixed together with a longitudinal Kirschner wire to promote fusion (Edmondson & Crenshaw, 1980, p. 1735).

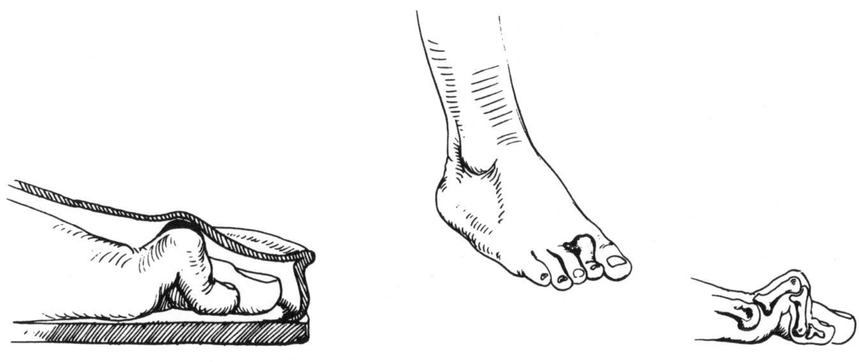

A B

Figure 8–19. A. Callosity formation caused by hammertoes. **B.** Hammertoes.

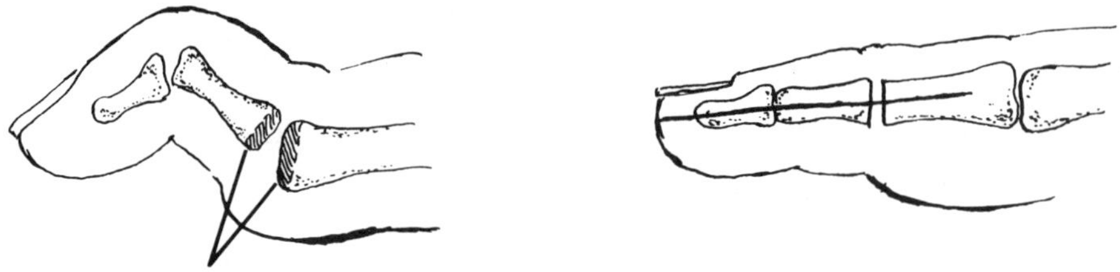

Figure 8–20. Correction of hammertoe. *(From Brantley, P., & Analla, M., 1980, p. 120. Courtesy of Howmedica.)*

After surgery the end of the wire is sealed with a collodion dressing and capped with a small sterile cork. If additional immobilization is required, the toe is strapped with adhesive tape to an adjacent toe. Weight bearing is allowed approximately 2 weeks after surgery, and the wire is removed 3 to 4 weeks after surgery. The patient should be aware that although the affected toe will be straightened, it will be shorter and fused at the middle phalangeal joint.

Ingrown Toenail

The term ingrown toenail is misleading. The nail does not grow in, but rather soft tissues overgrow and obliterate the medial and lateral side grooves of the nail. An ingrown toenail can be caused by an excessively short trimming of the nail or by a crowding of the toes in shoes or tight stockings. As the nail grows, its corner penetrates the overgrown soft tissue and infection with suppuration develops (Fig. 8–21). Ingrown toenails almost always involve the great toe (Edmondson & Crenshaw, 1980, p. 1740; Gartland, 1979, p. 448).

Conservative measures are to control infection by wet packs and rest, and to try and allow the nail to grow out beyond the obliterated groove by elevating it using a small bit of cotton, a metal shield, or even a plastic strip. Once the nail has grown out, the toenail must always be trimmed squarely across the end so that each corner always extends beyond the groove, or the condition with recur.

If conservative treatment is unsuccessful, surgery is indicated. In most operations for ingrown toenail part or all of the nail is excised. Some physicians, however, prefer to excise the soft tissue from the involved side of the toe, whereas others remove the nail, the medial and lateral wedges of the soft tissue, and the nailbed, and resect the distal phalanx dorsally.

After surgery, a light elastic dressing is usually applied over a thin layer of petroleum gauze. The foot is elevated, and pain is relieved by mild analgesics and warm moist dressings. Twenty-four to forty-eight hours after surgery, the dressing is changed, and the patient is allowed to walk in a shoe that has the

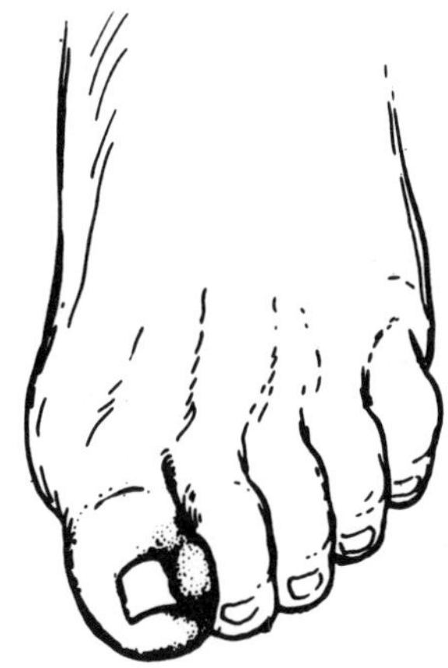

Figure 8–21. Ingrown toenail.

top cut out over the affected toe. The nail grows back to normal length in 4 to 8 months.

COMMON FOOT PROBLEMS

Hard Corns (Clavus Durum)

A hard corn is a thickening of the soft tissue over a bony prominence, and is usually caused by pressure over a period of time (Fig. 8–22). The most common hard corn on the foot is on the dorsolateral aspect of the proximal interphalangeal joint of the fifth toe. The hard corn is caused by a flexion–adduction deformity of the toe that causes the toe to press against the shoe (Edmondson & Crenshaw, 1980, p. 1733). A corn in that location can be permanently cured only by shortening the fifth toe and removing the osseous deformity.

Hard corns may also develop on the dorsum of the proximal interphalan-

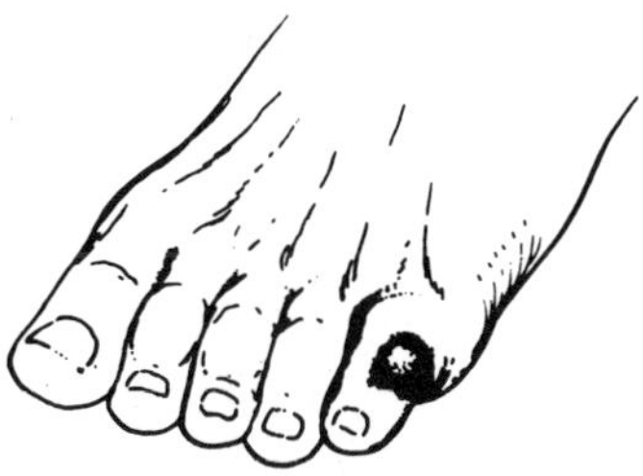

Figure 8–22. Hard corns.

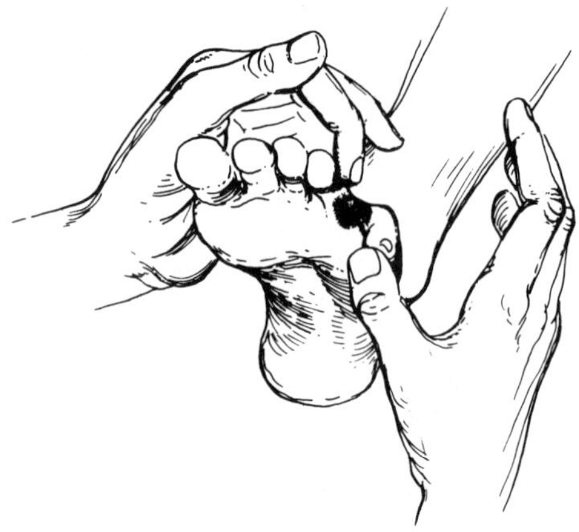

Figure 8–23. Soft corns.

geal joints of the other toes. One caused by a hammertoe or claw toe deformity spontaneously disappears after the toe has been shortened and the deformity has been corrected (Gartland, 1979, p. 449).

A corn may be softened with hot water or preparations containing salicylic acid and then trimmed with a scalpel. Steps should also be taken to relieve pressure on bony prominences from tight-fitting shoes.

Soft Corns (Clavus Mollum)

Soft corns typically develop between the toes, and are soft because of the moistness of the area. Although a soft corn may develop between any two toes, it

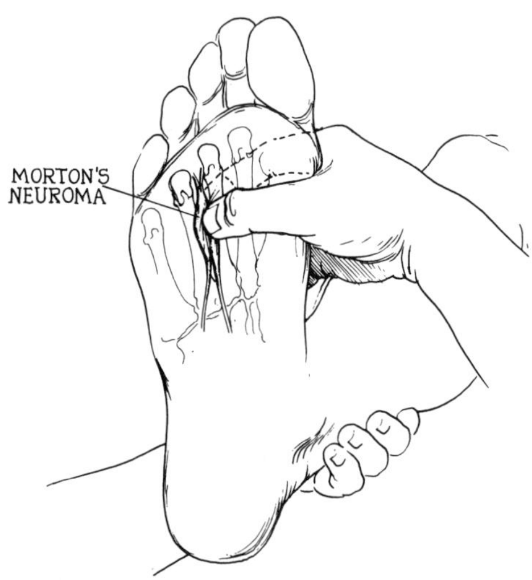

Figure 8–24. Morton's neuroma—a painful neuroma usually located between the third and fourth metatarsal heads.

develops most frequently on the lateral aspect of the base of the fourth toe, deep in the web between the fourth and fifth toes (Fig. 8–23). There it is usually caused by pressure on the base of the phalanx of the fourth toe by the proximal interphalangeal joint or the distal metaphysis of the proximal phalanx of the fifth toe. The corn is painful and often disabling. It is rare to find a soft corn between the fourth and fifth toes without also finding a hard corn on the dorsolateral aspect of the fifth toe (Edmondson & Crenshaw, 1980, p. 1724).

Callus

A callus is a growth composed of a hypertrophied horny layer of squamous epithelium in response to excessive pressure. It is similar to a corn, but generally larger in size. The usual sites are at the points of bony prominences, such as the plantar aspect of the first metatarsal head, the plantar surface of the second metatarsal head, the dorsal aspect and the tips of clawed toes, the dorsum of the foot at the base of the first metatarsal, the skin overlying a bunion, and over the os calcis at the insertion of the Achilles tendon.

The callus in itself is not painful. As a thickening over a bony prominence, it can increase pressure from the shoe on the tissues beneath, and in response, a bursa is likely to form beneath it. Traumatic bursitis then develops and is the most common cause of the discomfort associated with calluses. When a callus develops between the toes, perspiration softens it, and a soft corn results.

Removal of pressure is the essence of treatment. Shoes of adequate width with low heels should be worn. A felt pad behind or surrounding (but not over) the bony prominence may relieve some pressure. The callus can be trimmed down to a flat surface. Hot soapy foot soaks are often prescribed, followed by applications of a keratolytic agent, such as a 20 percent solution of salicylic acid in collodion (Turek, 1977, p. 1307).

Plantar Warts

A plantar wart is an extremely painful vascular papillomatous growth that may occur on any part of the skin of the sole of the foot. Plantar warts usually occur on the ball of the foot but are situated independent of points of pressure. The surface of the wart is flat and continuous with the adjacent skin and is pressed inward by weight bearing. Usually a large "mother wart" is surrounded by several smaller warts. Callus may form completely over the surface of the wart, increasing the degree of local tenderness. Warts are believed to be caused by viruses, and can appear, disappear, and reappear spontaneously. Some of the procedures that have been used to treat plantar warts are surgical removal by local excision with electrocoagulation and surgical excision with roentgenotherapy (Gartland, 1979, p. 449; Turek, 1977, p. 1307).

Morton's Neuroma

The most common interdigital neuritis is Morton's neuroma, a painful fusiform swelling of a digital nerve (Fig 8–24). The most common site is the nerve between the third and fourth toes, but it can occur also between the second and third metatarsals. The neuroma is usually located where the interdigital nerve branches to the two neighboring toes.

The condition occurs most often in middle-aged women. The patient usually gives a history of "desire to take off their shoes and massage the metatarsal area." Upon physical examination, pain is produced by pressure between the metatarsal heads. (In metatarsalgia, tenderness is found by pressure on the plantar surface of the metatarsal heads.)

Adequately broad shoes that permit the forefoot to spread may be sufficient treatment. A metatarsal pad behind the heads to elevate the transverse arch can sometimes be of benefit as well. Diagnostically, and frequently therapeutically, an injection of a local anesthetic with a steroid gives some relief. The injection is given from the dorsum of the foot directly into the interdigital area. Persistence of symptoms may warrant surgical excision of the neuroma (Cailliet, 1981, pp. 281–283).

AMPUTATION THROUGH THE FOOT

Amputation of a single toe, with few exceptions, usually causes little disturbance in stance or gait. Amputation of the great toe does not materially affect standing or walking at a normal pace. If the patient walks rapidly or runs, however, a limp appears because of the loss of push-off normally provided by the great toe. Amputation of the second toe is always followed by severe hallux valgus because the great toe tends to drift toward the third to fill the gap left by amputation. Amputation of any of the other toes causes little disturbance. Of these the fifth toe is most commonly amputated, usually because it overlaps the fourth toe. Amputation of all toes causes little disturbance in ordinary slow walking and usually requires no prosthesis other than a shoe filler. It is some-

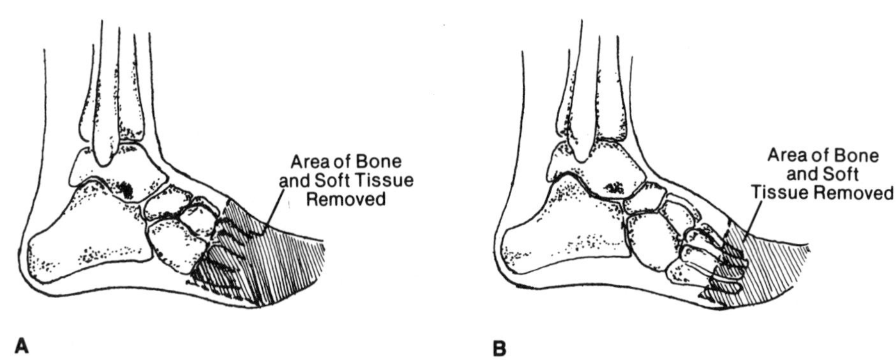

Figure 8–25. Amputation of the foot. **A.** Tarsometatarsal amputation. **B.** Transmetatarsal amputation. *(From Brantley, P., & Analla, M., 1980, p. 115. Courtesy of Howmedica.)*

what disabling for a more rapid gait, when spring and resilience in the foot are required, and when squatting or "tiptoeing."

An amputation through the metatarsals (Fig. 8–25) is disabling in proportion to the level of amputation. The more proximal the level, the greater the disability. The loss of push-off due to the absence of a positive fulcrum in the ball of the foot is chiefly responsible for the impairment of gait. Again, no prosthesis is usually required other than a shoe filler.

Amputations more proximal than the transmetatarsal level (e.g., tarsometatarsal) result in considerable awkwardness in walking because of the loss of support and push-off. Consequently, amputations of the forefoot have been largely replaced by amputations at the ankle or below the knee.

REFERENCES

Brantley, P., & Analla, M. *The nurse and orthopedic surgery.* Rutherford, N. J.: The Orthopedic Nurses' Association, Inc., in cooperation with Howmedica, Inc., 1980.

Cailliet, R. *Foot and ankle pain.* Philadelphia: F. A. Davis, 1981.

Edmondson, A. S., & Crenshaw, A. H. (Eds.). *Campbell's operative orthopaedics* (6th ed.). St. Louis: C. V. Mosby, 1980.

Fries, J. F. *Arthritis, a comprehensive guide.* Menlo Park, Calif.: Addison-Wesley, 1982.

Gartland, J. J. *Fundamentals of orthopaedics* (3rd ed.). Philadelphia: W. B. Saunders, 1979.

Hoppenfeld, S. *Physical examination of the spine and extremities.* New York: Appleton-Century-Crofts, 1976.

Iversen, L. D., & Clawson, D. K. *Manual of acute orthopaedic therapeutics.* Boston: Little, Brown, 1977.

Swinson, D. R., & Swinburn, W. R. *Rheumatology.* New York: Wiley, 1980.

Turek, S. L. *Orthopaedics, principles and their applications* (3rd ed.). Philadelphia: Lippincott, 1977.

Warwick, R., & Williams, P. L. *Gray's anatomy* (35th Brit. ed.). Philadelphia: W. B. Saunders, 1973.

BIBLIOGRAPHY

Abraham, E., & Stirnaman, J. E. Neglected rupture of the peroneal tendons causing recurrent sprains of the ankle. *Journal of Bone and Joint Surgery,* 1979, *61A* (8), 1247–1248.

Akhtar, M., & Levine, J. Dislocation of extensor digitorum longus tendons after spontaneous rupture of the inferior retinacubum of the ankle. *Journal of Bone and Joint Surgery,* 1980, *62A* (7), 1210–1211.

Albright, J. A., & Brand, R. A. (Eds.). *The scientific basis of orthopaedics.* New York: Appleton-Century-Crofts, 1979.

Alexander, A. H., & Lichtman, D. M. Surgical treatment of transchondral talar-dome fractures (osteochondritis dissecans). *Journal of Bone and Joint Surgery,* 1980, *62A* (4), 646–652.

Althoff, D. G. External fixation of the lower extremity: Care considerations. In N. E. Hill (Ed.), *Assessment and fracture management of the lower extremities.* Pitman, N. J.: Anthony J. Jannetti, 1984.

Arthritis Health Profession Section of the Arthritis Foundation. *Self-help manual for patients with arthritis.* Atlanta, Ga.: Arthritis Foundation, 1980.

Bartell, L. Bunionectomies. *Orthopaedic Nursing,* 1985, *4* (1), 21–28.

Beeson, P. B., & McDermott, W. *Cecil-Loeb textbook of medicine.* Philadelphia: Saunders, 1971.

Bechtel, S. L. Anatomy and assessment of the foot and ankle. In N. E. Hill (Ed.), *Assessment and fracture management of the lower extremities.* Pitman, N. J.: Anthony J. Jannetti, 1984.

Berger, M. R. Bunions: An overview. *Orthopaedic Nursing,* 1984, *3* (5), 17–22.

Berger, M. R. Morton's neuroma. *Orthopaedic Nursing,* 1982, *1* (1), 31–32.

Burgess, E. M. Amputations. *Surgical Clinics of North America,* 1983, *63* (3), 749–770.

Cailliet, R. *Soft tissue pain and disability* (5th ed.). Philadelphia: F. A. Davis, 1981.

Canale, S. T., & Belding, R. M. Osteochondral lesions of the talus. *Journal of Bone and Joint Surgery,* 1980, *62A* (1), 97–102.

Compere, E. L. *Orthopaedic surgery: A handbook of operative surgery.* Chicago: Year Book Medical, 1974.

Coventry, M. B., & Rathacker, G. W. Bilateral calcaneal fracture in a diabetic patient. *Journal of Bone and Joint Surgery,* 1979, *61A* (3), 462–464.

Dabezies, E., D'Ambrosia, R. D., & Shoji, H. Classification and treatment of ankle fractures. *Orthopedics,* 1978, *1* (5), 365–373.

DeGowin, E. L., & DeGowin, R. L. *Bedside diagnostic examination* (3rd ed.). New York: Macmillan, 1976.

Demottaz, J. D., Mazur, M., Thomas, W. H., et al. Clinical study of total ankle replacement with gout analyses. *Journal of Bone and Joint Surgery,* 1979, *61A* (7), 976–988.

Dennis, M. D., & Tullos, H. S. Blair tibiotalar arthrodesis for injuries to the talus. *Journal of Bone and Joint Surgery,* 1980, *62A* (1), 103–107.

Ghista, D. N., & Roof, R. *Orthopaedic mechanics: Procedures and devices.* San Francisco: Academic Press, 1978.

Gimple, K., Amspacher, J. C., & Kopta, J. A. Metatarsaphalangeal joint fusion of the great toe. *Orthopedics,* 1978, *1* (6), 462–467.

Harrington, K. D. Degenerative arthritis of the ankle secondary to long-standing lateral ligament instability. *Journal of Bone and Joint Surgery,* 1979, *61A* (3), 354–361.

Maale, G., & Seligson, D. Fractures through the distal weight-bearing surface of the tibia. *Orthopedics,* 1980, *3,* 517–521.

Manzella, J. P., Vanvaris, L. P., & Hrusker, J. F. Isolated calcaneal tuberculous osteomyelitis. *Journal of Bone and Joint Surgery,* 1979, *61A* (6), 946–947.

Marquis, A. M. Pes anserine bursitis. *Orthopedic Nurses' Association Journal,* 1979, *6* (10), 418–419.

Mayer, P. J., & Evarts, C. M. Fracture–dislocation of the ankle with posterior entrapment of the fibula behind the tibia. *Journal of Bone and Joint Surgery,* 1978, *60A* (3), 320–324.

Mazur, J. M., Schwartz, E., & Simon, S. R. Ankle arthrodesis. *Journal of Bone and Joint Surgery,* 1979, *61A* (7), 964–975.

Mock, M. S. Sprains and strains: Orthopedics in the emergency room. *Orthopedic Nurses' Association Journal,* 1979, *6* (8), 318–319.

Oh, I., Nahigian, S. H., Salas, A. S., & Zahrawi, F. B. Cerclage of the lateral malleolus in displaced fractures of the ankle. *Orthopedics,* 1978, *1* (5), 374–379.

Paules, L., Coleman, S. S., & Samuelson, R. M. Pes cavovarus. *Journal of Bone and Joint Surgery,* 1980, *62A* (6), 942–953.

Pusey, R. Pott's fracture. *Nursing Times,* 1978, *74* (31), 1293–1295.

Quigley, J. T. A glomus tumor of the heel pod. *Journal of Bone and Joint Surgery,* 1979, *61A* (3), 443–444.

Richter-Davies, L., Barnett, K., & Reid, D. Emergency management of lower extremity fractures. In N. E. Hill (Ed.), *Assessment and fracture management of the lower extremities.* Pitman, N. J.: Anthony J. Jannetti, 1984.

Roof, R., & Hodkinson, L. J. *Textbook of orthopaedic nursing* (2nd ed.). Oxford: Blackwell Scientific, 1975.

Robbins, S. L. *Pathologic basis of disease.* Philadelphia: W. B. Saunders, 1974.

Scranton, P. E. Metatarsalgia: Diagnosis and treatment. *Journal of Bone and Joint Surgery,* 1980, *62A* (5), 723–732.

Smith, C. L. Physical therapy management of patients with total ankle. *Physical Therapy,* 1980, *60* (3), 303–306.

Spiegel, P. G., Cooperman, D. R., & Laros, G. S. Epiphyseal fractures of the distal end of the tibia and fibula. *Journal of Bone and Joint Surgery,* 1978, *60A* (8), 1046–1050.

Steans, H. C. Principles of lower extremity fracture management. In N. E. Hill (Ed.). *Assessment and fracture management of the lower extremities.* Pitman, N. J.: Anthony J. Jannetti, 1984.

Stearns, C. M. Surgical implants used for fractures of the lower extremity. In N. E. Hill (Ed.), *Assessment and fracture management of the lower extremities.* Pitman, N. J.: Anthony J. Jannetti, 1984.

Waller, J. F. Physiology of the foot and the biomechanics of the flexible flat foot. *Orthopedic Nurses' Association Journal,* 1978, *5* (4), 101–105.

Warpus, J. M. Foot disorders. *Orthopedic Nurses' Association Journal,* 1978, *5* (3), 82–83.

Wassel, A. C. Sports medicine: Acute and overuse injuries. *Orthopaedic Nursing,* 1984, *3* (2), 29–33.

Waugh, T. Ankle replacement arthroplasty. *Orthopedic Nurses' Association Journal,* 1979, *6* (1), 15–18.

Yuan, H. A., Cody, R. B., & De Rosa, C. Osteochondritis dissecans of the talus associated with subchondral cysts. *Journal of Bone and Joint Surgery,* 1979, *61A* (8), 1249–1251.

9

THE SHOULDER AND UPPER ARM

Chapter 9 focuses on the treatment and associated nursing care of traumatic and pathological conditions of the shoulder including the clavicle and the upper arm. The major pathological conditions discussed are arthritis, infections, and neoplasms. Both common surgical procedures, such as repairs for recurrent dislocations of the shoulder and torn rotator cuffs, and less common procedures, such as arthrodesis and arthroplasty, are presented. The chapter begins with a review of the anatomy of the shoulder and the upper arm.

ANATOMY

The term shoulder is used clinically to encompass the entire shoulder girdle, which comprises the upper humerus, the scapula, the clavicle, and the sternum. These bones articulate through the glenohumeral, the acromioclavicular, and the sternoclavicular joints. The clavicle acts to hold the arm and the scapula outward and backward. Elevation of the arm is forward flexion, and abduction takes place through the glenohumeral joint, accompanied by rotation of the scapula on the thorax. Rotation of the scapula involves movement in the acromioclavicular joint and the rotation of the clavicle in the sternoclavicular joint (Gartland, 1979, p. 244). Thus the active range of motion of the arm involves the complete shoulder girdle.

BONES

Scapula

The scapula (or "shoulder blade") (Fig. 9–1) is a large, flattened, triangular bone on the posteriolateral aspect of the thorax, overlapping parts of the sec-

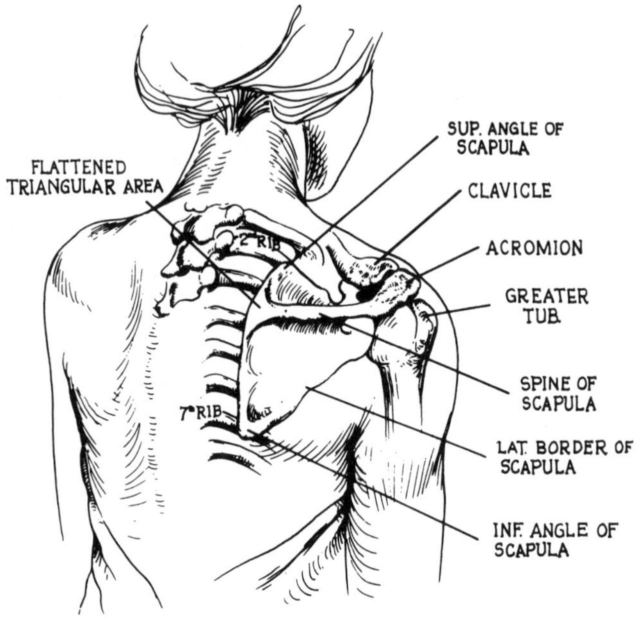

Figure 9–1. Posterior aspect of the bone structure of the shoulder. *(Figures 9–1, 9–2, 9–4, 9–8, 9–11, and 9–16 are reproduced from Hoppenfeld, S., 1976, with permission.)*

ond to the seventh ribs (Warwick & Williams, 1973, p. 318). It has costal and dorsal surfaces; upper, lateral, and medial borders; inferior, superior, and lateral angles; and three bony processes, the scapular spine, the acromion, and the coracoid process. The dorsal surface is divided by the scapular spine, a horizontal bony ridge that extends laterally past the glenoid fossa and ends in the bulbous acromial process. This process overhangs the head of the humerus, is the site where the clavicle attaches (the acromioclavicular joint), and contains the attachment of the coracoacromial ligament. The acromion and the coracoacromial ligament form part of the arch overlying the suprahumeral joint.

The scapula moves in a gliding manner in conjunction with the motion and the rotation of the clavicle. The motion of the scapula and the clavicle is primarily produced by two muscles, the trapezius and the serratus anterior. The upper fibers of the trapezius originate from the ligamentum nuchae in the lower cervical region, the posterior spinous process of the cervical spine, and the upper thoracic spine. They attach to the upper margin of the medial and central scapular spine, act to pull the scapula upward, and cause inward pivoting of the acromioclavicular joint. The middle fibers, which originate from the spinous processes of the upper thoracic vertebrae, attach to the medial border of the scapular spine, and "fix" the scapula during abduction of the arm. The lower fibers, which originate from the spinous processes of the lower thoracic vertebrae, attach to the medial portion of the spine of the scapula, and act to pull the medial border of the spine of the scapula down and in. The serratus anterior muscle, which originates from the upper eight ribs, attaches to the medial (vertebral) and inferior borders of the scapula, and acts to pull the scapula forward.

The trapezius muscle is supplied by the spinal accessory nerve (XI). The serratus is innervated by the long thoracic nerve formed by the anterior branches of the roots of C5, C6, and C7 (primarily C6) before entering the brachial plexus (Cailliet, 1981, p. 22–24).

Clavicle

The clavicle (or "collar bone") extends almost horizontally across the root of the neck laterally toward the point of the shoulder (Fig. 9–2). The lateral or acromial end of the bone is flattened and articulates with the medial side of the acromion, whereas the medial or sternal end is enlarged and articulates with the clavicular notch of the manubrium of the sternum. The shaft is gently curved with a shape that resembles the italic letter *f* (Warwick & Williams, 1973, p. 322).

Humerus

The humerus is the longest and largest bone of the upper extremity. The upper (proximal) end consists of a greater and lesser tuberosity and a rounded "head" that articulates with the glenoid cavity of the scapula to form a ball-and-

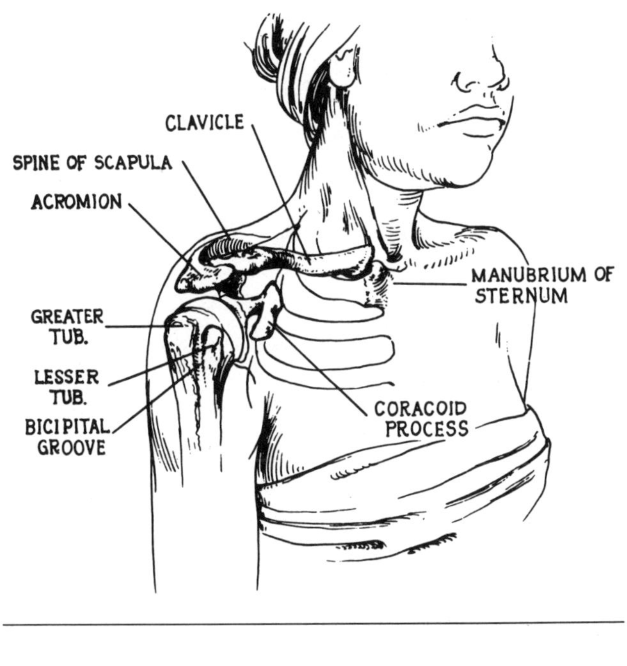

Figure 9–2. Anterior aspect of the bone structure of the shoulder.

socket joint (Fig. 9–3). The lower (distal) end is condylar, adapted to the forearm bones (the ulna and the radius) to form the elbow joint (Warwick & Williams, 1973, p. 324). (For further discussion of the distal portion, see Chap. 10.)

JOINTS

Sternoclavicular Joint

The sternoclavicular joint is formed by the sternal end of the clavicle articulating with the superior lateral portion of the manubrium of the sternum and the cartilage of the first rib (Fig. 9–4). The articular surface of the clavicle is covered with a layer of fibrocartilage. The joint is completely divided by an articular disc between the sternum and the clavicle. The ligaments that surround the joint are the anterior and posterior sternoclavicular, the interclavicular, and the costoclavicular ligaments (Warwick & Williams, 1973, p. 422). The anterior and posterior sternoclavicular ligaments reinforce the loose fibrous capsule of the joint, and the interclavicular ligament connects the two clavicles. The costoclavicular ligament, which originates from the medial portion of the first rib and attaches into the undersurface of the clavicle, acts as a fulcrum for all motion of the shoulder girdle and stabilizes the clavicle (Cailliet, 1981, p. 31).

The arteries supplying the joint are branches of the internal thoracic and supracapsular arteries. The nerves are from the anterior supraclavicular nerve and the nerve to the subclavius (Warwick & Williams, 1973, p. 423).

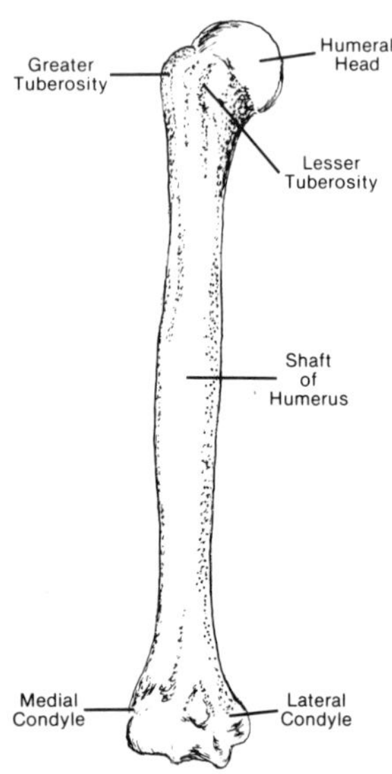

Figure 9–3. Humerus. *(From Brantley, P., & Analla, M.* The nurse and orthopedic surgery. *Rutherford, N.J.: Howmedica, Inc., 1980, p. 14. Courtesy of Howmedica.)*

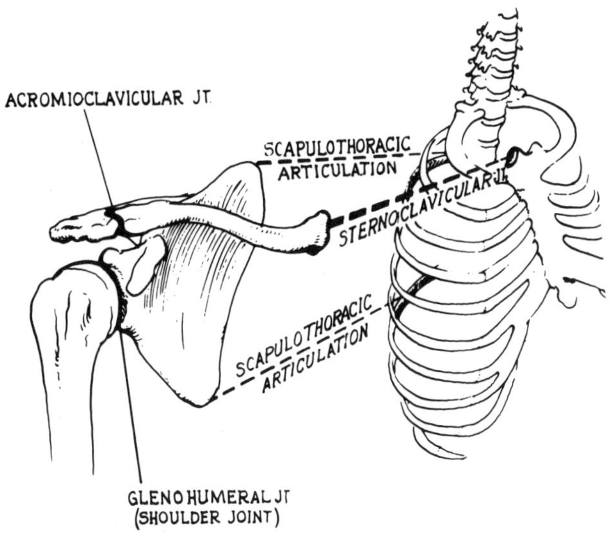

Figure 9–4. The shoulder girdle.

Acromioclavicular Joint

The acromioclavicular joint articulates between the lateral (acromial) end of the clavicle and the anterior medial portion of the acromial process of the scapula (see Fig. 9–4). Both articular surfaces are covered with fibrocartilage. On the acromial end of the clavicle is a narrow, oval area that is directed downward and laterally to overlap a corresponding area on the medial border of the acromion (Warwick & Williams, 1973, p. 422). The acromioclavicular joint has a weak, relaxed fibrous capsule that is reinforced by strong superior and inferior acromioclavicular ligaments that prevent posterior displacement of the clavicle upon the acromion. The clavicle is attached to the scapula by the coracoclavicular ligament, formed by the lateral trapezoid and the medial conoid ligaments (Cailliet, 1981, pp. 28–29).

The arterial supply to the acromioclavicular joint is derived from the supracapsular and thoracoacromial arteries. The nerve supply is from the supracapsular and lateral pectoral nerves (Warwick & Williams, 1973, p. 423).

Glenohumeral Joint

The glenohumeral or shoulder joint, the pivotal joint of the upper extremity, is a type of ball-and-socket joint (see Fig. 9–4). The ball, the humeral head, has only a small area of bony contact with the glenoid fossa, a shallow, ovoid socket that faces anteriorly, laterally, and upward. Both articular surfaces are covered with a layer of hyaline cartilage. The cartilage on the head of the humerus is thickest in the center and becomes thinner peripherally, whereas the reverse is true for the glenoid cavity. Surrounding the perimeter of the fossa, to deepen the cup, is a fibrous lip known as the glenoidal labrum. Compared to the ball-and-socket joint of the hip, the construction of the shoulder joint permits greater movement but provides less stability. Structurally the joint is weak because it depends on the support given by the surrounding muscles, not on its bone structure or the presence of strong ligaments.

The capsule of the glenohumeral joint is an extremely thin-walled, loose container that attaches to the entire perimeter of the glenoid rim. The capsule is attached medially to the glenoid cavity beyond the glenoidal labrum, laterally to the anatomical neck of the humerus close to the articular margin, and superiorly to the root of the coracoid process so as to include the origin of the long head of the biceps. Throughout the joint there is a synovial lining that blends with the hyaline cartilage of the head of the humerus but fails to reach the cartilage of the glenoid fossa.

Rotation of the arm around its longitudinal axis has an effect on the tautness and laxity of the capsule. The anterior portion of the capsule is reinforced by the superior, middle, and inferior glenohumeral ligaments. They are attached on the humerus and converge toward the glenoid rim to attach on the anterior superior portion of the glenoid and adjacent scapular bone. The external rotation of the humerus upon the glenoid fossa is limited by the coracohumeral ligament. The coracohumeral ligament originates at the coracoid process of the scapula and attaches to the front of the greater tubercle of the humerus, blending with the tendon of supraspinatus. The transverse humeral ligament functions as a retinaculum for the tendon of the long head of the biceps. It passes from the lesser to the greater tubercle of the humerus and attaches above the epiphyseal line. The fibrous capsule is strengthened above by the tendon of supraspinatus, below by the long head of the triceps, behind by the tendons of the infraspinatus and teres minor, and in front by the tendon of the subscapularis. The muscles and tendons of the subscapularis, the supraspinatus, the infraspinatus, and the teres minor are all intimately blended with the fibrous capsule forming a cuff, termed the rotator cuff. They reinforce the capsule and provide active support for the joint (Warwick & Williams, 1973, p. 425). Besides the muscles of the rotator cuff, the deltoid muscle is also important in joint movement. In conjunction with the muscles of the rotator cuff, contraction of the deltoid muscle elevates the humerus.

BURSA

There are numerous bursae in the neighborhood of the shoulder. The subscapularis bursa is between the tendon of the subscapularis and the joint capsule, communicating with the joint through an opening between the superior and the middle glenohumeral ligaments. There is a bursa that separates the tendon of infraspinatus and the capsule. The subacromial bursa lies between the deltoid muscle and the capsule. There is a bursa on the upper surface of the acromion, one between the teres major and the long head of the triceps, and one in front of, and another behind, the tendon of the latissimus dorsi. In addition, one is frequently found between the coracoid process and the capsule and another is sometimes found behind the coracobrachialis (Warwick & Williams, 1973, p. 426).

THE SHOULDER

Trauma

SCAPULA

A fracture of a portion of the scapula is an unusual injury. It is usually caused by a direct blow, and is often associated with bruising of muscles, fractures of underlying ribs, or other injuries in patients sustaining severe trauma. Persons with a fractured scapula tend to hold their arm in adduction. Although painful, displacement of the fragments is rare because the scapula is encased in a heavy muscular envelope (Gartland, 1979, p. 254; Roaf & Hodkinson, 1975, p. 80). Fractures of the scapula are almost always treated symptomatically. The arm is rested in a sling until the pain has disappeared. As a general rule there is a full restoration of movement and function (Donahoo & Dimon, 1977, p. 53; Gartland, 1979, p. 254; Roaf & Hodkinson, 1975, p. 80).

CLAVICLE

Fractures of the clavicle (collar bone) are one of the most common bony injuries, and are encountered much more frequently in children than in adults. The injury commonly occurs because of a fall on an outstretched hand, or a fall on the arm or shoulder, though it may be due to a direct injury. The clinical picture is of a patient who has a drooping of the shoulder, a hematoma over the site of the clavicle, an obvious protrusion of the inner half of the bone, and pain. The patient usually holds the arm against the chest in a protective manner. In some instances an undisplaced clavicular fracture may be overlooked.

The fracture is self-healing and does not require elaborate splinting. When the clavicle calcifies, however, there may be an unsightly enlargement at the fracture site unless steps are taken to keep the fragments in correct alignment during healing. It may be possible to reduce the fracture satisfactorily by moving the shoulders upward and backward. When displacement is minimal and ligaments are not torn, the reduced position, once obtained, may be maintained by the use of a sling to support the elbow. For most adults with fractured clavicles, that position may be maintained by a sling and a padded figure-of-eight bandage, a plaster of Paris figure-of-eight bandage, or even a shoulder spica cast. Some authorities advise the use of a Velpeau dressing for 10 to 14 days prior to the application of the figure-of-eight or spica (Gartland, 1979, p. 253; Roaf & Hodkinson, 1975, p. 77–79). Even though displaced fractures of the clavicle often cannot be reduced and maintained in perfect position, functional results are usually excellent. Healing time for fractrues of the clavicle is generally about 8 weeks.

Open reduction of clavicular fractures is rarely indicated in adults, except for complicated fractures or possibly for patients with multiple injuries (Fig. 9–5). Complications of clavicular fractures are relatively infrequent, and in particular, damage to the brachial plexus or the subclavian artery are rare (Roaf & Hodkinson, 1975, p. 77).

□ NURSING PROCESS (Table 9–1)

Assessment

The nursing assessment of a patient following a closed reduction of a fractured clavicle and the application of a figure-of-eight bandage, arm sling, or both, begins with a check of the neurovascular status of both upper extremities. Pulse, color, temperature, movement, and sensation must be determined. To assess the circulatory status, first note if there is any swelling of the hands or the fingers, and check for color (i.e., pallor or cyanosis) and temperature (i.e., coldness or increased warmth). Determine circulation to the fingers by blanching (i.e., pinching the end of the finger or thumb between your finger and thumb and then letting go). The patient's

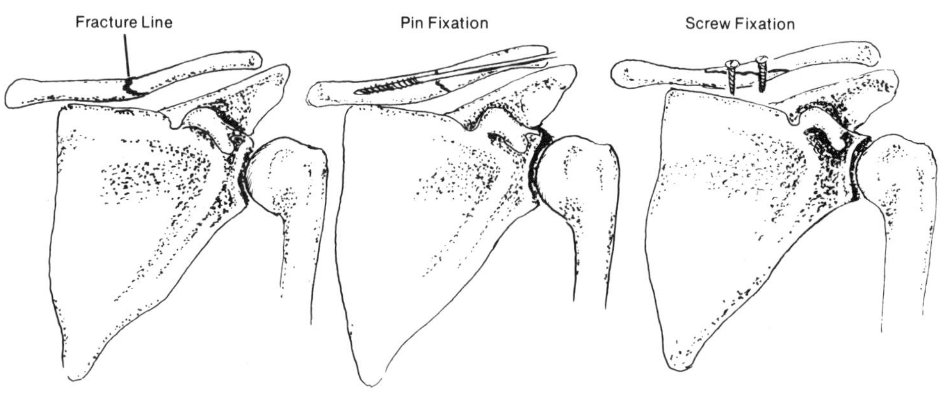

Figure 9–5. Open reduction and internal fixation, fractured clavicle. *(From Brantley, P., & Analla, M.* The nurse and orthopedic surgery. *Rutherford, N.J.: Howmedica, Inc., 1980, p. 5. Courtesy of Howmedica.)*

TABLE 9–1. NURSING PROCESS FOR FRACTURED CLAVICLE TREATED WITH CLOSED REDUCTION AND FIGURE-OF-EIGHT BANDAGE

Assessment	Nursing Diagnosis	Goal Formulation	Planning and Intervention	Evaluation and Reassessment
1. Assess the location, duration, and severity of pain. Check for areas of protrusion, swelling, or discoloration at the fracture site. Check the comfort of the figure-of-eight bandage.	1. Alteration in comfort: pain in the shoulder related to soft tissue trauma and bone instability.	1. Short-term goal: a relative state of comfort through the use of nursing measures and medications. Long-term goal: free of pain.	1. Alleviate Pain When lying supine, place a small folded towel or other soft item along the spinal column for support. Instruct on relaxation techniques. Support the arm on the affected side. Administer prescribed pain medications.	1. The patient should remain relatively free of pain.
2. Check that the shoulders are level. Check that the shoulders are pulled upward, outward, and backward from the thorax. Check the neurovascular status of both arms.	2. Impaired physical mobility: decreased shoulder function related to lack of bone stability.	2. Short-term goal: an increase in mobility through the use of controlled exercises. Long-term goal: a return of full function in the affected shoulder.	2. Increase Mobility *Position* Position the patient supine with the head of the bed elevated. Instruct patient not to elevate the affected arm above shoulder level. *Exercises* Instruct on active range-of-motion exercises for the elbows, wrists, and fingers as soon as possible after bandage application. Instruct on shoulder exercises under physician's direction (e.g., pendulum, external rotation, elevation, and internal rotation exercises). *Ambulation* Assist patient with initial ambulation.	2. The patient should follow the exercise regime without supervision.

(continued)

TABLE 9–1. *(Continued)*

Assessment	Nursing Diagnosis	Goal Formulation	Planning and Intervention	Evaluation and Reassessment
3. Assess the neurovascular status of both arms. Check for any tightness of the bandage at the axillary areas.	3. Potential for injury: neurovascular deficit related to soft tissue swelling and a tight bandage.	3. Short- and long-term goal: free of any neurovascular complication.	3. Prevent Complications *Circulatory and Neurological* Make sure the bandage does not become too tight with changes in position. Make sure that the bandage firmly holds the reduction. Report any abnormalities in neurovascular status.	3. The bandage should be secure but not too tight or too loose. Determine if there is any paresthesia in upper extremities that could indicate nerve injury or impending ischemia. There should not be any weakness or disappearance of the pulse, or swelling of the hands.

Check for any protrusion, swelling, or discoloration at the fracture site. Check if the bandage is pulling on the skin in the axillary areas. Check the edges of the bandage for possible skin irritation.	Potential for injury: impairment of skin integrity related to bandage and soft tissue swelling.	Short- and long-term goal: free of any break in skin integrity.	*Integumentary* Teach the patient to apply a slight amount of pressure to the skin alongside the bandage at the axilla. Pad the axillary area if needed. Instruct on cleansing the axillary area, relaxing skin tautness and using antiperspirant but not powder.	The skin under the bandage should be free from excoriation.
4. Assess patient's level of knowledge about the rehabilitation process and self-care with a figure-of-eight bandage in place.	4. Potential knowledge deficit related to the rehabilitation process and self-care.	4. Short- and long-term goal: a decrease in anxiety with an increase in knowledge.	4. Patient Teaching Go over the various steps in the rehabilitation process. Make sure the patient can demonstrate all of the exercises. Go over various methods of dressing and self-care. Go over restrictions (e.g., not to raise hands above shoulder level or lift heavy objects). Include family and significant others in teaching plan.	4. The patient should be aware that he or she should not use the upper extremities to lift or move heavy objects. The patient should know the appropriate clothing to wear and how to get in and out of the clothing, especially heavy coats, without applying stress to the fractured clavicle.

nail bed should first turn white and then return to pink. The unaffected side can usually be compared to the affected side, but not when a figure-of-eight bandage is used, as it may cause a neurovascular impairment on either side. Evaluate the radial pulse, and note if there is any weakness or disappearance. Check the neurological status of the upper extremities by testing the function of the radial, median, and ulnar nerves. To determine the motor function for the radial nerve, have the patient hyperextend the thumb or the wrist on both extremities; for the median nerve, have the patient oppose the thumb and the little finger (that is, do a pinch using the thumb and the little finger), or flex the wrist; and for the ulnar nerve, have the patient abduct all fingers. Assess for paresthesia of the sensory components of the radial nerve by pricking dully and then sharply at the first web space (the space between the thumb and the index finger). Assess the median nerve by pricking the distal surface of the index finger and assess the ulnar nerve by pricking the distal end of the little finger.

Note if there is any portrusion, swelling, or discoloration at the fracture site and if the shoulders are at the same level; that is, there should be no drooping of the shoulder on the affected side. Assess the amount, location, severity, and duration of pain, the comfort of the figure-of-eight bandage, and the position of the bandage.

Nursing Diagnosis and Goal Formulation

Nursing diagnoses for a typical patient with a closed reduction of a fractured clavicle and the application of a figure-of-eight bandage, arm sling, or both, are (1) alterations in comfort related to trauma and surgery, (2) alterations in mobility related to lack of bone stability, (3) potential complications related to surgical procedure and decreased arm mobility, and (4) alterations in psychological well-being related to anxiety and knowledge deficit about the injury and treatment methods.

Short-term goals are to have the patient experience (1) a decrease in the amount of pain through nursing measures and prescribed medications; (2) an increase in mobility through the use of controlled exercises; (3) an absence of complications from surgery and decreased activities; and (4) a decrease in anxiety through increased knowledge. Long-term goals are to have the patient free of pain and to have return of full function without supportive devices.

Planning and Intervention

In the treatment of the patient with a clavicular fracture, there is a need for nursing supervision. As the patient is usually an outpatient, he or she must understand the treatment, the rationale for the treatment, and the potential complications. In many instances, the patient may be asked to check with medical personnel at specific times to verify that the treatment is progressing satisfactorily.

Alleviate Pain. The assessment for pain must determine the cause, that is, whether the pain is from the fracture site, from muscle spasms, from the figure-of-eight bandage, or from nerve and/or circulatory impairment. The immobilizing device may be too loose and allow movement at the fracture, thus increasing pain. The figure-of-eight bandage may be too tight, causing discomfort at either or both axillae or impairing the neurovascular status of the upper extremities. In either case, the figure-of-eight bandage must be adjusted.

The patient will probably be most comfortable sleeping in the supine position, or supine with the head of the bed elevated a few degrees. Because the shoulders have been pulled up and back to reduce the clavicular fracture, a small folded towel or other soft item placed along the spinal column may be needed to give enough support to the center of the back to reduce stress and yet not interfere with the reduction. In changing position or in helping with activities of daily living, the patient should not attempt to utilize the overhead trapeze, even with the uninvolved arm, as that would apply stress to the fracture site.

If the fixation device is pulling on the skin in the axillary areas, the patient can be taught to apply a slight amount of pressure to the skin alongside the bandage. That releases the pull on the skin and allows a readjustment of the figure-of-eight bandage.

Pain medications should be administered only after other interventions have been explored. Because most patients are outpatients or have a short hospital stay, they need to know how to manage the pain.

Increase Mobility

Position. The clavicle helps to hold the shoulder upward, outward, and backward from the thorax. Therefore, when the clavicle is fractured the objective is to hold the shoulder in its normal position by means of a sling, clavicular strap, or a figure-of-eight bandage.

For patients with a fractured clavicle medial to the coracoclavicular ligament, usually a figure-of-eight bandage is used for immobilization. To apply the bandage, seat the patient on a stool. An assistant should stand behind the patient and place one knee between the patient's shoulder blades (scapulae) to apply traction to the shoulders to pull them back and upward as needed. Pads are then placed in the patient's axillae. To apply the bandage, start it in front of the unaffected shoulder, carry it under the patient's arm, across the back, over the affected shoulder, under the affected arm, and so on, so that the turns of the bandage cross over between the scapulae. Each turn of the bandage draws the shoulder upward and backward in a figure-of-eight fashion. The bandage is applied firmly but not so tight as to interfere with circulation to the arms. A roll of plaster over the bandage may be used to provide more security. The affected arm may also be placed in a sling for additional support (see p. 594).

There are other kinds of figure-of-eight bandages. One is a strip of tubular stockinette stuffed with splint-wool or other types of padding to form a thick sausage. The stuffed stockinette is placed under each arm at the axilla and around each shoulder and fastened together between the scapulae. The shoulders are then pulled up and back in the same manner as discussed above. Commercially prepared figure-of-eight bandages are also available.

When an undisplaced fracture occurs lateral to the coracoclavicular ligament, the shoulder is usually held in place with a sling. If proper reduction and immobilization cannot be maintained, an open reduction with internal fixation may be required.

Exercises. Patients are encouraged to begin active range-of-motion exercises of their elbows, wrists, and fingers as soon as possible after the application of the figure-of-eight bandage. These exercises help to maintain joint mobility and to prevent loss of joint motion. Patients are generally able to move their elbow, wrist, and finger joints the way they normally move them.

Exercises to regain full motion of the shoulder are not begun until prescribed by the patient's physician. The most common shoulder exercises are pendulum, external rotation, elevation, and internal rotation exercises. In beginning these exercises, the unaffected arm may be used to assist the affected arm. A wall climbing exercise, where the fingers "climb" up a wall, thus extending and lifting the arm and abducting the shoulder, may also be used.

Prevent Complications. Potential complications following clavicular fractures include trauma to the nerves of the brachial plexus or injury to the subclavian vein or artery from a bony fragment. When a clavicular strap or figure-of-eight bandage is used to pull the shoulders up and back and to hold them in that position, the axillae should be well padded to prevent a compression injury to the brachial plexus and axillary artery. The bandage is applied firmly to hold the reduction, but there should be no restriction of the circulatory or nerve function in either arm. If nerve or circulatory impairment should arise, the bandage can be loosened to release the obstruction.

The figure-of-eight bandage may cause skin irritation. When the bandage is too tight under the axillae, it can be readjusted by changing the position of the patient's arm and inserting a finger between the bandage and the skin to push the skin away from the tight edges. At times the bandage may be too loose, and allow rubbing at the axillae. Additional padding may be needed to prevent irritation. The patient may have skin excoriation develop from increased perspiration, especially during the summer months. Padding the bandage at the axillae with splint-wool should absorb most of the moisture. An antiperspirant would also be helpful. Do not have the patient apply powder to the area, as that is only a temporary measure and leads to the development of an undersirable paste-like substance.

Patient Teaching. Following a fractured clavicle and the application of a figure-of-eight bandage, the patient is cautioned not to elevate the affected arm above shoulder level until the fracture has united (approximately 3 weeks). The patient, the family, and significant others need to understand that the purpose of the figure-of-eight bandage, or the other supportive devices, is to maintain the shoulder in good posture. It is not possible to completely immobilize a fractured clavicle with a figure-of-eight bandage. When the patient changes position, he or she may feel the bones at the fracture site move for appoximately 7 to 10 days after immobilization, until they become "sticky" and begin to knit. The healing time for fractures of the clavicle is generally considered to be about 8 weeks.

The patient should not be afraid of the immobilization, and should be instructed on how to insert a finger to push the skin away from any tight edges and how to add additional padding at the axillae as needed. The patient should be taught how to readjust the bandage and reposition the arms to increase comfort. Go over activities of daily living with the patient, especially what to wear and how to get in and out of clothing.

Evaluation and Assessment

Check for paresthesia (a prickling or burning sensation) in the upper extremities, as that may indicate nerve injury or impending ischemia and requires early treatment to restore circulation before irreparable damage occurs. There should not be any weakness or disappearance of the pulse, or swelling of the hands. The fixation bandage must be secure but neither too loose nor too tight, and no adverse affects from the device should have developed. The skin under the bandage must be free from excoriation.

Determine how well the patient is doing with each of the exercises and in following the exercise regime. The patient must be aware that he or she should not be using the upper extremities to lift or move heavy objects. The patient should know the appropriate clothing to wear and how to get in and out of the clothing, especially heavy coats, without applying stress to the fractured clavicle. Once the patient returns home, he or she should understand that the physician should be notified if the treatment apparatus is causing serious discomfort or if any of the potential complications occur.

STERNOCLAVICULAR JOINT

Traumatic injuries of the sternoclavicular joint can result from a force applied to the arm, the shoulder, or the chest. Such injuries may vary from a first-degree sprain to a complete dislocation. A first-degree sternoclavicular sprain involves minor tearing of the sternoclavicular and costoclavicular ligament fibers. A second-degree sprain (a subluxation) involves a complete rupture of the sternoclavicular ligament and a partial tear of the costoclavicular ligament. A third-degree sprain (a dislocation) involves a complete rupture of the sternoclavicular and costoclavicular ligaments. The medial end of the clavicle can dislocate anteriorly and inferiorly so that it overlaps the first rib, or in rare instances, it can dislocate posteriorly (a retrosternal dislocation). The displaced clavicle rides upward causing a visible and palpable prominence of the joint. The prominence is apparent when the injured joint is compared with its counterpart joint on the opposite side (Donahoo & Dimon, 1977, p. 52; Gartland, 1979, pp. 249–250; Iversen & Clawson, 1977, pp. 129–130).

In most instances, a dislocation can be reduced by closed manipulation. Anterior dislocations are usually treated nonoperatively. Occasionally, a prominence may remain at the site of the dislocation. Posterior dislocations, on the other hand, may require immediate medical attention if the medial end of the clavicle is pressing upon the vital structures of the mediastinum, including the great vessels, trachea, esophagus, and thoracic duct. If that is the case, a sandbag placed between the scapulae of a patient lying supine, which allows them to retract, pulling the medial end of the clavicle out of the retrosternal area, may be administered as emergency care. Nonoperative medical treatment may consist of carefully injecting a local anesthetic into the area of the dislocation, placing the patient supine with a sandbag between the scapulae, and applying posteriorly directed pressure over the lateral end of the clavicle. If that does not succeed in reducing the dislocation, a second person might need to grasp the medial end of the clavicle with the fingers, or even a towel clip, to elevate it into position. The reduction is maintained with a figure-of-eight splint. Such treatment produces a stable joint, but most patients continue to have mild crepitation and discomfort during strenuous activity (Iversen & Clawson, 1977, pp. 129–133).

If close reduction is unsuccessful for an anterior or posterior dislocation, an open reduction can be performed and the reduction maintained by the temporary use of metallic pin fixation. Surgery is also advocated if there is severe damage to the joint capsule, articular disc, and periarticular ligaments. Such surgery consists of reconstructing torn ligaments to maintain the joint in proper alignment. Resection of a medial inch of the clavicle is recommended for an old unreduced sternoclavicular joint dislocation that is symptomatic. (Some authorities would also treat an acute dislocation by that method.) A recurrent sternoclavicular joint dislocation may be treated by stabilizing the joint with a fascial loop about and through the medial clavicle and the first rib. The shoulder is then protected with a Velpeau bandage for 3 to 4 weeks, followed by a similar period of restricted activity.

ACROMIOCLAVICULAR JOINT

The acromioclavicular (AC) joint, where the clavicle joins the scapula, is a synovial joint that has relatively weak capsular ligaments. The joint is usually injured by a direct fall on the point of the shoulder, i.e., a force applied to the lateral or superior aspect of the acromion, which is not uncommon in athletic and industrial accidents. Such an injury may tear the supporting ligaments and cause varying degrees of disruption of the AC joint. The weight of the arm may pull the acromion down, which then allows the lateral end of the clavicle to displace out of the joint and become prominent beneath the skin.

First- and Second-Degree Sprains

Depending on the force, the capsule and the ligaments around the AC joint may be stretched, sprained, or torn, with the degree of injury ranging from a sprain to a dislocation of the joint. That dislocation has been termed a shoulder separation, but it does not indicate any injury to the glenohumeral ("shoulder") joint. A first-degree AC sprain (shoulder pointer) is an incomplete tear of the AC ligament without subluxation of the joint. A second-degree sprain is a more severe disruption of the joint capsule that allows subluxation (partial separation) of the AC joint, but with the coracoclavicular ligaments remaining intact. With these sprains, the deformity is usually small and the swelling minimal. The diagnosis of second-degree sprain can be confirmed by using roentgenography to demonstrate subluxation of the AC joint. The usual procedure is to make a roentgenogram that includes both AC joints, with the patient erect and holding a 5- to 10-pound weight in each hand. (The weight tends to pull the acromion downward and allows some upper migration of the lateral end of the clavicle.) The stress roentgenogram for a first-degree sprain shows no separation, but for a second-degree sprain shows a small degree of displacement of the distal clavicle, or a widening of the joint space compared to that of the unaffected side (Donahoo & Dimon, 1977, p. 52; Gartland, 1979, p. 250; Iversen & Clawson, 1977, pp. 130–131).

First- and second-degree sprains of the AC joint may be treated symptomatically with a pressure strapping centered over the joint and a sling to support the arm (or only a sling to support the arm), until the ligaments and tissues have healed, usually 10 days to 3 weeks. Occasionally the strapping has to encircle both the shoulder and the elbow to elevate the acromion enough to bring about a reduction. Once reduction has been effected, the patient is started on an exercise program.

Surgery to resect the distal end of the clavicle is usually indicated if the patient continues to have symptoms after nonsurgical treatment or is dissatisfied with the cosmetic results. Some authorities recommend surgical treatment for all second-degree sprains.

Third-Degree Sprain

A third-degree sprain, i.e., a complete dislocation of the AC joint, occurs when the injury ruptures the joint capsule and overlying musculature along with the conoid and trapezoid ligaments. The deformity is obvious because the skin is pushed out by the lateral end of the clavicle, which has been displaced by the weight of the arm. An anteroposterior roentgenogram of the shoulder under stress (described previously) demonstrates the distance between the coracoid process and the clavicle.

Dislocations are treated by various methods, with those that do not disrupt the AC joint surfaces decreasing the chance of later degenerative joint changes. Nonoperative treatment utilizes some type of encircling bandage designed to reduce the dislocation and hold the parts together until healing occurs. A figure-of-eight bandage with adhesive strapping from the chest to the back together with a pad over the clavicle may be used. Easy-to-apply splints are now available from commerical manufacturers (Fig. 9–6A), and appear efficient in maintaining reduction of the dislocation. Immobilization must be maintained long enough to allow complete healing. On the other hand, better anatomical and functional results may be obtained with operative methods (Fig. 9–6B). Those methods are (1) open reduction with internal fixation using two Kirschner wires that usually pass through the AC joint, (2) fixation of the distal clavicle to the coracoid process with a screw (which has the disadvantage of requiring synchronous motion of the clavicle and scapula), (3) fixation by cerclage of the clavicle and coracoid process with fascia, nonabsorbable suture, or wires, (4) internal fixation of the AC joint itself using a heavy nonabsorbable suture, and (5) lateral clavicular resection arthroplasty (Edmondson & Crenshaw, 1980,

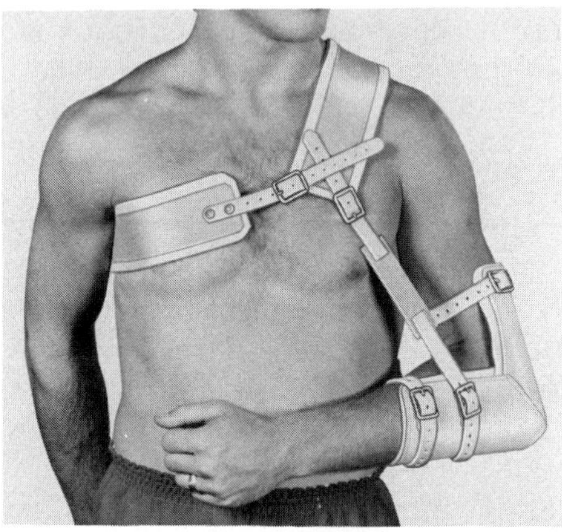

A

Figure 9–6. A. Acromioclavicular dislocation strap. *(Courtesy of Zimmer, Inc.)* **B.** Repair of acromioclavicular joint separation. *(From Brantley, P., & Analla, M.* The nurse and orthopedic surgery. *Rutherford, N.J.: Howmedica, Inc., 1980, p. 4. Courtesy of Howmedica.)*

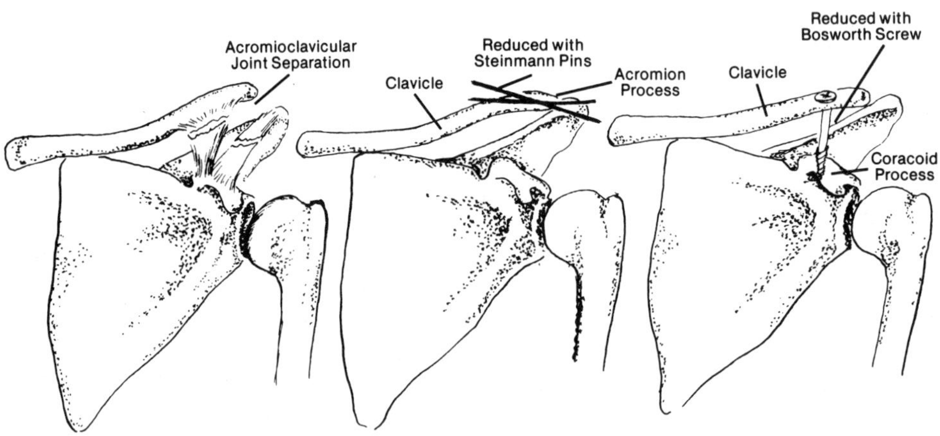

B

pp. 141–146; Iversen & Clawson, 1977, pp. 130–133). After the repair of the AC joint is completed, the patient will have a Velpeau dressing or a sling and swath. In chronic painful dislocations, the resection of the outer inch of the clavicle usually leads to relief of symptoms and restoration of function. Recovery occurs in about 3 weeks. Metallic fixation by a nail or Kirschner wire may also be used in some instances.

☐ NURSING PROCESS (Table 9–2)

Assessment

The first step in the nursing assessment of a patient following reduction of an AC separation and the application of a Velpeau bandage, or a sling and swath, is to check the neurovascular status of the affected arm. Pulse, color, temperature, movement, and sensation in the involved extremity are determined and compared with those of the uninvolved side. For further information on assessment, see pp. 494 and 498 and Chapter 2. If a commercially available Velpeau-type support is used, there should be no problem in completing every step of the neurovascular assessment. If a physician-made Velpeau bandage is used, however, the bandage may prevent a complete motor assessment by immobilizing the wrist. Record specifically what assessments were made. With a Velpeau bandage or a sling and swath, the neurovascular assessment of the involved arm is vital because the flexion of the elbow means that there is an added potential for neurovascular impairment. For a patient with a sling and swath, also check that the hand is higher than the elbow.

Assess the respiratory status for rate, depth, and rhythm, and determine whether it is affected by a change in position. Does the patient need to be in a sitting or semi-Fowler position to breathe comfortably? Is the Velpeau bandage too tight, or does it prevent the patient from taking deep breaths?

Determine the amount, location, and severity of pain. Check the upper trunk, affected arm, and immobilizing device for position and comfort. Note if there is any undue pressure or tautness to the skin from the immobilizing device.

Nursing Diagnosis and Goal Formulation

Nursing diagnoses for a typical patient following reduction of an AC separation and the application of a Velpeau bandage (Fig. 9–7A), a sling and swath, or shoulder immobilizer (Fig. 9–7B) are (1) alterations in comfort related to pain from the trauma and surgery on the joint and soft tissues, (2) alterations in mobility related to lack of joint stability, (3) potential complications related to surgical procedure and decreased arm mobility, and (4) alterations in psychological well-being related to anxiety and knowledge deficit about the injury and the rehabilitation process.

Short-term goals are to have the patient experience (1) a decrease in

TABLE 9–2. NURSING PROCESS FOR ACROMIOCLAVICULAR SEPARATION TREATED WITH VELPEAU BANDAGE

Assessment	Nursing Diagnosis	Goal Formulation	Planning and Intervention	Evaluation and Reassessment
1. Assess the location, duration, and severity of pain. Check the upper trunk, affected arm, and immobilizing device for position and comfort.	1. Alteration in comfort: pain in the shoulder related to soft tissue swelling and joint instability.	1. Short-term goal: a relative state of comfort with the use of an immobilizing device. Long-term goal: free of pain.	1. Alleviate Pain Make sure the bandage is positioned correctly. Reposition and instruct on muscle setting exercises. Apply ice to the joint (not directly over the joint).	1. The patient should remain relatively free of pain if the arm is correctly positioned and immobilized. Muscle setting exercises should help relieve muscle spasms.
2. Check the position of the trunk and affected arm. Assess the neurovascular status of the affected arm. Assess the ability to do exercises.	2. Impaired physical mobility: decreased shoulder and arm function related to lack of joint stability.	2. Short-term goal: an increase in mobility through immobilization and controlled exercises. Long-term goal: regain full function in the shoulder and arm.	2. Increase Mobility *Positioning* Position the patient so as to maintain the trunk of the body in correct alignment. Make sure the shoulders are level with the patient supine, place a small support at the side of the chest to keep the arm in the correct position. *Exercises* Instruct on finger exercises. Instruct on other exercises as determined by site of fracture and repair (see text). *Ambulation* Assist with ambulation (usually on the first day). Assist with getting out of bed.	2. The patient should find the most comfortable position to be supine; lying on the unaffected side may also be comfortable. The patient should do exercises without supervison. The patient is usually unsteady at first because of the lack of arm swing.

3. Assess the fit of the bandage. Assess the neurovascular status of the affected arm. Check for any areas of swelling.	3. Potential for injury related to inadequate maintenance of immobilization.	3. Short- and long-term goal: free of any injury.	3. Prevent Complications *Incomplete Reduction* Make sure the bandage fits properly and is safely secured in place with the hand and arm correctly positioned.	3. The patient should have proper immobilization and complete reduction.
Assess neurovascular status. Check for any area of swelling. Check that the bandage is not too tight.	Potential for injury: neurovascular deficit related to soft tissue swelling and tightness of the bandage.	Short- and long-term goal: free of any neurovascular deficit.	*Circulatory and Neurological* Check the neurovascular status every 2–4 hours or as indicated by the patient's condition. Instruct on finger exercises. Make sure bandage is not too tight. Make sure the elbow is not hyperflexed. Notify the physician of abnormal neurovascular status.	The patient should remain free of any neurovascular deficit.
Assess the skin for any possible break in integrity. Check the skin at the edges of the bandage. Check for any areas of swelling.	Potential for impairment of skin integrity related to swelling, irritation, and tight bandage.	Short- and long-term goal: free of any break in skin integrity.	*Integumentary* Make sure the edges of the bandage are not irritating the skin. Place pad between the patient's chest and arm (no skin to skin touch). Decrease the amount of perspiration (especially under the arm).	The patient should be free of any break in skin integrity.
4. Assess the patient's level of knowledge about the rehabilitation process and how to bathe, dress, and care for self.	4. Potential knowledge deficit related to lack of knowledge about the rehabilitation process and self-care.	4. Short- and long-term goal: decrease in anxiety through an increase in knowledge.	4. Patient Teaching Discuss the rehabilitation process with the patient, the family, and significant other. Instruct the patient how to do neurovascular checks and to report any abnormalities. Have an open discussion on activities of daily living. Stress that the immobilizing device should not be removed. Demonstrate methods of bathing, cleansing, and dressing.	4. The patient, the family, and significant other should feel comfortable about going home with a Velpeau bandage on. The patient should verbalize an understanding of the rehabilitation process and self-care.

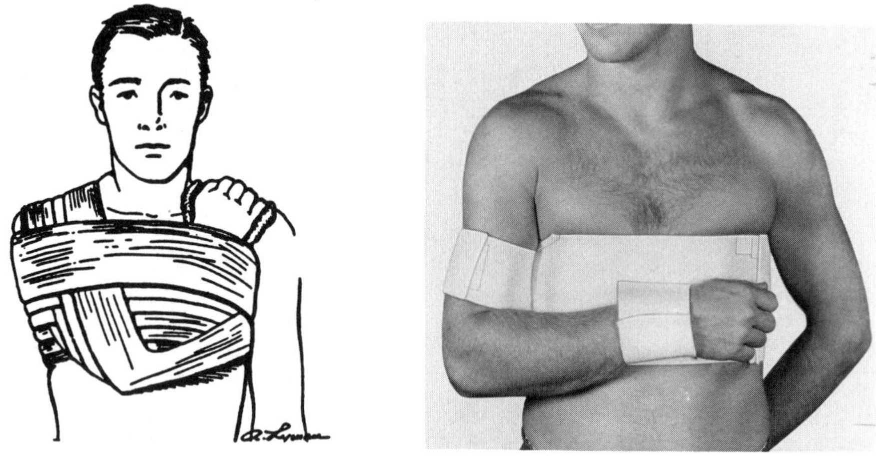

A B

Figure 9–7. A. The Velpeau bandage is used temporarily to immobilize the clavicle, shoulder, humerus, elbow, or forearm. A protective pad should be inserted wherever skin comes in contact with skin. *(From Larson, C.B., & Gould, M., 1978, p. 184, with permission.)* **B.** Shoulder immobilizer. *(Courtesy of Zimmer, Inc.)*

the amount of pain through the use of surgery, nursing measures, and prescribed medications, (2) an increase in mobility through exercise, (3) an absence of complications from surgery and decreased activities, and (4) a decrease in anxiety through increased knowledge. Long-term goals are to have the patient pain free and to have full return of motion and function in the involved arm.

Planning and Intervention

In the treatment of patients with an AC separation, there is a great need for the patient to understand the treatment, rationale, and potential for complications.

Alleviate Pain. Acromioclavicular joint pain may be due to muscle spasms, the surgical repair of the joint, incorrect positioning of the immobilizing device, neurovascular impairment, or skin impairment. The assessment must determine the source, location, and severity of the pain.

For muscle spasms, repositioning and muscle setting exercises that increase circulation to the area may help reduce pain, but medications may still be necessary. Position the patient so as to maintain the trunk of the body in correct alignment. Check that the level of the shoulders is equal. Check the position and neurovascular status of the arm. If a patient is in a sling, the arm may have moved to the side of the chest. Repositioning the arm to the front of the chest reduces discomfort. When the patient is lying supine, a small support at the side of the chest may be needed to keep the arm in the correct position. Check that the hand of the involved arm is level with or higher than the elbow, and readjust the sling accordingly. For patients in a commercial Velpeau bandage (or shoulder immobilizer), periodic readjustment of the immobilizer may be necessary. For instance, if the hand is not positioned properly, the edge of the strap may cut into the wrist. If the strap over the upper arm is slipping down, circulation may be impaired at the elbow. The chest strap of the shoulder immobilizer can be another source of discomfort to the patient if it is fastened too tight.

If swollen fingers occur, the patient must do finger exercises to increase the circulation and reduce the swelling. Excessive pain and swelling at the AC joint may be reduced by applications of ice. If ice is utilized, make sure the ice bags are not placed directly over the AC joint as that would cause pressure and add to the pain.

Increase Mobility. After the surgical repair of a separated AC joint, the amount of activity in the affected arm depends on the type of surgical procedure. Some procedures allow the patient to use the arm immediately, whereas others require the arm to have a period of immobilization.

When a patient has the end of the clavicle resected, the arm may have minimal or no immobilization, as the patient is encouraged to use the arm immediately after surgery. Patients with an AC separation repaired by the use of a screw usually have their arm immobilized in a sling. Patients with a Kirschner wire inserted for repair usually have the involved arm immobilized in a Velpeau bandage for at least 2 weeks.

The Velpeau bandage (see Fig. 9–7A) is a comfortable, effective method of bandaging the arm to the trunk of the body and immobilizing the shoulder girdle. It may be used in the treatment of a fracture of the surgical neck or shaft of the humerus, a fracture of the scapula or clavicle, and following the reduction of a glenohumeral, sternoclavicular, or acromioclavicular joint. There are a number of commercially developed Velpeau bandages, sometimes called Velpeau slings. Alternatively, a physician-made Velpeau bandage can be used. To apply such a bandage, the patient should sit on an examining table or stool, with someone supporting the affected arm in the position of immobilization. The axilla on the affected side should be clean and dry, and for female patients the area beneath the breasts should also be clean and dry. Padding is then placed in the axillae (and beneath the breasts of a woman) to prevent the skin of the arm from being pressed against the skin of the trunk. The arm is then placed across the patient's chest so that the fingers lie just below the shoulder. Padding may also be placed under the hand. Some 10 to 12 layers of rolled gauze bandage are applied smoothly around the chest to hold the arm against the trunk. The bandage may or may not be encased in a single layer of plaster of Paris. If the plaster is applied, care is taken to make sure that it does not come in contact with the patient's skin.

Position. Patients with a reduced AC separation will find the supine or supine with slight elevation of the head of the bed position the most comfortable position in bed. The patient is not allowed to turn to the affected side or lie prone, and will probably find lying on the unaffected side uncomfortable.

Exercise. The surgical repair determines the type of exercises allowed and when they should be started. If the end of the clavicle was resected, the use of the arm is encouraged immediately after surgery. Raising the arm above the horizontal is not permitted for 3 to 4 weeks, however. For patients whose AC separation was surgically repaired by the use of a screw, gentle active exercises are permitted and usually encouraged in the first week postsurgery. Motion above 90 degrees of abduction, heavy lifting, and strenuous exercises are avoided until the screw is removed (about 6 or 8 weeks after the surgery). Once the screw is removed, more vigorous exercises are permitted, and full activities may be resumed 10 weeks after surgery. Patients who have had Kirschner wires inserted as the method of repair have active motion exercises begun 2 weeks postsurgery. The wires are usually not removed until approximately 8 weeks after surgery, and then more vigorous exercises are begun.

The patient with a Velpeau bandage or with an arm in a sling must do finger exercises to increase circulation and maintain joint mobility. The more swollen the fingers, the greater the need for finger exercises. Recommended finger exercises include the following:

1. Fully extend the fingers and spread them into abduction.
2. Flex the fingers by touching the palm with the finger tips.
3. Flex the metacarpophalangeal joints by attempting to touch the front of the wrist.
4. Approximate the tip of the thumb to each finger in turn. The thumb must also be exercised.

Ambulation. The patient is usually allowed up the first day following surgery, but will probably need help at first. Once the patient is out of bed, make sure he or she is steady before starting to walk. With one arm immobilized across the chest, the patient may become unsteady when walking because of the change in balance and lack of arm swing.

Prevent Complications. The major complications following reduction of an AC separation are incomplete reduction and inadequate maintenance of immobilization. To help prevent complications, make sure the immobilization device is secured in place and properly positioned. The patient should not do exercises beyond those stipulated, or use the arm in activities that cause stress to the site. For some patients there may be reduced range of motion postsurgery if the patient is not diligent in doing the required exercises.

There is also the potential for infection at the surgical site. Utilize preventive measures, and be alert to the early signs and symptoms of infection. An infection may also occur as a secondary complication of skin irritation from the immobilizing device. The arm, which is supported by a sling supplemented by a modified Velpeau bandage, needs a soft pad placed in the axilla to help prevent skin excoriation. Check that the shoulder immobilizer straps do not cut into the skin of the patient's arm. Assess and implement nursing measures to prevent skin irritation.

Patient Teaching. Discuss with the patient, the family, and significant others the rehabilitation regime. Make sure the patient understands the surgical procedure, the need for an immobilizing device, the exercises that are allowed or encouraged, and the limitations that are required.

Teach the patient how to assess for neurovascular status in the affected arm by using the unaffected arm. Explain the importance of notifying the physician immediately if there is a change in neurovascular status. Include a discussion of the signs and symptoms of infection, the potential for developing one, and what to do if one seems to be developing.

Have an open discussion with the patient on activities of daily living: what the patient will realistically be able to do for him- or herself, and what others will need to do. Stress that the immobilizing device must not be removed. If the patient feels moisture from perspiration under the immobilizer or feels that he or she has body odor, the skin under the immobilizer can be washed and dried by lifting part of the immobilizer off the body, and cleansing under it. The patient will not be able to do this alone. Cleansing under the affected arm with a washcloth and soap may be difficult or impossible. Other ways to cleanse the body include the use of products like "handiwipes," alcohol swabs, or "tucks." Antiperspirants are suggested whenever possible. The patient will usually be taking a sponge bath, but may also sit in a bathtub that has only a couple of inches of water to prevent the bandage from getting wet. Help will probably be needed for safety even though the water should be drained from the tub before the patient starts to get out. Help may also be needed in washing hair, shaving, and eating.

Discuss with the patient what clothing to wear when the Velpeau bandage is on. Clothing may be modified by letting out seams, and Velcro straps may be used for closure. Clothing should not be tight over the chest and arm as that would add to discomfort.

Evaluation and Reassessment

Determine whether measures are effectively reducing the patient's pain. Is the patient trying to do too much on his or her own, leading to added stress and discomfort? Note how well the patient understands and follows the required exercise program. The patient should be free of any neurovascular impairment or infection.

GLENOHUMERAL (SHOULDER) JOINT

The glenohumeral joint is a ball-and-socket joint that allows greater range of motion but less stability than the ball-and-socket joint of the hip. Stability is augmented by the glenoid labrum, the rotator cuff, the coracoacromial arch, and the long heads of the biceps and triceps muscles. The branches of the brachial plexus nerve lie just anterior to the glenohumeral joint and the axillary nerve is immediately inferior to the joint.

Sprain

An injury to the glenohumeral joint caused by a twisting of the upper extremity of shoulder region can result in a stretching of the capsule or muscles surrounding the shoulder joint, and may produce a temporary painful disability. Such an injury is usually associated with bleeding into the joint that can give the shoulder region a swollen appearance. Roentgenographic examination is usually negative, except for possible capsular swelling. A simple sling to support the arm, combined with cold compresses, is helpful in relieving pain. Motion should be encouraged as soon as comfort permits. Moist heat treatments to the area are beneficial after joint motion begins to return (Gartland, 1979, pp. 254–255).

Dislocation

A dislocation of the glenohumeral joint is one of the most common upper extremity injuries and accounts for approximately 50 percent of all major joint dislocations (Fig 9–8). Of all shoulder dislocations, 95 percent are anterior, and of all anterior dislocations, 50 to 70 percent are in patients under 30 years of age. After a primary anterior dislocation, recurrent dislocations appear in 90 to 95 percent of patients under 20 years of age. For patients over 40 years of age the recurrence rate declines to 10 to 15 percent. Some authorities believe that with appropriate treatment, the recurrence rate can be reduced to 25 to 35 percent for patients in the under 20 age group. With anterior dislocations, damage to the major nerves to the arm and the axillary nerve occur some 5 to 14 percent of the time, and bony lesions (fractures of the humeral head or greater tuberosity in conjuction with the dislocation) some 38 percent of the time (Iversen & Clawson, 1977, pp. 135–136). With axillary nerve injury, the disability varies from slight weakness of the deltoid muscle and hypoesthesia over the upper outer aspect of the arm to complete paralysis of the muscle and anesthesia in the same area. Both usually clear up in a few weeks to several months (Turek, 1977, p. 840).

Posterior Dislocation

When the shoulder dislocates posteriorly, the humeral head slips out from behind the posterior edge of the glenoid at the level of the glenoid. Many, perhaps most, posterior dislocations are produced by a convulsion, which produces

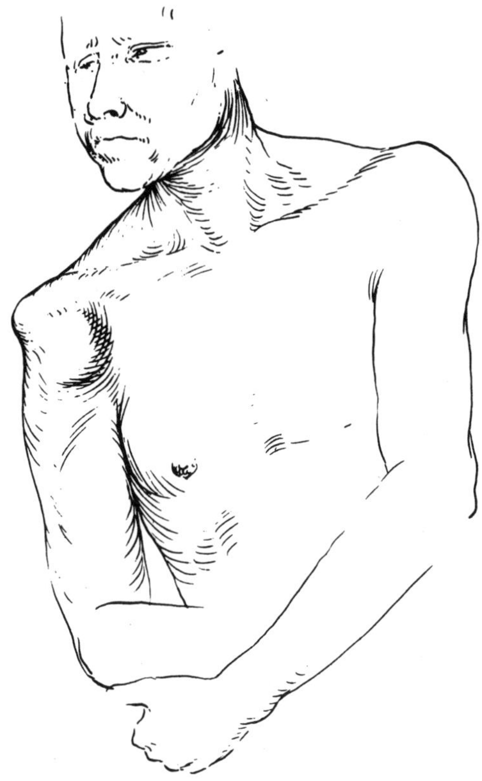

Figure 9–8. Dislocation of the shoulder.

a violent internal rotation (Iversen & Clawson, 1977, p. 139). Having regained consciousness, the patient usually complains of stiffness or pain in the shoulder and inability to raise that arm. Upon examination there is considerable limitation on abduction and external rotation and a defect can be palpated where the humeral head should be. Neurovascular function in the arm and the hand are usually normal.

Reduction is usually accomplished by relaxing the shoulder muscles and externally rotating the humerus by means of direct pressure on the posterior aspect of the shoulder joint. Once reduction is accomplished, the shoulder is immobilized with the use of a sling for 4 to 6 weeks.

Anterior Dislocation

An anterior dislocation of the shoulder joint usually results from a combination of abduction, extension, and external rotation of the shoulder. Examples are when a person dives into a pool, puts on a heavy overcoat, or falls on an outstretched arm. Abduction of the shoulder joint is possible to only 90 degrees. At that point, the humerus presses against the acromion process, which pushes the head of the humerus downward or forward. For the joint to dislocate anteriorly, the subscapularis muscle and the anterior joint capsule must be stretched or torn. The capsule of the joint is torn either anteriorly or at its attachment to the glenoid fossa. The head of the humerus enters the space below the glenoid fossa and rests under the coracoid process. In older persons, that usually results in a disruption of the anterior part of the joint capsule and associated soft tissues. For adolescents and young adults, the labrum of the glenoid is usually torn from its bony attachments, and the humeral head then rests in front of the neck of the scapula. The dislocation may be associated with a compression fracture in the humeral head, sustained as the head rolls out and over the edge of the glenoid. Anterior dislocations may be associated with damage to the nerves and, on rare occasions, to the blood vessels (Gartland, 1979, pp. 254–258; Iversen & Clawson, 1977, pp. 135–139; Roaf & Hodkinson, 1975, pp. 80–81).

Post-Trauma Assessment. The patient with an anterior dislocation seeks medical attention because of shoulder pain and severe disability. The patient usually resists any attempt at passive movement or active abduction of the arm. Clinical observation reveals a loss of symmetry of the shoulder. There is a flattening of the normally rounded shoulder contour when compared to the uninvolved side. The acromion is inordinately prominent, there is fullness anteriorly, and the humeral head can be palpated anteriorly in the subacoracoid region. (In very obese patients, however, those signs may be difficult to elicit.) Check the integrity of the axillary, radial, median, and ulnar nerves, and the arterial circulation to the arm. If the axillary nerve is involved, there will be paralysis of the deltoid muscle and an area of anesthesia on the lateral aspect of the arm. Locating an area of anesthesia is important in assessing the axillary nerve function because the dislocation itself is so painful that active abduction, i.e., voluntary contraction of the deltoid, might be impossible.

Roentgenography is an essential part of the assessment, as the standard anteroposterior view and an axillary view demonstrate whether the head of the humerus has been displaced forward or backward in relation to the glenoid fossa and also indicate the presence or absence of any accompanying bony injury (e.g., to the glenoid fossa, humeral head, neck, or tuberosities).

Medical Treatment. Treatment for a dislocated shoulder is to reduce the dislocation as soon as possible, immobilize the joint long enough for the damaged tissues to heal, and mobilize the joint soon enough to prevent permanent limitation of motion. Immediate reduction provides the patient with a great deal of relief. Reduction may be accomplished with or without general anesthesia. A reduction without general anesthesia requires muscle relaxation, possibly by means of 5 mg of diazepam intravenously, along with meperidine or morphine to reduce pain. The following are two of the numerous maneuvers that have been described to reduce a dislocated shoulder. First, after medication, the patient is placed prone with the involved arm and shoulder hanging over the edge of the stretcher or table. A weight (approximately 10 pounds) is secured to the patient's hand. The patient is reassured and placed in a quiet area to let the medication relax the muscles. In about 20 to 30 minutes, the combination of muscle relaxation and the weighted pull on the arm should bring about reduction. If not, the physician may then place a hand in the axilla and lift the humerus laterally, using 5 to 10 pounds of force with gentle internal and external rotation. If successful, the shoulder will snap quickly into position.

Reduction under general anesthesia may be the method of choice, or used if the first method fails. Once anesthesia is achieved, the physician applies traction to the arm and manipulates it to a position of approximately 30 to 45 degrees of abduction and 15 to 20 degrees of flexion, with the elbow flexed 90 degrees. If that is not sufficient to accomplish reduction, an assistant may place the palm of the hand in the axilla and gently provide lateral pressure.

Once the shoulder is reduced, the timing of immobilization varies with the age of the patient. In young people, the risk of habitual or recurrent dislocation is fairly high, so the shoulder is usually immobilized either by a collar and cuff or by binding the arm to the side by means of a Velpeau bandage. Immobilization is usually maintained for 3 to 6 weeks to allow soft tissues and muscles to heal and to minimize the danger of permanent stiffness. In patients over 50, the risk of recurrent dislocation is minimal but the risk of permanent shoulder stiffness is considerable, so the shoulder is immobilized for much less time, if at all. These patients are usually started on gentle active and assisted movements as soon as they can tolerate them. In the older patient, it may be difficult to restore full movement, and for such patients a course of treatment for a stiff shoulder may be necessary (see p. 545).

Complications following a dislocated shoulder include (1) damage to the nerves originating in the brachial plexus, (2) tears of the rotator cuff, (3) avulsion fractures of the greater tuberosity, and (4) recurrent dislocations of the shoulder.

Recurrent Dislocation

Dislocation of the shoulder joint in a young patient carries with it a high rate of recurrence. Recurrence is not nearly as frequent in middle-aged or elderly patients because of the normal tendency of the subscapularis muscle to tighten with age, thereby limiting the external rotation of the joint (Gartland, 1979, p. 258). Authorities do not agree on why recurrent dislocations occur, but undoubtedly some type of capsular or tendinous stretching occurs with the initial dislocation that does not completely heal. Most believe that the tendency for redislocation is related to the inherent anatomical instability of the shoulder joint.

Some persons experience multiple shoulder dislocations following unguarded movements of the arm (e.g., abduction and external rotation), and many become adept at reducing their own dislocations. Recurrence can become so frequent as to preclude vigorous physical activity in an otherwise healthy person, and no amount of immobilization will prevent that tendency. Operative repair is necessary for permanent correction for recurrent dislocations, and many different surgical techniques are performed to tighten the soft tissue components of the joint. Some of these procedures are:

1. The Bankart operation, in which the detached anterior structures (the glenoid labrum and the anterior part of the capsule) are reattached to the rim of the glenoid cavity using sutures passed through holes in the glenoid rim.
2. The staple capsulorrhaphy of du Toit and Roux, in which the detached capsule and labrum are stapled with no reconstruction of the muscles.
3. The Putti-Platt operation (Fig. 9–9A), in which the subscapularis tendon is overlapped and shortened and the capsule is overlapped and tightened.
4. The Magnuson and Stack operation (Fig. 9–9B), in which the anterior capsulomuscular wall is tightened by advancing the tendon of the subscapularis laterally on the humerus.
5. The Eden-Hybbinette operation, in which a bone graft is placed against the anterior aspect of the neck of the scapula and the rim of the glenoid cavity so that it blocks anterior displacement of the humeral head.
6. The Bristow procedure, in which the coracoid process is transplanted with the attached conjoined tendons of the short head of the biceps and coracobrachialis to the anterior rim of the glenoid (Edmondson & Crenshaw, 1980, pp. 476–489).

The choice of repair depends upon the patient's age and activity level, and the degree of damage to the glenoid. The most common are the Putti-Platt and Bristow repairs, the latter preferred for athletic individuals who want as much external rotation as possible.

□ NURSING PROCESS (Table 9–3)

Assessment

The first step in the nursing assessment of a typical patient, following surgical repair of a recurrent dislocated shoulder and the application of a Velpeau bandage or a sling and swath, is to check the neurovascular status of the affected arm (for details, see Chapter 2). Assess the respiratory status and the position of the upper trunk, affected arm, shoulder, and immobilizing device. Note if there is any undue pressure or tautness of the skin due to the immobilizing device. Assess the location, type, and severity of pain, and note if there is any drainage.

Nursing Diagnosis and Goal Formulation

Nursing diagnoses for a typical patient following the surgical repair of a recurrent dislocated shoulder are (1) alterations in comfort related to pain from the surgical procedure, (2) alterations in mobility related to lack of glenohumeral joint stability, (3) potential complications related to the sur-

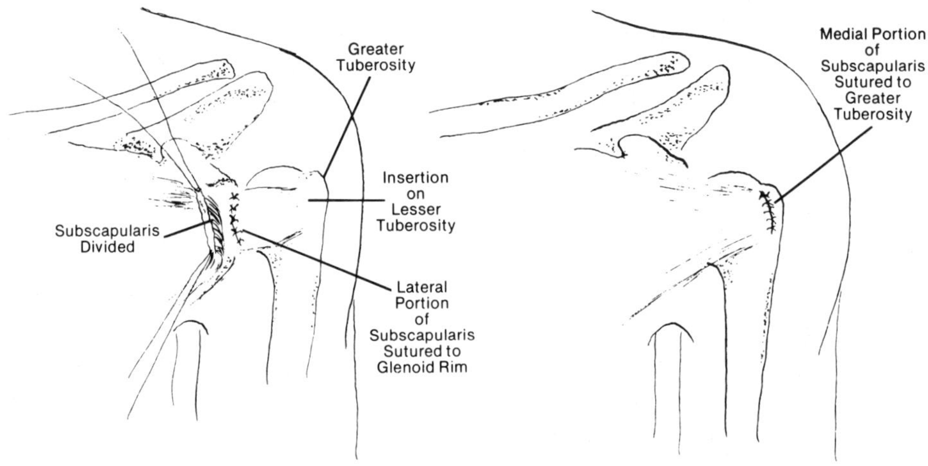

Figure 9–9. A. Open reduction anterior shoulder dislocation: Putti-Platt procedure. *(From Brantley, P., & Analla, M.* The nurse and orthopedic surgery. *Rutherford, N.J.: Howmedica, Inc., 1980, p. 9. Courtesy of Howmedica.)*

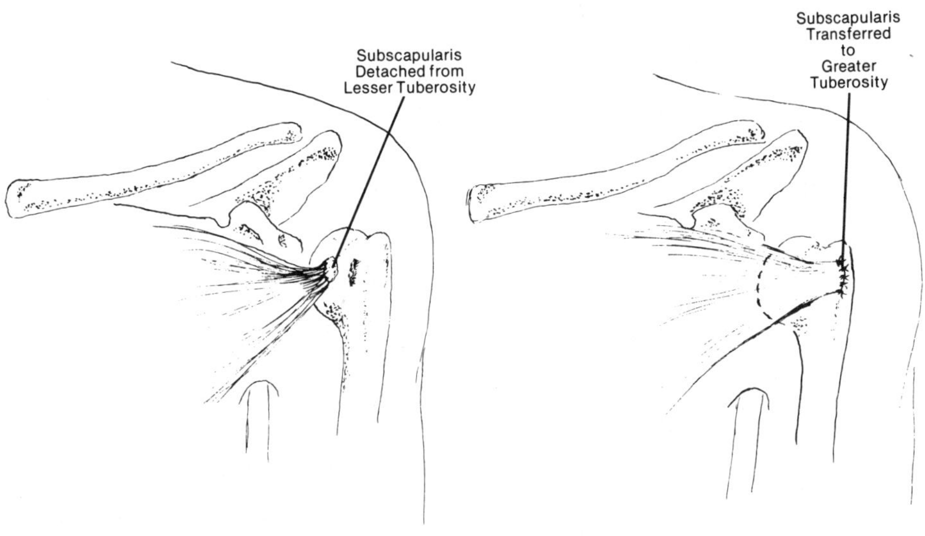

Figure 9–9. B. Open reduction anterior shoulder dislocation: Magnuson and Stack procedure. *(From Brantley, P., & Analla, M.* The nurse and orthopedic surgery. *Rutherford, N.J.: Howmedica, Inc., 1980, p. 8. Courtesy of Howmedica.)*

TABLE 9–3. NURSING PROCESS FOR DISLOCATED SHOULDER TREATED WITH OPEN REDUCTION AND VELPEAU BANDAGE

Assessment	Nursing Diagnosis	Goal Formulation	Planning and Intervention	Evaluation and Reassessment
1. Assess the location, duration, and severity of pain. Note if there is any undue pressure or tautness of the skin due to the immobilizing device. Assess neurovascular status.	1. Alteration in comfort: pain in the shoulder related to soft tissue trauma and joint instability.	1. Short-term goal: relative comfort through the use of immobilization and medications. Long-term goal: free of pain in the shoulder.	1. Alleviate Pain Make sure the arm, shoulder, and trunk are correctly positioned. Make sure the immobilizing device is properly applied and maintained. Apply ice to the incision site. Avoid jarring the shoulder. Teach relaxation techniques. Administer pain medication.	1. The patient should remain relatively comfortable with the use of immobilization and medications.
2. Assess the level of the shoulders. Check the position of the hand and arm. Check the ability to do exercises. Check the position and tightness of the bandage. Assess the patient's ability to get out of bed and ambulate alone.	2. Impaired physical mobility: decrease in arm function related to shoulder joint instability.	2. Short-term goal: an increase in mobility through immobilization and controlled exercises. Long-term goal: regain full function of the shoulder.	2. Increase Mobility *Position* Appropriate position for the shoulder depends on the surgical repair (see text). Maintain Velpeau bandage (2–4 weeks). Maintain sling for next 4–6 weeks. *Exercises* Instruct on finger exercises. Other exercises depend on surgical repair (e.g., pendulum, abduction and external rotation). Instruct on no exercise with weights, vigorous manual labor, or competitive athletics for 3 months or more.	2. The patient should maintain the proper position of the arm at all times. The exercise program should be followed with only a moderate amount of discomfort. There should be no problems with ambulating alone after the first few times the patient is up.

			Ambulation Assist the patient in getting out of bed and walking.	
3. Assess for any signs of infection. Check for any drainage. Check for any signs of pressure areas or skin breakdown.	3. Potential for injury: infection related to surgical incision and break in skin integrity.	3. Short- and long-term goal: free of any signs of infection.	3. Prevent Complications *Integumentary* Keep the dressing clean and dry. Keep the bandage from irritating the skin. Instruct on a well-balanced diet.	3. The patient should remain free of any signs of infection or neurovascular deficit.
Assess neurovascular status. Check the flexion of the elbow. Check the tightness of the immobilizing device.	Potential for injury: neurovascular deficit related to swelling and immobilization.	Short- and long-term goal: free of any injury.	*Neurological and Circulatory* Assess neurovascular status on a routine basis; report any abnormalities. Instruct on hand exercises. Use nursing methods to prevent swelling. *Other Complications* (see text)	
4. Assess the patient's level of knowledge concerning the rehabilitation process and self-care.	4. Potential knowledge deficit related to the rehabilitation process and self-care.	4. Short-and long-term goal: a decrease in anxiety through an increase in knowledge.	4. Patient Teaching Tell the patient that skin irritation under the immobilizer is probably inevitable, especially in hot weather or under heavy wool clothing. Instruct on methods to reduce skin irritation and on bathing and dressing with the immobilizer in place. Reinforce techniques to reduce pain that can be used at home. Discuss activity level. Discuss with patient, family, and significant other the goals of the rehabilitation process. Go over the home exercise program.	4. The patient should verbalize an understanding of activity limitations, self-care, and the goals of rehabilitation.

gical procedure and decreased mobility, and (4) alterations in psychological well-being related to anxiety and knowledge deficit about the injury and the rehabilitation process.

Short-term goals are to have the patient experience (1) a decrease in the amount of pain, (2) an increase in joint mobility and stability, (3) an absence of complications from surgery and decreased activity, and (4) a decrease in anxiety through increased knowledge. Long-term goals are to have the patient pain free and to have full return of joint motion without dislocation.

Planning and Intervention

Alleviate Pain. The amount of pain the patient has is related to the extent of the procedure and the physical condition of the shoulder before surgery. A patient with a very large shoulder and arm usually has more postoperative pain because more soft tissue is incised. A patient with an internal fixation usually has more postoperative pain than a patient with soft tissue suturing. Correct positioning, immobilization, and the application of ice around the incisional area may be helpful in reducing pain. The ice also helps to reduce any swelling that may occur postsurgery. Make sure the ice bags are not placed on the incision line.

Pain at the surgical site may be caused by stress from incorrect positioning or immobilization. Check to make sure that the patient is in correct body alignment, and that the immobilizing device is properly applied. The immobilizer can cause a pull on the skin, which leads to discomfort. Because of the awkwardness of having the arm and the shoulder immobilized, patients may suffer a painful "jar" to the shoulder when they first try to get out of bed alone. Give the patient pain medications as needed.

Increase Mobility

Position. The appropriate position for the shoulder following a surgical repair of a recurrent dislocation of the shoulder depends upon the surgical procedure. Patients who have had the Bankart, Putti-Platt, Magnuson and Stack, or Eden-Hybbinette operations have their shoulder immobilized for the first 2 to 4 weeks in a Velpeau bandage (see p. 509). The Velpeau bandage is then removed and gentle exercises started, but the shoulder and arm may still need to be supported in a sling until approximately 6 weeks postsurgery. With the Bankart procedure, the sling is worn at night only, whereas with the Magnuson and Stack operation it is worn all the time.

The Bristow and du Toit and Roux procedures usually require a sling and a swath dressing. Patients having the du Toit and Roux procedure may be placed in a simple triangular sling the day following surgery, and that sling is worn for approximately 1 week. With the Bristow procedure, the sling is usually worn for 4 to 5 weeks postsurgery.

Exercises. The type of exercises and when they are begun depend upon the type of surgical repair. Following a du Toit and Roux procedure, pendulum exercises without weights are usually begun at the end of the first week after surgery. At approximately 3 weeks postsurgery, gentle range-of-motion exercises with active abduction and external rotation are begun and are increased gradually over the next 3 weeks. By the sixth week postsurgery, all motion except external rotation has usually returned to normal. Increasingly active exercises for the shoulders are continued without weights so that by the end of 3 months normal motion has returned, except for some slight restriction of external rotation. Patients are not permitted to exercise with weights or to return to vigorous manual labor and competitive athletics for 3 or more months.

The patient having a Bristow operation usually begins circumduction exercises between the third and sixth week postsurgery. After 6 weeks, increasing range-of-motion exercises without weights are started. Passive elbow extension is allowed at 4 to 5 weeks, but active extension is not allowed for at least 6 weeks after surgery.

With the Bankart, Putti-Platt, Eden-Hybbinette, and Magnuson and Stack operations, active exercises are begun when the Velpeau bandage is removed. The exercises are very gentle and are gradually increased with the patient being instructed to avoid external rotation. Pendulum exercises are used, at first passive and later active. With the Bankart procedure, rehabilitative exercises are begun approximately 6 weeks postsurgery that allow the shoulder joint to be abducted to 90 degrees. At 8 to 12 weeks the motion in the shoulder should be at the maximum, except that abduction and external rotation may be somewhat limited. The Putti-Platt and Magnuson and Stack procedures usually allow the patient to begin an exercise program 3 to 4 weeks after surgery. At 6 weeks postsurgery, a vigorous rehabilitation program is begun to restore motion in the joint and strengthen the muscles of the shoulder girdle and the arm. For patients having a Magnuson and Stack procedure, external rotation of the shoulder will always be limited to about 50 percent of normal.

Ambulation. Because of the awkwardness resulting from not having the use of the involved arm, patients need assistance when first getting out of bed. In the beginning, they may also have problems in walking because of the lack of arm swing.

Prevent Complications. Infection is a potential threat following surgery and nursing procedures aimed at prevention should be implemented. The patient with a repair of a recurrent shoulder dislocation has the added potential complications of circulatory impairment, stiffness of the shoulder joint, and reduced range of motion of the glenohumeral joint, especially for external rotation. Following the prescribed exercise program rigorously helps prevent these complications.

Periodic roentgenograms are required following the Bristow procedure to note any change of position of the transferred coracoid or the screw utilized in the repair. To prevent further complications, a loose screw is usually removed. An osseous union only occurs in approximately 50 to 75 percent of the patients, and is difficult to determine even by roentgenograms. A fibrous union occurs in the remaining 25 to 50 percent.

Patient Teaching. Tell the patient that skin irritation under the immobilizer is probably inevitable, especially in hot weather or under heavy wool clothing. The immobilizer must be kept in place, but the skin underneath can be cleansed and dried (see p. 511). If possible, antiperspirants should be used under the affected arm to reduce body odor. Discuss sponge bathing and taking a tub bath with a minimal amount of water to maintain overall hygiene.

To help the patient reduce discomfort at home, reinforce techniques utilized in the hospital. Discuss the types of chairs that are best for the patient to sit in. The patient needs to evaluate how stressful to the shoulder it will be to get out of a comfortable living room chair before sitting in one. Long, uninterrupted car rides should be avoided because the motion of the car affects the shoulder.

Discuss with the patient, the family, and significant others the goals of the rehabilitation process. In the beginning the patient is usually taught to do pendulum or gentle range-of-motion exercises without weights or external rotation. The exercises are then gradually increased over time. Pendulum exercises are carried out by (1) having the patient lean forward, (2) allowing the arm to hang down and away from the body, and (3) slowly swinging the arm from side to side. In the beginning there may be very little pendulum swing, but it will gradually increase. Teach the patient what range of motion is and provide a routine to follow. Tell the patient not to do internal or external rotation movements until allowed to so by the physician. Joint movements help to maintain and increase muscle strength as well as to regain full joint motion. Later, internal rotation may be regained by having the patient place the hand behind the lower back and then reach upward toward the scapula.

There are a number of exercises that will help the patient regain external rotation. The following four exercises are done with the patient lying supine:

1. With the arms parallel to the body, the palms are alternatively pronated and supinated.
2. With the hands clasped behind the head, the elbows are alternatively raised and flattened against the bed.
3. With the shoulders abducted to a right angle, the top of the bed is touched with each hand.
4. The patient reaches over the head to touch the opposite ear.

These four exercises can also be performed with the patient standing with the back to a wall. Another exercise is to have the patient stand sideways to a wall, and have the fingers "climb" up the wall as far as possible. It is encouraging for the patient to mark the level reached each time, so that the amount of progress can be observed.

Evaluation and Reassessment

Determine the level of pain and whether nursing measures and drug therapy are effective in relieving it. Note whether the patient is able to maintain correct positioning in bed and when ambulating. Determine whether the immobilizing device is effectively immobilizing the shoulder and the arm. In discussions with the patient, the family, and significant others, determine the level of understanding about the exercise program and the total rehabilitation process. Supply information or correct misconceptions as needed. If the patient lives alone, make sure help is available. Discuss potential problems with the patient (and social worker) if indicated. Make sure the patient understands the importance of adhering to the physician's orders regarding follow-up visits and if problems arise.

FRACTURED PROXIMAL HUMERUS

Fractures of the proximal humerus in adults may be classified as (1) avulsion fractures of the tuberosities, (2) impacted fractures of the surgical or anatomical neck, (3) fracture–dislocations, and (4) displaced fractures of the neck of the humerus.

Avulsion fractures of the tuberosities may result from a variety of mechanisms, but they frequently occur as a result of seizures or secondary to glenohumeral dislocations. When related to shoulder dislocations, these fractures often reduce anatomically with reduction of the humeral head, and are usually treated nonoperatively. In some cases, the avulsed tuberosity is displaced more than 1 cm because the musculotendinous (rotator) cuff has retracted and pulled the tuberosity fragment toward or under the acromion. Such avulsion fractures, of either the lessor or greater tuberosity, are usually repaired through a standard deltopectoral approach and reduction and fixation of the tuberosity with a stainless steel wire suture or screw. When the tuberosity has been displaced and retracted, a significant tear in the rotator cuff mechanism may also exist, and a careful repair of the rotator cuff defect is required to produce optimal results.

Impacted fractures occur almost exclusively in older people (Edmondson & Crenshaw, 1980, p. 662). They are rarely manipulated or subjected to surgery to improve alignment because restoration of function would probably be made more difficult. Because people with impacted fractures tend to develop periarthritis of the shoulder, these fractures are treated with conservative methods that allow early motion and restoration of function. In most cases, the use of a sling to support the arm and progressive arm exercises are all that is required. Even when significant angulation is present in the impaction, the results are usually much better than one might expect from the appearance of the fracture on roentgenograms.

Fracture–dislocations of the shoulder are common injuries and occur in all age groups. They usually require only closed reduction, but occasionally open reduction and internal fixation are necessary (Fig. 9–10).

A fracture of the surgical neck of the humerus with a slight displacement is one of the most common fractures of the elderly. The fracture occurs when the elderly person falls directly against the shoulder with the arm against the chest or completely abducted, and immediate pain and disability are noted by the patient. After such a fracture, there is frequently a hemorrhage around the fracture site that works its way to the surface in approximately 24 to 72 hours, resulting in ecchymosis and discoloration around the shoulder, the breast, and the arm. The patient and the family needs to be informed in advance that this is likely to occur, and that it does not indicate a blood clot or any serious complication.

In a displaced fracture, the pectoral muscles pull the distal fragment inward and forward, and the deltoid pulls it upward. Although a roentgenogram may disclose varying degrees of comminution or displacement of the fragments, their position is usually such that no actual reduction is necessary (Gartland, 1979, pp. 254–255). These fractures are usually treated symptomatically with guided, active, assisted range-of-motion and pendulum exercises to prevent stiffness of the shoulder. There is very little danger of displacement of the fracture or damage from such early motion (Donahoo & Dimon, 1977, p. 54). In some cases, the arm and the shoulder are immobilized in a Velpeau

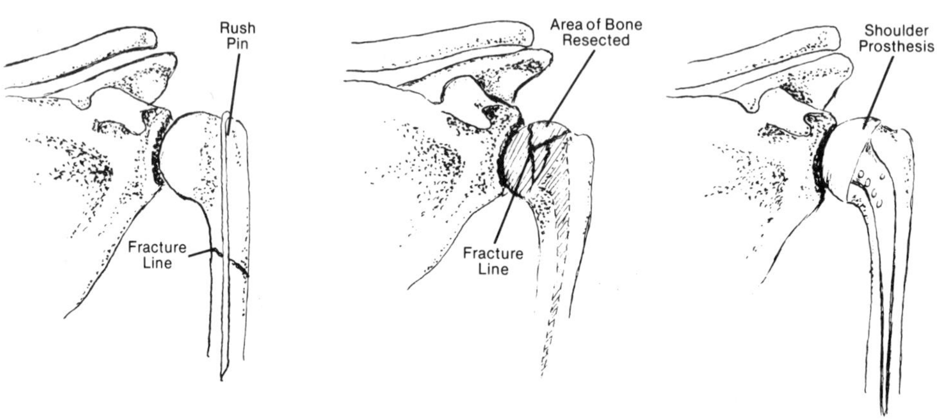

Figure 9–10. Open reduction and internal fixation or prosthetic replacement of fractured humeral head and neck. *(From Brantley, P., & Analla, M.* The nurse and orthopedic surgery. *Rutherford, N.J.: Howmedica, Inc., 1980, p. 7. Courtesy of Howmedica.)*

bandage (see p. 509) for 3 weeks, in a hanging arm cast (see pp. 551 and 554), or are placed in a lateral traction apparatus that maintains forward flexion and traction until a soft callus forms. A satisfactory range of shoulder motion is usually regained even if the fragments heal in a moderately deformed position.

If displacement of the fragments is too severe to expect return of function, an open reduction to replace the fragments is performed. If comminution is so severe that an open reduction is impractical, the fragments can be excised and replaced with a metallic humeral head prosthesis (hemiarthroplasty). A few patients with severe trauma resulting in extensive destruction of the shoulder joint, including the rotator cuff, may require a total shoulder arthroplasty (see pp. 537–538).

ROTATOR CUFF

The musculotendinous or rotator cuff of the shoulder, which acts to stabilize the humeral head in the glenoid cavity during shoulder abduction, normally undergoes some degenerative changes with advancing age. Asymptomatic "worn out" spots may appear in the cuff (Gartland, 1979, p. 259). A rupture of the rotator cuff can then occur if a sudden adduction force is applied to the cuff while the arm is being held in abduction. Traumatic tears of the cuff can also result from a fall on the shoulder, from throwing, from heavy lifting, or in conjunction with a glenohumeral dislocation. Such a tear in younger patients is usually the consequence of substantial trauma (Iverson & Clawson, 1977, pp. 139–140).

Patients with a tear of the rotator cuff have shoulder pain where the tear comes in contact with the coracoacromial ligament when the arm is in abduction. Local tenderness may be noted over the cuff, and the patient may be unable to initiate or maintain active abduction of the arm at the shoulder joint. The arm can be passively abducted at the shoulder, but the patient may be unable to sustain that position and the arm will drop to the side (Fig. 9–11). Full mobility of the shoulder joint is not lost because the scapula is not affected. Atrophy of the cuff muscles (i.e., the supraspinatus, infraspinatus, and teres minor) may be palpated (DeGowin & DeGowin, 1976, p. 698). Roentgenographic examination is often normal, but can show spur formation at the anterior edge of the acromion or a displaced fracture of the tuberosity. The diagnosis of a ruptured rotator cuff is confirmed by an arthrogram that demonstrates leakage of the contrast material from the shoulder joint capsule into the subacromial bursa.

Treatment of rotator cuff tears depends on the age of the patient and the size of the tear. A young patient with an ordinary or large tear is usually treated with immediate surgical repair (Fig. 9–12). In an older patient, or one with a small tear, the treatment is symptomatic, with the emphasis on maintaining good passive range of motion and on the return of abduction strength. Later surgical repair might be indicated if satisfactory abduction

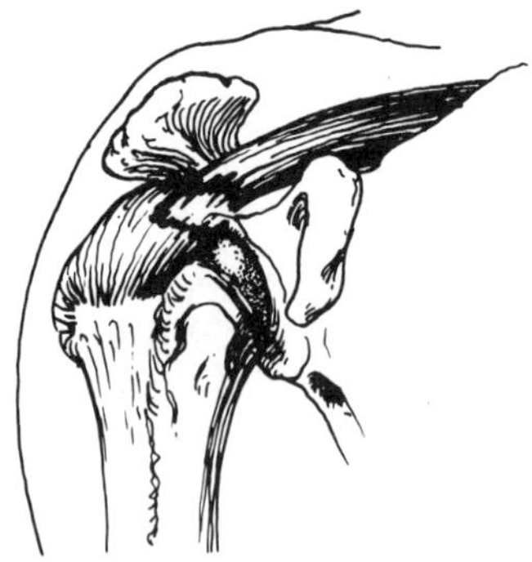

A

Figure 9–11. **A.** Tears in the rotator cuff. **B.** The drop arm test, to determine if there are tears in the rotator cuff. **C.** If there are tears in the rotator cuff, the arm drops and the patient is unable to lower his arm slowly to his side.

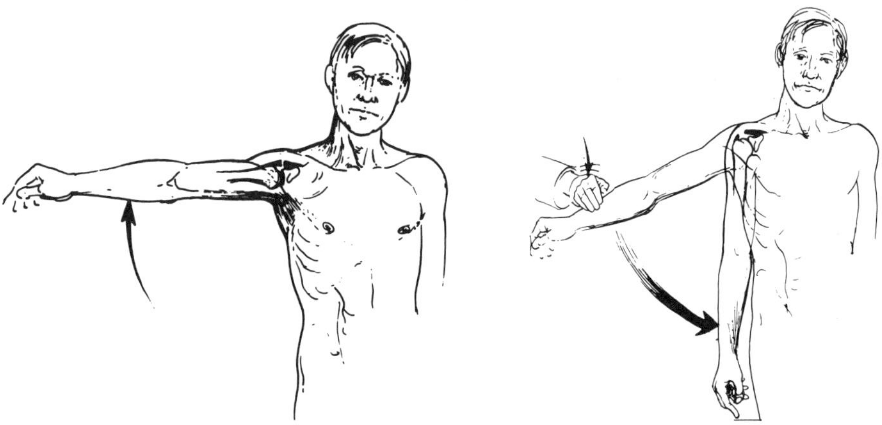

B C

strength does not return after at least 6 weeks of physical therapy (Iversen & Clawson, 1977, p. 140). Because many patients sustain only an incomplete rupture and gradually recover strength and motion spontaneously, initial treatment of a torn rotator cuff is usually conservative. The arm is supported in a sling, and hot applications may be used on the shoulder after the initial bleeding stops.

Surgical treatment of the rotator cuff area is used for patients who do not respond to a conservative program (see Fig. 9–12). Those patients have usually sustained massive tears or complete ruptures of the rotator cuff. Surgically, the torn edges are sutured together with heavy, nonabsorbable sutures. Massive tears may require attaching the torn edges to the humeral head through drill holes or a wedge-shaped osteotomy. Postoperatively, simple repairs are treated with a sling. Pendulum exercises are started on the third or fourth postoperative day and progressive, active exercises started in 2 weeks. More extensive repairs may require side arm suspension and restriction of abduction for 4 to 6 weeks. Active exercises are begun after that period.

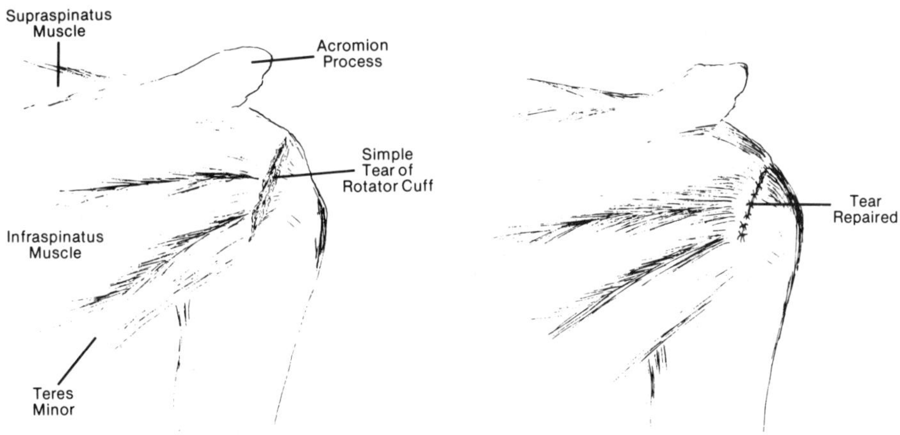

Figure 9–12. Posterior view, repair of rotator cuff tear. *(From Brantley, P., & Analla, M.* The nurse and orthopedic surgery. *Rutherford, N.J.: Howmedica, Inc., 1980, p. 12. Courtesy of Howmedica.)*

Pathology

ARTHRITIS AND INFECTIOUS DISEASES

Rheumatoid Arthritis

Rheumatoid synovial disease often involves the shoulder joint, and when it does it almost invariably extends beyond the confines of the joint to the subacromial bursa and the synovial sheath about the bicipital tendon. The main destructive force in rheumatoid arthritis is an inflamed, proliferating synovium. The three stages in joint destruction are the initial acute synovitis, the stage of synovial proliferation, and the final stage of destruction.

In the first stage there are episodes of acute synovial inflammation associated with effusions of a thin, cellular fluid. Eventually the subacromial bursa and bicipital synovial sheath become involved in the inflammatory process and are distended with a thin, turbid fluid. The subacromional bursal distention is almost always an extension of an intra-articular synovitis. In the second stage, the inflammation becomes less acute, and the synovial tissue proliferates and extends, destroying the joint capsule. The swollen mass of tissue then extends into the subacromial bursa and along the bicipital sheath. Slowly the capsule and surrounding muscles contract and produce an adduction and internal rotation deformity. In the last stage, destruction occurs when the proliferated synovium forms a pannus that destroys the articular cartilage and subchondral bone. The same process invades and destroys the bicipital tendon, which may rupture or become fixed in its groove by peritendinous adhesions. The rotator cuff and capsule are weakened by synovial distention and invasion, which cause them to rub against the coracoacromial arch. The resulting capsular defect provides a direct communication between the subacromial bursa and the glenohumeral joint. Disintegration of the glenohumeral articulation and the development of capsular adhesions and contractures permanently restrict shoulder motion (Turek, 1977, p. 859).

Rheumatoid disease of the shoulder assumes a wide variety of forms. The acute inflammation may be limited to the glenohumeral joint where it almost always starts, or it may appear as an acute subscromial bursitis and/or bicipital tenosynovitis, both of which are almost invariably associated with intra-articular disease. Recurrent acute inflammatory episodes may be interspersed with symptom-free intervals when the joint may appear normal. The condition may develop insidiously producing synovial proliferation that appears as persistent, painful, boggy swellings about the shoulder joint, extending along the course of the bicipital tendon. Capsule disease and disintegration are reflected in rotator cuff insufficiency. In about 10 percent of the cases of advanced disease, a disabling adduction and internal rotation contracture develops.

The aim of treatment is to halt the synovial inflammatory process before it proceeds to destroy the articular surfaces and para-articular structures. If the spread of the synovial disease process is unrelenting and cannot be controlled by conservative means, a synovectomy of the joint and removal of the subacromial bursa and bicipital tenosynovium sometimes stops or greatly retards the disease. However, such surgery needs to be done early in stage two for best results.

Because early diagnosis is not available in most cases, surgery is usually not done until the disease has advanced and involves tendinous structures, causing persistent pain and restricting glenohumeral motion by pain and contracture. In addition to a synovectomy, other surgical procedures are (1) excision of the subacromial bursa, (2) repair of the rotator cuff, (3) capsular release, and (4) resection of the intra-articular position of the biceps tendon. To overcome adduction and internal rotation contractures, the subscapularis tendon is lengthened, the adductors sectioned, and the coracoacromial ligament and the anterior portion of the acromion are removed. When rheumatoid arthritis of the shoulder has caused a deterioration of the joint, some function can be restored by a hemiarthroplasty (i.e., the insertion of a prosthesis for the humeral head) or a total shoulder joint replacement. Arthrodesis is rarely indicated because it completely restricts motion and may even encourage further deterioration of other joints of the extremity (Turek, 1977, pp. 860–861).

Degenerative Arthritis (Osteoarthritis)

Sternoclavicular Joint

Degenerative arthritis may affect the sternoclavicular joint and give rise to a painful thickening and swelling of the joint. A patient may seek medical attention because of a "lump" in the neck area. In the acute stage, the joint may be warm, thickened, and tender. Later, all signs and symptoms may subside, but the thickness and enlargement usually remain. Pain may be relieved by warm applications and by use of oral anti-inflammatory agents. Sometimes, if pain persists, hydrocortisone is injected into the sternoclavicular joint. Surgical treatment is usually not required (Gartland, 1979, p. 250).

Acromioclavicular Joint

Degenerative arthritis in the AC joint is a major cause of shoulder area pain, especially in older patients. The condition is more frequent in men, particularly those who have subjected the joint to repeated trauma from either athletic or occupational demands. Adduction of the arm across the chest and abduction above the horizontal are motions that cause shoulder pain when the AC joint is involved. Thus patients frequently experience pain in the affected shoulder when they sleep on that side.

In most patients, the joint margins become palpably enlarged and roughened, and visible enlargement of the joint is frequently observed. When direct pressure is applied to the joint, pain is felt by the patient. Often there is little damage to the joint that can be demonstrated on roentgenographic examination, because the majority of the changes involve the soft tissue and the cartilage components of the joint. The pain due to degenerative arthritis of the AC joint usually can be relieved by local heat applications, oral anti-inflammatory drugs, and in some instances injection of hydrocortisone into the joint. If the symptoms cannot be controlled by these measures, the distal end of the clavicle may be removed by surgery. This widens the joint and relieves the pain.

Glenohumeral Joint

Degenerative arthritis of the shoulder joint can result from wear and tear on the joint or from infection, trauma, fractures, or abnormalities of the joint. In the past, osteoarthritis of the shoulder tended to occur more frequently in men, because of repeated athletic and occupational demands. As the disease progresses, the articulating cartilage gradually becomes inelastic and develops a pitted irregular surface. Eventually those irregularities deepen, ulceration into the bone occurs, there is spurring around the edge of the joint, and destruction of surrounding soft tissues.

Pain is the main symptom, usually in the form of an ache associated with joint motions. Rest may relieve the pain for a short while, but stiffness usually follows. Range of motion is not affected but the patient may consciously restrict movement to avoid pain. This can lead to muscle, tendon, and soft tissue shortening. Treatment consists of heat applications, physical therapy, oral anti-inflammatory drugs, and in some instances local injection of hydrocortisone. If the symptoms cannot be controlled by these measures, a shoulder arthroplasty may be done.

Tuberculosis

Tuberculosis of the shoulder is rare. When present, tubercular lesions are usually found in the anatomical neck of the humerus and the glenoid of the scapula. A synovitis develops and the joint capsule becomes filled with masses of granular tissue. Early in the disease only osteoporosis is evident, cortical margins are indistinct, and the capsular shadow is expanded and denser than normal. The localized osteolytic lesions and a narrowing of the articular space become apparent when the disease is well advanced.

Muscle weakness, a sensation of heaviness, and pain on motion are the earliest symptoms. Later, the pain becomes severe, and muscle spasm fixes the shoulder in adduction. The soft tissues become swollen, thickened, and generally tender. Motion in all directions, particularly external rotation and abduction, is restricted. Marked muscle atrophy becomes evident, and the axillary lymph nodes become enlarged.

In the beginning, treatment focuses on conservative measures that include constitutional measures (i.e., rest and a nutritious diet), drugs, and immobilization by a shoulder spica cast, as a shoulder bony ankylosis will arrest the disease process. The shoulder is placed in a functional position, usually 90 degrees of abduction, 60 degrees of external rotation, and 30 degrees of forward flexion, in the event that ankylosis occurs while the shoulder is immobilized. In some adults, abduction may be limited to 60 to 70 degrees to allow the arm to be brought down to the side (Turek, 1977, pp. 862–863).

A surgical procedure that is used to treat tuberculosis of the shoulder is the resection of abnormal tissues and joint arthrodesis. Once the shoulder is fused, a shoulder spica cast is applied, and immobilization is continued until the bony bridging of the joint is demonstrated by roentgenograms. Under rare conditions, shoulder motion may be preserved by the resection of the upper end of the humerus, leaving a movable but weakened shoulder (Roaf & Hodkinson, 1975, pp. 371–372).

Arthrodesis

An arthrodesis (fusion) of the glenohumeral joint is an uncommon procedure. Both intra-articular and extra-articular arthrodesis may be done, either alone or in combination. Fusion by the intra-articular technique alone, however, is sometimes difficult to accomplish, so the combined intra-articular and extra-articular procedure is preferred by most physicians. Many different fixation devices and surgical techniques are utilized, including (1) long metal screws or Knowles pins to fix the humerus in the glenoid; (2) staples to anchor the acromion to the head of the humerus in the Gill technique; (3) a wire loop passed through the humerus and the scapula to maintain opposition; (4) compression clamps attached to two Steinmann pins, one inserted through the proximal humeral shaft and the other through the acromion and scapular neck to maintain stability; and (5) fixing the shoulder internally with a screw and inserting a muscle pedicle bone graft in the joint. After surgery, the most common position of the shoulder is 50 degrees abduction, 20 degrees flexion, and 25 degrees internal rotation. This position allows the arm to fall to the side and to have a range of motion of 90 to 95 degrees of abduction, up to 80 degrees of flexion, and 90 degrees of internal rotation. With that range of motion, the patient can reach any part of the face or head and place the hand in the front trouser pocket, and often even in the hip pocket. After skin closure, a shoulder spica cast is applied. After 8 to 12 weeks, motion of the elbow and the wrist may be instituted, although some form of support must be continued until osseous union is demonstrated by roentgenograms (Edmondson & Crenshaw, 1980, p. 1132).

□ NURSING PROCESS (Table 9–4)

Assessment

The first step in the assessment of a typical patient following an arthrodesis of the shoulder and the application of a shoulder spica cast is to check the respiratory status. The rate, depth, and rhythm of breathing need to be assessed as the cast may be constricting chest movements necessary for respiration. Make sure the patient is in correct alignment and that there are sufficient pillows to support the arm and the upper torso. Assess for possible nausea and potential vomiting because of the anesthesia and the possible tightness of the cast over a portion of the abdomen.

Check the neurovascular status of the involved arm and compare it to the uninvolved arm. (For further details on neurovascular assessment, see Chap. 2.) As the cast may impinge on the ulnar nerve, assess the status of that nerve by asking the patient to abduct the fingers and respond to a pricking of the little finger. Note any swelling of the hand or the fingers. Check the cast over the incisional area and posterior portion of the shoulder for bleeding into the cast. The patient may have wound catheters for the first 36 to 48 hours. If so, check the placement and the amount of drainage from the wound catheters. Assess for any bleeding at the bone graft donor site.

Nursing Diagnosis and Goal Formulation

Nursing diagnoses for a typical patient with a shoulder arthrodesis and a shoulder spica are (1) alterations in comfort related to pain from bone and joint surgery, (2) alterations in mobility related to joint instability, (3) potential complications related to surgical procedure and arm immobility, and (4) alterations in psychological well-being related to anxiety and knowledge deficit about surgical procedure, treatment method, and prognosis.

Short-term goals are to have the patient experience (1) a decrease in the amount of shoulder pain, (2) a stability of the arm through surgery and exercise, (3) an absence of complications from surgery and decreased activities, and (4) a decrease in anxiety through increased knowledge.

TABLE 9–4. NURSING PROCESS FOR SHOULDER ARTHRODESIS WITH A SHOULDER SPICA CAST

Assessment	Nursing Diagnosis	Goal Formulation	Planning and Intervention	Evaluation and Reassessment
1. Assess location, duration, and severity of pain. Assess the neurovascular status. Check for correct positioning.	1. Alteration in comfort: pain in the shoulder related to bone and soft tissue trauma.	1. Short-term goal: a decrease in shoulder pain through immobilization and pain medications. Long-term goal: free of pain.	1. Alleviate Pain Make sure patient is correctly positioned and supported with pillows. Help to change or correct positioning. Make sure there is no respiratory impairment. Administer pain medications as prescribed. Teach relaxation techniques.	1. Pain medications should relieve pain with no negative side effects.
2. Assess the neurovascular status of the affected arm. Check the hand grip on the affected side. Assess the ability to move self. Check for correct positioning.	2. Impaired physical mobility: decreased shoulder function related to shoulder fusion.	2. Short-term goal: regain shoulder function through immobilization and controlled exercise. Long-term goal: regain optimal function within the limits of a fused shoulder.	2. Increase Mobility *Position* Supine position with the head of the bed elevated. Upper torso propped with pillows. Head of bed elevation depends on cast. Assist with turn to unaffected side and support with pillows. *Exercises* Instruct on abdominal and breathing exercises, active range-of-motion exercises for all unaffected joints, and finger and thumb exercises (5 minutes every hour while awake).	2. Supine should be the most comfortable position when lying. When ambulating, the balance and gait should be safe, and the patient should be able to get in and out of a chair with the use of an arm rest. The patient should follow the exercise program without supervision.

			Ambulation Assist in getting the patient out of bed. Assist with ambulation.	
3. Assess the neurovascular status. Check for any tightness of the cast.	3. Potential for injury: neurovascular deficit related to soft tissue swelling and cast restrictions.	3. Short- and long-term goal: free of any neurovascular deficit.	3. Prevent Complications *Circulatory* Report abnormalities in neurovascular status. Listen for any complaints of pain or discomfort. Instruct on finger and thumb exercises.	3. The neurovascular status should remain good.
Assess the skin for any areas or irritation or pressure areas, especially over the medial epicondyle.	Potential for impairment of skin integrity: a break in skin integrity or pressure areas related to spica cast.	Short- and long-term goal: free of any break in skin integrity.	*Integumentary* Petal cast edges. Follow up complaints of pain over bony prominences *Other Complications* (See text.)	There should be no break in skin integrity.
4. Assess patient's level of knowledge of the rehabilitation process and self-care.	4. Potential knowledge deficit related to the rehabilitation process and self-care.	4. Short- and long-term goal: a decrease in anxiety with an increase in knowledge level.	4. Patient Teaching Discuss the rehabilitation process. Discuss how to do the exercises and their rationale. Discuss and demonstrate proper body mechanics with an arm spica cast on. Discuss methods of solving transportation problems. Demonstrate methods of bathing and dressing that are helpful at home. Include family and significant other in teaching plan.	4. The patient, the family, and significant other should verbalize confidence in home care and express support for the rehabilitation process. The patient should demonstrate proper body mechanics by picking up an article from the floor.

Long-term goals are (1) to have the patient free of pain, (2) to have stability in the shoulder joint, and (3) to have the return of partial function in the shoulder and the arm.

Planning and Intervention

Alleviate Pain. Immediately after the application of the shoulder spica the patient may be restless and appear quite uncomfortable. This does not necessarily mean that the patient is having a lot of pain. It may be that the patient finds it difficult to get into a comfortable position with the heavy cast on and the arm in abduction. Help the patient change or readjust position. Correct alignment helps to relieve stress to the surgical site and the arm.

Evaluate complaints of pain for possible neurovascular impairment. Specifically, there may be complaints of pain near bony prominences under the cast, especially the medial epicondyle and adjacent ulnar nerve. One way to help prevent or relieve that pressure is to encourage the patient to exercise the fingers and the thumb frequently. The cast edges are also a potential source of pain and skin irritation. Petal the edges as a preventive measure. Sources of bone pain are the incision site and the donor site of the bone graft. Medicate the patient as needed.

Increase Mobility

Position. When the patient is in bed, the head of the bed may be elevated or the patient's upper torso propped up with pillows. The amount of elevation of the head of the bed may be restricted by how far the cast extends down the trunk, and how much the patient can flex the back. The patient needs pillows to support the casted arm. The patient will probably find the supine position the most comfortable when in bed. However, the patient may turn to the unaffected side. He or she will then need help to do so, and will still need pillows to support the affected arm. Turning is essential for comfort and for cast drying.

Shoulder Spica Cast. The shoulder spica is a cast applied to the upper torso and may extend below the iliac crests (Fig. 9–13). The cast envelops the upper trunk and one arm, although the wrist and the hand of that arm may not be included. The arm is held in a position of abduction, and may be supported by a strut from the body portion of the cast. A spica cast is used to immobilize the shoulder following a disease, injury, or surgery affecting the shoulder or the humerus. Unless the patient is under anesthesia, a shoulder spica is applied with the patient standing or sitting on a stool. Padding is applied over bony prominences and under the breasts of female patients. After applying protective padding, the plaster is first applied in a circular fashion around the trunk of the body. Plaster is then applied in a spiral reverse that goes between the arm and the upper torso, thereby immobilizing the shoulder joint. The position of the shoul-

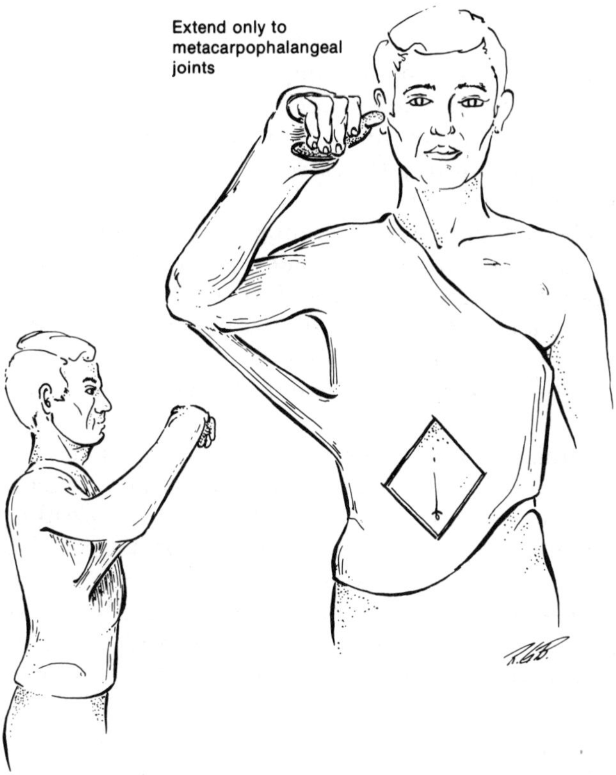

Figure 9–13. The shoulder spica cast is made in a similar manner to the hip spica, in that a support is necessary, extending from the body of the cast to the arm. The position of the arm in the cast depends upon the condition being treated and upon the personal preference of the physician. *(From Lewis, R.C.* Handbook of traction, casting and splinting techniques. *Philadelphia: Lippincott, 1977, p. 84, with permission.)*

der is determined by clinical signs, roentgenograms, and the patient's age and occupation. The most usual position for an adult without a shoulder arthrodesis is 70 degrees of abduction, 40 degrees of flexion, and enough external rotation to allow the mouth to be reached by the fingers when the elbow is flexed. Positioning following a shoulder arthrodesis varies depending on the surgical procedure. In all cases, the elbow is flexed at a right angle, the forearm is held in mid-rotation, and the wrist is dorsiflexed.

Exercises. The patient needs to be encouraged to exercise. The recommended exercises include chest and abdominal exercises, active range-of-motion exercises for all unaffected joints, and finger and thumb exercises to stimulate circulation in the involved arm. Once the cast is removed, other exercises are begun.

Ambulation. At first, the patient needs assistance in getting out of bed. Once the patient is out of bed, some support is needed until he or she is able to adjust to the weight of the cast and strengthen the abdominal and back muscles.

Prevent Complications. The most common complication following an arthrodesis and spica cast application is neurovascular impairment due to pressure from the cast at the medial epicondyle. An impairment of the ulnar nerve is indicated if the patient has decreased or no ability to abduct the fingers or feel pricking at the distal end of the fifth (little) finger. If that should occur, notify the patient's physician immediately. To help prevent nerve impairments, have the patient do finger and thumb exercises on a regular basis. At times the patient may have decreased circulation to the affected hand because of a lack of activity and slow arterial flow caused by the elevated position of the arm. The decreased circulation may lead to numbness or whiteness of the fingers, which should be relieved by finger exercises.

Another potential complication is respiratory impairment. The cast may be too tight and prevent or decrease respiratory movement, which can lead to pneumonia. Have the patient turn, cough, and deep breathe. Incentive spirometry may also be used. Be alert for the possiblity of fat emboli.

Skin irritation and breakdown may develop at the cast edges and where the cast rubs on bony prominences. Listen to the patient's complaints to become aware of early problems, and petal the cast edges even before problems occur.

Not infrequently, some patients become depressed at the prospect of living with a fused shoulder. Others have difficulty in adjusting to the temporary change in body image brought about by wearing the cast for 2 to 3 months. Spend time with the patient. Let him or her express feelings and concerns. Be honest, realistic, and help the patient obtain answers to questions.

Patient Teaching. Make sure the patient is able to do abdominal and respiratory breathing exercises and understands the rationale behind them. Go over range-of-motion exercises for all uninvolved joints and why they are necessary. Exercises for the fingers and the thumb (see p. 510) are to be done 5 minutes every hour the patient is awake. If the patient awakens during the night, the finger exercises should be done then as well. The patient should continue all of these exercises until the cast is removed. A different set of exercises for the arm and the upper torso will then be prescribed so that the patient can regain as much function as possible in the involved shoulder.

Instruct the patient on the proper ways to ambulate, get in and out of a chair, pick up items from the floor, and go up and down stairs. Discuss possible problems that may arise in using public transportation, e.g., hitting somebody with the casted arm in a crowded bus. The patient should not attempt to drive a car even if the dominant arm is unaffected, because the casted arm may interfere with steering, shifting, and reacting to emergencies.

The patient should be taught how to bathe and dress at home. Sponge baths are recommended, although the patient may need help in washing the unaffected arm and hair. Because the patient has the cast on for a number of weeks, a plastic hair washing board may be helpful. Dressing the upper torso can be a problem. Opening seams on the affected side of blouses or shirts and using Velcro straps for closure is the best approach. Once the cast is removed, the seams can be repaired. Patients living in cold climates will probably be unable to wear a coat even if there is no strut supporting the arm. Wearing a poncho, cape, or large wool shawl is suggested. Discuss with the patient the availability of such items from family or friends before suggesting they buy them.

Evaluation and Reassessment

The patient should have good neurovascular status in the affected arm and no respiratory complications. There should be a decrease in the amount of pain and no side effects from pain medications. The patient should be able to demonstrate good balance and gait when ambulating, and know how to safely get in and out of a bed or chair, and go up and down stairs. He or she should be able to pick up objects from the floor with good body mechanics and no bending of the upper trunk. The patient should feel confident about the ability to perform activites of daily living and to move about and care for self after going home. Exercises should be incorporated into a schedule for home care. The patient should accept the temporary restrictions imposed by the cast and the permanent limitations of a fused shoulder.

Arthroplasty

Lesions about the shoulder requiring arthroplasty are much less common than those of weight-bearing joints such as the hip and the knee. An arthroplasty of the shoulder may be a prosthetic humeral head replacement (hemiarthroplasty) or a total shoulder arthroplasty, where the humeral head is replaced and the glenoid cavity resurfaced. A hemiarthroplasty is usually indicated for the treatment of certain acute fractures or painful, chronic glenohumeral incongruities. Replacement of the proximal humerus is done for fracture–dislocations and for the treatment of fractures in which reduction is almost impossible and the articular fragment is likely to undergo avascular necrosis. These patients usually need surgery as soon as possible after the injury. A delay of 10 to 14 days or longer results in increased scarring, contractures of the muscles and other soft tissue structures, and increased osteoporosis of the bone fragments.

A total shoulder arthroplasty is indicated when there is severe destruction of the joint from trauma or a disease process such as rheumatoid arthritis. The total shoulder arthroplasty replaces the humeral head with a metallic component and resurfaces the glenoid cavity with a polyethylene unit. Prostheses for the humerus are available in a range of stem lengths, neck lengths, and head diameters that allow the normal anatomy of the shoulder to be closely approximated. A number of different types of such prostheses are presently available, and developmental work is continuing.

During a total shoulder replacement procedure the tip of the coracoid may be resected, and the subscapularis muscle and capsule are divided to expose the glenohumeral joint (Fig. 9–14). The humerus is then dislocated and the humeral head is resected. The glenoid cavity and the humeral canal are reamed in preparation for the prosthesis. The humeral and glenoid components are then cemented into place with methyl methacrylate cement. The glenohumeral joint is reduced, and the capsule and subscapularis are closed. Once the procedure is completed and the wound closed, a sling and swath bandage are applied. If the musculotendinous (rotator) cuff has required reconstruction, an abduction humeral splint or a spica shell may be used.

□ NURSING PROCESS (Table 9–5)

Assessment

The first step in the nursing assessment of a typical patient following a shoulder arthroplasty with a sling or a sling and swath is a neurovascular assessment of the affected arm (see Chap. 2). Make sure the patient is in correct body alignment and that the sling and swath are supporting the arm and relieving the pull on the shoulder. As the patient will probably have wound catheters in place, check the amount and color of the drainage. Note if there is any drainage on the incisional dressing. Check the depth, rate, and rhythm of respirations. Determine the location, type, and severity of pain.

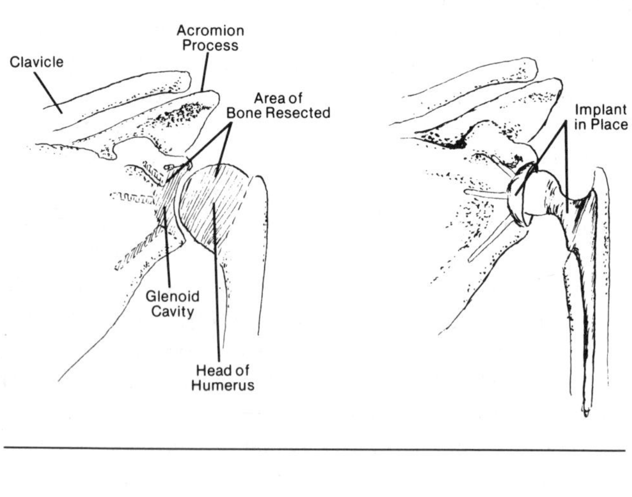

Figure 9–14. Total shoulder arthroplasty. *(From Brantley, P., & Analla, M.* The nurse and orthopedic surgery. *Rutherford, N.J.: Howmedica, Inc., 1980, p. 3. Courtesy of Howmedica.)*

Nursing Diagnoses and Goal Formulation

Nursing diagnoses for a typical patient following a shoulder arthroplasty are (1) alterations in comfort related to surgery involving bone and soft tissue, (2) alterations in mobility related to lack of joint stability and decreased muscle strength, (3) potential complications related to surgical procedure and decreased arm mobility, and (4) alterations in psychological well-being related to anxiety and knowledge deficit about the surgical procedure and the rehabilitation process.

Short-term goals are to have the patient experience (1) a decrease in the amount of pain, (2) an increase in joint mobility through controlled exercise, (3) an absence of complications from surgery and decreased mobility, and (4) a decrease in anxiety through increased knowledge. Long-term goals are to have the patient free of pain and able to have full function in the glenohumeral joint.

Planning and Intervention

Alleviate Pain. Following a shoulder arthroplasty, the patient may have pain during the first few days after surgery even through the arm is immobilized. Check the patient for correct body alignment to reduce the stress on the shoulder. Pillows may be necessary to help keep the shoulder aligned while the patient is lying in bed. Ice may be applied near the incision to reduce swelling and discomfort.

Pain medications are administered after nursing interventions for specific problems. Do not wait until the patient asks for medications but assess and intervene before the pain becomes severe. When the patient begins a shoulder exercise program, give medication before beginning the exercise.

Increase Mobility

Position. Nursing interventions after a shoulder arthroplasty are based on maintaining the proper position of the affected arm to reduce pain, promote healing, and prevent complications. A sling or a sling and swath bandage is usually employed to immobilize the arm unless the musculotendinous rotator cuff required reconstruction during the arthroplasty. If so, an adduction humeral splint or a spica cast shell may be used. If the arm is immobilized in a sling or a sling and swath, the arm should be in a sling at all times, except when exercising.

The head of the bed is elevated for comfort. The patient usually lies supine but may turn onto the uninvolved side. After the turn, pillows are necessary to help support the affected arm.

Exercises. Exercises of all the joints, except those of the involved arm, are encouraged from the day of surgery. Finger and thumb exercises with the involved arm may also be started immediately. After 4 to 5 days, and under supervision, the patient begins gentle passive exercises consisting

TABLE 9–5. NURSING PROCESS FOR SHOULDER ARTHROPLASTY WITH A SLING AND SWATH

Assessment	Nursing Diagnosis	Goal Formulation	Planning and Intervention	Evaluation and Reassessment
1. Assess the location, duration, and severity of pain. Check for any areas of swelling. Assess the neurovascular status.	1. Alteration in comfort: pain in the shoulder related to bone and soft tissue trauma.	1. Short-term goal: remain relatively free of pain. Long-term goal: free of pain.	1. Alleviate Pain Make sure that the arm is correctly positioned and that the body is in correct alignment. Instruct on finger exercises. Discuss methods of relaxation. Administer pain medications.	1. The patient should remain relatively pain free with the use of nursing measures and prescribed medications.
2. Assess the neurovascular status. Assess the ability to do active range of motion of all unaffected joints. Assess the ability to do exercises with the affected arm. Check for any areas of swelling. Check for ability to ambulate safely without assistance.	2. Impaired physical mobility: decrease in shoulder and arm function related to instability of the shoulder joint.	2. Short-term goal: an increase in mobility through arm support and controlled exercises. Long-term goal: regain as much function in the arm as is possible.	2. Increase Mobility *Position* Properly position the affected arm in the sling and swath. Elevate the head of the bed for comfort. Keep the patient supine or on the unaffected side with the arm supported by pillows. *Exercises* Instruct on gentle finger and thumb exercises to the affected arm and on active exercises for all unaffected joints. Start gentle passive forward flexion and external rotation shoulder exercises 4–5 days after surgery. Start pendulum type exercises 10 days after surgery (other exercises depend on type of prosthesis).	2. The patient should follow the exercise program without supervision. There should be only a moderate amount of pain during and after exercise.

			Ambulation Assist patient in getting out of bed and with ambulation.	
3. Assess the neurovascular status. Assess the respiratory status.	3. Potential for injury: neurovascular deficit related to soft tissue swelling.	3. Short- and long-term goal: free of any neurovascular deficit.	3. Prevent Complications *Circulatory* Report abnormalities in neurovascular status. Instruct on exercise program. Administer anticoagulant medications.	3. The patient should remain free of any signs of complications from surgery or immobility.
Check for any areas of redness or swelling and for other signs of infection.	Potential for injury: infection related to surgical incision and break in skin integrity.	Short- and long-term goal: free of any signs of infection.	*Integumentary* Keep the dressing clean and dry. Keep pressure off any bony prominences. Instruct the patient on signs and symptoms of infection. *Other Complications* (See text.)	
4. Assess the patient's level of knowledge about the rehabilitation process, self-care, and prognosis.	4. Potential for knowledge deficit related to the rehabilitation process, self-care, and prognosis.	4. Short- and long-term goal: a decrease in anxiety through an increase in knowledge.	4. Patient Teaching Discuss the steps in the rehabilitation process. Go over the rationale for each exercise and why the exercise program needs to continue for at least a year. Record progress in the exercise program. Discuss exercising to music and to specific radio or television programs. Include the family and significant other in the education program. Discuss methods of doing activities of daily living and dressing.	4. The patient should verbalize an understanding of the rehabilitation process, self-care activities, and prognosis.

mainly of forward flexion and external rotation shoulder exercises (see pp. 521–523). For many patients pendulum type exercises (see p. 500) are not started until approximately 10 days postsurgery. The gentle passive and active-assisted exercises progress according to the patient's pain tolerance. Some patients may utilize a shoulder exerciser (Fig. 9–15). To a great degree, functional recovery depends on implementing a comprehensive postoperative rehabilitation regime. The patient needs to do the exercise program for up to a year after surgery.

The prescribed exercises may vary with the patient's condition and the type of prosthesis. For example, a patient with a Neer prosthesis who has had few muscles severed and a fully functional rotator cuff has more muscle power than a patient who has undergone a total glenohumeral replacement. Both have had their deltoid muscles cut, so neither should attempt to actively elevate their arm to the side until the deltoid muscle has healed, usually 6 to 8 weeks after surgery. Other patients may begin the pendulum exercises as early as the second postoperative day. Because that would be the first time the affected arm has been extended and lowered in some time, the patient will usually complain of tingling. Once the exercise program is begun, the role of the nurse includes encouraging the patient and reinforcing the instructions.

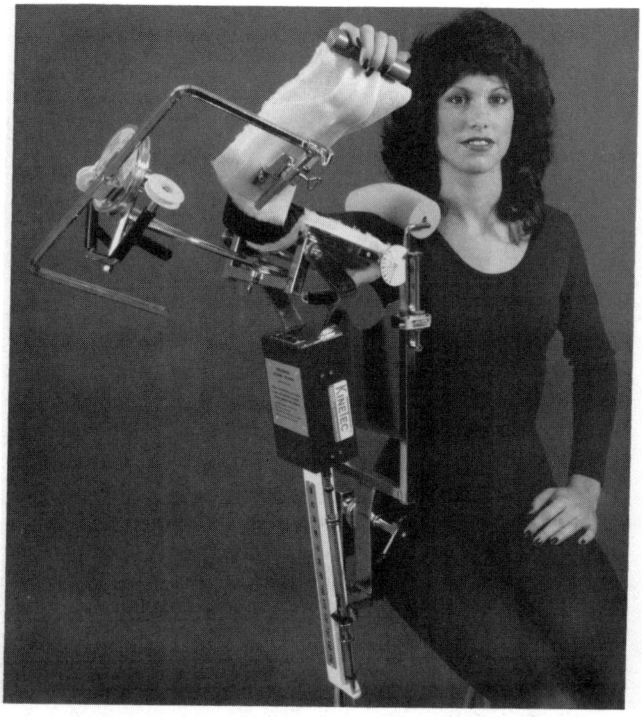

Figure 9–15. The Kinetic shoulder exerciser provides passive motion and exercise for physical therapy of the shoulder. The unit features automatic control of all passive exercise motions, including external rotation, with the speed and range of motion programmed by the physician. The exerciser may also be operated manually by the patient within range limits preset by the physician. Postoperative treatment with the exerciser aids in preventing stiffness of the shoulder joint. *(Courtesy of Richards Medical Company. KINETIC is a registered trademark of CO-GEMO, an affiliate of Richards Medical Company.)*

Ambulation. Ambulation may begin early. At first the patient needs assistance in getting out of bed, balancing after standing, and taking the first few steps because wearing a sling changes the patient's center of gravity. When supporting the patient, do not take hold of the affected arm or shoulder. The patient also needs instruction in getting into and out of a chair.

Prevent Complications. Complications involving the prosthesis or implant include loosening, bending, breaking, or dislocating the prosthesis. Fractures may occur in the bone around the prosthesis. The patient may have adverse reactions to the implant itself or to the bone cement. Other complications are similar to those that exist in any surgical procedure, namely infection, bleeding, thromboemboli, and adverse reactions to anesthesia, blood transfusions, or medication.

The risk of surgical infection is reduced by routine antibiotic therapy, at first intravenous and then oral. Respiratory infections may arise because of decreased respiratory depth and the patient's hesitancy to cough and deep breathe because of a fear of increasing pain in the glenohumeral joint. Continue to encourage coughing and deep breathing exercises and educate the patient on the need to do so.

The patient will have wound catheters connected to suction, and if the amount of drainage exceeds 100 ml in the second 12 hours, notify the physician. To decrease the risk of thrombus formation, most patients are placed on anticoagulant therapy (i.e., aspirin 650 mg four times a day).

Although the humerus is a much smaller bone than the femur or tibia, there is still a danger of fat emboli because of the reaming of the medullary canal of the humerus. The nurse needs to be alert to any chest pain, shortness of breath, confusion, or other signs of a fat embolism (see p. 72).

Patient Teaching. Educate the patient, the family, and significant others about the early signs and symptoms of infection and nerve and vascular impairment. Never underestimate the need for encouragement and evaluation of the exercise program. In any exercise program, progress will be slow and deliberate. Careful records help to document the patient's accomplishments. Use them to encourage the patient and set realistic goals. Some patients may feel the exercises are boring, time consuming, and often painful. Work out a program with the patient to facilitate exercising. For example, suggest exercising to music, while listening to or watching a specific radio or television program, or with others. To help reduce pain in the initial stages, suggest doing exercises after showering, using warm packs, or taking pain medications. Remember, the patient may need to follow a rigid exercise program for up to a year to regain maximum shoulder function. Help the patient, the family, and significant others with potential problems in activities of daily living.

Evaluation and Reassessment

Determine the patient's ability to understand and accomplish the required exercises. The amount of pain at the incisional site should decrease over time, but there should still be some pain after exercising as the patient continues to regain joint function. The patient should be free of any complications from the surgery and decreased mobility.

THE PAINFUL SHOULDER

Pain in the shoulder may be caused by various conditions, including diseases of the internal organs. Apart from traumatic lesions, 85 to 90 percent of painful disabilities of the shoulder are due to nonarticular disorders of tendons, bursae, tendon sheaths, and the musculotendinous cuff.

Calcific Tendinitis (Subacromial Bursitis)

Bursitis is an inflammation of the sac (bursa) covering a bony prominence. When the underlying tendon is also inflamed, tendinitis is combined with bursitis. There tends to be an increase in calcium content with degenerative changes in the tendon, and calcific deposits in and about the rotator tendon are the most frequent abnormality encountered in the subacute or acutely painful shoulder. As calcific granules accumulate, they cause no symptoms in the relatively avascular tendon. When they extend to vascular areas, however, and in particular to the underlying subdeltoid or subacromial bursa, they cause an acute inflammation. When the calcium salts break into the bursa, they take up water, and the potential bursal space enlarges, causing severe pain, occasional warmth, and redness to the overlying skin (Beeson & McDermott, 1980, p. 1418; Iversen & Clawson, 1977, pp. 140–142).

The patient usually seeks medical attention because of pain, tenderness, and limitation of motion. The onset may be sudden, without known injury, and the pain severe and agonizing. The patient may complain of pain at the upper humerus and in the subacromial area, which may radiate to the insertion of the deltoid, and in severe cases up to the neck and down to the fingertips. Pain is increased with motion, particularly abduction and external rotation. Extreme tenderness is felt at the lateral area of the humeral head, below the acromion, and above at the insertion of the deltoid. Acute symptoms may persist for several days and then diminish abruptly or gradually.

Treatment usually consists of resting the shoulder with a sling, with complete or partial immobilization if necessary. Ice bags are applied during the acute stage, which lasts approximately 2 days, and then heat applications are used. Anti-inflammatory and pain-relieving drugs are usually prescribed, and in some instances a local anesthetic and corticosteroids are injected into the bursa. As the pain subsides. physical therapy and exercises are started to restore function as rapidly as possible to prevent residual subacute or chronic progression (Beeson & McDermott, 1980, p. 1418; Cailleit, 1981, pp. 53–73;

Donahoo & Dimon, 1977, p. 113). In the beginning, exercises may be the Codman or pendular passive exercises that add traction to the glenohumeral joint, stretch the capsule, avoid active abduction, and minimize scapular shrugging.

Adhesive Capsulitis (Frozen Shoulder)

Adhesive capsulitis is a condition in which fibrous tissues develop in the shoulder joint capsule, causing progressive loss of movement and pain, particularly during abduction and rotation. The pain can become constant and disabling, and may radiate down the arm and the back to the scapula. Motion in abduction and external rotation is limited, and atrophy of the muscles of the shoulder girdle may occur (Fig. 9–16). There is an obliteration of the subdeltoid bursa and adhesive inflammation between the joint capsule and the peripheral articular cartilage. Adhesive capsulitis is distinct from calcific tendinitis in that adhesive capsulitis has a gradual onset, slowly increasing pain and stiffness, little or no localized tenderness, and progressive limitation of motion. No specific cause is known, but prolonged bedrest or immobilization of the shoulder joint appear to be predisposing factors. Secondary causes tend to include fracture–dislocations and arthritic conditions.

Widely accepted treatments are physical therapy with heat and assistive exercises, and analgesics and anti-inflammatory drugs to relieve pain and joint inflammation. A periarticular or joint injection of a local anesthetic and corticosteroids, ice packs, and manipulation of the shoulder are controversial treatments (Beeson & McDermott, 1980, p. 1418; Cailliet, 1981, pp. 82–89; Roaf & Hodkinson, 1975, p. 372).

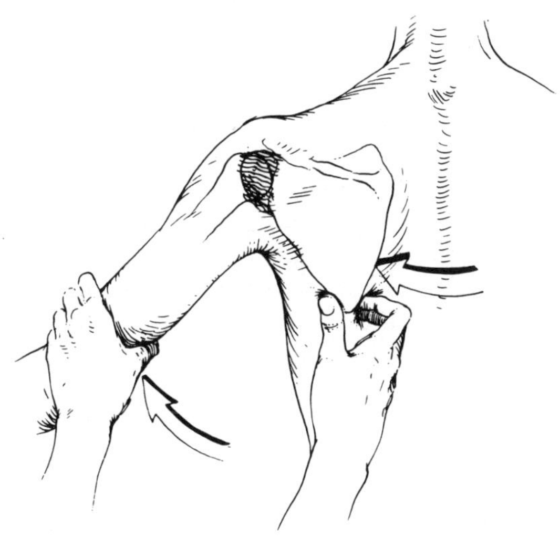

Figure 9–16. Frozen shoulder syndrome. No glenohumeral motion—only scapulothoracic motion.

Tendinitis

Tendinitis, an inflammation of a tendon, is associated with both chronic trauma and the degenerative changes that occur with aging. Because tendons are less vascular than other structures in the shoulder, tendinitis often leads to calcific deposits that can lead to calcific tendinitis, calcific tenosynovitis, and bursitis.

The tendon of the supraspinatus muscle is the one most commonly affected by tendinitis and the one most likely to be associated with calcific deposits. The patient complains of a deep ache in the shoulder region with referral of pain to the deltoid, and has difficulty in lying on the affected side. There is tenderness at the site of inflammation and difficulty with abduction and internal rotation movements (Iversen & Clawson, 1977, pp. 140–141).

Treatment is based on relieving the inflammatory process and maintaining functional range of motion in the shoulder. Oral anti-inflammatory and analgesic drugs are given to help reduce pain and inflammation. The use of prednisolone is controversial.

NEOPLASMS

Malignant bone tumors grow rapidly, are hard to diagnose early, and are frequently fatal. The following are examples of bone tumors that occur in the shoulder region.

Osteosarcoma

Osteosarcoma is a rapidly growing, extremely malignant tumor characterized by producing neoplastic osteoid directly from anaplastic, osteoblast-like cells. Osteosarcoma is found predominantly in the metaphysical region of a large, long bone, occasionally in the midshaft. It is most common in the distal femur, proximal tibia, and proximal end of the humerus. It is slightly more common for men than for women, and its incidence peaks in the second decade of life, decreasing with advanced age.

The onset is gradual and spontaneous but occasionally trauma precipitates symptoms or, infrequently, a pathological fracture. Pain is intermittent at first but eventually becomes continuous and incapacitating. In approximately 80 percent of the patients progressive pulmonary metastases develop (Turek, 1977, p. 556). Sometimes the metastases extend to other skeletal sites. If untreated the median time for survival after the onset of pulmonary metastases is 2 to 3 months. Treatment consists of radical amputation, chemotherapy, high voltage irradiation, and pulmonary resection of large tumors.

Chondrosarcoma

Primary chondrosarcoma is a virulent, malignant tumor, composed of cartilage and myxomatous tissue and occurring subperiosteally, at first without involvement of the cortex of the bone. It is usually found at points where muscles attach to the bone near a joint and where cartilage formation continues throughout life. The most common areas are the knees, the shoulders, and the pelvis.

Patients are usually 14 to 21 years of age, with pain in the affected area that becomes progressively more severe. The pain is worse at night than during the day. Upon examination, there is swelling at the site. The course of the disease is one of rapid growth of the tumor and severe and persistent pain. A fatal outcome within a year is usual (Turek, 1977, p. 543). The tumor is not radiosensitive, so that most radical form of amputation is usually attempted (e.g., forequarter amputation).

Secondary Chondrosarcoma

Secondary chondrosarcoma is a very slow-growing malignant tumor, occuring as a result of malignant degeneration of a enchondroma or a cartilaginous exotosis. Long bones, especially the proximal end of the humerus, the ribs, and the innominate bone are the usual sites.

The onset is usually third decade or later in life. The patient usually gives a history of mild, intermittent ache and swelling that suddenly increases in severity. There may be persistent pain, pain at night, and edema due to venous and lymphatic obstruction.

Treatment usually consists of amputation, as local removal and irradiation are ineffective (Turek, 1977, p. 544).

Amputations About the Shoulder

Shoulder amputations are usually necessitated by malignancy or severe trauma. The types of amputations are (1) through the anatomical neck of the humerus, (2) disarticulation at the shoulder, and (3) forequarter amputation. Any amputation performed at the level of the axillary fold or more proximally requires the same prosthetic fitting as a shoulder disarticulation. Although prosthetic devices are available for these amputees, they are only able to perform limited functions.

An amputation at the neck of the humerus is usually done for severe trauma. The humerus is resected at the level of the anatomical neck and the end of the humerus is smoothed with a rasp. The long head of the triceps, both heads of the biceps, and the coracobrachialis are then sutured over the end of the humerus. Other muscles are then sutured and a skin closure that allows accurate opposition of the skin edges is done. Disarticulation is a very similar procedure, except that the head of the humerus is also removed, and in some instances a partial excision of an unduly prominent acromion process may be done to give the shoulder a more smooth and rounded contour.

A forequarter (shoulder girdle or interscapulothoracic) amputation consists of the removal of the entire upper extremity and shoulder girdle in the interval between the scapula and the thoracic wall. It is performed only for the removal of malignant tumors when the tumor extends to or through the region of the shoulder joint, or extensively infiltrates the deltoid, pectoral, or subscapular muscles. Because of the nature of the operation and the disease for which it is performed, an atypical skin flap is often done. Closure is somewhat difficult and often requires auxillary skin grafts (Edmondson & Crenshaw, 1980, p. 863).

The primary focus of nursing care in all three of these amputations is to help the patient adjust to a change in body image, assist in rehabilitation with or without a prosthesis, and, depending on the prognosis, help the patient adjust to impending death.

UPPER ARM

Trauma

The upper arm region includes the shaft of the humerus and its covering muscles, principally the biceps brachii and the triceps brachii. The proximal end of the humerus is included with the shoulder, and the distal end with the elbow.

FRACTURES OF THE HUMERAL SHAFT

Fractures of the shaft of the humerus may be due to a direct force, such as a blow to the side of the arm, an indirect force such as a fall on an outstretched hand, or pathology, such as a secondary malignancy. Fractures of the shaft of the humerus do not produce as much overriding of the fragments as do fractures of the femur, because the muscles of the arm are not as powerful as those in the leg, and their retraction is inhibited by the weight of the arm. The possibility of overriding is greatest in humeral fractures when the fracture is above the attachment of the deltoid muscle.

Humeral shaft fractures are usually easily corrected by manipulation and treated nonoperatively. When a closed reduction is completed, the arm may be placed in a sugar-tong splint with a Velpeau bandage, an arm cylinder cast with a collar and cuff sling, an abductor splint, a shoulder spica cast, or most commonly, a hanging arm cast. Although most of these methods do not secure complete immobilization, they rest the arm in a satisfactory anatomical position that allows union to occur with good cosmetic and functional results. Other nonsurgical methods of treatment, which provide more complete immobilization and better alignment but require bedrest, are skin and skeletal traction.

In some instances an open reduction with internal fixation is indicated. These include circumstances where (1) satisfactory position and alignment cannot be achieved by conservative measures, (2) associated arm injuries require early mobilization, (3) the fracture is pathological, (4) the fracture is associated with major vascular injuries, (5) there is a spiral fracture of the distal humerus in which radial nerve palsy develops, and (6) treatment of associated injuries makes bedrest necessary. It is often difficult to maintain both upper and lower extremities in traction. Thus in multiple injury situations, elective open reduction with internal fixation of the humerus may be indicated.

Fractures of the humeral shaft may be repaired internally by plates and screws, medullary nails, or external fixation devices (Fig. 9–17). Methods of repair are usually (1) for transverse of short oblique fractures, a compression plate with the arm supported in a sling for 3 to 4 weeks postoperatively; (2) for long oblique and spiral fractures, transfixation lag screws with external support such as an abduction humeral splint until the fracture heals; (3) for open fractures of the humerus in which the insertion of internal fixation may lead to infection or other complications, external fixation appliances such as the Wagner or Hoffman device; and (4) for pathological fractures secondary to malignant tumors, medullary fixation, possibly in conjunction with methyl methacrylate cement for increased stability. Occasionally a segmental fracture in which satisfactory position cannot be obtained by closed methods may be treated by medullary fixation (Küntscher) (Edmondson & Crenshaw, 1980, p. 670).

The two major complications of fractures of the humeral shaft are nonunion of the bone and radial nerve palsy. Nonunion occurs in 5 to 12 percent of patients and requires a bone graft operation. Injury to the radial nerve ad-

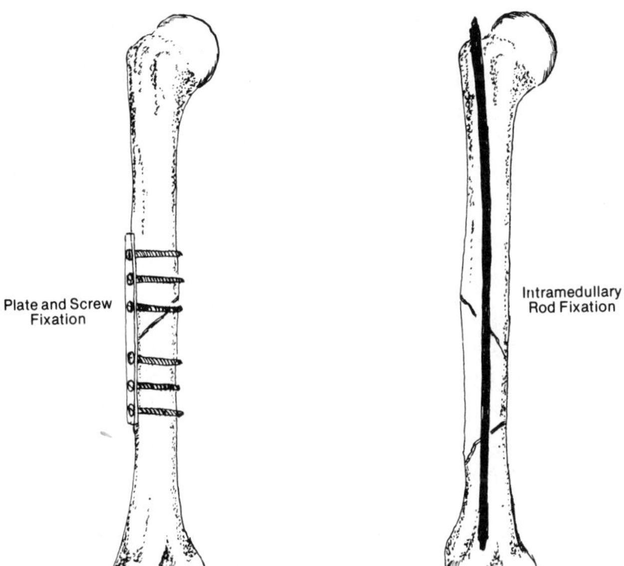

Figure 9–17. Open reduction and internal fixation, fractured humerus. *(From Brantley, P., & Analla, M.* The nurse and orthopedic surgery. *Rutherford, N.J.: Howmedica, Inc., 1980, p. 24. Courtesy of Howmedica.)*

jacent to the musculospiral groove may accompany humeral shaft fractures and cause the patient to lose the power to actively dorsiflex the wrist and elevate the thumb. The condition, known as "wrist drop," occurs in about 12 percent of the patients with humeral shaft fractures (Gartland, 1979, pp. 270–271). Because in most instances the radial nerve is only bruised and not severed, nerve function usually returns within 3 to 9 months, unless there is further trauma from the treatment itself. The wrist is usually splinted in the dorsiflexed (functional) position while awaiting nerve regeneration. Complete severance of the radial nerve requires surgical repair, or if that is not possible, wrist fusion with tendon transfers to restore wrist dorsiflexion and thumb elevation (Gartland, 1979, p. 272).

□ NURSING PROCESS (Table 9–6)

Assessment

The first step in the assessment of a patient with a hanging arm cast applied following a fractured humerus is to note the position of the affected arm in relation to the patient's body. The humerus should be in correct alignment. When the patient is in bed, the head of the bed must be elevated high enough so that the casted portion of the arm applies downward traction to the proximal humerus. The strap that is attached to the cast and goes around the patient's neck must support the distal portion of the cast, but should not reduce the downward pull on the humerus. Note if there is any protrusion, swelling, or discoloration near the fracture site in the proximal humerus.

Check the neurovascular status of the affected arm (Chap. 2). Compare the involved arm with the uninvolved arm to check for deficiences. Determine the amount, location, and severity of pain. Check the patient for the possibility of other injuries, especially skin abrasions and contusions. Remember, most patients will be older adults, as the fracture usually results from a fall.

Nursing Diagnosis and Goal Formation

Nursing diagnoses for a typical patient with a fractured humerus and a hanging arm cast are (1) alterations in comfort related to pain from trauma to the humerus and soft tissues, (2) alterations in mobility related to instability of the humerus, (3) potential complications related to decreased arm mobility, and (4) alterations in psychological well-being related to anxiety and knowledge deficit about the injury and the treatment methods.

Short-term goals are to have the patient experience (1) a decrease in the amount of pain, (2) an increase in mobility in the arm through the use of traction and controlled exercise, (3) an absence of complications from decreased activities, and (4) a decrease in anxiety through increased knowledge. Long-term goals are to have the patient free of pain and able to regain function in the arm and the shoulder.

Planning and Intervention

Alleviate Pain. In the treatment of a patient with a fractured humerus and a hanging arm cast, pain relief may be the patient's most important goal. The hanging arm cast is not a method of immobilizing a fracture but a means of applying traction. The traction helps to realign the fracture and reduce muscle spasms, thus reducing the amount of pain in the arm. Do not place the casted arm on a pillow as that reduces the pull, manipulates the fracture site, and increases muscle spasm.

The patient may hold the affected arm protectively against the body, and be afraid to relax and let the hanging arm cast support the arm. In the beginning the patient may keep the muscles of the arm so tense that they are actually working against the pull of the cast, thus increasing the pain in the arm. Spending time with the patient and explaining the purpose of the cast are the best nursing interventions.

Determine whether pain is from the fracture site or from neurovascular impairment. Administer pain medications as needed.

Increase Mobility

Position. Immediately after the application of a hanging arm cast, the patient should be sitting upright in bed with the head of the bed elevated so that the casted arm pulls downward on the humerus. That position is to be maintained at all times. Occasionally the patient's arm may drop back and move out of alignment. That may be due to kyphosis of the thorax, which does not allow the patient's shoulders to lie flat against the bed. In that event, a small towel or other support may be placed under the patient's arm along the chest to correct the alignment of the humerus. Usually, the patient cannot have the bed flat or turn to either side. Some patients may be allowed to have their bed flat, and if so, traction must be applied to the cast using a pulley and weights at the foot of the bed.

Hanging Arm Cast. The hanging arm cast (Fig. 9–18) is used in the treatment of humeral fractures when the weight of the arm is not sufficient to correct the displacement. It is a long arm cast with a loop on the radial surface between the wrist and the elbow, usually close to the wrist. A strap is placed around the patient's neck and attached to the cast through the loop. The strap is usually padded with felt, foam, or other substances that help relieve the pressure on the skin at the back of the neck. The hanging arm cast may actually be heavier than a normal long arm cast because its purpose is to exert traction. A second loop is attached just below the elbow on the ulnar side. If the patient is allowed to lie flat in bed, mechanical traction may be applied using the ulnar loop. A common practice is to use 5 pounds of weight.

TABLE 9–6. NURSING PROCESS FOR FRACTURED HUMERUS TREATED WITH A HANGING ARM CAST

Assessment	Nursing Diagnosis	Goal Formulation	Planning and Intervention	Evaluation and Reassessment
1. Assess the location, duration, and severity of pain. Check the position of the arm. Assess the neurovascular status.	1. Alteration in comfort: pain in the upper arm related to soft tissue swelling and bone instability.	1. Short-term goal: pain reduction with the use of traction and pain medications. Long-term goal: free of pain.	1. Alleviate Pain Make sure the arm is in correct alignment. Make sure the traction is maintained at all times. Discuss relaxation techniques. Administer pain medications.	1. The patient should remain in a relative state of comfort with continuous traction. Periods of pain should be relieved by repositioning and pain medications.
2. Assess the neurovascular status of the affected arm. Assess the ability to follow instructions and do the exercises. Assess the patient's ability to ambulate safely without assistance.	2. Impaired physical mobility: decreased arm function related to bone instability.	2. Short-term goal: an increase in mobility through traction and exercise. Long-term goal: regain bone stability and optimal arm function.	2. Increase Mobility *Position* Instruct the patient to lie supine with the head of the bed high enough to maintain a downward pull on the humerus at all times. Place a small towel or other support under the patient's arm alongside the chest to correct alignment. Apply mechanical traction before allowing the patient to lie flat.	2. The patient should maintain the traction at all times. The patient should follow the exercise program, get out of bed with minimal assistance, and ambulate safely.
			Exercises Instruct on finger and pendulum exercises (shoulder exercises depend on age, location, and type of fracture).	The patient should remain free of any stiffness.
			Ambulation Assist the patient in getting out of bed and ambulating for the first couple of times.	

3. Assess the neurovascular status. Check for any areas of swelling.	3. Potential for injury: neurovascular deficit related to soft tissue swelling and tightness of the cast.	3. Short- and long-term goal: free of any signs of neurovascular deficit.	3. Prevent Complications *Circulatory* Report any abnormalities in neurovascular status. Instruct on finger exercises. Maintain traction and correct positioning.	3. The patient should remain free of any signs of complications.
Check the skin around cast edges, at the back of the neck, and areas of the chest where the cast rests.	Potential for impairment of skin integrity related to utilization of a hanging arm cast.	Short- and long-term goal: free of any signs of a break in skin integrity.	*Integumentary* Trim and petal cast edges. Utilize measures to prevent swelling. Intervene when complaints are made of pressure over bony prominences. *Other Complications* (See text.)	
4. Assess the patient's knowledge of the rehabilitation process, the purpose of the hanging arm cast, and self-care.	4. Potential knowledge deficit related to the rehabilitation process and self-care.	4. Short- and long-term goal: a decrease in anxiety through increase in knowledge.	4. Patient Teaching Discuss the steps in the rehabilitation process. Go over the rationale and the need for each exercise (especially the shoulder exercises). Go over the purpose of the hanging arm cast. Discuss methods of bathing, dressing, and sleeping while maintaining traction with the hanging arm cast. Discuss limitations on activities. Include the family and significant other in teaching plan. Explore the need for an extended care facility or living with others.	4. The patient should verbalize an understanding of the rehabilitation process and self-care.

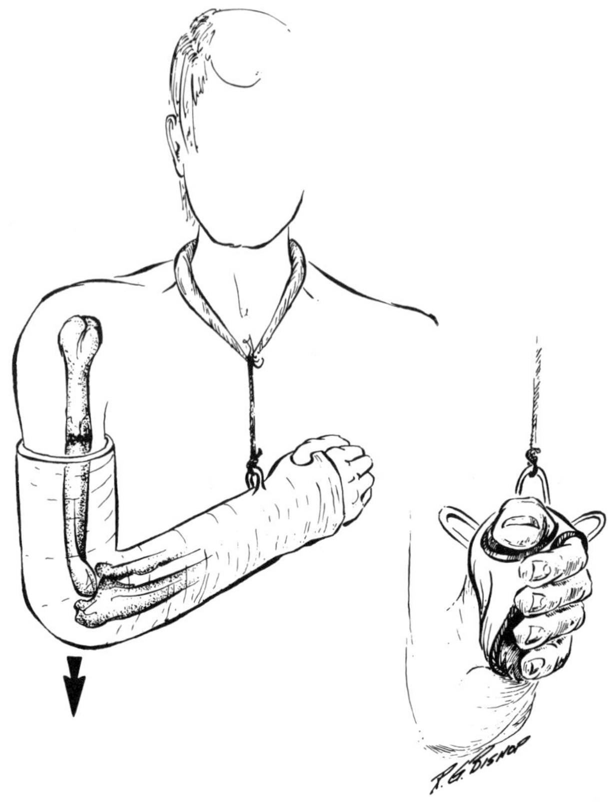

Figure 9–18. Hanging cast traction for the humerus or shoulder. The cast must be precisely applied to be effective. The cast does not necessarily need to come above the fracture site per se since it supplies weight and traction rather than immobilization. *(From Lewis, R.C.* Handbook of traction, casting and splinting techniques. *Philadelphia; Lippincott, 1977, p. 34, with permission.)*

Exercises. Exercises are needed to prevent stiffness of the joints, especially the shoulder. The location and type of fracture, and the age and physical condition of the patient, determine the kind of exercises and when they are to be started. Finger exercises (see p. 510) are usually started as soon as the cast is applied, however, and pendulum exercises (see p. 500) are done as directed to prevent adhesions of the shoulder joint capsule. After the cast is removed, a sling is applied and exercises of the shoulder, the elbow, and the wrist are begun.

Ambulation. At first, the patient needs assistance in getting out of bed. Do not support the patient on the affected side or apply pressure to the affected arm or shoulder. Patients may initially find it difficult to keep their balance with the heavy arm cast, so do not hurry them. The arm is usually properly positioned when the patient is standing or sitting in a straight-backed chair.

Prevent Complications. The major complications following a fractured humerus treated with a hanging arm cast are (1) skin irritation, (2) radial nerve injury, (3) decreased shoulder function, and (4) malunion of the fracture. Skin irritation is likely to develop in a patient with a hanging arm cast. Although the strap that goes around the patient's neck is padded, it is a source of pressure. The cast presses against the ribs and the chest. Women with large breasts may be particularly affected. The edges of the cast may be rough and irritating. Pad the axilla with a thick dressing and petal the cast edges as needed. All of those areas require observation and meticulous skin care, especially in the elderly.

There is the potential for damage to the radial nerve, which more or less wraps itself around the humerus. An injury or edema near the radial nerve may cause wrist drop. When a hanging arm cast is used, it immobilizes the wrist, making a complete motor assessment impossible. If the radial nerve has been injured, however, the thumb will not be able to offer resistance to pressure, nor will extension of the thumb be possible.

A stiff or "frozen" shoulder from a contracture is a real danger when motion in the shoulder is limited for a period of time. Shoulder exercises (see pp. 500 and 521–523) can prevent that complication, and there is little danger of their displacing the fracture.

Malunion of the fractured humerus may also occur, but does not appear to be a severe problem. A satisfactory range of shoulder motion is usually regained even if the fragments heal in a moderately deformed position.

Patient Teaching. Patients with a fractured humerus treated by a hanging arm cast are not usually hospitalized for very long, so it is important that discharge planning start as soon as possible. Although having an arm immobilized is not necessarily disabling, the patient's ability to perform self-care will depend on his or her response to the trauma and whether the dominant arm was affected. Because many patients are elderly and live alone, they may be anxious about their ability to care for themselves or to continue to live alone. Some may need to stay with relatives or friends, whereas others may require a period of time in an extended care facility or the services of a home health professional. Not being able to return home may lead to a period of depression and a feeling of helplessness.

During the period of hospitalization, the focus is on the patient's strengths and the ability to do as many of the activities of daily living as possible. The nurse can help the patient make a start toward resolving some of the difficulties of home care by encouraging the patient to be as independent as possible in the hospital. Let the patient wash the face, comb the hair, and brush the teeth. Because the unaffected arm has to do the work of two arms, muscle fatigue may occur in that arm, and rest periods should be planned with the patient.

Discuss with the patient, the family, and significant others the best positions for sleeping, sitting, bathing, and dressing. Sitting is best done in a straight-backed chair. The patient needs to be aware of the problems in sitting up and, more importantly, of getting out of a comfortable living room chair or couch. Patients are able to bathe themselves. Sponge baths are easiest. With a plaster of Paris cast, a plastic cast cover or even a garbage bag will protect the cast in the shower, but the strap will still get wet. Tub baths can be taken, with minimal water in the tub and someone to help the patient in and out. Hospital gowns are fine for day wear in the hospital but clothing for home should be discussed, as wearing a gown at home may make the patient feel like an invalid. Make sure that the patient knows how to care for a cast (Appendix B) and how to check for neurovascular impairment.

Evaluation and Reassessment

Determine that the hanging arm cast is properly aligned, and that the patient knows that the arm must not be elevated. Have the patient assess the neurovascular status to make sure he or she can perform the assessment correctly.

The patient should have a decrease in pain over time. When pain does occur, nursing measures and medications should relieve or at least reduce it. The patient should demonstrate the correct method of doing the required exercises. The patient should show an absence of complications from the fracture and the traction.

Bicipital Tenosynovitis

Tenosynovitis involves an inflammation of the tendon and the tendon sheath. The mechanical gliding mechanism of the tendon of the long head of the biceps in the bicipital groove of the humerus is a common cause of shoulder pain. The smoothness of this gliding is readily disturbed by excessive activity of the arm, particularly under stress, or by direct trauma to the area of the bicipital groove. Once the gliding mechanism is disturbed, abduction and external rotation, as well as internal rotation and extension (e.g., the motions involved in combing hair, putting on a shirt or jacket, fastening a bra, reaching for a telephone, or shoveling snow), are likely to irritate the biceps tendon and cause pain.

In seeking medical attention the patient, usually a woman 45 to 65 years old, gives a history of either gradual onset of pain or acute onset following vigorous arm activities. The pain usually originates in the anterior and medial aspects of the shoulder, and may radiate down the biceps muscle, and on to the fingers, or up to the shoulder and neck. Pain in the bicipital groove may be elicited by a combination of abduction, external rotation, and extension of the arm at the shoulder. Forced flexion of the elbow against resistance, and forced supination of the forearm against resistance with the elbow flexed will also cause pain in the bicipital groove (Gartland, 1979, pp. 164–165; Iversen & Clawson, 1977, p. 141).

Treatment may include resting the arm and shoulder in a sling, moist heat applications, diathermy and ultra-sound treatments, oral anti-inflammatory drugs, and a hydrocortisone injection into the tendon sheath. In some patients, however, a hydrocortisone injection may cause degenerative lesions in and eventual rupture of the biceps tendon (Gartland, 1979, p. 265).

Rupture of the Biceps Brachii

A rupture of the biceps brachii muscle can occur in the tendon of the long head of the muscle, in the muscle itself, or in the distal tendon. Usually a rupture is preceded by degenerative changes in the tendon and the tendon sheath, and occurs as a result of chronic bicipital tenosynovitis or acute stress to the arm, such as from lifting a heavy weight. A sudden force to the weakened tendon may cause it to fray apart, with resulting pain and weakness. The distal fragment, with the attached muscle belly, retracts toward the elbow, giving a ball-like appearance to the arm muscle. When the patient "makes a muscle" the biceps bunches up closer to the elbow than normal because the long head at the upper end has pulled loose. The lower shoulder and upper arm area is tender to palpation and a muscular gap can be felt. There is soft tissue swelling and the overlying skin becomes ecchymotic. The patient may also note weakness in the elbow flexion and forearm supination (Gartland, 1979, pp. 258–259; Iversen & Clawson, 1977, p. 142).

The treatment for a rupture of the biceps brachii long head tendon may be conservative or surgical. An elderly patient, or one not involved with heavy lifting, may be treated conservatively. For others, surgical attachment of the ruptured tendon to the bicipital groove or to the coracoid process is indicated. A rupture of the biceps brachii muscle is much less common than a tendon rupture, and is usually treated conservatively by means of a Velpeau bandage with the elbow held at more than 90 degrees of flexion. Least commonly, a rupture or avulsion may occur at the elbow, where the biceps tendon inserts distally on the bicipital tuberosity of the radius. In this instance, the muscle belly retracts toward the shoulder. Such a rupture or avulsion is treated surgically by attaching the tendon to the bicipital tuberosity of the radius. The arm is then positioned with the forearm moderately supinated and the elbow flexed to 110 degrees, and held in position by a posterior splint. After 5 to 6 weeks, progressive active exercises are begun.

Pathology

NEOPLASM

Chondroblastoma

A chondroblastoma is a cellular, vascular, and cartilaginous tumor of young adults, which occurs about the epiphyseal lines, destroys cancellous bone, and characteristically contains multiple calcium deposits. It typically occurs about the knee or the upper humerus, and in men between the ages of 10 and 20.

The patient usually gives a history of trauma, pain, tenderness, swelling, and joint effusion. Conservative surgical treatment is usual, and consists of curettage and obliteration of the tumor cavity by the use of bone grafts.

AMPUTATIONS

Amputations through the arm, or above-elbow amputations, are defined as those between the axillary fold and the distal supracondylar region of the humerus. Those amputations are usually done because of trauma or malignancy. Arm prostheses contain an elbow-lock mechanism to allow movement and stabilize the joint in flexion and extension, and a turntable mechanism to substitute for humeral rotation (Edmondson & Crenshaw, 1980, p. 860; Turek, 1977, p. 1495). The elbow-lock mechanism usually extends 3.8 cm distally from the end of the prosthetic socket and should be at the level of the elbow on the opposite arm. Therefore the above-elbow amputation should be at least 3.8 cm proximal to the elbow joint. Nursing care should focus on helping the patient and significant other adjust to the change in body image, and assisting with rehabilitation.

Cineplastic Procedure

A cineplastic amputation is one in which the stump is formed so that the patient may activate the prosthesis by muscular action. The cineplastic procedure consists of surgically constructing a canal transversely through a muscle, usually the biceps brachii. A rod is inserted into the canal and attached to an external cable, which connects with the mechanism of the artificial hand. Contraction of the muscle is effective in producing flexion in the artificial hand (Edmondson & Crenshaw, 1980, p. 867; Turek, 1977, p. 1497). Because of the advances in prosthetic techniques, however, the procedure is rarely used at present.

REFERENCES

Beeson, P. B., & McDermott, W. *Cecil-Loeb textbook of medicine.* Philadelphia: W. B. Saunders, 1980.

Cailliet, R. *Shoulder pain* (2nd ed.). Philadelphia: F. A. Davis, 1981.

DeGowin, E. L., & DeGowin, R. L. *Bedside diagnostic examination* (3rd ed.). New York: Macmillan, 1976.

Donahoo, C. A., & Dimon, J. H. III. *Orthopedic nursing.* Boston: Little, Brown, 1977.

Edmondson, A. S., & Crenshaw, A. H. (Eds.). *Campbell's operative orthopaedics* (6th ed.). St. Louis: C. V. Mosby, 1980.

Gartland, J. J. *Fundamentals of orthopaedics,* (3rd ed.). Philadelphia: W. B. Saunders, 1979.

Hoppenfeld, S. *Physical examination of the spine and extremities.* New York: Appleton-Century-Crofts, 1976.

Iversen, L. D., & Clawson, D. K. *Manual of acute orthopaedic therapeutics.* Boston: Little, Brown, 1977.

Roaf, R., & Hodkinson, L. J. *Textbook of orthopaedic nursing* (2nd ed.). Oxford: Blackwell Scientific, 1975.

Turek, S. L. *Orthopaedics, principles and their applications.* (3rd ed.) Philadelphia: Lippincott, 1977.

Warwick, R., & Williams, P. L. *Gray's anatomy* (35th Brit. ed.). Philadelphia: W. B. Saunders, 1973.

BIBLIOGRAPHY

Albright, J. A., & Brand, R. A. (Eds.). *The scientific basis of orthopaedics.* New York: Appleton-Century-Crofts, 1979.

Arthritis Health Profession Section of Arthritis Foundation. *Self-Help manual for patients with arthritis.* Atlanta, Ga.: Arthritis Foundation, 1980.

Beller, R. D., Grana, W. A., & O'Donoghue, D. H. Recurrent posterior dislocation of the shoulder: A method of reconstruction. *Orthopedics,* 1978, *1* (5), 384–388.

Bert, J. M., Lenscheld, D. L., & McElfresh, E. C. Rotatory contracture of the forearm. *Journal of Bone and Joint Surgery,* 1980, *62A* (7), 1163–1168.

Cailliet, R. *Soft tissue pain and disability* (5th ed.). Philadelphia: F. A. Davis, 1981.

Carini, G. K., & Birmingham, J. J. *Traction made manageable, A self-learning module.* New York: McGraw Hill, 1980.

Cafield, R. H., & Briggs, B. T. Glenohumeral arthrodesis. *Journal of Bone and Joint Surgery,* 1979, *61A* (3), 668–677.

Coughlin, M. J., Morris, J. M., & West, W. F. The semiconstrained total shoulder arthroplasty. *Journal of Bone and Joint Surgery,* 1979, *61A* (4), 574–581.

Farrell, J. Casts, your patients and you, Part 2: A review of arm and leg cast procedures. *Nursing 78,* 1978, *8* (11), 57–61.

Fries, J. F. *Arthritis, A comprehensive guide.* Menlo Park, Calif.: Addison-Wesley, 1982.

Gallagher, L. L. When your patient has a shoulder arthroplasty. *Nursing 80,* 1980, *10* (7), 46–49.

Ganel, A., Horaczowski, H., Heim, M., et al. Persistent dislocation of the shoulder in elderly patients. *Journal of American Geriatric Society,* 1980, *28* (6), 282–284.

Ghista, D. N., & Roaf, R. *Orthopaedic mechanics: Procedures and devices.* San Francisco: Academic Press, 1978.

Herndon, J. H., & Hubbard, L. F. Total joint replacement in the upper extremity. *Surgical Clinics of North America,* 1983, *63* (3), 715–736.

Hovelius, L., Thorling, J., & Fredin, H. Recurrent anterior dislocation of the shoulder: Results after the Bankart and Putti-Platt operations. *Journal of Bone and Joint Surgery,* 1979, *61A* (4), 566–569.

Jewsbury, C., et al. The hinged longarm cast brace: An alternative to longarm casts. *Orthopedic Nurses Association Journal,* 1979, *6* (7), 275–280.

Karadimas, J., Rentist, G., & Varouchas, G. Repair of recurrent anterior dislocation of the shoulder using transfer of the subscapularis tendon. *Journal of Bone and Joint Surgery,* 1980, *62A* (7), 1147–1149.

Kerr, A. *Orthopedic nursing procedures: Part 1. Initial and emergency care.* New York: Springer, 1980.

Larson, C. B., & Gould, M. *Orthopedic nursing* (9th ed.). St. Louis: C. V. Mosby, 1978.

Linson, M. A. Axillary artery thrombosis after fracture of the humerus. *Journal of Bone and Joint Surgery* 1980, *62A* (7), 1214–1215.

Porter, S. F., & Hersey, S. L. Supporting the subhexated shoulder joint with a pajama-bottoms sling. *Nursing 79,* 1979, *9* (4), 56–58.

Post, M., Haskell, S. S., & Jablon, M. total shoulder replacement with a constrained prosthesis. *Journal of Bone and Joint Surgery,* 1980, *62A* (3), 327–335.

Powell, M. *Orthopaedic nursing.* New York: Churchill Livingstone, 1976.

Prietta, C. A. Supracondylar fractures of the humerus: A comparative study of Dunlop's traction versus percutaneous pinning. *Journal of Bone and Joint Surgery,* 1979, *61A* (3), 425–428.

Protzman, R. R. Anterior instability of the shoulder. *Journal of Bone and Joint Surgery,* 1980, *62A* (6), 909–918.

Reeder, J. M. Help your disabled patient be more independent. *Nursing 84,* 1984, *14* (11), 43.

Spickler, L. Shoulder dislocations. *Orthopedic Nurses' Association Journal,* 1979, *6* (9), 374–375.

Stright, P. A. How to help the patient with a dislocated shoulder. *American Journal of Nursing,* 1979, *79* (4), 666–669.

Swinson, D. R., & Swinburn, W. R. *Rheumatology.* New York: Wiley, 1980.

Wu, K. K., Guise, E. R., Frost, H. M., & Mitchell, C. L. The surgical technique for forequarter amputation: A clinical analysis of 10 cases. *Orthopedics,* 1978, *1*(6), 457–461.

10

THE ELBOW AND FOREARM

Chapter 10 focuses on the care of patients with traumatic and pathological conditions of the elbow and the forearm, with emphasis on nursing care and the process of rehabilitation. This chapter discusses minor but limiting conditions like tennis elbow and major trauma, including dislocations and fractures. The chapter begins with a review of the anatomy of the elbow and the forearm.

ANATOMY

The elbow is a uniaxial or hinge joint that permits flexion and extension between the lower end of the humerus and the upper ends of the radius and the ulna.

BONES

Humerus

The lower end of the humerus is basically a broad condyle with articular and nonarticular parts. The articular parts adjoin the radius and the ulna to the elbow joint. The humerus is divided by a faint groove into a lateral, convex surface, the capitellum, and a medial, pulley-shaped surface, the trochlea. The capitellum is a rounded, convex projection formed by the anterior or inferior surfaces of the lateral part of the condyle of the humerus. It articulates with the disc-like head of the radius, which lies in contact with its inferior surface when the elbow is in full extension. The trochlea is a grooved surface that covers the anterior and posterior surface of the condyle of the humerus. The trochlea of the humerus articulates with the trochlear notch of the ulna.

The nonarticular part of the condyle of the humerus includes the medial and lateral epicondyles, together with the olecranon, coronoid, and radial fossae (Fig. 10–1). The medial epicondyle is a blunt projection on the medial side of the condyle. Its posterior surface is smooth and crossed by the ulnar nerve, which runs down into the forearm, and its anterior surface has the attachment of the superficial group of the forearm flexor muscles. The lateral epicondyle is the lateral part of the condyle and its anterior surface has the origin of the superficial group of forearm extensor muscles. A deep hollow situated on the posterior surface of the condyle, immediately above the trochlea, is the olecranon fossa. The olecranon fossa contains the tip of the olecranon of the ulna when the elbow is extended. A similar but smaller hollow, the coronoid fossa, lies immediately above the trochlea on the anterior surface of the condyle. A very slight depression situated above the capitellum on the lateral side of the coronoid fossa is the radial fossa, which articulates with the head of the radius when the elbow is fully flexed.

Radius

The radius is the lateral bone of the forearm (Fig. 10–2). It is wider at its proximal and distal ends, especially the latter. The proximal end of the radius includes a head, neck, and tuberosity. The head is disc-shaped and its upper surface is a shallow cup for articulation with the capitellum of the humerus. The articular circumference of the radial head is smooth and deepest medially

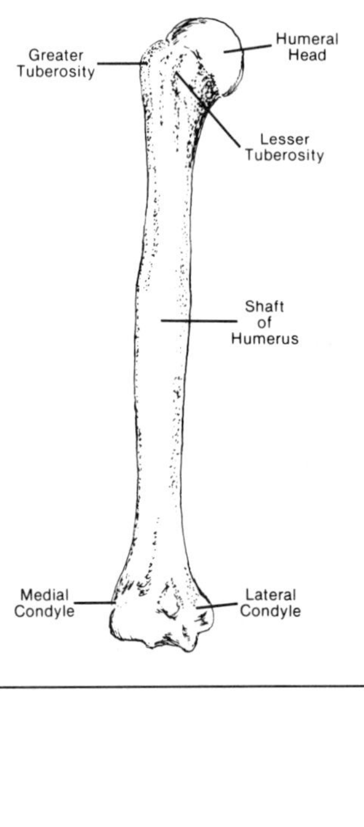

Figure 10–1. Skeletal anatomy of the upper extremity, humerus. *(From Brantley, P., & Analla, M., 1980, p. 14. Courtesy of Howmedica.)*

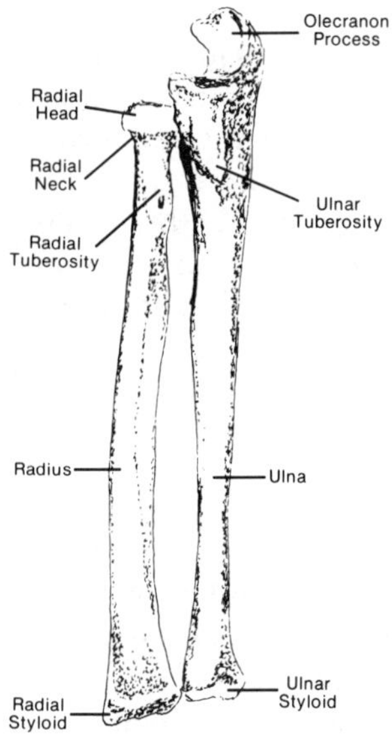

Figure 10–2. Skeletal anatomy of the upper extremity, ulna and radius. *(From Brantley, P., & Analla, M., 1980, p. 14. Courtesy of Howmedica.)*

where it articulates with the radial notch of the ulna. The neck of the radius is the constricted part below the head, and the tuberosity is located just below the medial part of the neck.

Ulna

The ulna is the medial bone of the forearm and is parallel with the radius when the forearm is supine (see Fig. 10–2). Its proximal end is thick, strong, and hook-like, with the concavity of the hook directed forward. The proximal end of the ulna has two substantial processes, the olecranon and the coronoid, and two articular areas, termed the trochlear and the radial notches, which articulate with the humerus and the radius.

The olecranon is the uppermost part of the ulna. It forms a prominent beak that projects into the olecranon fossa of the humerus when the forearm is extended. The coronoid process is a bracket-like projection from the front of the ulna immediately below the olecranon. The upper part of the lateral surface contains the shallow radial notch that articulates with the side of the head of the radius, and the bone below it is indented to make room for the tuberosity of the radius during movements of pronation and supination. The anterior surface of the coronoid process is triangular in shape, and its lower part becomes the rough tuberosity of the ulna. The trochlear notch, formed by the anterior surface of the olecranon and the superior surface of the coronoid process, articulates with the trochlea of the humerus.

ELBOW JOINT

The elbow is a compound hinge joint (Fig. 10–3) that includes the humeroulnar joint between the trochlea of the humerus and the trochlear notch of the ulna, the humeroradial joint between the capitellum of the humerus and the head of the radius, and the radioulnar joint between the head of the radius and the radial notch of the ulna. Flexion is produced by the brachialis, biceps, and brachioradialis muscles. Extension is accomplished by the triceps and the anconeus muscles. The joint has a fibrous articular capsule and ulnar and radial collateral ligaments.

ARTICULAR CAPSULE

The anterior portion of the fibrous capsule is a broad and thin layer. The proximal part is attached to the front of the medial epicondyle of the humerus, and the distal part is attached above the coronoid and radial fossae of the ulna and to the annular ligament. Posteriorly the fibrous capsule is very thin. The proximal portion is attached to the humerus behind the capitellum and to the lateral margins of the trochlea. The distal portion is attached to the rim of the olecranon fossa and to the medial epicondyle of the ulna. The capsule is sup-

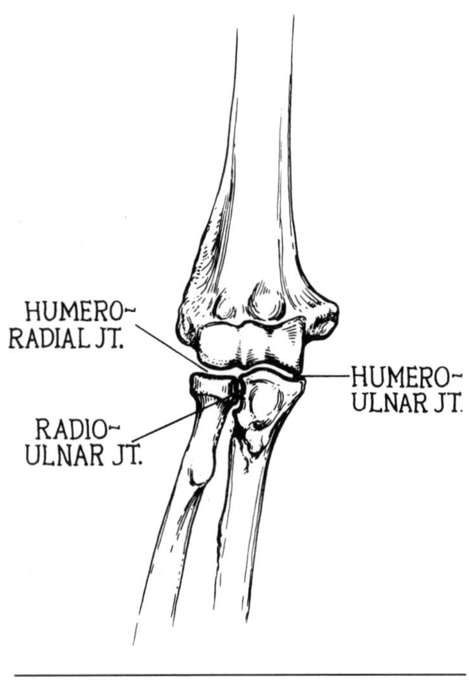

Figure 10–3. The three elbow articulations. *(Figures 10–3, 10–4, 10–13, and 10–14 are reproduced from Hoppenfeld, S., 1976, with permission.)*

ported laterally by the ulnar and radial collateral ligaments. A synovial membrane surrounds the articular surfaces of the humerus, the radius, and the ulna.

LIGAMENTS

The ulnar collateral ligament of the elbow is a thick triangular band that consists of an anterior and a posterior portion. The anterior part is attached above to the medial epicondyle of the humerus, and below to a tubercle on the upper part of the medial margin of the coronoid process of the ulna. The posterior part is attached above to the lower and back part of the medial epicondyle of the humerus and below to the medial margin of the olecranon. The ulnar collateral ligament is related to the triceps and flexor carpi ulnaris and the ulnar nerve.

The radial collateral ligament of the elbow is attached above to the lower

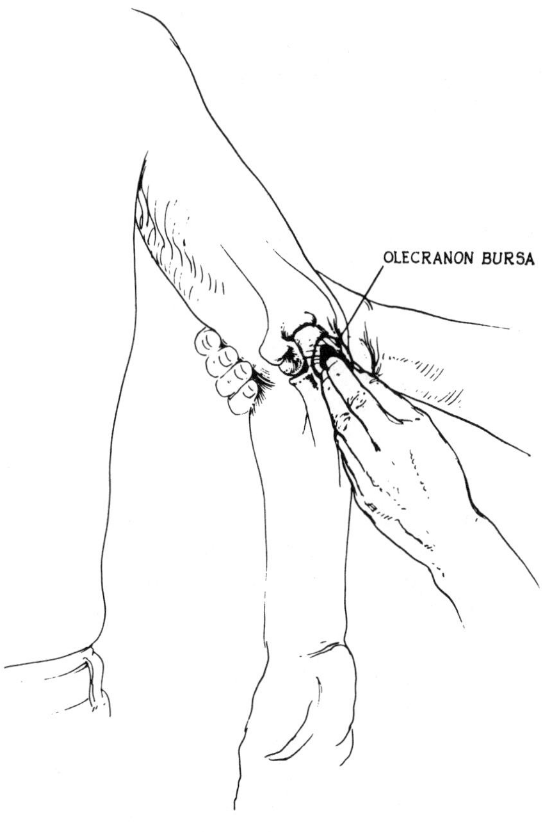

Figure 10–4. The olecranon bursa.

part of the lateral epicondyle of the humerus and below to the annular ligament. The radial collateral ligament is related to the brachialis, the triceps, and the anconeus muscles. Laterally it is related to the common tendon of the extensor muscles, and medially to the common tendon of the flexor muscles and the flexor carpi ulnaris.

The annular ligament is composed of transversely disposed fibers that encircle the radial head, and it attaches distally to the radial neck and medially to the anterior and posterior margins of the lesser sigmoid fossa of the ulna.

The major artery of the elbow is the brachial artery, which divides just below the elbow into the radial and ulnar arteries. The veins are laterally the cephalic, and medially the basilic veins. The articular nerves are mainly from the musculocutaneous and radial nerves, but the ulnar, the median, and sometimes the anterior interosseous nerves also contribute to the articular branches.

BURSAE

Two bursae lie in relation to the triceps insertion. One lies between the triceps tendon and the upper surface of the olecranon. The other, the larger and more important one, lies between the skin and the dorsal surface of the olecranon (Fig. 10–4). Another bursa lies between the neck of the radius and the biceps tendon as the latter approaches the bicipital tuberosity. Other bursae are located about the lateral collateral ligament.

THE ELBOW

Trauma

SPRAIN

A sprain of the elbow is a forced movement of the joint beyond full extension, or a forced abduction or adduction of the forearm that tears the fibrous capsule and its reinforcing ligaments. A sprain of the elbow may involve the radial collateral ligament, the ulnar collateral ligament, or the anterior capsule. When the radial collateral ligament (which extends from the lateral epicondyle to the side of the orbicular ligament) is sprained, there is tenderness below the lateral epicondyle, and pain is accentuated by forcing the elbow into varus. When the ulnar collateral ligament (which extends from the medial epicondyle to the side of the annular ligament) is sprained, there is tenderness below the medial epicondyle, and pain is accentuated by forcing the elbow into valgus. The more common injury of the strong ulnar collateral ligament, however, is an avulsion and displacement downward of the medial epicondyle (Turek, 1977, p. 872). With a sprain of the anterior capsule, caused by a violent hyperextension of the elbow short of actual posterior dislocation, there is pain and tenderness over the attachment of the capsule to the lower anterior aspect of the humerus. Pain can be reproduced by attempting to extend the elbow joint. The treatment of sprains of the elbow usually consists of immobilizing the elbow in flexion for a few days.

DISLOCATION

A dislocation of the elbow occurs when the humerus, the ulna, and the radius are forced out of correct anatomical position. A fall on the outstretched hand is the usual cause of a traumatic dislocation. An anterior dislocation of the elbow is quite rare. A posterior dislocation typically involves the lower end of the humerus being driven over the coronoid process of the ulna and out through the torn anterior capsule. The ulna and the radius are then forced backward, and the ulna ends up being lodged behind the lower end of the displaced humerus. There is usually an avulsion of the brachialis anticus muscle from the coronoid process, a stripping of the periosteum, and the development of a subperiosteal hematoma. There may also be an injury to the median and radial nerves or damage to the brachial artery.

The dislocation results in a painful deformity of the elbow that is marked by swelling. The olecranon process is unusually prominent. The point of the olecranon, which normally lies ahead of the line connecting the medial and lateral humeral epicondyles, typically lies behind that line following a posterior dislocation. The patient's arm assumes an attitude of 40 degrees of flexion, and the joint is immovable, either actively or passively. Dislocations can be distinguished from supracondylar fractures because in dislocations the forearm does not require support from the opposite hand and the prominence of the bony triangle is shortened or abolished (DeGowin & DeGowin, 1976, p. 689).

Closed manipulative reduction under anesthesia is carried out as soon as possible. In adults, if reduction is delayed for several hours, permanent limitation of movement usually results. Once muscle relaxation has been achieved, reduction of the elbow may be accomplished by the elbow being flexed over the physician's knee. The elbow is then immobilized in a posterior plaster splint in a safe degree of flexion for 3 weeks. The elbow joint has poor tolerance for injury and immobilization, and it may be months before full motion returns. There may be associated median or radial paralysis, damage to the brachial artery, and traumatic myositis ossificans may also follow.

Recurrent Dislocation

Unlike the shoulder joint, the entire elbow joint rarely has problems with recurrent dislocations. When the radial head is dislocated without dislocation of the humeroulnar joint, the radial head is displaced anteriorly and can usually be reduced by closed manipulation. That dislocation does tend to recur, however, and if so, an open reduction and repair of the annular ligament may be necessary. Postoperatively the elbow joint is splinted or casted for 3 weeks with the elbow in 90 degrees of flexion and the forearm in neutral rotation. Gentle active motion and especially rehabilitation of the muscles are then begun. The elbow must not be manipulated, nor must motion be passively forced in any attempt to restore function. After motion and strength have been actively restored, slight displacement may sometimes recur, but if so, it does not interfere significantly with function (Edmondson & Crenshaw, 1980, p. 446).

☐ NURSING PROCESS (Table 10–1)

Assessment

The first step in the assessment for a typical patient following a reduction of a dislocated elbow and the application of a long arm cast or posterior splint is to check the neurovascular status of the affected arm and compare it with the unaffected arm (Chap. 2). There may be associated median or radial paralysis or damage to the brachial artery. Note any swelling, discoloration, or change in the temperature of the affected hand. When a cast or a posterior splint is too tight, it compresses the blood vessels and nerves. The neurovascular assessment must be repeated every 15 minutes for the first few hours and then every 2 hours for the first 24 hours. After the first 24 hours, the checks usually can be reduced to once every shift if the patient is not complaining of any symptoms.

Check the upper and lower edges of the cast or splint for possible skin irritation. In the assessment for pain, try to determine whether the pain is due to soft tissue trauma or to neurovascular impairment. For example, an arm that "ached" all night and ceases to do so in the morning may have a muscle with a decreased supply of oxygenated blood. Check for possible pressure points around the styloid and olecranon processes, and the lateral and medial epicondyles.

Nursing Diagnosis and Goal Formulation

Nursing diagnoses for a typical patient are (1) alterations in comfort related to pain from the trauma and soft tissue injury, (2) alterations in mobility related to lack of joint stability, (3) potential complications related to joint trauma and decreased arm mobility, and (4) alterations in psychological well-being related to anxiety and knowledge deficit about the injury and the treatment methods.

Short-term goals are to have the patient experience (1) a decrease in the amount of pain through the use of immobilization, nursing measures, and prescribed medications, (2) an increase in mobility through the use of controlled exercises, (3) an absence of complications from trauma and decreased activities, and (4) a decrease in anxiety through increased knowl-

TABLE 10–1. NURSING PROCESS FOR DISLOCATED ELBOW TREATED WITH A LONG ARM CAST

Assessment	Nursing Diagnosis	Goal Formulation	Planning and Intervention	Evaluation and Reassessment
1. Assess the location, duration, and severity of pain (continuous dull ache or periods of severe pain?). Assess the neurovascular status of the affected arm.	1. Alteration in comfort: pain in the elbow related to soft tissue trauma.	1. Short-term goal: a decrease in pain through the use of immobilization. Long-term goal: free of pain.	1. Alleviate Pain Keep the arm elevated on pillows. Apply ice bags at the elbow. Instruct on finger exercises. Continue to assess pain to determine if it follows a nerve path or is over a bony prominence.	1. The patient should be in a state of relative comfort; medication should relieve severe pain. The arm should be kept elevated.
2. Check the position of the arm. Check the sensory and motor function of the hand and arm. Assess the range of motion at the shoulder. Assess finger movement. Check the positioning of the cast (or splint).	2. Impaired physical mobility: decreased range of motion related to lack of elbow joint stability.	2. Short-term goal: an increase in mobility by controlled exercises. Long-term goal: regain full range of motion and function of the elbow.	2. Increase Mobility *Position* Keep the arm elevated whether patient is supine or lying on unaffected side. *Posterior Splint* Assure that the arm is securely immobilized. Teach how to use the trapeze. *Exercises* Instruct on respiratory and abdominal exercises. Demonstrate range of motion of all unaffected joints. Demonstrate isometric, shoulder and finger exercises for the affected arm. *Ambulation* Apply a sling to support the affected arm. Assist patient in getting out of bed.	2. The arm should be elevated at all times. The patient should do exercise routines correctly without supervision. The patient should verbalize an understanding of rationale for exercises. Expect the patient to ambulate safely with arm supported in a sling.

(continued)

TABLE 10–1. *(Continued)*

Assessment	Nursing Diagnosis	Goal Formulation	Planning and Intervention	Evaluation and Reassessment
3. Assess neurovascular status. Check the amount of swelling. Check tightness of cast (or splint).	3. Potential for injury: neurovascular deficit related to soft tissue swelling and trauma.	3. Short- and long-term goal: no neurovascular impairment.	3. Prevent Complications *Circulatory* Do neurovascular assessments after surgery, every 15 minutes for first 2 hours, every 30 minutes for next 2 hours, every 60 minutes for next 2 hours, every 2 hours for next 18 hours and then at the beginning of every shift. Apply nursing measures to prevent swelling. Report any neurovascular deficit. Bivalve cast as indicated.	3. Neurovascular status should be good without any signs of swelling.
Check for skin irritation at the edges of the cast Assess for pressure over bony prominences.	Potential for impairment of skin integrity related to rough cast edges and pressure from the cast.	Short- and long-term goal: free of any skin disruption.	*Integumentary* Trim and petal cast edges. Keep the arm elevated on soft surface. Avoid pressure at the elbow. Listen to complaints of pain and discomfort.	Expect no break in skin integrity. If irritation over bony prominences occurs, the cast may need to be removed.

Assess range of motion of the shoulder. Assess strength of arm.	Potential for injury: stiffness of shoulder and elbow related to immobilization.	Short- and long-term goal: no decrease in shoulder function.	*Shoulder and Elbow Stiffness* Demonstrate shoulder exercises. Develop an exercise program for the shoulder. Develop an exercise program for the elbow once the immobilization is removed. *Other Complications* (See text.)	Expect no restriction in the range of motion or decrease in strength of the shoulder or elbow.
4. Assess for level of understanding of rehabilitation process and cast care. Assess for possible problems with home care.	4. Potential knowledge deficit related to rehabilitation process and cast care.	4. Short- and long-term goal: a decrease in anxiety through increase in knowledge level.	4. Patient Teaching Explain cast care. Demonstrate how to do prescribed exercises. Go over methods of bathing and dressing. Include family and significant others in teaching plan.	4. The patient should verbalize confidence in going home and caring for self. The patient should verbalize an understanding of the rehabilitation process and be able to do activities of daily living with only a minimum of assistance.

edge. Long-term goals are to have the patient pain free and with full return of motion and function in the involved arm.

Planning and Intervention

Alleviate Pain. Measures for relief of pain following the reduction of a dislocated elbow and the application of a long arm cast or a posterior splint are to keep the arm elevated on pillows and to apply ice bags at the elbow to prevent or reduce swelling from soft tissue trauma. If the arm and the hand are elevated but the swelling is still increasing, lower the head of the patient's bed so the hand and the elbow are higher than the heart. Later, shoulder and finger exercises may also help to reduce swelling.

Do not hesitate to give pain medication after assessing and applying nursing measures. However, a nurse should keep in mind the location and description of all pain before analgesics are given. Is the pain at the fracture site or does it follow a nerve path? Is it over a bony prominence and could it be due to pressure, necrosis, or the formation of a decubitus ulcer? Is the cast "green" or has it been on for several days, while the location and description of the pain are new? Never ignore complaints of pain or pressure.

Increase Mobility

Position. Most patients with a long arm cast or a posterior splint find the supine position with the head of the bed slightly elevated the most comfortable. The patient can turn from side to side as necessary, but should not stay on the affected side for any length of time. The affected arm should be elevated on a pillow. The patient should be instructed to use the trapeze with the unaffected arm to help with movement in bed and to strengthen the unaffected arm.

Posterior Splint. The posterior splint is basically the posterior half of a long arm cast. The splint is held in place by roller gauze or an elastic bandage, and is less rigid than a long arm cast.

Exercises. The patient is encouraged to exercise all uninvolved joints with active range-of-motion, respiratory, and abdominal exercises. Exercises specific for the affected arm are isometric, shoulder, and finger exercises. Elbow exercises for short periods are started once the splint is removed. The patient's physician should be consulted, however, before beginning any exercises on the affected extremity. The patient is taught muscle setting or isometric exercises using the uninvolved extremity so that they can be done on the involved arm under the immobilizer. Shoulder exercises are encouraged to prevent stiffness of the shoulder joint. The patient can abduct the arm until the plaster touches the side of the head, and the arm can then be externally rotated so that the hand is behind the head. The arm may also be lowered and internally rotated so it is behind the patient's back with the fingers pointing to the mid-scapular region. Finger exercises help prevent stiffness and swelling of the fingers (see p. 510).

Ambulation. The patient is usually allowed up with a sling (see p. 594) once he or she has recovered from the anesthetic. At first, the patient probably needs help in getting out of bed and learning to balance with the immobilizer because of the awkwardness and weight of the cast or posterior splint.

Prevent Complications. Potential complications following an elbow dislocation and the application of a long arm cast or a posterior splint include neurovascular impairment, skin disruption, shoulder stiffness, and decreased function in the elbow joint. There may be an impairment of the median or radial nerve or the brachial artery at the time of injury or from an excessively tight cast or splint. Nursing interventions that improve the neurovascular status of the arm are to elevate the arm, apply ice as indicated, have the patient do finger exercises, and continue to assess complaints of pain or pressure.

Disruption of the skin is apt to occur at the splint or cast edges or over bony prominences. Effective nursing interventions require early detection. Feel the surface of the cast over the area where the pain has been reported. If necrosis or infection has developed, the cast or splint is likely to feel warm. For skin irritation at the splint or cast edges, trim and petal the edges. For skin irritation over bony prominences, notify the patient's physician for a possible removal or alteration of the cast or splint.

Stiffness of the shoulder should be reduced by the shoulder exercises discussed above. Once the cast or splint is removed, usually after 3 weeks, elbow exercises (see pp. 607 and 610) are started to restore function in the elbow. Because the elbow has a low tolerance for injury and immobilization, it may be months before full function returns.

Patient Teaching. Explain the care of the cast or splint (Appendix B), how to do the prescribed exercises, and how to dress and do the other activities of daily living. Bathing can be done in a tub or shower after covering the cast or splint with a plastic bag or cast cover.

Dressing can be less of a problem if the sleeves of shirts and blouses are ripped at the seams and velcro strips used for closure. A cape or poncho may be used as a coat if the patient's regular coat will not fit over the immobilized arm.

Once the patient is ready to go home, the patient, the family, and significant others must know the signs and symptoms of neurovascular impairment and pressure ulcers. Patients need to have a clear understanding of the rehabilitation process and their role in that process.

Evaluation and Reassessment

Determine whether the patient feels confident about going home in a long arm cast or a posterior splint. If not, ask specific questions to determine what the patient does not understand, and explain it again. Pain should have been reduced by nursing measures and medications. The patient should be able to demonstrate required exercises and explain how often each is to be done. The patient should be able to do activities of daily living with a minimum amount of assistance.

FRACTURE–DISLOCATION

A fracture–dislocation of the elbow is a serious injury in which a dislocation is combined with a fracture of the olecranon, the head of the radius, or the internal epicondyle. Treatment consists of reduction of the dislocation and the treatment of the individual fracture or fractures.

FRACTURES

Supracondylar Fracture of the Humerus

The supracondylar area of the humerus is the lower flared end of that bone just above the elbow joint. Fractures in this area occur more commonly in children and the elderly, but they can occur at any age. The mechanism of injury is trauma when the elbow is in either extension or flexion. The extension injury is produced by a fall on the extended elbow, and before repair the arm is stable only in significant flexion. (Such fractures may also be accompanied by intracondylar or intracapsular injuries.) The flexion injury is produced by a fall on the flexed elbow, and the arm is relatively stable in extension.

Normally the lower end of the humerus, which contains the condyles, is at an angle of approximately 30 degrees to the shaft of the humerus (Gartland, 1979, p. 276). A fracture through the supracondylar area breaks the bone into two major fragments. The smaller distal fragment is the lower flared condylar portion of the humerus, which articulates with the forearm. The larger proximal fragment is the remainder of the humeral shaft. Following the fracture, the small distal fragment is usually displaced backward, through it may be displaced forward depending on the direction of the fracturing force. Displacement results in a lowering of the normal forward angulation of the lower end of the humerus, and the smaller distal fragment usually rotates relative to the larger proximal fragment. Immediate deformity may superficially resemble that caused by a posterior dislocation of the elbow, except that the relationship between the olecranon and the epicondyles is not disturbed.

A neurovascular assessment is necessary to determine if there is any circulatory embarrassment or nerve damage before reduction. Immediate attention to treat the fracture is essential. With delay, swelling about the elbow increases rapidly, and enhances the danger of bony or vascular complications. Reduction of a displaced supracondylar fracture involves restoring the normal forward angulation of the distal end of the humerus and correcting the rotational spin of the distal fragment. If the correct forward angulation is not restored, the flexion and extension of the elbow will be impaired. If the rotational displacement is not corrected, it will result in a permanent abnormality with the appearance of a cubitus varus or cubitus valgus deformity.

The choice of a method of reduction depends on the severity of the fracture. Many of these fractures are successfully reduced by closed manipulation, but others may require skin or skeletal traction. Open reduction is usually not necessary. Postreduction fixation of the reduced fracture may be by percutaneous pinning or by immobilization in a cast for 6 weeks to insure adequate bone healing. The prognosis for return to normal function is excellent in a well-reduced fracture that heals without complications. Complications that may arise following a supracondylar fracture of the humerus are usually due to (1) inadequate or incomplete reduction of the fracture, (2) damage to nerves passing over the fracture site, or (3) circulatory impairment, signaled by a weak or absent radial pulse (Gartland, 1979, p. 277).

□ NURSING PROCESS (Table 10–2)

Assessment

The first step in the assessment of a typical patient in sidearm traction following a supracondylar fracture of the humerus is to determine the neurovascular status of the affected arm and hand and compare it with the unaffected side. Because of the potential for circulatory impairment, the radial pulse must be checked immediately after the application of traction and then at least every 3 to 4 hours while the patient is in traction. Check for any swelling at the shoulder, elbow, or hand, for cyanosis or pallor of the hands or fingers, and for numbness or decreased function of the fingers (see p. 510). Fingers that have good color, sensation, and movement may be cold because the hand is elevated and immobile.

Assess for pain. If the patient complains of pain under the traction tapes, you can run your fingers gently under the tapes and wrapping to assess whether the pain is from skin breakdown or neurovascular impairment. To detect painful pressure points under the skin traction, palpate the area over the traction tapes at least daily. When skin traction is applied to the arm, check that the area around the elbow where the ulnar nerve is located is not wrapped too tightly. Check the areas near the shoulder, the anterior surface of the elbow joint, and the wrist for any irritation, reddened areas, skin breakdown, or macerations. Check for any slipping of the traction tapes or loosening of the wrapping as that can lead to skin problems. If the patient has skeletal traction, check the pin site for any signs of inflammation. With overhead 90-90 traction, check the sling or cast edges for possible skin irritation. Always follow up patient's complaints

TABLE 10–2. NURSING PROCESS FOR SUPRACONDYLAR FRACTURE OF THE HUMERUS TREATED WITH SIDEARM TRACTION

Assessment	Nursing Diagnosis	Goal Formulation	Planning and Intervention	Evaluation and Reassessment
1. Assess the location, duration, and severity of pain. Assess the neurovascular status of the affected arm. Check the amount of swelling.	1. Alteration in comfort: pain in the elbow and arm related to bone and soft tissue trauma.	1. Short-term goal: a relative state of comfort through the use of traction. Long-term goal: free of pain.	1. Alleviate Pain Maintain traction in correct alignment. Instruct on how to do gentle finger exercises. Teach relaxation technique. Administer prescribed medications. Maintain correct body alignment.	1. The patient should be in a relative state of comfort. Medication should be effective in relieving severe pain; at other times, traction and relaxation alone should be effective.
2. Check the alignment of the traction. Check the traction tapes or boot straps for possible loosening or tightness. Check body alignment in relation to traction pull. Check traction for possible mechanical problems.	2. Impaired physical mobility: decreased arm function related to lack of bone stability.	2. Short-term goal: an increase in bone stability through immobilization. Long-term goal: complete bone stability and return of full function in the arm.	2. Increase Mobility *Position* Keep the patient supine. Do not allow the patient to turn. Allow no shifting toward the head or foot of the bed. Raise knee gatch periodically to allow knee flexion. *Exercises* Active range of motion for all uninvolved joints. Finger exercises with affected hand. Breathing and abdominal exercises. *Traction* Maintain arm outward at the humerus and upward for side arm traction.	2. Traction should be maintained in correct alignment. Active range-of-motion exercises should be done with all unaffected joints. Expect no decrease in range of motion and no muscle atrophy. Hand exercises should be done every hour while awake without need for supervision.

			Maintain correct alignment. Maintain correct poundage. Maintain countertraction by elevating the side of the bed on the affected side.	
3. Check that traction is maintained. Assess for bone stability.	3. Potential complications related to inadequate fracture reduction.	3. Short- and long-term goal: free of complications.	3. Prevent Complications *Inadequate Reduction* Maintain traction in correct alignment at all times.	3. There should be no interruption in traction.
Assess neurovascular status. Assess ability to do finger exercises. Assess complaints of pain or aches.	Potential for injury: neurological deficit related to bone and soft tissue trauma.	Short- and long-term goal: free of nerve deficit.	*Neurological* Assess nerve status every 4 hours while traction is maintained. Report any abnormal response.	Neurological status should remain normal.
Assess neurovascular status. Check for any swelling. Assess the flexion of the elbow. Assess tightness of traction tapes (especially in area around the elbow).	Potential for injury: impaired circulation related to pressure and soft tissue swelling.	Short- and long-term goal: free of circulatory complications.	*Circulatory* Do neurovascular assessments every 15 minutes for first 2 hours, every 30 minutes for next 2 hours, every 60 minutes for next 2 hours, every 2 hours for next 18 hours, and then at the beginning of every shift. Check neurovascular status. Maintain comfortable tightness in traction tapes. Keep elbow at correct amount of flexion. Apply nursing methods to prevent swelling. Instruct patient on hand exercises.	Expect good circulation to arm and hand.

(continued)

TABLE 10–2. *(Continued)*

Assessment	Nursing Diagnosis	Goal Formulation	Planning and Intervention	Evaluation and Reassessment
Assess for possible skin breakdown (especially in areas near the shoulder, the anterior surface of the elbow joint, the wrist and back. Check for slipping of traction tapes.	Potential for impairment of skin integrity related to pressure and slippage of traction tapes.	Short- and long-term goal: free of any skin complications.	*Integumentary* Detect pressure points under skin traction by palpating area over the traction tapes. Maintain correct tightness of traction. Administer back care every 2 hours while patient is awake and every 4 hours at night. Keep linen free of wrinkles. Keep skin along traction tapes clean, dry, and free of irritation.	The patient should have no skin breakdown.
Assess activity level. Assess interest and cooperation in daily activities.	Potential diversional activity deficit related to boredom of confinement secondary to immobilization devices.	Short- and long-term goals: positive mental attitude.	*Psychological* Find activities that the patient enjoys (listening to music, reading, playing cards or other games). Utilize prism glasses. Try to find mentally stimulating activities. Utilize patient social support system. Develop a schedule for activities. *Other Complications* (See text.)	The patient should be doing activities that stimulate mental activity.
4. Determine level of knowledge about rehabilitation process.	4. Potential knowledge deficit related to the rehabilitation process.	4. Short- and long-term goal: free of anxiety.	4. Patient Teaching Discuss the various steps in the rehabilitation process. Work with occupational and physical therapists. Help identify "can do" activities.	4. The patient should verbalize an understanding of the rehabilitation process.

of pain. Check the patient's body alignment, make sure that the pull of the traction is at the proper angle in relation to the patient's body. Check the traction for possible mechanical problems.

Nursing Diagnosis and Goal Formulation

Nursing diagnoses for a typical patient in a sidearm traction following a supracondylar fracture of the humerus are (1) alterations in comfort related to arm pain from trauma to the humerus and soft tissue, (2) alterations in mobility related to lack of bone stability, (3) potential complications related to trauma and decreased mobility, and (4) alterations in psychological well-being related to anxiety and knowledge deficit about the injury and the treatment methods.

Short-term goals are to have the patient experience (1) a decrease in the amount of pain, (2) an increase in bone stability, (3) an absence of complications from the trauma and decreased activity, and (4) a decrease in anxiety through increased knowledge. Long-term goals are to have the patient pain free and to have full return of arm function.

Planning and Intervention

Alleviate Pain. The amount of pain the patient has is related to the type of fracture, the amount of soft tissue trauma, and the degree of fracture site immobilization. Nursing measures to help reduce pain are to maintain the traction in correct alignment and have the patient do gentle finger exercises to increase circulation. Other noninvasive measures for pain relief may be utilized. Nonetheless, the patient will almost certainly require prescribed medications for pain relief.

Increase Mobility

Position. Arm traction is designed for a patient who is supine in bed and the bed level or flat when the traction is applied. Any shift of the patient toward the foot or the head of the bed changes the line of pull of the traction. The head of the bed may be elevated *only* when the sidearm traction pulley has been attached to the basic frame that clamps to the bed under the mattress, so that the traction apparatus moves with the head of the bed. This allows a change in position of the head of the bed without disrupting the traction. If the head of the bed *cannot* be elevated, the knee gatch may be raised periodically to flex the patient's knees. That maneuver helps relieve strain on the patient's back.

Exercises. Active range-of-motion exercises for all uninvolved joints should be stressed. Active range-of-motion finger exercises with the affected hand are to be done frequently as they increase the circulation to the elevated hand and assist with arterial flow. This activity also helps prevent muscle atrophy that can occur during immobility. Breathing exercises and abdominal exercises should also be encouraged.

Traction. Fractures of the humerus, with or without shoulder involvement, may be treated with traction attached to the skin or the skeleton, with an overhead or sidearm pull, and with the arm in flexion or extension, depending on the location of the fracture and associated injuries. Skin sidearm traction is accomplished by the use of two sets of two traction tapes that are secured by an elastic bandage wrap at separate sites on the arm (Fig. 10–5). One set is applied to the upper arm and extends past the elbow where it is attached to a spreader and pulley-weight setup, and it exerts a horizontal (or outward) pull on the humerus. The weights are determined by the needs of the individual patient based on the size and the age of the patient and the type of fracture, but it rarely exceeds 6 pounds. The other set is applied to the forearm and extends beyond the hand where it is attached to a spreader and pulley-weight setup. It exerts a lateral (or upward) pull to support and suspend the arm vertically. The

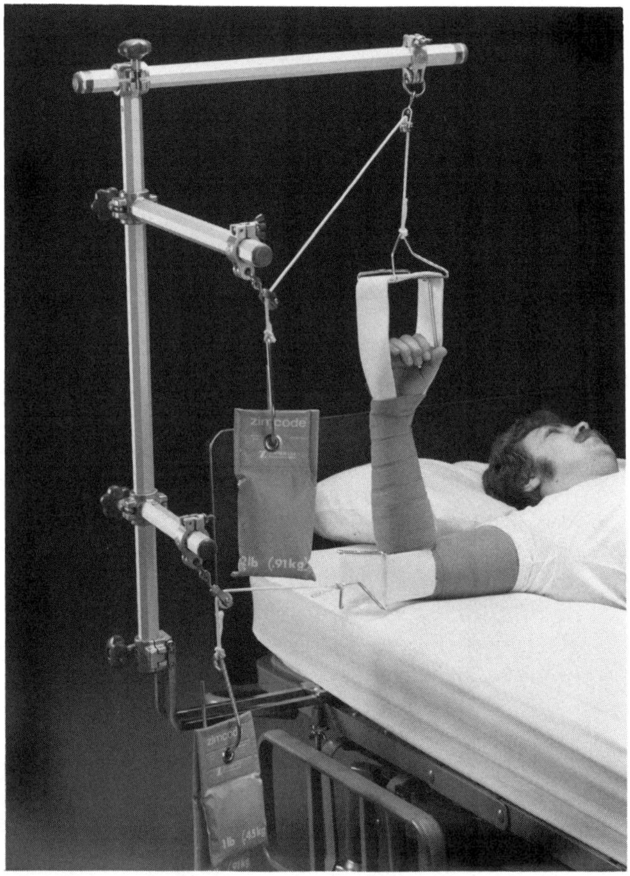

Figure 10–5. Side arm skin traction. *(Courtesy of Zimmer, Inc.)*

weights rarely exceed 3 pounds. A suspended handle within the forearm apparatus allows the patient to flex and extend the fingers and exercise the wrist. The elbow is usually flexed, although some authors discuss sidearm traction that uses a Thomas arm splint to hold the elbow in extension. Many physicians prefer not to place the elbow in extension however, because immobilization in that position causes muscle strain and discomfort at the elbow.

Countertraction, to provide additional resistance to the traction, can be provided by elevating the side of the bed on the affected side. That can be accomplished in two ways. One is to place shock blocks under the legs of the bed on the side where the traction is attached. However, that may cause the patient to slide too far away from the traction apparatus. The second method is to place a folded blanket between the mattress and the bedframe on the affected side.

Skeletal sidearm traction is obtained by placing a pin through the olecranon process at the elbow and attaching weights that rarely exceed 12 pounds (Fig. 10–6). The forearm still has traction tapes and the positioning of the forearm probably is the same as in skin sidearm traction. Skeletal traction is utilized instead of skin traction when the traction is in place for a longer period of time or requires more weight, or an elastic bandage wrap over the upper arm is inappropriate.

In overhead (or 90–90) traction (Fig. 10–7), the shoulder and the elbow are in 90 degrees of flexion. The forearm is suspended over the patient's chest with the upper arm perpendicular to the body. The forearm is usually supported by a sling suspended from an overhead pulley. Skin overhead traction is possible but skeletal overhead traction with a pin or a Kirschner wire through the olecranon process is more common. In that case, the sling may be replaced by a long arm cast applied over the pin, with the pin attached to a loop and pulley. Overhead traction allows the patient more freedom than sidearm traction, and there is also less edema and other circulatory problems. The weight of the patient's body provides sufficient countertraction.

Prevent Complications. The major complications that may arise following a supracondylar fracture of the humerus are (1) inadequate or incomplete reduction of the fracture, (2) neurological damage, (3) circulatory impairment, (4) integumentary disruption, and (5) psychological distress.

Inadequate Reduction. Inadequate or incomplete reduction of the humeral fracture can result in a permanent limitation of motion or an obvious physical deformity such as cubitus valgus or cubitus varus.

Neurological Damage. Stretching or contusion injuries to the median, the ulnar, or the deep muscular branch of the radial nerve have been reported in approximately 6 percent of patients sustaining a supracondylar fracture of the humerus. The nerve injury may be of varying degrees of severity:

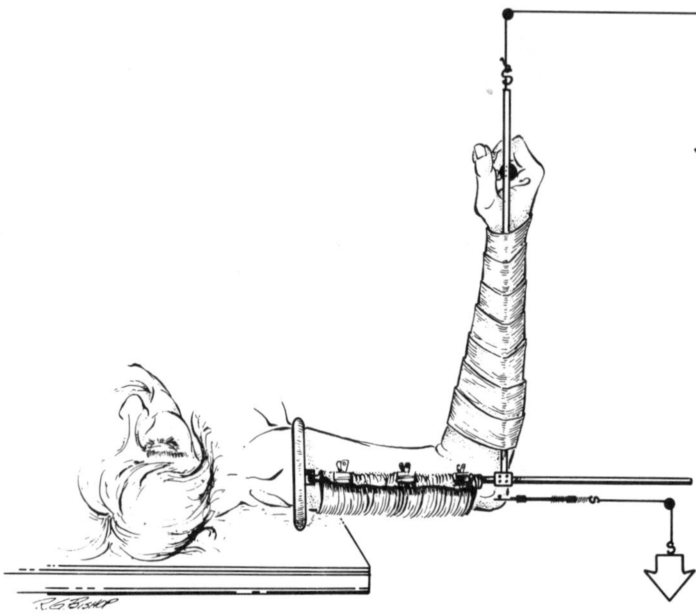

Figure 10–6. Balanced side arm traction. The arm is passed through the ring, which is then passed up so that it encompasses the shoulder. The upright attachment for the forearm may be moved in either direction to accomodate the length of the humerus. A cloth sling is placed on the horizontal segment to provide a surface on which the arm may rest. The olecranon extends just past the vertical limb, so that the pin drilled through the olecranon will be clear and allow unimpeded traction. The forearm is placed between the two upright supports, and usually held there with a circumferentially applied elastic bandage. A rope is attached to the vertical section and is passed through pulleys. A weight is attached to exactly counterbalance the weight of the arm and the frame. Skeletal traction is then applied in the desired amount through the pin in the olecranon. The entire extremity is counterbalanced so that a balanced traction system is created. *(From Lewis, R.C.* Handbook of traction, casting and splinting techniques. *Philadelphia: Lippincott, 1977, p. 30, with permission.)*

(1) a neurapraxia involves minimal damage to nerves, which recover spontaneously within a few weeks; (2) an axonotmesis involves peripheral nerve degeneration due to axon damage with spontaneous regeneration occurring after many months; and (3) a neurotmesis involves nerve destruction due to severing or scarring that is correctable only by excising the damaged section and anastomosing the ends. The nerve damage in most patients with supracondylar humeral fractures proves to be only temporary but nurses should still be alert to the possibility of serious nerve damage.

Circulatory Impairment. The most dreaded complication of a supracondylar fracture is Volkmann's ischemic contracture, a severely deforming condition of the hand and arm. If present before reduction, this circulatory

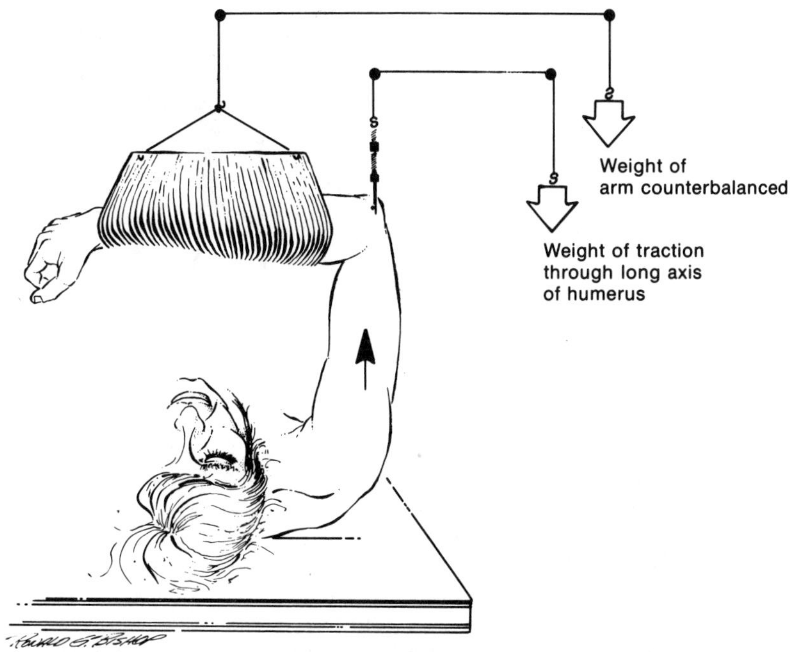

Figure 10–7. 90–90 arm traction. *(From Lewis, R.C.* Handbook of traction, casting and splinting techniques. *Philadelphia: Lippincott, 1977, p. 32, with permission.)*

impairment is usually due to antecubital edema, impingement of a bone fragment against the brachial artery, or, rarely, a torn or lacerated brachial artery. If the impairment appears after reduction, it is probably due to a vascular obstruction secondary to tight bandages or to a position of acute or extreme flexion of the elbow. The absence of a radial pulse in the presence of a supracondylar fracture of the humerus demands immediate attention. If it is not corrected within a 4- to 8-hour period, Volkmann's ischemic contracture may result.

VOLKMANN'S ISCHEMIC CONTRACTURE. This deformity is most common in supracondylar fractures of the humerus, dislocations of the elbow, or fractures of the proximal third of the forearm. The ischemic contracture develops as a result of an irritation or injury to the brachial artery, which causes a reflex spasm of the main brachial artery and collateral vessels, severely diminishing the blood supply to the muscles of the arm (Fig. 10–8). Volkmann's ischemic contracture may follow slight or severe injuries, and may even be caused by constriction from a bandage, splint, cast, or tourniquet, or by compression of the artery by swelling in an immobilized flexed elbow. For that reason, patients with injuries to the elbow or the

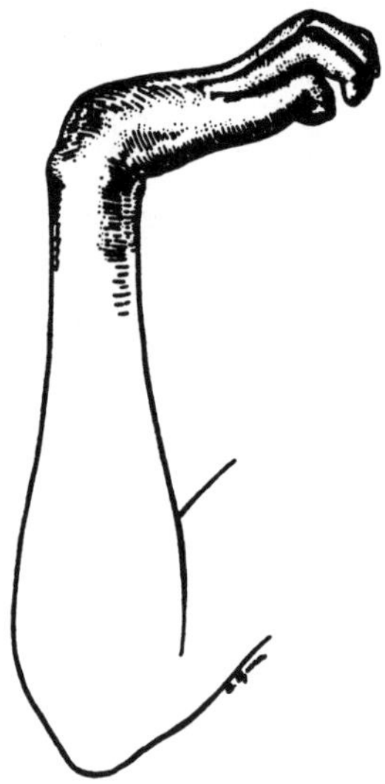

Figure 10–8. Volkmann's contracture with claw-hand and flexion of the wrist and fingers. Note atrophy of the forearm. *(From Larson, C.B., & Gould, M., 1978, p. 188, with permission.)*

forearm are frequently kept in the hospital for observation until it is clear that circulation in the involved arm is unimpaired.

One of the first signs of an impending Volkmann's ischemic contracture is an absence of the radial pulse. The radial artery should be palpated before an immobilizing device is applied, at 15-minute intervals for 2 to 4 hours, and then hourly for the first 24 hours following application. Other neurovascular checks should also be done at those times (Chapter 2). If ischemia develops the fingers may become cooled, swollen, and either cyanotic or pale, and are held in slight flexion and *cannot be completely extended.* Any attempt to passively straighten the fingers causes pain in the front of the forearm. Once ischemia develops, the patient may complain of severe burning pain in the forearm and the hand, but the onset is often painless. If the arterial spasm is not relieved within 6 to 8 hours, the muscles die and become matted, fibrosed, and contracted. Their functional ability is then permanently lost. The nerves of the arm and the hand degenerate, even if previously uninjured, and the fingers become anesthetic and fixed in a flexed position. A typical Volkmann's contracture includes a combined median and ulnar palsy, hyperextension of the metacarpophalangeal joints, flexion of the interphalangeal joints, and wasting of the intrinsic muscles of the hand and the thenar and hypothenar eminences.

Immediate measures to relieve the ischemia are essential. Inform the physician *at once* if any of the above signs are observed. Delay is dangerous. Keep the patient warm but do not attempt to warm the fingers by applying a hot water bottle or heating pad. Do not elevate the arm. If the arm is elevated, reducing the elevation may help increase the arterial flow to the hand.

Treatment to relieve the ischemia consists of (1) removal of the front half of the cast or loosening of the encircling bandage, (2) further manipulation of any still unreduced fracture, (3) reducing the degree of flexion to less than 90 degrees, (4) if those measures fail to relieve the symptoms promptly, doing a sympathetic nerve block, or (5) exploratory surgery of the brachial artery to excise the damaged portion of the artery. After the arterial spasm is relieved, rehabilitation is aimed at improving the function of the arm by correcting any residual deformity and reeducating the muscles that remain functional.

OTHER CIRCULATORY COMPLICATIONS. Because of immobility, the patient in traction for a supracondylar fracture has the potential for developing a thrombus or thrombophlebitis. Most patients should wear elastic stockings and do active range-of-motion exercises of all unaffected joints to increase circulation and help reduce that risk. Some patients may also be placed on a low dose of aspirin. Circulation can be impeded by vessel trauma, edema, or pressure from the immobilization device. In older patients, circulatory impairment may be a greater problem because the blood flow to the extremities may be compromised by arteriosclerotic disease.

Integumentary. Because the patient is unable to turn, there is a potential for skin breakdown of the patient's upper back. Problems with the lower trunk and extremities are much less frequent as patients are able to lift their trunk and move their legs. Measures to prevent skin breakdown are: (1) keep linen wrinkle free, dry, and free of food crumbs; (2) have two persons change the linen with care so as not to disrupt the traction; (3) give skin care to the back at least every 3 to 4 hours. Avoid use of lotions as they soften the skin and leave it sticky. Alcohol leaves the skin dry and also helps to toughen the skin and prevent further trauma. Gentle rubbing is essential to increase circulation to the area. Take care that the skin along the traction edges is kept dry, clean, and free of irritation. Make sure the affected hand has lotion applied to help prevent dryness, but apply alcohol rubs to the bony prominences of the wrist to toughen the skin where the traction tapes might rub.

Psychological. To help prevent or reduce boredom and self-centeredness, find activities that the patient likes to do and still can do. Listening to music is one example. Reading is another. The nurse may need to obtain prism glasses or a device to hold a book or newspaper so the patient can read comfortably in bed. The nurse may be able to get reading books or "talking books" from the local library. Other possible activities include games or cards. There are card holders available that allow the patient to play with one hand. Try to make the activities mentally stimulating, as a change from the passive role of a television viewer. Because the patient may be immobile for some time, a social support system can increase the patient's feelings of competence and self-worth.

Patient Teaching. The patient lying supine in traction because of a fractured humerus may have a feeling of helplessness because of an unrealistic understanding of the severity of the injury and the potential for recovery. Once the initial pain is reduced, the patient should be encouraged to begin doing simple activities of daily living, with assistance as needed from the nurse. How much the patient is able to do depends on whether the dominant arm was affected. Occupational therapy may be needed to help with assistive devices. Schedule self-help activities when the patient is not tired. Many patients fear that any motion, including self-care, will disturb the traction. Educate the patient about the purposes and the principles of traction. Tell the patient what movements are allowed. The "can't do" activities should be discussed, but if too much emphasis is placed on them the patient is less likely to engage in any activity.

Most patients benefit psychologically from understanding the rehabilitation program, especially (1) when and whether they will get return of function in the arm, (2) how long they will be in traction, (3) whether they will need to be in a cast after the traction is removed, (4) what kind of exercises they will need to do, and when, and (5) whether they will be able to return home when they leave the hospital. Because the answers to those questions depend on the age of the patient, the location and type of fracture, the length and type of treatment, and the patient's response to that treatment, they must be answered by the physician. Help the patient obtain that information, for example, by suggesting that he or she prepare a list of questions to discuss with the physician.

Evaluation and Reassessment

Determine whether a patient's pain has been reduced by the application of sidearm traction, nursing measures, and pain medications. The patient should have normal neurovascular status with no circulatory impairment. The fingers and the hand should have good color, be warm, and have sensory and motor function.

There should be no signs of complications from bedrest or traction. Patients should be doing activities that stimulate their minds as well as their bodies. The exercise program should have become a routine part of their daily activities. They should have a good overall knowledge of the rehabilitation process and how they will regain function in their arm.

Intercondylar Fractures

Intercondylar fractures are usually due to direct violence. There is considerable comminution of the bony fragments and damage to the articular surface. The most common are T or Y type fractures of the lower end of the humerus with a vertical component running into the elbow joint, but any combination of fractures may be included. The elbow is often grossly swollen and painful and can look like a "bag of bones" (Roaf & Hodkinson, 1975, p. 93). The treatment of intercondylar fractures varies with the extent of the damage. If the fracture is one in which reduction and firm fixation can be achieved by open reduction and internal fixation, that may be done (Fig. 10–9). There are many different methods of internal fixation that can hold the fragments after reduction, but they all are likely to lead to extensive fibrosis of the muscles and periarticular tissues, and ultimately to stiffness of the elbow joint. In addition, a fracture treated by open reduction and internal fixation is often not stable enough to allow early movement. If the degree of comminution of the fracture is so great that internal fixation cannot be satisfactorily achieved, the fracture may be treated by olecranon pin traction and early motion. Movements of the hand and the fingers are usually begun immediately, but shoulder movement is not allowed for 2 to 3 weeks. If it appears that the bony fragments cannot be restored to their proper positions, the aim is to develop what joint movements are possible by putting the arm in a splint or a collar and cuff and beginning gentle, early, active exercises. If traction is not used, active flexion from the position of the immobilization is encouraged if it does not cause pain. Tenderness will probably disappear in 4 to 6 weeks, the splint is then discarded, and further active elbow movement is encouraged. The average end result is full flexion, full rotation, and loss of extension of not more than 30 degrees.

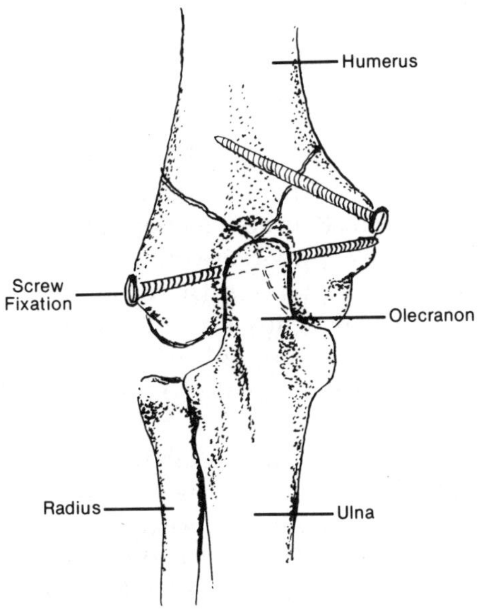

Figure 10–9. Open reduction and internal fixation, intracondylar fracture of the humerus. *(From Brantley, P., & Analla, M., 1980, p. 23. Courtesy of Howmedica.)*

Fractures of the Olecranon

Fractures of the olecranon are more common in adults than in children. They are usually caused by direct violence from a fall on the elbow or by muscular violence from a contraction of the triceps muscle following a fall on the hand with the elbow flexed. Many times associated laceration of the lateral aponeurosis of the triceps tendon allows marked separation of the fragments. The patient is unable to extend the elbow actively, and a gap can be felt between the olecranon and the rest of the shaft of the ulna (Gartland, 1979, p. 282). Because the fracture involves the humeroulnar component of the joint, an inadequate reduction may result in limitation of extension at the elbow.

Many olecranon fractures can be reduced satisfactorily and then immobilized in a cast from the shoulder to the wrist, with the elbow in 90 degrees of flexion. It may take 2 or 3 months for the fracture to heal, however, and several more months for the patient to regain elbow joint motion. Thus, when possible, operative treatment is preferred because it offers the advantage of earlier motion. Many authorities tend to treat undisplaced olecranon fractures in a posterior splint with the elbow flexed 90 degrees (Iversen & Clawson, 1977, pp. 161–162). Pronation and supination movements are then started 2 or 3 days after splinting, and flexion–extension movements are started 2 weeks after splinting. The protective splinting is continued until there is evidence of union (usually about 6 weeks). Displaced fractures are usually reduced and internally fixed. The procedure usually used is either (1) open reduction and fixation with a figure-of-eight (Kirschner) wire loop, used when the fracture is not comminuted and is proximal to the coronoid process, (2) medullary fixation when the olecranon is comminuted and its distal fragments and the head of the radius are dislocated anteriorly (Fig. 10–10), or (3) excision of the proximal fragment of the olecranon when a comminuted fracture extends as far distally as the coronoid process (Edmondson & Crenshaw, 1980, pp. 684–685). When the olecranon is excised, the triceps muscle is resutured to the ulnar shaft.

After an internal fixation and closure, the elbow is usually immobilized in a posterior splint with elbow in 90 degrees of flexion. In approximately 7 to 10 days, active and active-assisted exercises are started. Between exercise periods, the elbow is still supported with the splint. Usually support is continued until the fourth week, though maximum function may not return for 6 to 12 months. Pronation and supination are seldom permanently limited to any extent, although flexion and extension may be. The speed with which motion returns, and the final range of motion, depend on the extent of injury to the joint surfaces.

Patients who have an olecranon excised have the affected elbow immobilized in a posterior splint with 70 degrees of flexion. Motion is begun approximately 7 to 10 days after surgery, but the patient continues to wear the splint between exercise periods for approximately 3 weeks. The arm is then placed in a sling for another 10 days. The patient is instructed to avoid forceful extension of the elbow for at least 3 months.

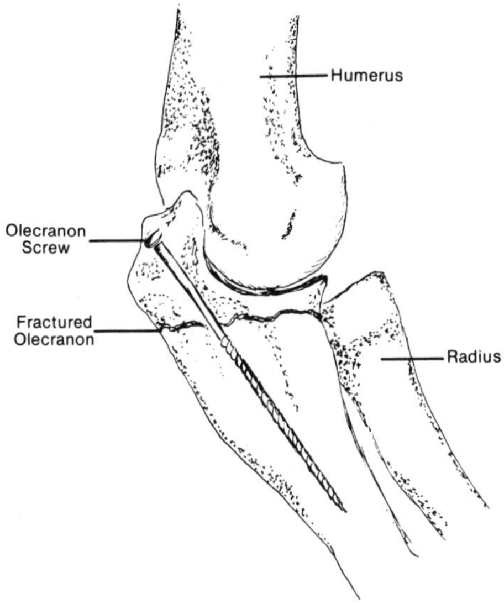

Figure 10–10. Open reduction and internal fixation, olecranon. *(From Brantley, P., & Analla, M., 1980, p. 21. Courtesy of Howmedica.)*

Fractures of the Head of the Radius

Fractures of the head of the radius are common in adults and usually occur as a result of a fall on the outstretched hand. There is swelling at the elbow joint, tenderness over the head of the radius, and limitation of elbow function, especially painful pronation–supination. Because these fractures tend to cause joint stiffness if immobilized, the key to successful treatment is to allow early motion. The treatment method and ultimate prognosis depends on the amount of damage to the joint articular cartilage, the type of fracture, and the degree of displacement. Fractures of the head and neck of the radius are classified as (1) undisplaced fractures, (2) marginal fractures, (3) comminuted fractures, and (4) fractures associated with dislocations of the elbow. Undisplaced or impacted fractures are usually treated by supporting the elbow in a comfortable degree of flexion in a collar and cuff or in a posterior splint until the pain disappears (usually several days to a week). The arm may then be placed in a sling, and active movement of the elbow started. Displaced fractures involving less than a third of the articular surface are treated by reduction and early motion. Marginal fractures with displacement, and comminuted fractures, are treated by early excision of the radial head. The end result of excision of the radial head is good, but a normal elbow is not achieved. Some 50 percent of those patients later develop subluxation and pain at the distal radioulnar joint (Iversen & Clawson, 1977, p. 164). With recent developments and improvements in implants, those patients may have a Silastic radial head prosthesis inserted.

☐ NURSING PROCESS (Table 10–3)

Assessment

The first step in the nursing assessment of a patient with an undisplaced or impacted fracture of the head of the radius supported by a collar and cuff is to determine the neurovascular status of the affected arm (Chap. 2). Check the elbow for the amount of swelling and determine whether there is any swelling of the hand. Check that the affected arm is in the correct position, with the elbow at the proper degree of flexion and the hand safely elevated and supported. Make sure that there is a cloth support between the patient's arm and chest, i.e., that there is no skin-to-skin contact. Elicit information on the location, duration, and severity of pain. Note that the edges of the collar and cuff are not irritating the skin around them.

Nursing Diagnosis and Goal Formulation

Nursing diagnoses for a typical patient with a fracture of the head of the radius and a collar and cuff support are (1) alterations in comfort related to pain from the trauma to the soft tissue and bone, (2) alterations in mobility related to lack of bone stability, (3) potential complications related to trauma and decreased arm mobility, and (4) alterations in psychological well-being related to anxiety and knowledge deficit about the injury and the rehabilitation process.

Short-term goals are to have the patient experience (1) a decrease in the amount of pain, (2) an increase in bone stability, (3) an absence of complications from trauma and immobilization, and (4) a decrease in anxiety through increased knowledge. Long-term goals are to have the patient pain free and to have full return of arm function.

Planning and Intervention

Alleviate Pain. Nursing measures that help to reduce pain are applying ice to reduce swelling, maintaining correct flexion at the elbow, and having the patient do exercises as allowed. Medicate for pain as needed.

Increase Mobility

Position. The patient usually finds that the most comfortable position in bed is the supine position with the head of the bed slightly elevated. The patient can turn from side to side as necessary for care, but will probably not find lying on a side for any period of time comfortable as then it is next to impossible to keep the arm in the correct position. The patient should be encouraged to use the trapeze with the unaffected arm to readjust and change position in bed and to help with daily care.

Exercises. When allowed by the physician, the patient should start finger exercises and muscle setting or isometric exercises to the affected arm

TABLE 10–3. NURSING PROCESS FOR FRACTURE OF THE HEAD OF THE RADIUS TREATED WITH A COLLAR AND CUFF

Assessment	Nursing Diagnosis	Goal Formulation	Planning and Intervention	Evaluation and Reassessment
1. Assess the location, duration, and severity of pain. Assess neurovascular status. Check for any swelling.	1. Alteration in comfort: pain in the elbow related to bone and soft tissue trauma.	1. Short-term goal: a relative state of comfort. Long-term goal: free of pain.	1. Alleviate Pain Maintain correct flexion at the elbow. Apply ice to fracture site. Instruct on finger and isometric exercises. Administer prescribed pain medications. Teach relaxation techniques.	1. The arm should be maintained in correct position. The patient should be in a relative state of comfort; medication should reduce severe pain.
2. Assess neurovascular status of affected arm. Assess ability to do exercises. Check the position of the collar and cuff (or sling). Assess ability to ambulate alone.	2. Impaired physical mobility: decreased arm function related to lack of bone stability.	2. Short-term goal: an increase in arm function through controlled exercises. Long-term goal: return of full arm function.	2. Increase Mobility *Position* Supine position with the head elevated (when in bed). Encourage use of trapeze to change position. *Exercises* Instruct on finger and muscle setting exercises with affected arm. Maintain collar and cuff support (until pain decreases). Instruct on active elbow exercises after pain decreases. *Collar and Cuff* Maintain correct collar and cuff position. Keep hand level with or above the elbow. *Ambulation* Maintain arm support. Assist with ambulation on the unaffected side.	2. When in bed, the patient should be in the supine position with head of bed elevated. Doing exercises should not increase pain. The arm should be kept elevated with a collar and cuff (or sling). Expect no problem with ambulation.

(continued)

TABLE 10–3. *(Continued)*

Assessment	Nursing Diagnosis	Goal Formulation	Planning and Intervention	Evaluation and Reassessment
3. Assess neurovascular status. Assess activity level in affected arm. Check flexion at the elbow and tightness of the collar and cuff.	3. Potential for injury: neurovascular deficit related to soft tissue swelling.	3. Short- and long-term goal: free of any neurovascular complications.	3. Prevent Complications *Circulatory* Do neurovascular assessments every 15 minutes for first 2 hours, every 30 minutes for next 2 hours, every 60 minutes for next 2 hours, every 2 hours for next 18 hours, and then at the beginning of every shift. Instruct patient and family on how to do a neurovascular assessment. Apply nursing methods to reduce swelling. Keep elbow at proper degree of flexion. Report any abnormal findings.	3. The patient should be free of any neurovascular deficit. The patient should be able to demonstrate how to do neurovascular assessment.
Assess for any swelling. Check the skin at the back of the neck, around the wrist, and between the arm and chest.	Potential for impairment of skin integrity related to irritation from collar and cuff.	Short- and long-term goal: free of any complications.	*Integumentary* Follow-up any complaints of pain by checking the skin area. Maintain collar and cuff with comfortable tightness. Apply nursing methods to reduce swelling. Pad area at the back of the neck. Place a small pad between the patient's chest and arm.	The patient's skin should remain free of any irritation.

4. Assess the patient's level of understanding of the steps in the rehabilitation process.	4. Potential for knowledge deficit related to the rehabilitation process.	4. Short- and long-term goal: a decrease in anxiety with an increase in knowledge.	4. Patient Teaching Explain the steps in the rehabilitation process. Include the family and significant others in the teaching. Go over the various exercises. Go over methods of bathing and dressing.	4. The patient should verbalize an understanding of the rehabilitation process. The patient should be able to demonstrate exercises and how to do some activities of daily living. The patient and the family should verbalize methods of bathing and dressing with a collar and cuff (or sling) in place.

while in the collar and cuff support. The patient is usually in the support until the pain disappears, usually several days to a week. The arm may then be placed in a sling and active movement of the elbow started (see pp. 607 and 610).

Collar and Cuff. This form of support involves a collar or sling around the patient's neck that is attached to a cuff around the wrist of the affected arm. The length of the connection between the collar and the cuff determines how much the hand is elevated, and thus the amount of flexion obtained at the elbow. There can be minimal flexion if there is gross swelling of the elbow, but it can later be increased when the swelling subsides.

Sling. A sling is used to support the arm with the hand level to or about the elbow, and the hand and the wrist in a functional position. Such support is often desirable if there is edema in the hand, the wrist, or the elbow, shoulder pain or an excessive pull on the shoulder, or if a cast or splint is used on the arm. The use of a sling promotes comfort and, in some cases, helps to protect the extremity.

There are many commercial slings available, or a properly fitting sling can be made. Obtain a triangular piece of cloth or bandage. Place the top corner of the triangular cloth sling over the front of the patient's affected shoulder, with the sling hanging between the patient's body and affected arm, and the point of the triangle toward the patient's affected elbow. Bring the bottom corner of the triangle over the affected arm, up and over the unaffected shoulder, and behind the neck to the affected shoulder. Tie the sling at the side of the patient's neck, and fold the point of the triangle over the front of the patient's elbow, securing it with a safety pin. Check to make sure the patient's forearm and hand are level with or slightly higher than the elbow. Make sure that the hand is well supported. Assess the patient for comfort and support of the affected arm. Monitor for adequate circulation every 2 hours.

A sling should not be used continuously. The position of the extremity should be changed frequently to prevent tightness and discomfort in the muscles of the arm and the shoulder. Check the sling to insure that (1) no pull is exerted on the shoulder joint, (2) the patient is not trying to protect the muscles of the neck and upper torso by contracting them, (3) excessive pressure is not exerted on the neck, and (4) the shoulder does not droop forward. The weight of the arm should be evenly distributed across the back of the neck.

Ambulation. The patient is usually allowed up shortly after the application of the collar and cuff, but needs assistance in getting out of bed at first. Do not support the patient under the affected elbow, and do not change the degree of flexion of the arm.

Prevent Complications. The most common complications for a patient with a radial head fracture in a collar and cuff support are neurovascular impairment and skin irritation. Neurovascular impairment may be due to an injury at the time of the trauma, swelling at the elbow following trauma, acute flexion of the elbow, or tightness of the cuff portion of the collar and cuff support. Nursing interventions to reduce swelling, and early detection and reporting of any neurovascular impairment, are essential. Immediately report any neurovascular irregularity to the patient's physician. If the cuff is too tight and is restricting circulation to the hand, it can be loosened, but there should be no change in flexion at the elbow.

Skin irritation can occur at the edges of the collar and cuff. If the cuff is too loose, place some padding (e.g., sheet wadding) between the patient's wrist and the cuff. The collar portion may need extra padding at the back of the neck because of pressure from the weight of the arm. A small pad should be placed between the patient's arm and chest to prevent skin irritation.

Patient Teaching. Teach the patient how to do the prescribed exercises. Try to work out a schedule that fits into the patient's daily activities. After the collar and cuff are removed, the patient will begin active exercises of the affected elbow. Make sure the patient understands that he or she is not to force the elbow to straighten, as too much force can damage the elbow. It will take time to regain complete function of the elbow.

Help the patient, the family, and significant others learn to do a neurovascular assessment of the affected arm and compare it with the unaffected arm. Make sure the patient understands the purpose and objectives of the collar and cuff and the sling. Once the patient begins to wear a sling, make sure it is removed for exercises.

The patient may need help in doing activities of daily living and with dressing. Most of the activities described for a patient with a Velpeau bandage or shoulder immobilizer (see p. 509) apply to a patient in a collar and cuff.

Evaluation and Reassessment

Following a reduction of a fractured radial head and the application of a collar and cuff, the patient should have a decrease in pain. If pain persists, nursing measures and medications should relieve it. The patient should be free of any neurovascular impairment, swelling, or skin irritation from the collar and cuff. Determine how comfortable the patient is in administering self-care and whether he or she needs help when returning home.

Rupture of the Biceps Tendon at the Elbow

The biceps tendon may be ruptured or avulsed at or near its insertion to the bicipital tuberosity of the radius. The injury is usually associated with forcible flexion of the elbow against strong resistance, for example, when a worker who is assisting in lifting a heavy object and suddenly has to bear its full weight alone. The worker will feel a painful snap or tearing sensation at the elbow, followed immediately by weakness during active flexion of the elbow and supination of the forearm. The biceps tendon is normally a flexor for supination or semisupination of the forearm, but provides little or no flexor power when the forearm is pronated. The antecubital space will be tender, but swelling is usually minimal because of the strong overlying fascia. When attempting active flexion, a bulbous swelling forms on the upper arm, caused by the retracted belly of the biceps.

A rupture of the biceps tendon is usually preceded by degenerative changes in the tendon, often associated with advanced age and arteriosclerosis. The bicipital tuberosity often develops an irregular jagged ridge that wears on the tendon and makes it more susceptible to rupture under stress. If the tendon is partially torn, but not yet completely ruptured, it may produce symptoms of localized pain during motions requiring lifting and supination. Tenderness and a sensation of fine crepitus may be palpable over the tuberosity. Following an acute rupture of the distal biceps tendon, marked flexor weakness and partial loss of supinator power is temporary, and function can be restored by a program of muscle-strengthening exercises. Unless strong flexion and supination are needed by someone engaged in strenuous occupations or sports, surgical repair is usually unnecessary.

The surgical procedure is to recover the retracted tendon and suture it to the insertion of the brachialis. This results in restoration of strong flexion, but supination remains weak. When the occupation of the patient demands good rotary power of the forearm, an attempt must be made to resuture the tendon to the bicipital tuberosity. Postoperatively, the elbow is immobilized in a posterior splint with the elbow flexed just beyond a right angle and the forearm in moderate supination. After 5 to 6 weeks, exercises are instituted.

Pathology

ARTHRITIS AND INFECTIOUS DISEASES

Rheumatoid Arthritis of the Elbow

Rheumatoid arthritis of the elbow develops insidiously, is tenacious and progressive, and often proceeds toward joint destruction in spite of local and systemic treatment. Rheumatoid arthritis of the elbow is often associated with rheumatoid arthritis of the shoulder, the wrist, and the hand. As a general rule, other joints are already involved, and the diagnosis established before elbow involvement.

Early in the disease process, the elbow is painful and somewhat limited in movement, particularly in the morning and at the extremes of motion. There is minimal diffuse soft tissue swelling, tenderness about the joint margins, and slight restriction of flexion, extension, and forearm rotation. Later in the disease process, the pain becomes more intense and persistent, movement is voluntarily restricted to guard against provoking pain, the soft tissue swelling about the joint becomes more pronounced, and the joint becomes extremely tender. The joint is warm and usually held in a semiflexed position. Soft tissue swelling usually develops adjacent to the medial and lateral humeral condyles.

Remissions and exacerbations are the rule. Repeated effusions into the joint occur, but gradually lessen as the inflammatory process becomes less intense and the course of the disease more chronic. As destruction and deformity develop, marked grating and crepitus reflect articular disintegration. Motion in flexion, extension, and forearm rotation become increasingly limited, and mediolateral instability occurs with destruction of the capsuloligamentous structures. In the latter stages of joint destruction, the muscles of the arm and forearm atrophy. The disease process may involve the capsule at various sites. When it proceeds posteromedially, it may encroach on the ulnar nerve, and unless that is recognized and the nerve decompressed, permanent nerve damage may ensue.

Subcutaneous rheumatoid nodules that develop over the proximal aspect of the ulna and recurring olecranon bursitis (see p. 613) are both characteristic of rheumatoid arthritis of the elbow. Rheumatoid arthritis causes bursal swelling and distention, and a thickening of the bursal wall.

In the elbow joint, the intra-articular destruction may predominantly affect the humeroradial joint or the humeroulnar joint, either of which will interfere with flexion and extension. The synovial extension may invade the radioulnar articulation, and rotation movement of the forearm may become impeded and painful. Pressure may cause the radial head to collapse, and the articular fossa of the ulna to become ragged and deeply excavated. Destruction of the capsuloligamentous structures results in subluxations and dislocations. When the annular ligament has been destroyed, the radius is displaced anteriorly by the pull of the biceps creating a mechanical block to flexion and preventing extension. The tendons, particularly the biceps and the brachialis, become elongated and may even rupture. Despite severe destructive changes that can be observed on a roentgenogram, and fibrous ankylosis, some degree of motion is usually preserved.

Rheumatoid arthritis of the elbow is but one part of a generalized disease, therefore the patient will be on a generalized medical regime. Local treatment for the elbow may consist of rest, a splint to prevent deformity, and intra-articular injection of corticosteroids. With advanced disease, reconstructive surgical procedures may be indicated. These procedures may be a synovectomy, a resection of the radial head, or even the removal of the distal end of the ulna. For an extensively destroyed and markedly unstable joint, a total joint replacement of the elbow may be done.

Tuberculosis of the Elbow

Osseous tuberculosis of the elbow, like tuberculosis of other bony structures, may be mild or severe, depending upon the intensity of the disease and the body's response to it. At first there is an acute exudative inflammation that produces a clinical picture of pain, muscle spasm, generalized joint tenderness, swelling that consists of boggy edema of the periarticular tissues, increased synovial effusion, and marked limitation of motion. The infection slowly spreads, destroying the intra-articular tissues, but the body may be able to seal it off by means of a fibrous ankylosis (or rarely, a bony ankylosis). If not, destructive changes continue, with the formation of persistent draining sinuses in the bones and the loss of all joint motion (Turek, 1977, pp. 880–881).

When roentgenograms reveal diffuse osteoporosis and the exudative reaction, conservative treatment by immobilization and antituberculous drugs may be sufficient. Surgical procedures to excise the focus of the disease may be necessary to halt the destructive process. If the infection has spread to the coronoid process, or joint destruction has been extensive, an arthrodesis may be required.

After an arthrodesis, the position of immobilization depends upon the functional needs of the patient. Ankylosis in a position of approximately 120 degrees presents the best cosmetic result. One can type, reach into a back pocket, and have the arm hang naturally at the side. For eating, however, fusion at not more than a right angle is best (for arthrodesis of the elbow, see pp. 599–604).

Synovectomy

For limitations of motion and pain in an elbow that has rheumatoid arthritic changes, surgical procedures such as synovectomy, resection of the radial head, and anterior transplantation of the ulnar nerve have satisfactorily decreased pain and increased motion without the need for further reconstructive procedures.

A synovectomy is the removal of the synovium, and it relieves pain in almost all patients with rheumatoid arthritis and, at least temporarily, halts the progression of the disease in the elbow. A synovectomy removes sites of immunoglobulin synthesis, thereby preventing the formation of the immune complexes that cause tissue destruction by activating lysosomal hydrolases. For best results, a synovectomy needs to be done before destruction in the joint is evident. After removal, the synovium will regenerate, usually within 60 days, and is then once again capable of secreting synovial fluid, but it is more fibrous and less vascular, and its secretory function is considerably reduced. The regenerated synovium is again susceptible to rheumatoid arthritis.

The synovium is usually removed through longitudinal incisions both medially and laterally to the elbow. The joint is then surgically opened and the elbow dislocated for the complete removal of the synovium. If necessary, the radial head can also be resected at that time. Closure is accomplished, the arm is placed in a plaster splint for a few days, and then guarded exercises are started.

Although a synovectomy is most applicable to joints that have not undergone cartilaginous destruction, the disease is usually long standing and no longer suitable for a synovectomy alone. Involvement of the radioulnar joint can limit not only supination and pronation but also flexion and extension of the elbow. The removal of the radial head usually markedly reduces pain and increases the range of motion. The head of the radius may, in some instances, be replaced with a prosthesis. If rotary movement of the forearm is still limited, the distal end of the ulna may also be resected, because rheumatoid arthritis often affects the distal radioulnar joint.

Arthrodesis

A surgical fusion (or arthrodesis) of the ulnohumeral joint is rare. Indications for an elbow arthrodesis are instances of chronic osteomyelitis that have invaded the joint, severe fractures followed by infection and, occasionally, tuberculosis. One method of doing an arthrodesis is to make a posterior midline incision over the lower end of the humerus and then extend it over the olecranon. The ulnar nerve is isolated from its groove between the olecranon and the medial epicondyle and retracted. The flat triceps tendon is severed at the musculotendinous junction, and the flap remaining attached to the olecranon is retracted downward, exposing the posterior joint capsule. The capsule is then cut longitudinally, and the soft tissues are elevated from the medial and lateral aspects of the joint and retracted forward, giving access to the anterior regions. The elbow is then flexed, exposing the articular cartilage of the radius, the ulna, and the humerus. All cartilage, granulation tissue, abnormally appearing bone, and thickened capsule are removed until normal cancellous bony structures remain. If the radial head is subluxated, it is also removed. It is important to preserve the function of the radiohumeral joint to insure pronation and supination in the forearm. A bed is then made for a bone graft in the posterior surface of the distal humerus and the superior part of the tip of the olecranon. With the elbow in flexion, the graft is fit into the olecranon bed and then, after extending the elbow to the position of fusion, into the humeral bed. One or two screws may be placed through the graft into the humerus to make it secure, and the ulnohumeral joint is then packed with cancellous bone from the proximal end of the tibia. (The graft, obtained from the upper half of the tibia, is usually 1.3 cm wide and 9 cm long.) A cast is then applied. For a unilateral arthrodesis of the elbow, an arm position of about 90 degrees is desirable. For a bilateral arthrodesis, one elbow should be at 65 to 90 degrees to permit the patient to reach the mouth, and the other should be approximately 110 to 120 degrees. These positions may be varied to meet the requirements of the patient's occupation (Edmondson & Crenshaw, 1980, p. 1137; Turek, 1977, p. 881).

□ NURSING PROCESS (Table 10–4)

Assessment

The first step in the assessment of a typical patient following an elbow arthrodesis and the application of a long arm cast is to check the neurovascular status of the affected arm and compare it with the unaffected arm (Chapter 2). Becuase of the potential for ulnar nerve damage, check the motor and sensory function of the ulnar nerve. The sensory function can

TABLE 10–4. NURSING PROCESS FOR ARTHRODESIS OF THE ELBOW WITH A LONG ARM CAST

Assessment	Nursing Diagnosis	Goal Formulation	Planning and Intervention	Evaluation and Reassessment
1. Assess for duration, location, and severity of pain. Assess the neurovascular status of the affected arm. Check the elevation of the arm.	1. Alteration in comfort: pain in the elbow and donor site related to bone trauma.	1. Short-term goal: a decrease in pain through immobilization and prescribed medications. Long-term goal: free of pain.	1. Alleviate Pain Elevate the arm. Apply ice to elbow. Instruct on finger exercises. Make sure cast is not too tight. Administer pain medications. Teach relaxation techniques.	1. Expect the patient to complain of more pain at the donor site than at the elbow. The patient should remain relatively free of pain with the use of medications.
2. Check the position of the cast. Assess the patient's ability to do exercises. Assess neurovascular status of the affected arm. Assess function at the shoulder and wrist. Check ability to ambulate without assistance.	2. Impaired physical mobility: decreased arm function related to lack of elbow joint stability.	2. Short-term goal: an increase in joint mobility through immobilization and exercises. Long-term goal: stability of the elbow joint with reduced range of motion.	2. Increase Mobility *Position* Keep the patient supine with arm elevated or turned to the unaffected side with arm supported on pillows. Head of bed may be elevated. Teach how to use the trapeze. *Exercises* Instruct on isometric finger and shoulder exercises for the affected arm, and active range of motion to all unaffected joints. *Ambulation* Support the arm with a sling. Assist patient with getting out of bed and ambulating.	2. The patient should keep the affected arm elevated at all times and do finger exercises every 1–2 hours while awake and active range of all other joints without supervision. The patient should be able to ambulate with the arm in a sling without difficulty.

3. Check skin at cast edges for any irritation. Assess for complaints of pain over bony prominences. Check for any signs of swelling. Check for signs and symptoms of infection. Check donor site.	3. Potential for impairment of skin integrity related to rough cast edges and pressure from cast. Potential for injury: infection related to surgical incision.	3. Short- and long-term goal: free of any skin complication.	3. Prevent Complications *Integumentary* Prevent possible contamination of incision. Make sure patient eats a well-balanced diet and gets adequate rest. Keep skin area at cast edges from irritation; petal cast edges.	3. The patient should be free of any added break in skin integrity or any sign of infection.
Assess neurovascular status of the affected arm (especially the ulnar nerve).	Potential for injury: neurovascular deficit related to soft tissue swelling and cast.	Short- and long-term goal: no neurovascular complications.	*Neurological* Do neurovascular assessments every 15 minutes for first 2 hours, every 30 minutes for next 2 hours, every 60 minutes for next 2 hours, every 2 hours for next 18 hours, and then at the beginning of every shift. Utilize nursing measures to reduce swelling. Be alert to patient's complaints of pain. *Other Complications* (See text.)	The patient should be free of any neurovascular complications.
4. Assess the patient's level of knowledge concerning self-care and the steps in the rehabilitation process.	4. Potential for knowledge deficit related to the rehabilitation process.	4. Short- and long-term goal: a decrease in anxiety through an increase in knowledge.	4. Patient Teaching Discuss the steps in the rehabilitation process. Clarify instructions on exercises. Demonstrate self-care and dressing with a long arm cast on. Discuss with patient the feelings and reactions to having the elbow fused in a flexed position. Include family and significant others in teaching plans.	4. The patient should be able to verbalize the reaction to a fused flexed elbow and demonstrate self-care and the ability to dress.

be checked by pricking the distal end of the patient's little finger, and the motor function can be checked by asking the patient to abduct all the fingers. Check for any swelling or any bleeding into the cast. The patient is prone to bleeding because of the large amount of joint reconstruction. Note the amount of bleeding at the donor site of the bone graft.

Assess for pain. Expect the patient to complain more about the pain at the donor site than at the elbow. Check the patient's body alignment and the position of the affected arm.

Nursing Diagnosis and Goal Formulation

Nursing diagnoses for a typical patient following an arthrodesis are (1) alterations in comfort related to pain from the surgical procedure, (2) alterations in mobility related to lack of elbow joint stability, (3) potential complications related to surgical procedure and decreased arm mobility, and (4) alterations in psychological well-being related to anxiety and knowledge deficit about the surgical procedure and the treatment methods.

Short-term goals are to have the patient experience (1) a decrease in the amount of pain, (2) an increase in joint stability, (3) an absence of complications from surgery and decreased activity, and (4) a decrease in anxiety through increased knowledge. Long-term goals are to have the patient pain free and to have a return of function in the arm.

Planning and Intervention

Alleviate Pain. Measures that help to relieve and prevent pain following an elbow arthrodesis and the application of a long arm cast are elevation of the arm to prevent or reduce swelling, application of ice at the site of the arthrodesis, and having the patient do finger exercises when allowed.

The location, duration, and severity of pain should be determined and nursing interventions specific to the pain implemented, before the administration of medication. Include measures specific to the donor site.

Increase Mobility

Position. The patient's arm is normally elevated on a pillow. The most comfortable position in bed for the patient is supine with the head of the bed elevated. The patient will be able to turn to the unaffected side for short periods of time with support to the affected arm. The patient can turn to the affected side, but will find it difficult. If the bone graft was taken from the patient's iliac crest, the patient will not want to turn to that side.

Long Arm Cast. The long arm cast extends from as high as the upper level of the axillary fold to the proximal palmar crease, with the elbow immobilized in a flexed position. The long arm cast is used to immobilize unstable fractures of the carpals and fractures of the distal humerus, the radius, the ulna, or both. For patients with an arthrodesis of the elbow, the elbow ordinarily is flexed up to 90 degrees, and the forearm is in a neutral position. Once the long arm cast is dry, the cast is bivalved and held together with an elastic wrap to allow for swelling at the elbow. Approximately 2 weeks after surgery, when the sutures are removed, the patient will have a new, snugly fitting cast applied.

Exercises. With the patient in a bivalved cast, check with the physician about having the patient do isometric, finger (see p. 509), or shoulder (see pp. 500 and 521–523) exercises with the affected arm. Encourage active range-of-motion exercises for all uninvolved joints. Even with the elbow fused, the objective is to preserve the pronation and supination movements of the forearm.

Ambulation. Ambulation will be allowed, however, the patient will probably need a sling (see p. 594) to help support the affected arm. In the beginning, the patient will also need assistance in getting out of bed and ambulating because of the awkwardness and weight of the long arm cast.

Prevent Complications. The major complications following an arthrodesis are ulnar nerve injury, infection, and nonunion of the arthrodesis. To prevent ulnar nerve damage, continue to assess the neurovascular status of the arm and the hand, utilize nursing measures to reduce swelling, and be alert to patient complaints.

To prevent infection, check for the signs and symptoms of infection, prevent possible contamination, and make sure the patient eats a well-balanced diet and gets adequate rest. Many patients will be placed on IV antibiotics following surgery. Such therapy is especially important if the initial reason for the arthrodesis was osteomyelitis or tuberculosis, and it may be followed by oral antibiotic therapy. Even when the incision site heals properly, there is always a chance of infection. An infection can also develop at the donor graft site or from skin irritation caused by the cast rubbing on bony prominences.

Nonunion usually occurs if there is poor blood supply to the joint or if there is an unstable fusion. Make sure the cast fits properly. If there was swelling when the cast was applied, there may be some play between the arm and the cast when the swelling subsides.

Following an arthrodesis the patient will have an elbow that is permanently in a flexed position. Even though the patient was aware of that before surgery, the patient will go through the stages of adjusting to a disability. Spend time with the patient to facilitate open and realistic discussions.

Patient Teaching. The patient will go home with a long arm cast and a sling. The most important points for the patient, the family, and significant others to understand are the signs and symptoms of neurovascular impairment and infection. It is essential that the patient know how to do neurovascular checks on the affected arm and compare it with the unaffected arm. The patient should understand the purpose of elevating the arm and how to elevate the arm effectively and safely.

For casts without stockinette, demonstrate how to petal a cast and explain the purpose of petalling. Teach the patient how to protect and cleanse the surface of the cast (Appendix B). Time must be spent helping the patient, the family, and significant others develop a plan for bathing and other activities of daily living. Discussions about how to modify present clothing for a long arm cast are essential.

Patients need to know when to return to the clinic or physician's office and who should be notified if they have any problems. About 8 weeks after surgery, a leather laced corset, extending from the upper arm to the heads of the metacarpal bones and reinforced by steel bars, is usually fitted and worn by the patient until osseous union takes place.

Evaluation and Reassessment

Determine whether nursing measures and pain medications have relieved the pain in the elbow and at the donor site of the bone graft. The patient may complain of increased pain when doing the required exercises, but that pain will usually subside shortly after stopping the exercises. If not, medicate the patient and try to determine whether the exercise period was too long or too vigorous.

Make sure the patient receives sufficient information to have a feeling of confidence about going home with a cast. Evaluate whether the patient, the family, and significant others have accepted that the patient will have a permanently flexed elbow. More time with the patient in a stress-free environment may be needed to allow for full and open discussion about the patient's changed body image.

Arthroplasty

An arthroplasty of the elbow may be considered in instances of painful limitation of motion or ankylosis caused by trauma, rheumatoid arthritis, or acute infectious arthritis. An arthroplasty is indicated when motion is more important than strength and stability (Edmondson & Crenshaw, 1980, p. 1419). In one form of arthroplasty, bone is resected and the joint surfaces are covered with a membrane, such as fascia or skin, which permits satisfactory motion but lacks stability. In an effort to restore both motion and stability, hinge and surface replacement devices have been designed for a total elbow arthroplasty. The total arthroplasty requires considerable resection of bone so that the components may be cemented into place.

Fascial Arthroplasty of the Elbow

Fascial arthroplasty of the elbow is done by first exposing the joint. The triceps aponeurosis is incised at the midline and retracted medially and laterally. If the joint is ankylosed, an osteotomy of the fusion between the olecranon and the humerus and between the radial head and the humerus is done while protecting the ulnar nerve. The articular surfaces of the elbow joint are remodeled, forming one humeral condyle. From the lateral side of the thigh a long rectangle of fascia lata large enough to cover the remodeled joint is obtained. The fascia lata is then interposed between the articular surfaces of the ulna and the humerus and the radius and the ulna. The joint is then reduced, the elbow flexed to approximately 90 degrees, and the joint capsule closed (Edmondson & Crenshaw, 1980, p. 2421).

After surgery, the arm is immobilized by two devices. The elbow is held in 90 degrees of flexion by an elbow splint or cast, and the arm is placed in an abduction humerus splint for 10 to 14 days to prevent rotation. After that time, when the wound has completely healed, both the abduction humerus splint and the elbow splint or cast are discarded, and a posterior elbow splint with straps and buckles is applied. That splint is removed for periods of 1 to 2 hours, three or four times a day, to permit active exercises to develop the flexors and extensors of the elbow and the flexors of the fingers. At 3 weeks after surgery, the splint may be discarded during the day, and a sling is used as necessary for support. The splint should be worn at night until a useful range of motion in the elbow and good strength in the muscles have been regained, usually at 8 weeks after surgery. The patient must continue active exercises for at least 6 months, and maximum strength and motion are usually regained approximately 2 years after surgery.

Total Elbow Arthroplasty

In a total elbow arthroplasty (Fig. 10–11), the central portion of the humeral head is cut away and the humeral canal reamed. The articular surface of the olecranon is cut away and the ulnar canal is also reamed. The radial head is excised. With some devices the radial head is replaced, but with others it is not. Both humeral and ulnar components are seated into their respective canals and held in place with methyl methacrylate cement. The humeral and ulnar components are metal with an inserted articulating surface of polyethylene. A wound suction is placed into the wound before closure (Brantley & Analla, 1980, p. 22).

□ NURSING PROCESS (Table 10–5)

Assessment

The first step in the assessment of a typical patient in a long arm posterior splint following an elbow arthroplasty is to determine the neurovascular status of the arm (Chapter 2). Check the position of the arm and make sure it is elevated on a pillow. The wrist should not be flexed, as that would

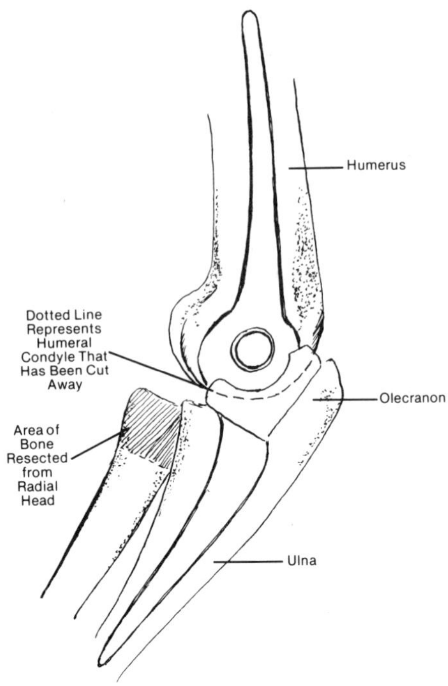

Figure 10–11. Total elbow arthroplasty, lateral view. *(From Brantley, P., & Analla, M., 1980, p. 22. Courtesy of Howmedica.)*

put pressure on the arm at the distal end of the splint. Check for skin irritation under or at the edges of the splint. Look for drainage from the incision and observe for signs of infection. Assess the location, duration, and severity of pain.

Nursing Diagnosis and Goal Formulation

Nursing diagnoses for a typical patient following an arthroplasty are (1) alterations in comfort related to pain from the surgical procedure, (2) alterations in mobility related to surgical procedure and lack of joint stability, (3) potential complications related to the surgical procedure and decreased arm mobility, and (4) alterations in psychological well-being related to anxiety and knowledge deficit about the surgical procedure and the rehabilitation process.

Short-term goals are to have the patient experience (1) a decrease in the amount of pain, (2) an increase in joint stability, (3) an absence of complications from surgery and decreased activity, and (4) a decrease in anxiety through increased knowledge. Long-term goals are to have the patient pain free with full return of function in the elbow.

Planning and Intervention

Alleviate Pain. Most patients with an arthroplasty have had rheumatoid arthritis or an infection in the elbow before surgery. During surgery, there is considerable resection of bone, so that the prosthetic components can be cemented into place. Nonetheless, the pain following surgery may be less than that experienced before surgery. Determine measures that the patient has used in the past to relieve pain in the elbow, and use those measures as well as elevating the arm, applying ice as needed, and having the patient do finger and hand exercises when allowed. Medicate as needed.

Increase Mobility

Position. The position that is usually most comfortable for the patient is supine with the head of the bed elevated. The patient may turn to either side but will probably not be comfortable on the affected side. The affected arm will usually be in a posterior splint with 40 degrees of flexion, with the splint supported by a sling (see p. 594). The patient should be encouraged to use the trapeze with the unaffected arm to change position.

Exercises. Only mild finger exercises are allowed until the wound catheters are removed, approximately 2 to 3 days after surgery. Once the catheters are removed, the exercises are gradually increased, and by 2 weeks after surgery the patient is encouraged to do active exercises of the hand (see p. 510) and shoulder (see pp. 500 and 521–523). At that time, the posterior splint is removed for short periods, and gentle active controlled exercises of the elbow are begun. Passive exercises, using an elbow exerciser, may also be started (Fig. 10–12).

To overcome shortening of arm muscles, active exercises of the elbow, the wrist, and the forearm are usually done twice a day. To help loosen the muscles before beginning the exercises, the patient can place hot packs over the biceps and triceps and then massage the arm muscles with long rhythmic strokes toward the shoulder. The following are some exercises for elbow extension and flexion that prevent compensatory shoulder movement and produce a reflex relaxation of antagonistic muscles that makes active motion of the elbow easier. To promote elbow flexion, place the patient in a supine position on a firm surface with the affected arm extended. Place a folded towel under the affected triceps and stabilize the affected shoulder by placing your palm over the shoulder with your thumb on the insertion of the biceps. Tell the patient to try to flex the affected elbow while you supply slight resistance by holding the wrist with your other hand. To promote elbow extension, place the patient in the same position but have the patient flex the arm with the wrist toward the shoulder. Then, have the patient attempt to extend the forearm while you provide slight resistance on the back of the wrist and the forearm. The amount of exercise is increased gradually, but if there is even the slightest

TABLE 10–5. NURSING PROCESS FOR ELBOW ARTHROPLASTY WITH A POSTERIOR SPLINT

Assessment	Nursing Diagnosis	Goal Formulation	Planning and Intervention	Evaluation and Reassessment
1. Assess the location, duration, and severity of pain. Assess the neurovascular status of the affected arm. Check for signs of swelling. Check the position of the arm.	1. Alternation in comfort: pain in the elbow related to bone and soft tissue trauma.	1. Short-term goal: a relative state of comfort. Long-term goal: free of pain.	1. Alleviate Pain Elevate the hand and elbow. Apply ice to surgical site. Have the patient do finger and hand exercises when allowed. Utilize measures for pain relief that the patient has found helpful in the past. Administer pain medications. Teach relaxation technique.	1. Even though patients have experienced surgery with considerable bone trauma, they may have less pain than before surgery. Pain medications should relieve episodes of severe pain.
2. Assess the neurovascular status of the affected arm. Check the patient's ability to do finger exercises. Check the position of the arm and wrist. Assess mobility of the unaffected joints.	2. Impaired physical mobility: decreased arm function related to elbow joint instability.	2. Short-term goal: an increase in arm function through controlled exercises. Long-term goal: regain maximum function in the affected arm.	2. Increase Mobility *Position* The most comfortable position is supine with the head of the bed elevated. The patient may turn to either side but is generally more comfortable on unaffected side. The arm is kept in splint with 40 degrees of flexion. Teach how to use trapeze. *Exercises* Mild finger exercises should be started 2–3 days after surgery. Start active finger and shoulder exercises 2 weeks after surgery. Start elbow exercises when splint is removed. Use hot packs and massage before doing elbow exercises.	2. The patient should be able to lie supine with the arm elevated. The wrist should not be flexed at the edge of the splint. The patient should be able to do mild finger exercises without an increase in pain. The patient should do the exercises without direct supervision. Using hot packs and massage before doing elbow

			Ambulation Assist the patient with getting out of bed. Start ambulation the second day.	exercises should help to reduce muscle spasms that occur when the elbow is extended. The patient should have no problem with ambulation unless she or he has pathology of the lower extremity.
3. Assess for any signs of infection. Check for any swelling or complaints of pain at the surgical site.	3. Potential for injury: infection related to surgical incision.	3. Short- and long-term goal: free of any complications.	3. Prevent Complications Keep the dressing clean and dry. Observe for signs of infection. Administer antibiotics. *Other Complications* (See text.)	3. The patient should be free of any complications.
4. Assess level of knowledge concerning rehabilitation process and self-care.	4. Potential knowledge deficit related to rehabilitation process and self-care.	4. Short-term and long-term goal: decrease in anxiety through increased knowledge.	4. Patient Teaching Explain the various steps in the rehabilitation process. Write down the various exercises. Discuss the importance of not forcing the elbow to flex or extend all at once but to gradually increase flexion and extension. Discuss methods of bathing and dressing at home.	4. The patient should verbalize an understanding of the rehabilitation process. The patient should realize that time and effort are needed to regain function of the elbow. Only prescribed exercises should be done.

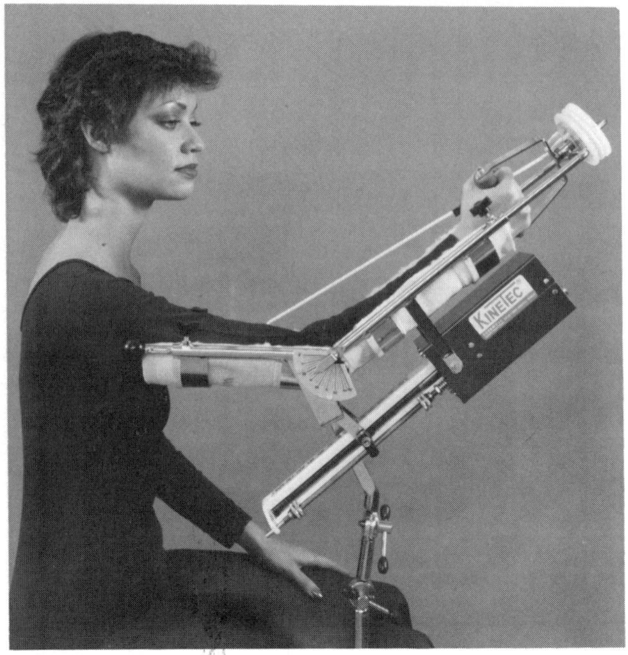

Figure 10–12. The Kinetic elbow exerciser provides passive motion for the elbow. *(Courtesy of Richards Medical Company. KINETIC is a registered trademark of CO-GEMO, an affiliate of Richards Medical Company.)*

pain, the exercises should be stopped. If the elbow becomes stiff and sore, the arm should be placed back in the sling, and splinting may be necessary for a few days. In addition to those exercises, some daily activities that increase elbow flexion are eating, hair combing, writing, and turning the pages of a book. Walking with the arm at one's side increases elbow extension. Active range-of-motion exercises of the shoulder, the wrist, and the fingers, however, should be continued.

Ambulation. Ambulation is usually allowed by the second day after surgery, but may be postponed until the wound catheters are removed. At first, the patient will need assistance in getting out of bed and in balancing during ambulation.

Prevent Complications. The major complications following an elbow arthroplasty are (1) infection, (2) loosening of one or both components, (3) breakage of a component, (4) rupture of the triceps, (5) a fracture of the bone surrounding the prosthesis, and (6) contractures of the elbow.

Observe for signs of possible infection. Most patients will be on antibiotic therapy immediately after surgery. Infection at the sites where the prosthesis is inserted can cause a loosening of the prosthesis, which can necessitate surgical removal and an elbow arthrodesis. Patients who have sustained a rupture of the triceps or a fracture of the surrounding bone may need added or extended immobilization. The elbow does not tolerate surgery and immobilization well. Following the prescribed exercise regime is necessary to prevent elbow contractures.

Patient Teaching. Following an arthroplasty of the elbow, the patient must know how to recognize the signs and symptoms of infection and whom to notify if one should occur. Discuss with the patient the results to be gained from an elbow arthroplasty. The patient must realize that time and effort are needed before he or she can regain function in the elbow. Only the prescribed exercises should be done, and the patient should not force the elbow to bend or straighten.

Evaluation and Reassessment

The patient should have minimal pain that responds to medication and exercise. A slow return to normal function in the elbow is to be expected. The patient should be encouraged to continue with the required exercises and should understand that he or she should not try to rush the progress by increasing the level of exercise or by forcing the elbow to flex or extend.

SPECIAL CONDITIONS

Tennis Elbow

The syndrome of chronic disabling pain in the region of the lateral epicondyle of the humerus, which radiates down the extensor surface of the forearm, is referred to as "tennis elbow." Tennis elbow is brought on by activities that combine excessive pronation and supination of the forearm with an extended wrist. The condition is particularly frequent after such activities as playing tennis or racquetball, or using a screwdriver, especially among persons not used to those activities. However, it is also common in individuals whose occupations require the frequent rotary motion of the forearm (e.g., tennis players, plumbers, and carpenters). It is often associated with tendinitis of the shoulder, fibrositis of the back, and other collagenous degenerative conditions occurring in young and middle-aged adults (Turek, 1977, pp. 871–872).

Although the movements producing tennis elbow are fairly well understood, the actual cause of the pain has never been clearly established. Some of the possible causes are radiohumeral bursitis, tendinitis at the common extensor origin, and traumatic epicondylitis or periostitis at the lateral epicondyle. The syndrome is not called epicondylitis or radiohumeral bursitis because of the lack of specificity regarding its origin.

The onset of the condition is usually gradual. An ache appears over the outer aspect of the elbow and is referred into the forearm. It is persistent and intensified by grasping or twisting motions. Grasping requires setting of the extensor carpi radialis brevis and longus muscles while rotary or twisting motions of the forearm toward supination require active contraction of the supinator longus and brevis. Those muscles originate from the lateral epicondyle and epicondylar ridge and the anterior capsule of the elbow joint. A well-localized point of tenderness exists at one of the following sites: the epicondylar ridge, lateral epicondyle, anterior lower edge of the capitellum, over the lateral radiohumeral interval, or near a portion of the circumference of the radial head. Most commonly, it is over the anterior aspect of the radial head when the forearm is in full supination. Swelling is rarely present, and the range of motion is normal. The patient complains of weakness of grasp, particularly with the forearm pronated. A clinical test consists of reproducing the pain by completely extending the elbow, pronating the forearm, and forcibly flexing the wrist (Fig. 10–13). Active attempts to dorsiflex the wrist and supinate the forearm against resistance will also intensify the discomfort. Roentgenographic examination of the elbow is usually negative, but on rare occasions calcium deposits have been noted.

Conservative treatment is effective most of the time, but recurrences are common. One of the best ways to prevent a recurrence is to identify the movements that brought on the tennis elbow, and then to have the patient avoid them. Most patients respond to moist heat, short-wave diathermy, and analgesics. Some authorities utilize local injections of corticosteroids at the site of maximum tenderness. Occasionally it may be necessary to rest the extensor tendons. To maintain relaxation of the extensors, the arm is placed in a posterior molded cast or splint with the elbow in flexion, supination, and extension at the wrist. In some instances the wrist may be left free for movement. If the patient has on a cast or splint, it should be removed at least daily for gentle exercises to avoid elbow stiffness.

For a few patients, conservative treatment will be unsuccessful and an op-

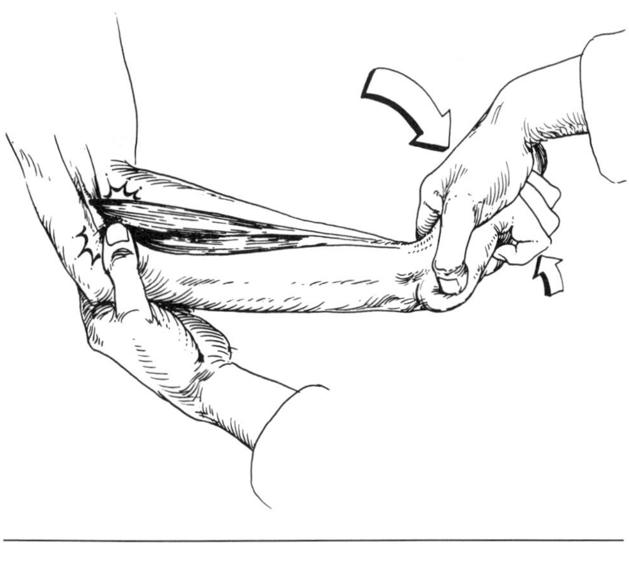

Figure 10–13. The tennis elbow test.

erative procedure will become necessary. One surgical procedure is to transversely divide the fascial covering of the tendons and then divide the intramuscular septum. The conjoined tendons are then severed at the epicondyle and the epicondylar ridge, and the remaining fibers are detached from the anterior joint capsule. The tendons and the extensor muscles are then allowed to displace distally. An optimal addition to the procedure is the resection of a portion of the annular ligament. The closure is only of subcutaneous tissues and skin. An elastic compression bandage is then applied and immediate motion of the joint is permitted.

Another surgical procedure for tennis elbow is the elevation of the conjoined tendons at the epicondyle and the curretage of cortical bone to expose cancellous bone. Crisscross sutures of heavy silk are then made through the tendons, which are then sutured to the cancellous bone through holes that have been drilled into the bone. The procedure helps to avoid weakening of the extensor muscles by reducing the distance between origin and insertion. Postoperatively the arm is immobilized for 6 weeks with the elbow flexed, the forearm supinated, and the wrist dorsiflexed.

Medial Epicondylitis

On rare occasions, the region of the medial epicondyle of the humerus may become painful as a result of activity that puts excessive strain on the common flexor pronator tendon. Pain is aggravated by the forced palmar flexion of the wrist against resistance, which places tension on the common flexor pronator tendon. Discomfort is intensified by strong grasping involving active flexion of the wrist, and by pronation of the forearm against resistance. The same measures used in treating tennis elbow can be used for a patient with medial epicondylitis.

Olecranon Bursitis

A bursitis is an inflammation of the sac (bursa) covering a bony prominence (Fig. 10–14). Trauma to the point of the elbow often results in marked swelling of the olecranon bursa, giving rise to a large knob (or goose-egg) at the elbow. Following trauma, the fluid contained in the bursal sac is frequently bloody. Tenderness and swelling of the bursa may also be seen with gout, rheumatoid arthritis, and infections, all of which lead to a thickening of the bursal walls.

Treatment consists of aspiration of the fluid and local instillation of corticosteroids, followed by application of a pressure dressing. If the problem cannot be controlled conservatively, surgical removal of the thickened bursa may be necessary.

Traumatic Ulnar Neuritis

Because of its vulnerable position in the ulnar groove behind the medial epicondyle of the humerus, the ulnar nerve may be impinged upon, giving rise to a traumatic ulnar neuritis. The ulnar nerve is unusually mobile in some people,

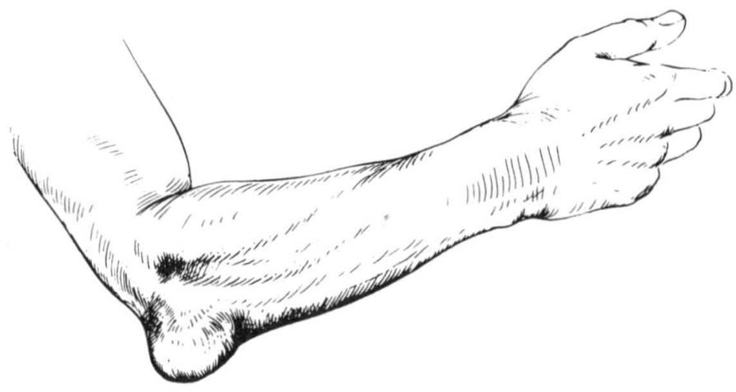

Figure 10–14. Localized swelling of the olecranon bursa.

and dislocates across the tip of the medial epicondyle on flexion, returning to its normal location when the elbow is extended. In some patients, a traumatic ulnar neuritis develops from that friction alone. Other causes of traumatic ulnar neuritis are osteoarthritis spur formation in the ulnar groove, scarring following laceration or contusion of the soft tissues near the medial epicondyle, and any congenital deformity that increases the carrying angle of the elbow. The most common cause of traumatic ulnar neuritis, however, is residual deformity of the elbow from a previous fracture, specifically a cubitus valgus deformity following a supracondylar fracture of the humerus or displaced fracture of the medial epicondyle of the humerus.

The patient with ulnar neuritis usually complains of numbness, tingling, and pain over the ulnar nerve distribution, particularly the fourth and fifth fingers. A feeling of clumsiness in the affected hand may also be noted by the patient. The condition can progress from the stage of muscle weakness to muscle wasting and complete paralysis.

The treatment for traumatic ulnar neuritis is the displacement of the ulnar nerve from the area of irritation, preferably before motor changes occur and while sensory complaints are still reversible. That can be accomplished by surgically transposing the nerve anteriorly to the front of the medial epicondyle and burying it beneath the mass of soft flexor muscle tissue.

Osteochondritis Dissecans of the Elbow

Osteochondritis dissecans of the elbow is the condition in which one or more fragments of articular cartilage, with or without subchondral bone, become partially or completely separated from the parent bone and intrude into the joint cavity. The source of the fragments is usually the capitellum of the humerus. The incidence of osteochondritis dissecans in the elbow is second only to that in the knee, which is affected in 85 percent of the cases.

The condition usually appears in adolescence, and in men more often than women. The right elbow is involved more frequently than the left, but occasionally the condition is bilateral. Authorities have hypothesized that repeated minor injuries are the cause of osteochondritis dissecans, but that is not universally accepted because individuals in occupations that involve stress and trauma to the elbow display no greater than the usual incidence. Early in the condition, the overlying intact articular cartilage appears normal, or slightly discolored. Later, the surface of the capitellum of the humerus becomes ragged, and a deep crater may develop. There are typically several loose bodies within the joint cavity, especially anteriorly or in the supratrochlear fossa posteriorly. The largest loose body usually consists of a center of bone and a covering of hyaline cartilage, whereas the smaller ones usually consist entirely of cartilage and thus are not visible in roentgenograms. Features of osteochondritis dissecans specific to the elbow are an enlargement of the radius (characteristically in a posterolateral direction), a funnel-shaped metaphysis, and a premature fusion of the epiphyseal lines, usually beginning on the lateral aspect and proceeding medially.

The presence of osteochondritis dissecans in an elbow joint may cause pain, joint swelling, and restriction of motion. The first indications may be swelling in the joint, a dull ache, and a slight stiffness. If a fragment becomes wedged between the bones of the joint, it can lock the elbow in one position or block the full extension of the elbow.

If a diagnosis is made before the fragments completely separate, healing may take place if the joint is immobilized (e.g., in a sling). If healing does not occur or the fragments separate, surgical excision by an arthrotomy or arthroscopy is indicated. However, the irregular articulation between the radial head and the capitellum usually continues to shear off fragments of cartilage which, lying free within the joint, continue to grow and enlarge. Therefore, removal of the radial head may be necessary to prevent the recurrence of loose bodies and to halt the spread of degenerative changes. Removal of the radial head may also be indicated to improve motion.

Loose Bodies

Joints, on occasion, have been found to contain loose fragments of bone, cartilage, or calcified tissue that, by their presence and mobility, cause pain, irritation, and locking of the joint. These loose fragments are known as loose bodies or "joint mice." Loose bodies are found in the knee, the elbow, the shoulder, the hip, and the ankle joints. They arise as a result of trauma or disease, such as osteochondritis dissecans, fractures of the articular surface, fractures of an osteoarthritic spur, fractures of the articular hyaline cartilage, and osteochondromatosis. Treatment is surgical removal to relieve the symptoms caused by those fragments and to save the joint from further damage. The surgical procedure is usually an arthrotomy or an arthroscopy.

NEOPLASM

The largest group of benign bone tumors are osteochondromas, which are composed of spongy bone covered by a cartilaginous cap. Osteochondromas appear and grow during the individual's growth period, but rarely thereafter.

The tumor typically occurs in long tubular bones, especially about the knee, the ankle, the hip, the shoulder, and the elbow. It is usually located in the bone at the site of tendinous attachments of strong muscles.

Pain is usually mild and due to an overlying bursitis. Surgical removal is indicated if there is interference with joint function, repeated painful bursitis, a fracture of the bone through the tumor, or a suspicion of malignant change. The tumor is not sensitive to radiation.

AMPUTATION AT THE ELBOW

A disarticulation of the elbow is the removal of the arm at the level of the distal condyles of the humerus. The elbow joint amputation is believed to be an excellent level for an amputation because the broad flair of the humeral condyles can be firmly grasped by the prosthetic socket and humeral rotation can be transmitted to the prosthesis. In more proximal amputations humeral rotation cannot be transmitted, and a prosthetic elbow turntable is necessary (for amputation at the shoulder, see pp. 547–548). Most authorities believe that disarticulation of the elbow is preferable to a more proximal amputation. The focus of nursing care is to help the patient adjust to a change in body image, and assist in rehabilitation with or without a prosthesis.

THE FOREARM

Trauma

FRACTURES OF THE FOREARM

Fractures of the forearm include fractures of the radius, fractures of the ulna, fractures of the shaft of the ulna with a dislocation of the head of the radius (Monteggia fracture–dislocation), and fractures of the radius with a dislocation of the lower end of the ulna (Galeazzi fracture). If there is a fracture of only one bone, angulation and overriding is usually prevented by the other, but if angulation or overriding occurs, it indicates that there is a dislocation of one of the radioulnar joints. The displacement of the fragments depends upon the relationship of the fracture site to the attachments of the pronator and supinator muscles.

Fractures of the Radius

Fractures of the radius are the most common fractures of the forearm. In fractures of the upper third of the shaft of the radius, the proximal fragment is supinated and the distal pronated. Treatment therefore involves immobilizing the forearm, the wrist, and the hand in full supination so that the lower fragment is aligned with the upper one. Fractures of the middle and lower thirds of the radius are immobilized with the hand, the wrist, and the forearm midway between full supination and full pronation. If that procedure is not followed, there may well be permanent limitation of supination and pronation.

Fractures of the Radius and Ulna

Forearm fractures of the ulna alone are rare, but fractures of both the ulna and the radius can occur at any age. In children they may be greenstick fractures but in adults they are usually associated with considerable displacement. Pronation and supination are the essential functional motions of the forearm. To preserve those functions after a fracture, the two bones must be replaced so that they will be in correct relative alignment. The width of the interosseous space varies according to the tension or relaxation of the muscles that rotate the forearm from pronation to supination. Therefore, the governing factor determining the position in which the distal fragments of the fractures are placed in relation to the proximal fragments is the location of the muscle attachments in relation to the fracture site. In fractures above the pronator radii teres, there is outward rotation of the upper fragment of the radius by the biceps tendon. Therefore, the forearm must be placed in outward rotation (supination). In fractures below the pronator radii teres, the forearm must be placed in a position of inward rotation (pronation) to match the muscle action above (Edmondson & Crenshaw, 1980, p. 698). When there is a fracture of both bones it is usually difficult to achieve and maintain a satisfactory reduction by closed manipulation and immobilization in a long arm cast. This is especially true for the ulna, which is not as well supplied with blood as the radius. Unsatisfactory results from closed treatment have been reported in 38 to 74 percent of all cases (Iversen & Clawson, 1977, p. 165). A surgical procedure that involves bone grafting and the possible use of bone plating or intermedullary nailing may be necessary to repair the fractures.

Closed Fractures

In adults, when there is a closed fracture of both the ulna and the radius, or a displaced, isolated closed fracture of the ulna or the radius, the treatment is by open reduction with internal fixation. This can be accomplished by the use of plates and screws (e.g., the AO standard compression plate, the dynamic compression plate [DCP], or the semitubular plate) or by medullary fixation (e.g., Sage nails) (Fig. 10–15). Normally, the radius is repaired by the application of a plate and the ulna fixed by inserting an intramedullary nail. In a plate and screw repair, there is frequently a bone graft at the fracture site, and the plate is secured by four to five screws that engage the cortices of the bone above and below the fracture site. If closed fractures are left displaced, they lead to deformity and limitation of the rotation movements of the forearm. As with other fractures of the forearm, there is a risk of ischemic damage to the

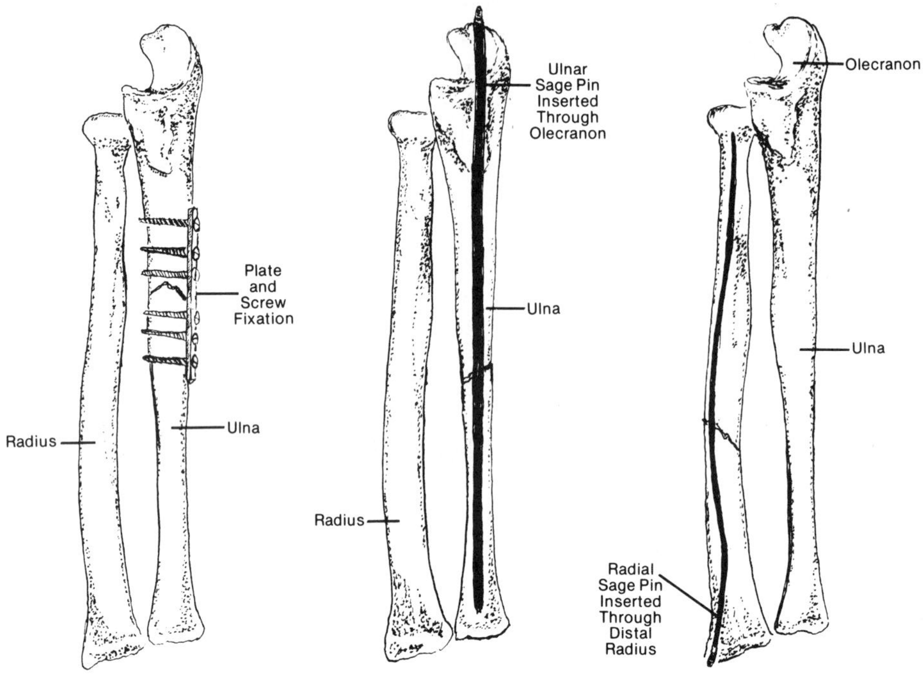

Figure 10–15. Open reduction and internal fixation, fractured radius or ulna. *(From Brantley, P., & Analla, M., 1980, p. 17. Courtesy of Howmedica.)*

forearm muscle, leading to severe loss of function of the hand (Edmondson & Crenshaw, 1980, pp. 698–699).

□ NURSING PROCESS (Table 10–6)

Assessment

The first step in the assessment of a typical patient with a compression dressing following an open reduction and internal fixation of a fracture of the ulna and the radius is to evaluate the neurovascular status of the affected arm and compare it with the unaffected arm (Chapter 2). Check the tightness of the dressing and the position of the arm. The arm should be elevated with the hand above the elbow. Check the dressing for any drainage and assess the location, duration, and severity of pain.

Nursing Diagnosis and Goal Formulation

Nursing diagnoses for a typical patient with a compression dressing following an open reduction and internal fixation of a fracture of the ulna and

TABLE 10–6. NURSING PROCESS FOR FRACTURES OF THE ULNA AND THE RADIUS TREATED WITH OPEN REDUCTION AND INTERNAL FIXATION

Assessment	Nursing Diagnosis	Goal Formulation	Planning and Intervention	Evaluation and Reassessment
1. Assess the location, duration, and severity of pain. Assess the neurovascular status of the affected arm. Check for tightness of the dressing and elevation of the affected arm.	1. Alteration in comfort: pain in the arm related to bone and soft tissue trauma.	1. Short-term goal: a relative state of comfort in the affected arm. Long-term goal: to be free of pain.	1. Alleviate Pain Elevate the affected arm. Apply ice bags to the fracture site. Instruct on finger and hand exercises. Utilize distraction and relaxation techniques. Administer pain medications.	1. The patient should remain relatively free of pain. Severe pain should be relieved by pain medications.
2. Check the position of the arm. Check the patients's ability to do gentle active exercises. Assess the patient's ability to ambulate without assistance. Assess the neurovascular status in affected arm.	2. Impaired physical mobility: decrease in arm function related to bone instability.	2. Short-term goal: an increase in mobility through the use of controlled exercises. Long-term goal: return of full range of motion with no reduction in muscle function.	2. Increase Mobility *Position* Keep the arm elevated. Keep the hand above the elbow. The patient can turn to any position of comfort. *Exercises* Instruct on gentle active exercises of the elbow, wrist, and hand. *Ambulation* Ambulate with the arm elevated. Start ambulation on the second day after surgery.	2. The patient should keep the arm elevated at all times. By 10–12 days after surgery, the patient should have good elbow, wrist, and forearm function. The patient should be able to ambulate with no problems with arm in a sling.

(continued)

TABLE 10–6. ***(Continued)***

Assessment	Nursing Diagnosis	Goal Formulation	Planning and Intervention	Evaluation and Reassessment
3. Assess neurovascular status in affected arm. Check for signs of swelling. Check the flexion of the elbow.	3. Potential for injury: neurovascular deficit related to soft tissue swelling.	3. Short- and long-term goal: free of any complications.	3. Prevent Complications *Circulatory* Do neurovascular assessments every 15 minutes for first 2 hours, every 30 minutes for next 2 hours, every 60 minutes for next 2 hours, every 2 hours for next 18 hours, and then at the beginning of every shift. Utilize methods to reduce swelling. Prevent acute flexion at the elbow. Prevent tightness of cast or dressing. Report any abnormal neurovascular change.	3. The patient should remain free of any neurovascular deficit.

Assess for signs of infection. Check for signs of swelling. Assess for any change in the amount of pain.	Potential for injury: infection related to surgical incision.	Short- and long-term goal: free of any complications.	*Integumentary* Assess for signs of infection. Keep dressing clean and dry. Administer antibiotics. *Other Complications* (See text.)	The patient should remain free of infection.
4. Assess knowledge level about the rehabilitation program and self-care activities.	4. Potential knowledge deficit related to rehabilitation process and self-care.	4. Short- and long-term goal: a decrease in anxiety through increased knowledge.	4. Patient Teaching Teach specific exercises to increase range of motion. Discuss the steps of the rehabilitation process. Caution the patient against lifting or doing strenuous arm activities until the fractures have healed. Discuss methods of self-care and dressing.	4. The patient should verbalize an understanding of the rehabilitation process and imposed restrictions on activity. The patient should demonstrate confidence in doing exercises and self-care.

the radius are (1) alterations in comfort related to pain from the surgical procedure, (2) alterations in mobility related to lack of bone stability, (3) potential complications related to surgery and decreased arm mobility, and (4) alterations in psychological well-being related to anxiety and knowledge deficit about the surgery and the treatment methods.

Short-term goals are to have the patient experience (1) a decrease in the amount of pain, (2) an increase in bone stability, (3) an absence of complications from trauma and immobilization, and (4) a decrease in anxiety through increased knowledge. Long-term goals are to have the patient pain free and to regain full arm function.

Planning and Intervention

Alleviate Pain. Measures that help to relieve pain are elevating the affected arm, applying ice as needed to reduce swelling, having the patient do the prescribed exercises, using noninvasive measures to relieve pain, and medicating for pain as needed.

Increase Mobility

Position. The patient's arm needs to be on pillows. It is especially important that the patient's hand be above the elbow to prevent or reduce swelling. The patient can turn to any position of comfort while in bed.

Exercises. When the fractures are uncomminuted, good compression and rigid fixation have been achieved, and the patient is cooperative, external fixation is usually unnecessary. The compression dressing is applied for the first few days after surgery, and gentle active exercises of the elbow, the wrist, and the hand are started immediately. In instances of severely comminuted fractures or when the cooperation of the patient is questionable, however, external protection in the form of a cast may be used. The cast can be bivalved and removed to allow early range-of-motion exercises. In either case, a cast is applied prior to the patient's discharge from the hospital. By 10 to 12 days after surgery, motion in the wrist, the forearm, and the elbow is usually good. The better the range of motion before cast application, the more rapid the return of function once the fracture has healed and the cast is removed.

Ambulation. Ambulation is allowed within 1 to 2 days after surgery. The patient will initially need assistance in walking because of awkwardness due to the compression dressing or the bivalved cast and the restrictions on the used of the affected arm. The patient may or may not utilize a sling while in the hospital.

Prevent Complications. The most common complications for a patient with an open reduction and internal fixation of a fractured ulna and radius are neurovascular impairment and infection. Neurovascular impairment may be due to an injury at the time of the trauma, swelling at the elbow following trauma or surgery, acute flexion of the elbow, or tightness of the cast or compression dressing. Nursing interventions to reduce swelling, and early detection and reporting of any neurovascular impairment, are essential. Immediately report any neurovascular irregularity to the patient's physician. If the dressing or bivalved cast is too tight and is restricting circulation, it can be loosened, but there should be no change in the degree of flexion of the elbow.

To prevent infection, check for the signs and symptoms of infection, avoid contamination of the incision site, and make sure the patient eats a well-balanced diet and gets adequate rest. Many patients will be placed on IV antibiotics immediately following surgery.

Patient Teaching. The patient should be taught specific exercises to increase the range of motion of the shoulder and the hands, but cautioned against lifting or doing strenuous arm activities until the fractures have healed. The healing period varies considerably with the amount of soft tissue damage, the age of the patient, and individual differences in the speed of healing. Solid union cannot be expected in adults in less than 8 to 12 weeks. In some patients, because of delayed union, immobilization must be maintained for 3 to 4 months. This causes a considerable delay in the return of motion and function to the elbow and the muscles of the arm after the cast is removed.

The plates and screws used in the internal fixation are not removed unless they cause symptoms, except in young persons or those resuming vigorous contact athletics. In those cases the plates and screws are removed after 12 months, and in most cases after 18 months. If the plates and screws are removed too soon, or if the arm is not supported by a splint for about 6 weeks after their removal, the bones may refracture.

Even when the incision site heals properly, there is always a chance of infection. An infection can also develop from skin irritation due to the cast rubbing on bony prominences. Make sure the patient, the family, and significant others understand the signs and symptoms of infection and neurovascular impairment, and the procedures for cast care (Appendix B).

Evaluation and Reassessment

The patient should have minimal pain except for a short period immediately after exercising. There should be no complications from surgery or immobility. The patient should understand the purpose of the long arm cast and the need to exercise to regain arm function. The patient, the family, and significant others should understand how to prevent complications from the cast. The patient should feel confident about carrying out activities of daily living while in a long arm cast with minimal help from others.

Open Fractures

As a general rule, internal fixation is not used initially in the treatment of open fractures of the forearm.To reduce complications, the wound is usually first treated by irrigation and debridement. This allows the wound to either reveal itself as infected or heal. Once the wound is healed (10 to 21 days in the absence of infection), surgery may be done to insert an appropriate internal fixation device (e.g., a compression plate) or an external fixation device may be utilized.

In single bone fractures of the forearm, a cast with a window over the open wound may be used, because it can provide sufficient external fixation until the wound is healed and internal fixation can be inserted. Shortening from overriding, resulting from delay inserting internal fixation, is not a problem in a single bone fracture. To prevent shortening in both bone open fractures, pins are inserted through the proximal ulna and the bases of the second and third metacarpals, traction is applied to restore length, and the pins are then incorporated in a plaster cast that is windowed to allow treatment and inspection of the wounds. An external fixation apparatus, such as a Wagner or Hoffman device, is also satisfactory for reduction and skeletal fixation when extensive soft tissue wounds are involved or skin grafts may be necessary. A medullary nail through the ulna is another means of stabilizing the forearm. Skin grafting and similar procedures on soft tissues are almost impossible to carry out unless the forearm is stabilized by either external or internal methods.

Monteggia Fracture–Dislocation

A Monteggia fracture–dislocation is the combination of a fracture of the ulna with a dislocation of the proximal end of the radius, with or without a fracture of the radius. There are two different types. One is an anterior dislocation of the radial head with the accompanying ulnar fracture producing an anterior and lateral angulation. The other, less common type, is a posterior dislocation of the radial head with the ulnar fracture producing a posterior angulation.

Monteggia fracture–dislocations are fairly rare, but extremely difficult to treat. Manipulative reduction may be successful, but open reduction and internal fixation of the ulna is generally necessary. If there is an open reduction of the ulna, a compression plate is utilized for fixation. A closed reduction of the radius is then attempted by supining the forearm and applying pressure on the head of the radius. If that is not successful, an open reduction is done to reduce the radius. If an open radial reduction is needed, it is usually necessary to do a reconstruction of the annular ligament (Edmondson & Crenshaw, 1980, p. 691; Iversen & Clawson, 1977, pp. 164–165).

Postoperatively, the patient's arm is either placed in a posterior splint for 2 weeks and then in a cast, or is immediately placed in a long arm cast. In both procedures the patient's arm is immobilized for 4 to 6 weeks in a position of 100 to 120 degrees of flexion at the elbow, which relaxes the biceps and helps keep the radial head reduced. The cast is then removed and the arm is supported with a collar and cuff sling, still maintaining the elbow at 100 to 120 degrees of flexion. Gentle pronation and supination motions are permitted, but extension beyond 90 degrees is not allowed, until at least 6 weeks after surgery.

Galeazzi Fracture of the Radius

Galeazzi fracture is a fracture in the middle or distal thirds of the radius combined with a subluxation–dislocation of the inferior (distal) radioulnar joint. The triangular fibrocartilage of the radioulnar joint and the tip of the ulnar styloid process may be avulsed, and the ligaments of the inferior radioulnar joint torn. Galeazzi fracture occurs in about 5 percent of all forearm fractures (Iversen & Clawson, 1977, p. 166).

Treatment usually involves nonoperative manipulative reduction followed by a cast from the upper arm to the metacarpal heads. The elbow is flexed at a right angle, the forearm is held in mid-position, and the hand is held in full ulnar deviation. An alternative method is to treat Galeazzi fracture as a displaced fracture of the radius. The arm is immobilized in supination for 6 weeks, and then immobilized in a neutral position for another 6 weeks, or until the fracture has united. The inferior radioulnar joint must be kept reduced during the immobilization period. If the cast becomes loose after the swelling subsides, a new cast should be applied. If closed reduction is not effective, an open reduction and internal fixation with a plate and screws is used. The arm is then immobilized in a cast until the fracture heals.

AMPUTATIONS THROUGH THE FOREARM (BELOW ELBOW)

Amputations through the forearm are the result of neoplasms or trauma. Such amputations usually preserve as much length as possible, because today almost any well-constructed, well-healed, and satisfactorily padded stump can be fitted with a functional prosthesis. The more distal underlying soft tissues consist primarily of relatively avascular structures such as fascia and tendons, thus with few exceptions an amputation at the junction of the middle and distal thirds of the forearm is preferable to a more proximal amputation. Even a very short (3.8 cm) below-elbow stump is preferable to an amputation through or above the elbow. From a functional standpoint, preserving the patient's elbow joint is extremely important. Improved prosthetic fitting techniques, such as the Munster or a split socket with step-up hinges, can provide even a very short below-elbow stump with an excellent prosthetic device (Edmondson & Crenshaw, 1980, pp. 859–860). The focus of nursing care is to help the patient adjust to a change in body image and assist in rehabilitation with or without a prosthesis.

REFERENCES

Brantley, P., & Analla, M. *The nurse and orthopedic surgery.* Rutherford, N. J.: The Orthopedic Nurses' Association, Inc., in cooperation with Howmedica, Inc., 1980.

DeGowin, E. L., & DeGowin, R. L. *Bedside diagnostic examination* (3rd ed.). New York: Macmillan, 1976.

Edmondson, A. S., & Crenshaw, A. H. *Campbell's operative orthopaedics* (6th ed.). St. Louis: C. V. Mosby, 1980.

Gartland, J. J. *Fundamentals of orthopaedics* (3rd ed.). Philadelphia: W. B. Saunders, 1979.

Iversen, L. D., & Clawson, D. K. *Manual of acute orthopaedic therapeutics.* Boston: Little, Brown, 1977.

Roaf, R., & Hodkinson, L. J. *Textbook of orthopaedic nursing* (2nd ed.). Oxford: Blackwell Scientific, 1975.

Turek, S. L. *Orthopaedics, principles and their applications* (3rd ed.). Philadelphia: Lippincott, 1977.

BIBLIOGRAPHY

Albright, J. A., & Brand, R. A. (Eds.). *The scientific basis of orthopaedics.* New York: Appleton-Century-Crofts, 1979.

Arthritis Health Profession Section of the Arthritis Foundation. *Self-help manual for patients with arthritis.* Atlanta, Ga.: Arthritis Foundation, 1980.

Burgess, E. M. Amputations. *Surgical Clinics of North America,* 1983, *63* (3), 749–770.

Cailliet, R. *Soft tissue pain and disability* (5th ed.). Philadelphia: F. A. Davis, 1981.

Cochran, G. Van B. *A primer of orthopaedic biomechanics.* New York: Churchill Livingstone, 1982.

During, M., Müller, W., Rüldi, T. P., & Gauer, S. F. The operative treatment of elbow dislocation in the adult. *Journal of Bone and Joint Surgery,* 1979, *61A* (2), 239–244.

Fries, J. F. *Arthritis, A comprehensive guide.* Menlo Park, Calif.: Addison-Wesley, 1982.

Ghista, D. N., & Roaf, R. *Orthopaedic mechanics: Procedures and devices.* San Francisco: Academic Press, 1978.

Grace, T. G., & Eversmann, W. W. Forearm fractures. *Journal of Bone and Joint Surgery,* 1980, *62A* (3), 433–438.

Grace, T. G., & Eversmann, W. W. The management of segmental bone loss associated with forearm fractures. *Journal of Bone and Joint Surgery,* 1980, *62A* (7), 1150–1155.

Green, D. P., & McCoy H. Turnbuckle arthitic correction of elbow flexion contractures after acute injuries. *Journal of Bone and Joint Surgery,* 1979, *61A* (7), 1092–1095.

Herndon, J. H., & Hubbard, L. F. Total joint replacement in the upper extremity. *Surgical Clinics of North America,* 1983, *63* (2), 715–736.

Hoppenfeld, S. *Physical examination of the spine and extremities.* New York: Appleton-Century-Crofts, 1976.

Kerr, A. *Orthopedic nursing procedures: Part 1. Initial and emergency care.* New York: Springer, 1980.

Kudo, H., Inano, K., & Watanabe, S. Total replacement of the rheumatoid elbow with a hingeless prosthesis. *Journal of Bone and Joint Surgery,* 1980, *62A* (2), 277–285.

LaFrenier, J. G. Tennis elbow: Evaluation, treatment and prevention. *Physical Therapy,* 1979, *59* (6), 742–746.

Larson, C. B., & Gould, M. *Orthopedic nursing* (9th ed.). St. Louis: C. V. Mosby, 1978.

Mansli, A. Medial displacement of the shaft of the radius with a fracture of the radial neck. *Journal of Bone and Joint Surgery,* 1979, *61A* (5), 788–789.
Morrey, B. F., Chao, E. Y., & Hui, F. C. Biomechanical study of the elbow following excision of the radial head. *Journal of Bone and Joint Surgery,* 1979, *61A* (1), 63–68.
Nirschi, R. P., & Pettrone, F. A. Tennis elbow: The surgical treatment of lateral epicondylitis. *Journal of Bone and Joint Surgery,* 1979, *61A* (6), 832–839.
Odenheimer, K., & Harvey, J. P. Internal fixation of fracture of the head of the radius. *Journal of Bone and Joint Surgery,* 1979, *61A* (5), 785–787.
Protzman, R. R. Dislocation of the elbow joint. *Journal of Bone and Joint Surgery,* 1978, *60A* (4), 539–541.
Robbins, S. L. *Pathologic basis of disease.* Philadelphia: W. B. Saunders, 1974.
Ross, N. Volkmann's ischaemic contracture: A complication following elbow injuries. *Orthopedic Nurses' Association Journal,* 1979, *6* (5), 211–215.
Shahriaree, H., Sajadi, K., Silver, C. M., & Shukholesleslamzadeh, S. Excisional arthroplasty of the elbow. *Journal of Bone and Joint Surgery,* 1979, *61A* (6), 922–927.
Swinson, D. R., & Swinburn, W. R. *Rheumatology.* New York: Wiley, 1980.
Zimmer. *The traction handbook.* Warsaw, Ind.: Zimmer, USA, 1980.

11

THE WRIST AND HAND

Chapter 11 focuses on the treatment and associated nursing care of patients with traumatic and pathological conditions of the wrist and the hand, from minor sprains to amputations and reconstructive surgery. The chapter begins with a review of the anatomy of the wrist and the hand.

ANATOMY

BONES

The skeleton of the wrist and hand has four main segments: (1) the distal radius and the ulna, (2) the carpal or wrist bones, (3) the metacarpal bones of the palm, and (4) the phalanges or bones of the fingers (Fig. 11–1).

Distal Radius and Ulna

The distal portion of the radius, its widest end, is four-sided. With the arm in pronation, the medial surface of the radius is slightly rough and projects downward beyond the rest of the bone to form a styloid process. Its lateral surface is the ulnar notch, a smooth strip, concave for articulation with the head of the ulna in the inferior radioulnar joint. The anterior surface is a thick prominent ridge, and the posterior surface is marked by the dorsal tubercle. The most distal surface of the radius is smooth and articulates with the wrist bones.

The distal ulna is slightly enlarged and comprises a rounded head and a styloid process. With the arm in pronation, the head forms a surface elevation on the lateral part of the posterior aspect of the wrist. The styloid process is then a short, rounded projection from the lateral aspect of the distal ulna.

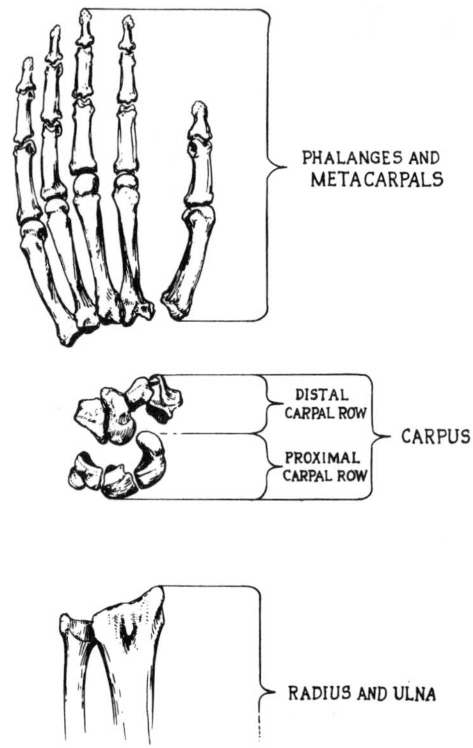

Figure 11–1. The bony anatomy of the wrist and hand. *(Figures 11–1 through 11–4, 11–14 through 11–16, 11–19, and 11–22 through 11–25 are reproduced from Hoppenfeld, S., 1976, with permission.)*

Carpal Bones

The carpus (wrist) is composed of eight carpal bones that are arranged in proximal and distal rows, each containing four bones. With the arm in supination, the bones of the proximal row from lateral to medial are the scaphoid (navicular), lunate, triquetral, and pisiform. The bones of the distal row are the trapezium, trapezoid, capitate, and hamate (Fig. 11–2). In the proximal row the pisiform is on the palmar surface of the triquetral bone and is separated from the other carpal bones (Fig. 11–3). The other bones of the proximal row form an arch that articulates with the radius and the articular disc of the distal radioulnar joint.

Metacarpal Bones

The metacarpus (palm) consists of five metacarpal bones, conventionally numbered from lateral to medial (with the arm in supination). The metacarpals are miniature long bones, each possessing a rounded head, a shaft, and an expanded base. The heads are the distal ends and articulate with the proximal

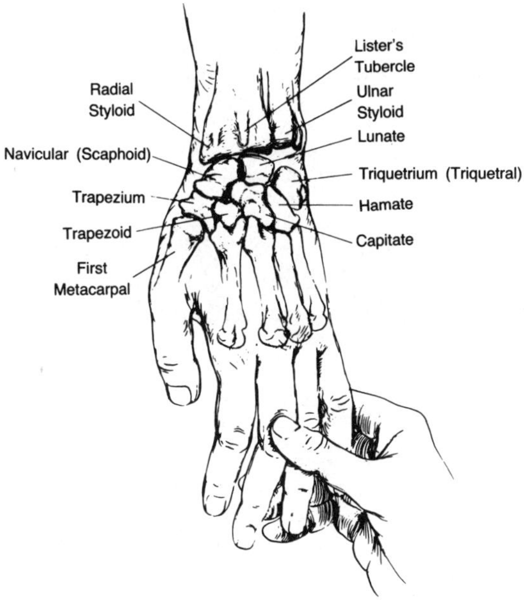

Figure 11–2. The bones of the wrist, dorsal aspect.

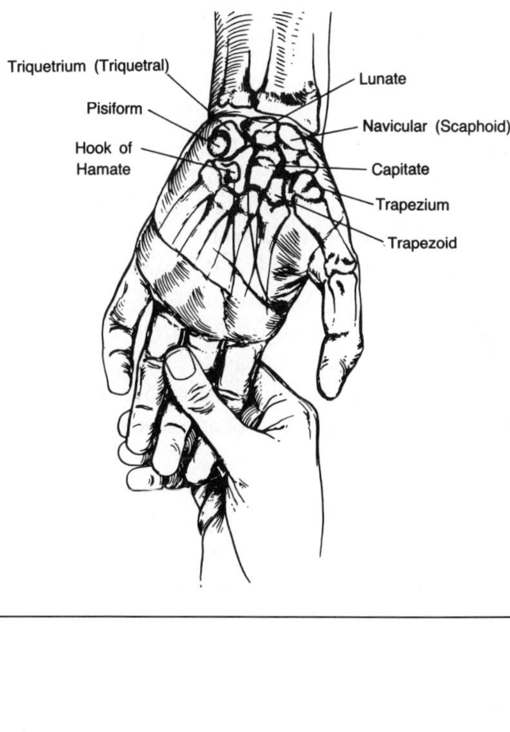

Figure 11–3. The bones of the wrist, volar aspect.

phalanges. The prominence of the knuckles is produced by the metacarpal heads. The bases are the proximal ends and articulate with the distal row of the carpal bones and with one another except that the first metacarpal bone (for the thumb) is isolated and does not articulate with the second metacarpal bone.

Phalangeal Bones

There are 14 phalanges, two in the thumb and three in each of the other digits. Each has a head, a shaft, and a base or proximal end. The bases of the proximal phalanges articulate with the heads of the metacarpal bones.

JOINTS OF THE WRIST AND HAND

The Distal Radioulnar Joint

The distal radioulnar joint is a uniaxial pivot joint between the distal end (head) of the ulna and the ulnar notch of the distal end of the radius. The joint surfaces are enclosed in an articular capsule and held together by an articular disc.

The movements that take place at the radioulnar joint result in pronation and supination of the hand. The muscle producing pronation is the pronator quadratus, which is aided during rapid movement and movement against resistance by the pronator teres. The muscle producing supination in slow unresisted movements and when the elbow is extended is the supinator. It is assisted by the biceps in fast movements with the elbow flexed, especially when resistance is encountered.

The Radiocarpal or Wrist Joint

The radiocarpal or wrist joint is a biaxial joint. Proximally, it is formed by the distal end of the radius and the lower surface of the articular disc between the radius and the ulna, and distally by the scaphoid, the lunate, and the triquetral bones.

The fibrous articular capsule of the radiocarpal joint is lined by a synovial membrane. The joint capsule is strengthened by a number of ligaments, specifically the palmar radiocarpal and ulnocarpal, the dorsal radiocarpal, and the radial and ulnar collateral. The movements of the radiocarpal joint are closely associated with those in the intercarpal joints.

The arteries supplying the joint are the anterior interosseous, the anterior and posterior carpal branches of the radial and ulnar, the palmar and dorsal metacarpals, and some recurrent branches of the deep palmar arch. The nerves are derived from the anterior and posterior interosseous nerves.

Intercarpal Joints

The intercarpal joints connect the carpal bones to one another and may be subdivided into (1) joints between the bones of the proximal row of the carpus, (2) joints between the bones of the distal row, and (3) a somewhat complicated and extensive joint between the two rows, termed the midcarpal joint. The carpal bones are connected by an extensive system of ligaments.

Carpometacarpal Joints

The five carpometacarpal joints connect the carpal bones to the metacarpal bones. The first is the carpometacarpal joint of the thumb, which is a saddle-shaped joint between the first metacarpal bone and the trapezium and is held together by lateral, anterior, posterior, and capsular ligaments. The second through fifth are the joints between the carpus and the second, third, fourth, and fifth metacarpal bones. The bones of each of those four joints are united by articular capsules, and are strengthened by dorsal, palmar, and interosseous ligaments.

Metacarpophalangeal Joints

The five metacarpophalangeal joints connect the articulating heads of the metacarpals with shallow concavities on the bases of the proximal phalanges. Each joint has a palmar, a deep transverse metacarpal, and two collateral ligaments.

Interphalangeal Joints

The interphalangeal joints in each digit are uniaxial hinge joints. In addition to a fibrous capsule, each has a palmar and two collateral ligaments (Fig. 11–4). Extensor tendons take the place of dorsal ligaments.

CARPAL ARCH

The carpal bones form an arch that is concave on its palmar surface. The ligament that spans the arch and maintains it is called the flexor retinaculum or the transverse carpal ligament. The ligament is composed of a proximal and a distal band. The proximal band attaches from the tubercle of the scaphoid to the pisiform. The distal band connects the tubercle of the trapezium to the hook of the hamate.

The space between the arched carpal bones and the spanning transverse carpal ligament is termed the carpal tunnel. The tunnel contains the tendons of the flexor digitorum profundus, which lie upon the carpal bones, and the tendons of the flexor digitorum superficialis. Also within the tunnel are the

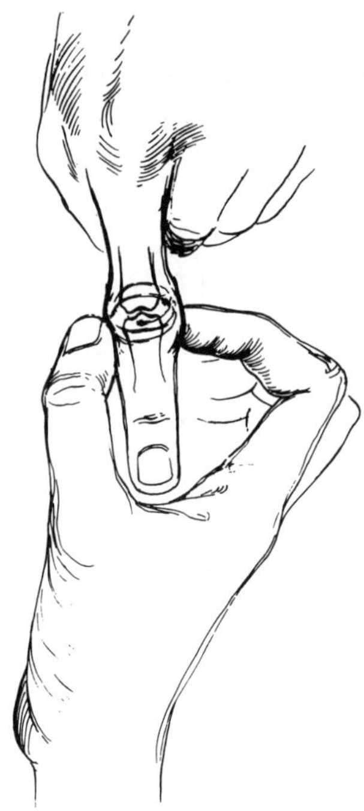

Figure 11–4. The proximal interphalangeal joint is covered by a thick joint capsule and the collateral ligaments.

flexor carpi radialis tendon, the flexor pollicis longus tendon, and the median nerve. The transverse carpal ligament protects the median nerve from external pressure (Cailliet, 1981, pp. 10–11).

THE WRIST

Trauma

The wrist, because of its mobility and exposed position, is frequently subjected to trauma, including lacerating injuries, sprains, dislocations, and fractures.

LACERATIONS

The wrist is the narrowest part of the arm. The tendons, nerves, and blood vessels of the hand must all pass through that narrow neck. Lacerating injuries at the wrist, therefore, can sever tendons, arteries, and nerves and inflict serious damage to the hand. With prompt medical attention, a lacerated or severed artery can usually be repaired or ligated (sutured) without danger of compromising the circulation. The repair of severed tendons and nerves is much more difficult, and successful restoration of the hand may depend upon sound surgical judgment and, frequently, the use of microsurgical techniques.

SPRAINS

Wrist sprains can give rise to pain, swelling, and loss of function of the hand. Most sprains of the wrist are momentary subluxations that spontaneously reduce. In a subluxation, as in a complete dislocation, the capsule and the collateral ligaments may be torn. Sprains are usually not detected on roentgenograms and thus tend to be ignored or minimized. Still, many authorities believe sprains of the wrist should be diagnosed as reduced subluxations. In the absence of complications, therefore, they should be treated by immobilization in a slightly flexed position for a period of 2 or 3 weeks, followed by the initiation of progressive active exercises. Despite treatment, limitation and swelling of the wrist may persist for months following a sprain. If pain and discomfort are not quickly reduced by immobilization, however, further investigation is required to eliminate more serious conditions, for example, a fracture of the scaphoid.

DISLOCATIONS

Dislocations of the wrist may occur at the radiocarpal joint or involve the bones of the carpus (Figs. 11–5A and B). Dislocations of the radiocarpal joint are commonly caused by a fall on the palm, which displaces the hand dorsally. Usually a dislocation of the radiocarpal joint can be readily treated by closed manipulation followed by immobilization for 3 to 4 weeks. If a closed reduction is unsuccessful, an open reduction may be necessary.

A dislocation of the lunate bone of the carpus is common, and may be caused by a fall on the palm that forces the wrist into sudden extension (Fig. 11–6). In some instances there may not be any other damage to the wrist, but in others it may dislocate anteriorly and proximally, tearing the capsule and coming to rest in the carpal tunnel. In that position, the lunate bone presses against the flexor tendons and causes the hand to be held with the wrist and the fingers in semiflexion. Motion of the wrist and the fingers is painful. The dislocated lunate bone may also press against the median nerve, causing a median neuritis characterized by pain, paresthesia, atrophy, and weakness or paralysis of the muscles of opposition. The injury may be difficult to detect on a roentgenogram.

If diagnosis is made early, closed reduction may be successful. A closed reduction may be accomplished under general or regional anesthesia by pro-

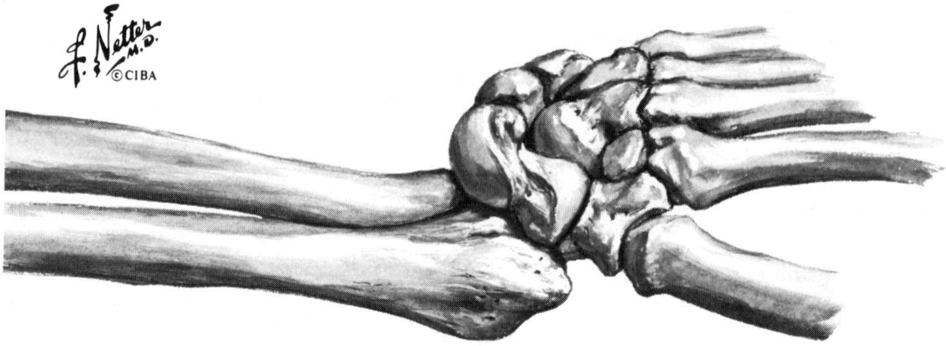

Figure 11–5. A. Dorsal dislocation of the carpus at the radiocarpal joint. *(Copyright © 1970, CIBA Pharmaceutical Company, Division of CIBA-GEIGY Corporation. Reprinted with permission from* Clinical symposia, *illustrated by Frank H. Netter, M.D. All rights reserved.)*

longed heavy traction or by direct pressure upon the palmar aspect of the lunate with simultaneous traction to the thumb and the fingers. A cast is then applied, or the wrist is immobilized in a dorsal splint with the hand in a compression dressing for the first 24 to 72 hours. After 24 to 72 hours, active range-of-motion exercises of the fingers are begun. The wrist is usually immobilized for 4 to 6 weeks. If closed reduction is not successful, an open reduction is necessary to reduce the dislocated lunate and repair the capsular tear. Some authorities favor excising a lunate bone if the bone is dislocated for a period longer than 3 weeks before reduction, because of the likelihood that avascular necrosis of the bone will develop.

Scapholunate dissociation is characterized by a vertical displacement of the scaphoid relative to the lunate and by a gap between the lunate and the proximal pole of the scaphoid. Roentgenographic examination, which includes

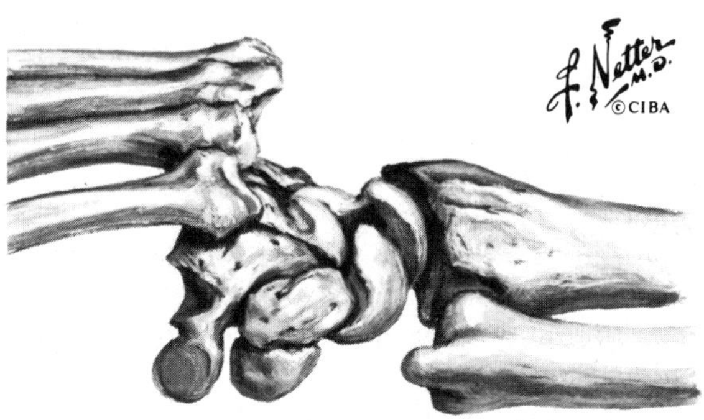

Figure 11–5. B. Dorsal metacarpocarpal dislocation. *(Copyright © 1970, CIBA Pharmaceutical Company, Division of CIBA-GEIGY Corporation. Reprinted with permission from* Clinical symposia, *illustrated by Frank H. Netter, M.D. All rights reserved.)*

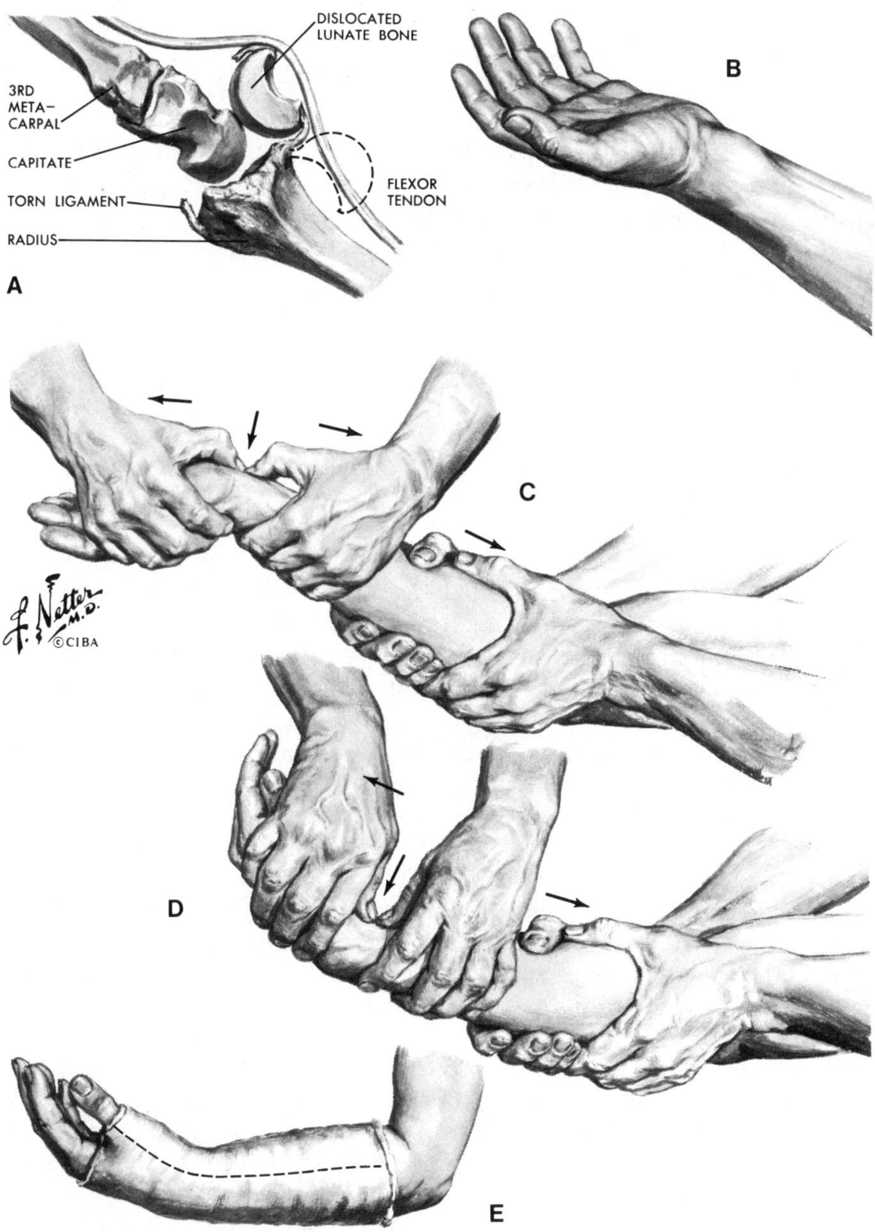

Figure 11–6. A. Dislocation of lunate bone: Broken line indicates more severe dislocation. **B.** Typical deformity in dislocation of lunate bone. **C.** Reduction: With traction applied to dorsiflexed hand and countertraction to forearm, pressure is made by operator's thumbs over the dislocated lunate bone to push it dorsally into position. **D.** As the bone is felt to relocate, the hand is brought into flexion while maintaining thumb pressure as well as traction and counteraction. **E.** The wrist is immobilized in about 20 degrees flexion for 3 to 4 weeks by posterior splint or forearm cast, which may be bivalved as indicated to allow for swelling. *(Copyright © 1970, CIBA Pharmaceutical Company, Division of CIBA-GEIGY Corporation. Reprinted with permission from* Clinical symposia, *illustrated by Frank H. Netter, M.D. All rights reserved.)*

stress views of the wrist, usually demonstrates a gap wider than the normal 2 mm. Treatment for an acute scapholunate dissociation usually involves an open reduction, often with fixation by Kirschner wires and a volar ligament repair. A long arm cast is used for approximately 8 weeks to keep the wrist immobilized. With a chronic dissociation, a reduction may be accomplished by prolonged heavy traction or by hyperextension of the wrist in traction with pressure directed dorsally over the scaphoid. If that fails, a fusion or Silastic implant may be indicated.

FRACTURES

Fractures of the Distal Radius

Colles' Fracture

A Colles' fracture is a nonarticular fracture of the distal radius, with or without a fracture of the ulnar styloid (Fig. 11–7). There is a volar angulation of the radius and a dorsal displacement of the distal fragment. Colles' fractures are commonly produced by a fall on an outstretched hand, and may be accompanied by a fracture of the elbow or shoulder. They are often seen in elderly women.

Clinically, the wrist appears puffy and deformed. The distal radial fragment gives rise to the characteristic hump ("silver fork" or "dinner fork") deformity seen when the wrist is viewed from the side. Backward displacement of the distal radial fragment causes shortening of the radius and an alteration in the normal position of the radial styloid in relation to the ulnar styloid. There is tenderness over the distal radius and over the ulnar styloid or medial ligament of the wrist. The normal volar concavity of the radius is lost and the area feels distended to the touch. Roentgenographic examination confirms the diagnosis and also shows if impaction or comminution of the fragments is present.

Many Colles' fractures can be adequately reduced by closed manipulation with or without anesthesia. The goal of the reduction is to restore distal length and replace the distal radial fragment in its normal anatomical position. After reduction, the wrist and elbow are immobilized to prevent pronation and supination, and a hand pressure dressing may be applied during the first 24 to 48 hours to help prevent swelling of the fingers. Immobilization can be achieved by the use of a forearm (sugar-tong) splint or a long arm cast. Still other patients may be treated with an external fixation device (Fig. 11–8). Although a cast is generally used, a forearm splint is appropriate when (1) the individual is debilitated or elderly; (2) an incomplete reduction is accepted; (3) no reduction is attempted; and (4) the impacted position of the fragments is accepted. In older patients with badly comminuted fractures, early excision of the distal ulna and acceptance of radial shortening is also considered.

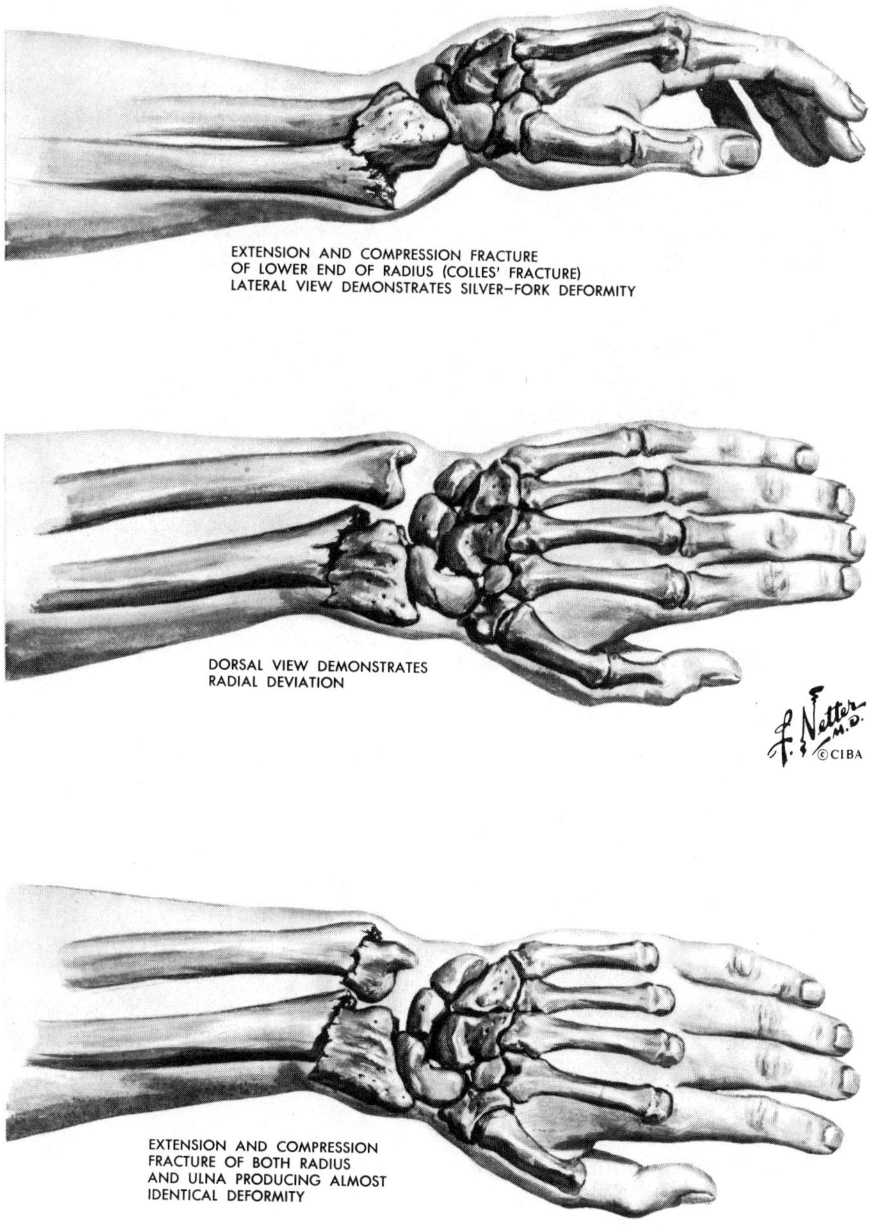

Figure 11–7. Extension and compression fracture of lower end of radius (Colles' fracture). Lateral view demonstrates silver-fork deformity. *(Copyright © 1970, CIBA Pharmaceutical Company, Division of CIBA-GEIGY Corporation. Reprinted with permission from* Clinical symposia, *illustrated by Frank H. Netter, M.D. All rights reserved.)*

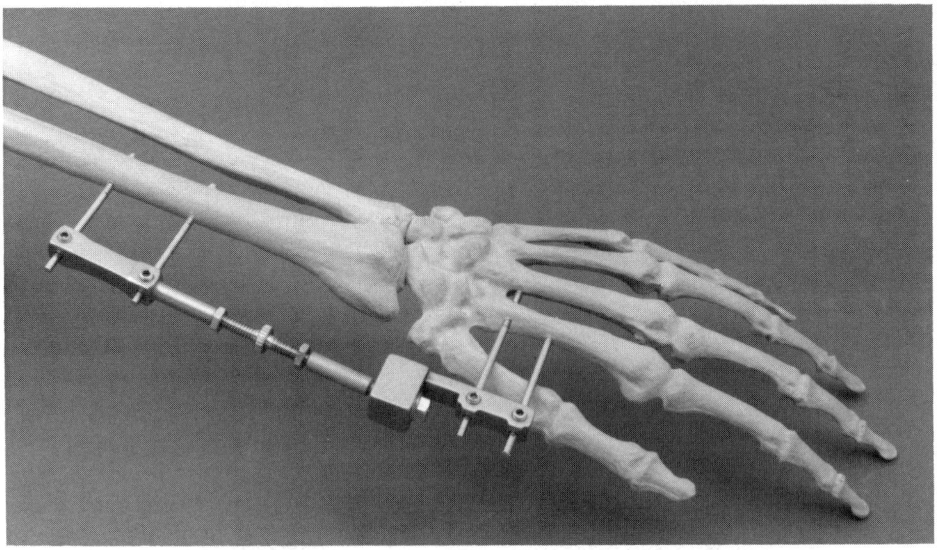

Figure 11–8. Richards Colles' fracture frame. *(Courtesy of Richards Medical Company.)*

□ NURSING PROCESS (Table 11–1)

Assessment

The initial step in the assessment of a typical patient in a long arm cast following the reduction of a Colles' fracture is a neurovascular assessment of the affected hand and arm and a comparison with the unaffected hand and arm (Chapter 2). It will probably be impossible to assess the radial pulse because the wrist and the palm are covered by the cast or a pressure dressing. The cast also impedes a complete motor assessment of the arm. Most patients have swelling at the fracture site, with edema and discoloration of the fingers and the thumb.

Check the position of the arm. The affected arm must be elevated with the hand higher than the elbow. Determine the location, duration, and severity of pain. Check the plaster of Paris cast for drying (Appendix B).

Nursing Diagnosis and Goal Formulation

Nursing diagnoses for a typical patient with a closed reduction of a Colles' fracture and cast application are (1) alterations in comfort related to pain from trauma, (2) alterations in mobility related to lack of bone stability in the arm, (3) alterations in psychological well-being related to anxiety and knowledge deficit about the treatment method and rehabilitation process, and (4) potential complications related to injury and decreased mobility.

TABLE 11–1. NURSING PROCESS FOR COLLES' FRACTURE TREATED WITH A LONG ARM CAST

Assessment	Nursing Diagnosis	Goal Formulation	Planning and Intervention	Evaluation and Reassessment
1. Assess the location, duration, and severity of pain. Assess the neurovascular status of the affected arm (impossible to assess pulse because of cast).	1. Alteration in comfort: pain in the wrist related to bone instability and soft tissue swelling.	1. Short-term goal: a decrease in the amount of pain through the use of nursing measures and prescribed medications. Long-term goal: free of pain.	1. Alleviate Pain Elevate the affected arm. Place ice bags at the fracture site. Instruct on finger exercises. Instruct on relaxation techniques. Administer prescribed medications.	1. The amount of pain should be reduced. Medications should be effective in reducing the pain. Swelling should be reduced and neurovascular status should be good.
2. Check the position of the affected arm. Assess motor and sensory functions in the affected arm; compare with unaffected arm. Assess ability to do finger and shoulder exercises.	2. Impaired physical mobility: lack of arm function related to bone instability.	2. Short-term goal: an increase in mobility through the use of controlled exercises. Long-term goal: return of full range of motion with no reduction in muscle function.	2. Increase Mobility *Position* Keep the hand elevated above the heart. Keep the arm and wrist immobilized in cast; reposition every 2 hours. Teach how to use trapeze. *Exercises* Instruct on finger and shoulder exercises. After the long arm cast is removed, instruct on elbow exercises. Active range of motion for all unaffected joints. *Ambulation* Assist patient in ambulating. Apply sling to support arm.	2. The arm and wrist should be elevated high enough to prevent or reduce any swelling of the fingers. The cast should not be so tight as to interfere with circulation, but not so loose as to allow movement of the bone fragments. Exercises should be done effectively and the rehabilitation program should be followed.

(continued)

TABLE 11–1. *(Continued)*

Assessment	Nursing Diagnosis	Goal Formulation	Planning and Intervention	Evaluation and Reassessment
3. Assess the affected hand for swelling, temperature, color, and capillary filling. Assess for tightness of cast.	3. Potential impairment in circulation: circulatory deficit related to trauma and swelling of soft tissue.	3. Short-term goal: only minimal swelling. Long-term goal: no circulatory impairment.	3. Prevent Complications *Circulatory* Keep the affected hand and arm elevated. Apply ice bags to fracture site. Instruct on finger and shoulder exercises. Report any deficit in circulation or excessive swelling.	3. The hand and arm should be elevated at all times and there should be only minimal swelling with good color and capillary filling. The cast should be bivalved if neurovascular deficit occurs.
Assess sensory and motor function of the radial, median, and ulnar nerves. Assess ability to move arm through range of motion.	Potential for impairment of neurological function: neurological deficit related to trauma ands soft tissue swelling.	Short- and long-term goal: no neurological deficit.	*Neurological* Keep the affected hand and arm elevated. Apply ice bags to fracture site. Report any neurological deficit.	

Assess site on cast over area of pain for warmth. Check skin at edges of cast. Assess for signs of infection.	Potential for impairment of skin integrity related to rough edges and pressure from cast.	Short- and long-term goal: no break in skin integrity.	*Integumentary* Apply nursing measures to reduce swelling. Petal cast edges as indicated. *Other Complications* (See text.)	There should be no pressure areas (especially at styloid processes, the olecranon, and the epicondyles). There should be no blisters caused by severe edema and no increase in pain.
4. Assess patient's level of understanding about how to do exercises and why they are necessary. Assess for understanding of fracture healing, cast care, and the ability to do activities of daily living with a long arm cast.	4. Potential knowledge deficit related to exercises, cast care, fracture healing, and home care.	4. Short- and long-term goal: a decrease in anxiety through an increase in knowledge level.	4. Patient Teaching Instruct on finger and shoulder exercises. Discuss the process of fracture healing and the rehabilitation process. Instruct on cast care. Go over ways to do activities of daily living with a long arm cast on. Include the family and significant others in teaching plan.	4. The patient should verbalize an understanding of cast care and the rehabilitation process, and do exercises correctly. Determine self-care abilities by observing self-care and dressing before discharge.

Short-term goals are to have the patient experience (1) a decrease in the amount of pain through nursing measures and prescribed medications, (2) an increase in mobility through the use of controlled exercises, (3) an absence of complications, and (4) a decrease in anxiety through increased knowledge. Long-term goals are to have the patient free of pain and to have a return of full arm function.

Planning and Intervention

Alleviate Pain. Following a Colles' fracture, the patient usually has pain and swelling of the affected wrist and hand. Some patients have their hand in the long arm cast, whereas others have a pressure dressing over the hand for 24 to 48 hours to prevent or reduce swelling of the fingers. Measures that help relieve pain and swelling are to elevate the arm, put ice at the fracture site, and have the patient do finger exercises. Once these measures have been implemented, and the neurovascular status of the affected arm is good, give pain medications as needed.

Increase Mobility

Position. The affected arm must be kept elevated to control swelling. One of the easiest ways to do that is to elevate the arm on one or more pillows. Another method is to use roller gauze or stockinette to encircle the cast at the patient's wrist, and then attach the casted arm to an intravenous pole (Fig. 11–9). Make sure the gauze or stockinette does not cause

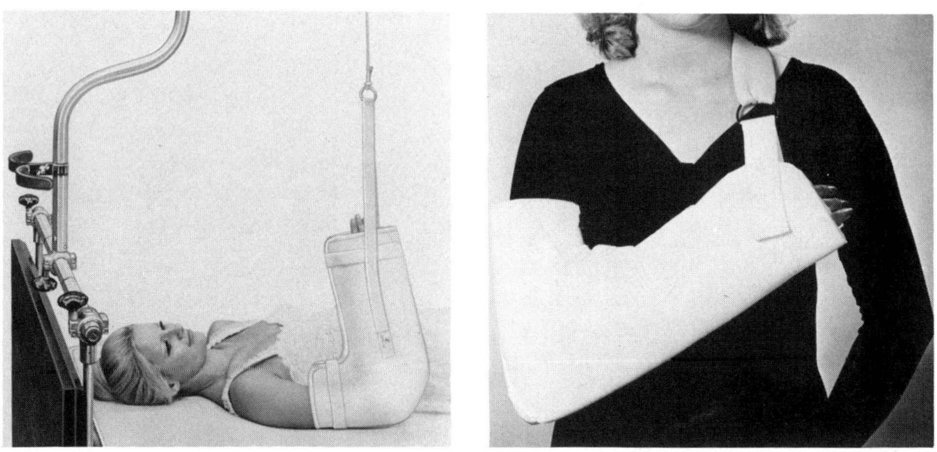

A B

Figure 11–9. A. Method of elevating arm and applying ice. **B.** Method of elevating arm: sling. *(Courtesy of Zimmer, Inc.)*

an indentation in a plaster of Paris cast. If the cast is not completely dry, the stockinette may be placed over the cast and then attached to the pole.

The arm and wrist of a patient with a Colles' fracture may be immobilized in a long arm cast, a short arm cast, or a forearm (sugar-tong) splint. In most patients, there is a closed reduction and immobilization in a long arm cast that includes the elbow and the distal half of the upper arm to help prevent rotation of the wrist. After 2 to 3 weeks in less severe fractures, and 3 to 4 weeks in more severe cases, the cast may be shortened to below the elbow. In patients with a closed reduction and percutaneous pinning with Kirschner wires through the radial styloids, the arm is immobilized in a long arm cast, with the wrist in neutral position. The Kirschner wires are removed after 6 weeks and the wrist is then supported by a removable splint. In patients with a traction cast, the pins and cast are left in place for 8 weeks. After the pins are removed, the wrist is supported by a removable splint (Edmonson & Crenshaw, 1980, p. 703). In all instances, the cast extends distally to the palmar crease. The casted arm is supported with a sling when the patient is out of bed (see p. 594).

Exercises. Exercises of the fingers (see p. 510) and shoulder (see pp. 500 and 521–523) are to be encouraged during the entire period of immobilization to minimize residual stiffness. If the cast is a short arm cast, include exercises for the elbow (see pp. 607 and 610).

Ambulation. The patient will probably be allowed to ambulate soon after recovering from anesthesia. Assistance is needed at the beginning because of the awkwardness of the cast.

Prevent Complications. The major complications following a Colles' fracture are circulatory impediment, neurological impairment, integumentary disruption, the recurrence of the prereduction deformity, and persistent pain. It is important that patients understand these potential complications as the hospital stay is usually very short. Patients are generally discharged when they have full active movement of the fingers and shoulder, minimal pain that is readily controlled with mild analgesics, and a satisfactory and comfortable immobilization.

Circulatory. Colles' fractures with displacement usually produce a large extravasation of blood and great swelling, which begins quickly and may involve the hand, the fingers, and the entire forearm. The swelling may be so extensive before reduction that the nature of the displacement is difficult to determine. Once the reduction is accomplished and the cast applied, the cast may need to be split to accommodate continued swelling. The patient is instructed to elevate the hand to help reduce swelling, to notify the physician if there is any neurovascular deficit or increase in pain, and to schedule appointments after discharge so that the swelling and the neurovascular status of the arm can be evaluated.

Neurological. The sensory branch of the radial nerve, which supplies the dorsum of the thumb and the radial side of the hand, may be stretched or even torn at the time of injury or reduction. Usually the anesthesia and paresthesia that occurs clears spontaneously within a few weeks. The median nerve is rarely injured, but a condition called Sudeck's Atrophy may develop. This condition is suspected if the patient has unduly persistent pain after reduction and immobilization. In Sudeck's Atrophy, the hand is typically warm, moist, and purplish in color from dilation of superficial blood vessels. The condition is apparently due to a hyperemia set up by nerve irritation, possible from an injury to the median nerve in the carpal tunnel. The symptoms usually subside, but some patients may require anesthetic blockage of the inferior cervical or stellate ganglion or small doses of deep x-ray therapy to relieve them. The end result of Sudeck's Atrophy is usually a very stiff hand, and roentgenograms usually show evidence of bone destruction in the hand and the wrist.

Integumentary. Possible pressure points are over the styloid processes, the olecranon, and the epicondyles. The surface of the cast should be felt over areas where pain has been reported. If necrosis or infection is developing, the cast usually feels warm. Severe edema often causes blisters and adds to the discomfort of patients in casts. That is particularly true over and around bony prominences where there is little tissue to absorb the fluid. Check the skin around the cast edges and petal the cast as indicated (Appendix B).

Recurrence of Deformity. Despite a good initial alignment by closed reduction and an adequate plaster immobilization of a Colles' fracture, the prereduction deformity may recur if the cancellous bone of the distal fragment of the radius does not return to its normal location. In that event, muscle pulls tend to produce shortening and angulation in the distal fragment that produce a deformity resembling the initial injury. This complication is particularly common in the elderly. In spite of the deformity, the function of the hand may be quite good after healing is complete. In patients with considerable deformity and painful restriction of motion, excision of the distal ulna may not only afford relief of pain but improve function and give a better cosmetic result.

Persistent Pain. Pain over the distal radioulnar joint on supination of the forearm is a common complaint after the cast is removed. The pain usually subsides gradually and disappears within 6 months. If the pain persists even after full return of function of the hand, excision of the distal ulna may be necessary.

Patient Teaching. Teach the patient that added discomfort in the form of tingling and numbness any time after cast application may be due to pressure on nerves or blood vessels, and must be reported to the physician immediately. As compression on a nerve continues, it causes localized and constant pain, numbness of increasing depth, and finally loss of feeling and paralysis. Teach the patient, the family, and significant others how to check for possible neurovascular impairment (Chap. 2).

Time is needed to discuss problems in going home and doing activities of daily living with the patient, the family, and significant others, especially if the patient is elderly and lives alone. Discuss cast care, how to do personal care, and dressing (Appendix B). With the arm casted it is especially important that the patient give attention to the hand of the casted arm, which should be cleansed without getting the cast wet. Alcohol swabs may be used to cleanse between the fingers. The patient may need to apply lotion to the hand if the skin becomes too dry.

Evaluation and Reassessment

There should be a reduction in swelling from the application of ice, elevation of the arm, and finger exercises. If nerve or circulatory impairment should occur due to swelling, the cast should be split. There should be a reduction in the amount of pain with the immobilization of the fracture. The patient should be able to demonstrate exercises for the fingers and the shoulder, and verbalize an understanding of the rehabilitation process.

Smith's Fracture

A Smith's fracture is a nonarticular fracture of the distal radius with a dorsal angulation of the radius and with the distal fragment and accompanying carpal row of bones displaced volarly (i.e., toward the palm) (Figs. 11–10A and B). A Smith's fracture is also known as a reverse Colles' fracture. Smith's fracture is usually secondary to a blow on the dorsum of the wrist or distal radius with the forearm in pronation.

Treatment usually involves closed reduction under anesthesia. In that procedure, with the hand in pronation and flexion, longitudinal traction is applied in line with the deformity until any impacted fragments are dislodged (Fig. 11–10C). Supination of the hand and application of dorsal pressure on the distal fragment usually reduces the fracture. Immobilization is accomplished using a long arm cast with the forearm in supination and the wrist in extension (Iversen & Clawson, 1977, p. 170) (Fig. 11–10D). Follow-up care is the same as for a Colles' fracture.

Stabilizing Distal Radial Fractures

Most nonarticular distal radial fractures can be successfully treated nonoperatively. When maintenance of the reduction of a Colles' or Smith's fracture requires prolonged immobilization in an extreme position, particularly if the patient is elderly with osteoarthritic changes in the joints of the hand, closed reduction followed by percutaneous pinning of the distal radius through the radial styloid is usually indicated. This method is particularly applicable when there is a large radial styloid fragment, but may be used for many comminuted fractures of the distal radius. After the fracture is manipulated and reduced, two large Kirschner wires are inserted through the radial styloid across the fracture and into the opposite metaphyseal cortex. The wires usually provide

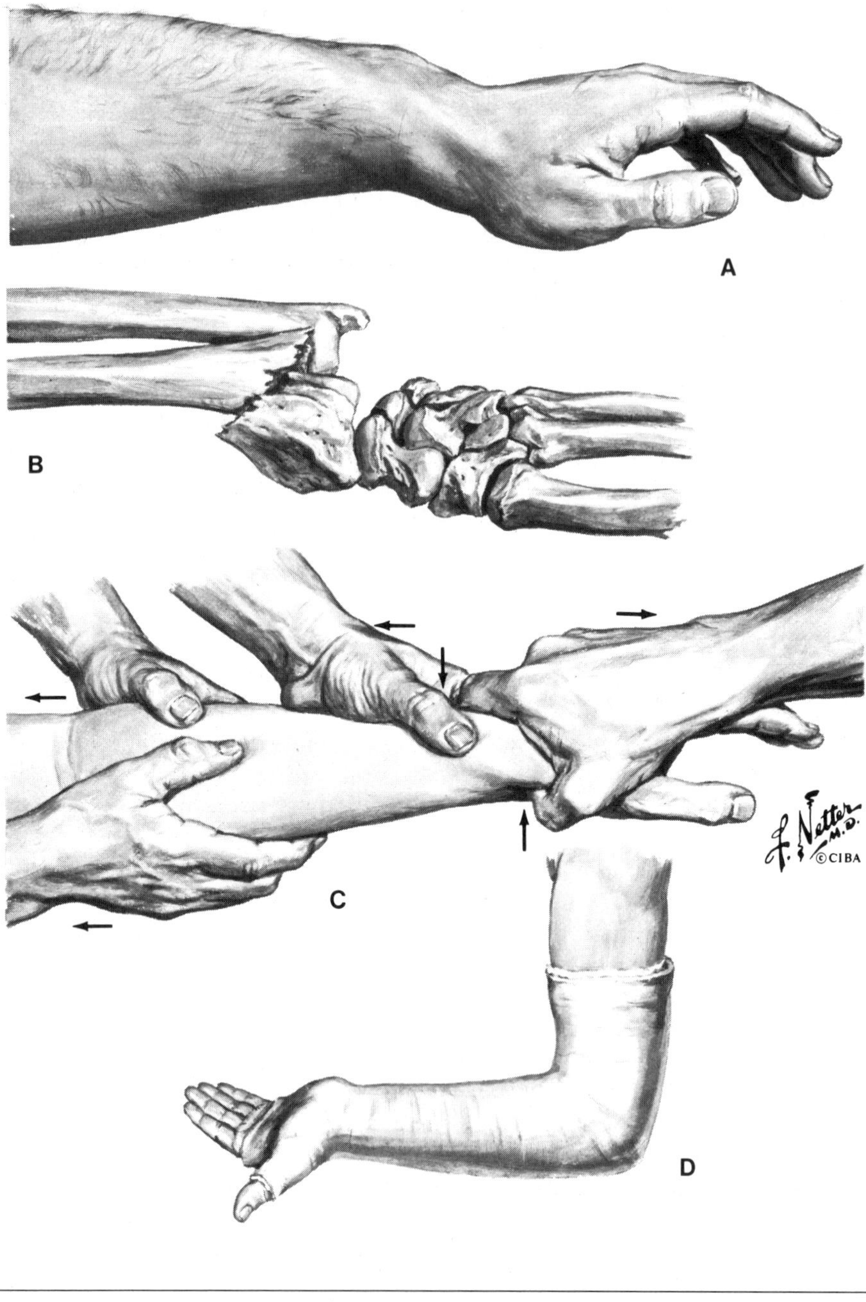

Figure 11–10. A. Garden-spade deformity in flexion–compression fracture of radius with anterior displacement of lower fragment (Smith's fracture). **B.** Flexion–compression fracture of radius. **C.** Reduction by traction and countertraction with backward pressure on distal fragment and forward pressure on proximal fragment. **D.** Immobilization in plaster with elbow flexed, forearm supinated, hand adducted (ulnar flexed) and moderately extended, and thumb widely abducted. *(Copyright © 1970, CIBA Pharmaceutical Company, Division of CIBA-GEIGY Corporation. Reprinted with permission from* Clinical symposia, *illustrated by Frank H. Netter, M.D. All rights reserved.)*

sufficient fixation to minimize radial collapse and radial shortening and allow immobilization in a cast with the wrist in a neutral position (Edmondson & Crenshaw, 1980, pp. 702–703).

For fractures that are not suitable for percutaneous Kirschner wire stabilization through the radial styloid, pins and plaster or a traction cast are often used, and produce good results. Following anesthesia, those fractures are reduced by suspending the forearm from the fingers in Chinese finger traps. After approximately 5 minutes of traction, gentle manipulation helps to reduce the fracture. A Steinmann pin is then inserted transversely through the proximal ulna 7.5 to 10 cm distal to the olecranon, and a second pin is inserted transversely through the bases of the second and third metacarpals. A plaster cast is then applied above the elbow, incorporating the two pins. The palm of the cast, once it is dry, is cut back proximal to the flexion crease in the hand to allow full active motion of the fingers. The cast and pins remain in place for a minimum of 8 weeks, as removing the pins earlier may allow the distal radius to shorten or reimpact. Open reduction of Colles' and Smith's fractures is almost never required (Gartland, 1979, p. 293).

Intra-Articular Fractures of the Distal Radius

Barton's fractures are distal radial fractures into the joint that involve the dorsal or volar margins of the articular surface. They may be reduced by closed reduction and, when the marginal fracture is small, immobilized satisfactorily with a cast. Dorsal margin fractures are usually more stable when the wrist is dorsiflexed and the forearm pronated, whereas volar margin fractures are usually more stable with volar flexion of the wrist and supination of the forearm. Stability is promoted by the intact carpal ligament opposite the fracture (Iversen & Clawson, 1977, p. 170).

When the marginal fracture involves a large portion of the distal articular surface of the radius, closed reduction may be achieved, but not maintained because of subluxation of the carpus. Accordingly, many authorities treat volar marginal Barton's fractures with a small buttress plate, and dorsal marginal Barton's fractures with Kirschner wires. The Kirschner wires are used for dorsal fractures instead of a plate and screws because of the location of the extensor tendons. Following the insertion of a small buttress plate and screws, immobilization may not be required, as simple limitation of activity until the fracture heals is sufficient. In other cases, however, a plaster sugar-tong splint is used, with gentle active exercises performed two or three times a day for the following 2 weeks. The splint is removed after 4 weeks, and progressive motion continued until union is solid.

Fractures of the Carpals

Fractures of the Scaphoid

A fracture of the carpal scaphoid bone is the most common fracture of the carpus and the most commonly undiagnosed fracture of the upper extremity

(Edmondson & Crenshaw, 1980, p. 176). Acute fractures of the scaphoid are difficult to view on roentgenograms for the first 10 to 14 days after trauma. Fractures of the scaphoid occur in persons 10 to 70 years old, but most commonly in young adult males. The fracture usually occurs as a result of a fall on an outstretched palm, which causes severe hyperextension and slight radial deviation of the wrist. Limitation of extremes of wrist motion are usually present because of pain and tenderness in the wrist near the styloid process of the radius (Figs. 11–11A and B).

Immediate closed reduction and immobilization in a cast for 6 to 12 weeks is the preferred treatment. The arm is placed in a cast with the wrist at 20 to 45 degrees of dorsiflexion and a slight (20-degree) radial deviation (Fig. 11–11C). The cast usually extends from the uppermost portion of the forearm to the distal joint of the thumb. The thumb is maintained in a functional position, and the fingers are left free to move distally from the metacarpophalangeal joints. However, if the fracture is displaced, the diagnosis delayed, or the fracture located in the proximal third of the scaphoid, delayed union and nonunion are common. If the fracture has not healed within 4 months after a closed reduction, an open reduction with a Kirschner wire fixation and a cancellous bone graft is needed. The open reduction procedure involves a short volar or transradial incision made at the base of the thumb. The fracture is then fixed with two Kirschner wires inserted across the fracture site and extended as far as the lunate and scaphoid joints. Cancellous (iliac) bone is placed in the fracture site to promote calcification. Postoperative care includes a short arm scaphoid cast. Internal fixation is removed at 10 to 12 weeks, and the cast is discontinued after the fracture is healed (approximately 4 months).

□ NURSING PROCESS (Table 11–2)

Assessment

The initial step in the assessment of a patient in a cast following an open reduction and internal fixation of a fractured scaphoid is a neurovascular assessment (Chap. 2). The assessment of the thumb is difficult, as the thumb is enclosed in the cast. Check that the casted arm is properly elevated, look for any drainage into the cast, and assess the location, duration, and severity of pain.

Nursing Diagnosis and Goal Formulation

Nursing diagnoses for a typical patient following an open reduction and internal fixation of a fractured scaphoid are (1) alterations in comfort related to pain from surgery, (2) alterations in mobility of the wrist and hand related to lack of bone stability, (3) potential complications related to surgery and decreased mobility in the wrist and the hand, and (4) alterations in psychological well-being related to anxiety and knowledge deficit about the treatment methods and the future prognosis.

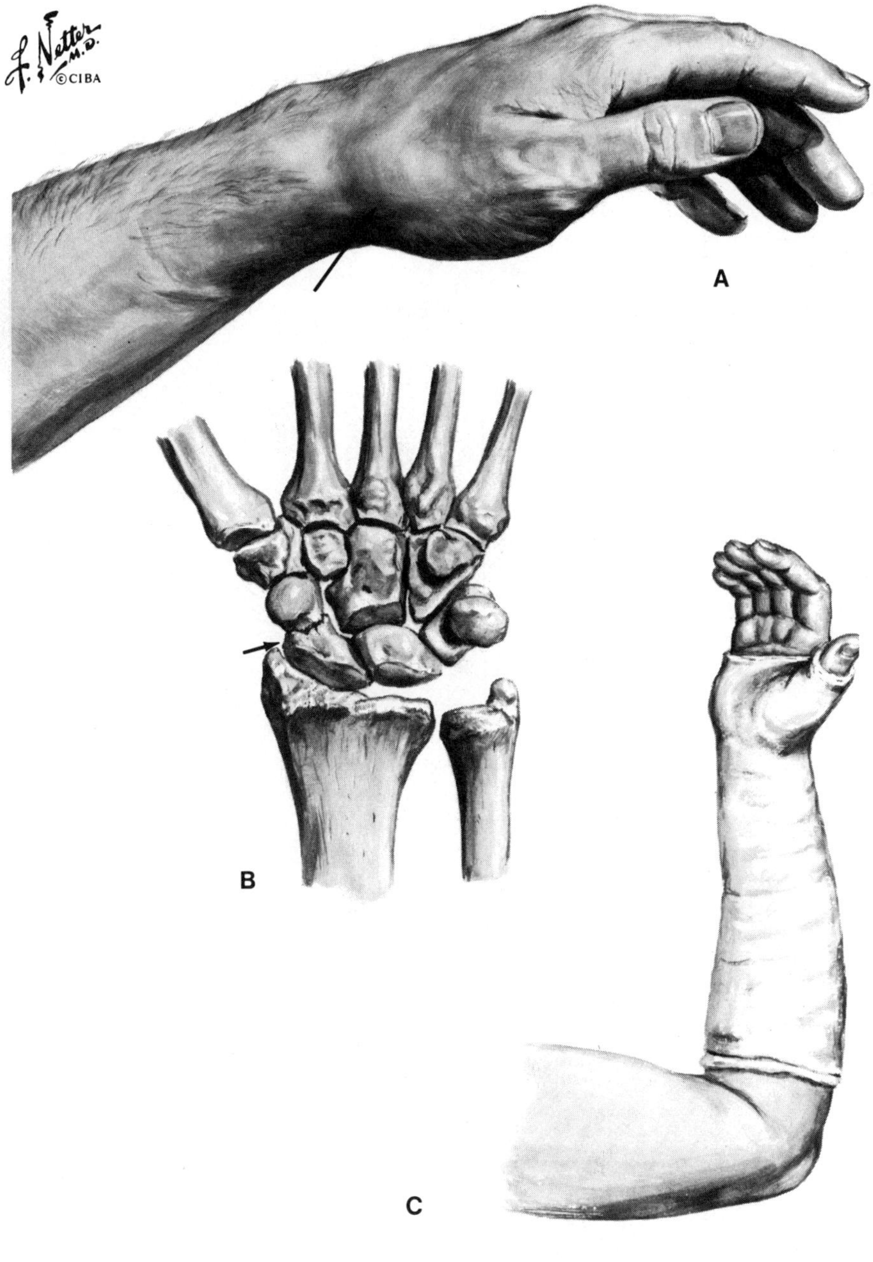

Figure 11–11. A. Typical clinical findings in fracture of scaphoid bone: swelling and tenderness in region of "anatomical snuff box." **B.** Fracture of scaphoid bone. **C.** Immobilization of 20-degree dorsiflexion with slight radial deviation. Thumb is extended in functional position. *(Copyright © 1970, CIBA Pharmaceutical Company, Division of CIBA-GEIGY Corporation. Reprinted with permission from* Clinical symposia, *illustrated by Frank H. Netter, M.D. All rights reserved.)*

TABLE 11–2. NURSING PROCESS FOR FRACTURE OF THE SCAPHOID TREATED BY OPEN REDUCTION, INTERNAL FIXATION, AND CAST APPLICATION

Assessment	Nursing Diagnosis	Goal Formulation	Planning and Intervention	Evaluation and Reassessment
1. Assess the location, duration, and severity of pain. Assess the neurovascular status of the affected hand and arm (impossible to assess for pulse or motor function of the affected thumb).	1. Alteration in comfort: pain in hand and wrist related to bone instability and soft tissue swelling.	1. Short-term goal: a relative state of comfort with only minimal pain. Long-term goal: free of pain.	1. Alleviate Pain Elevate the affected hand and arm. Place ice bags at the fracture site. Instruct on finger exercises. Teach relaxation techniques. Administer prescribed medications.	1. The amount of pain should be reduced. Medication should be effective in reducing the pain. There should be no swelling and the neurovascular status should be good.
2. Check the position of the affected arm. Assess sensory and motor function. Assess the patient's ability to do finger, shoulder, and elbow exercises.	2. Impaired physical mobility: lack of wrist function related to bone instability and utilization of an arm cast.	2. Short-term goal: an increase in mobility through the use of controlled exercises. Long-term goal: return of premorbid range of motion and function in the arm.	2. Increase Mobility Elevate the affected arm. Instruct on finger, shoulder and elbow exercises. Reposition every 2 hours. Avoid any pressure at the elbow. Teach how to use trapeze. Assist with first ambulation.	2. The arm should be kept elevated with no pressure at the elbow. Exercises should be done correctly.

3. Assess neurovascular status. Assess for tightness of cast. Assess for any swelling.	3. Potential for injury: neurovascular deficit related to soft tissue swelling.	3. Short- and long-term goal: free of neurovascular deficit.	3. Prevent Complications *Circulatory* Do neurovascular checks after surgery, every 15 minutes for first 2 hours, every 30 minutes for next 2 hours, every 2 hours for next 24 hours, and then at the beginning of every shift. Report any neurovascular deficit. Keep the affected arm elevated. Keep ice at the fracture site for the first 24 hours. Report any excessive swelling.	3. Neurovascular status should be good and there should be no swelling.
Assess for any signs of infection at the pin site. Assess for any signs of pressure areas under the cast.	Potential for infection related to utilization of a skeletal pin and surgical incision. Potential impairment of skin integrity related to pressure from cast over bony prominences.	Short- and long-term goal: free of any skin complications.	*Integumentary* Assess pin and incisional site for any drainage. Do dressing changes as indicated. Petal edges of cast. Keep casted arm elevated and on a soft surface.	Expect no signs of infection or skin breakdown due to pressure from the cast.
4. Assess the patient's level of understanding of the rehabilitation process. Assess patient's understanding of exercises and cast care.	4. Potential knowledge deficit related to exercises, cast care, fracture healing, and home care.	4. Short- and long-term goal: a decrease in anxiety through increase in knowledge.	4. Patient Teaching Instruct on exercises. Instruct on cast care and rehabilitation process. Include the family and significant others. Discuss how to do activities of daily living.	4. The patient should be able to do exercises correctly and be able to verbalize an understanding of the rehabilitation process and cast care.

Short-term goals are to have the patient experience (1) a decrease in the amount of pain through nursing measures and prescribed medications, (2) an increase in mobility through the use of controlled exercises, (3) an absence of complications from surgery and decreased arm activities, and (4) a decrease in anxiety through increased knowledge. Long-term goals are to have the patient free of pain and to have a return of hand function.

Planning and Intervention

Alleviate Pain. The measures used to relieve pain in a patient following a Colles' fracture apply here (see p. 644).

Increase Mobility. Measures to increase mobility are to elevate the affected arm to reduce swelling, and to do exercises of the fingers, the shoulder, and the elbow. The scaphoid cast is a short arm cast with the thumb casted in abduction. The cast is sometimes referred to as a thumb spica, and may be worn for 4 to 6 weeks following the surgery.

Prevent Complications. Complications following an open reduction of a fractured scaphoid are potential stiffness of the thumb and the wrist following cast removal and infection. Infection control measures are necessary and exercises to regain function in the thumb and the wrist are started when the cast is removed. Exercises for the fingers (see p. 510), elbow (see pp. 607 and 610), and shoulder (pp. 500 and 521–523) may be instituted immediately.

Patient Teaching. The major points are those discussed for a patient with a Colles' fracture (see pp. 646–647).

Evaluation and Reassessment

The patient should have a reduction in pain and swelling and no neurovascular impairment or infection. Patients should understand the rehabilitation process and feel comfortable in caring for themselves at home. The patient, the family, and significant others should be able to verbalize the signs and symptoms of potential complications and how to prevent them.

Other Carpal Fractures

Fractures of other carpal bones are less common but may occur when there is wrist trauma. Because they receive a good blood supply, most fractures of the other carpal bones heal satisfactorily with 6 to 8 weeks of immobilization. If there is significant displacement, reduction is indicated. Of special note is the fracture of the hook of the hamate, which can cause a neurological deficit.

Pathology

ARTHRITIS AND INFECTIOUS DISEASES

Rheumatoid Arthritis

Rheumatoid arthritis of the wrist is often associated with arthritis of the hands and the fingers. Synovial inflammation and proliferation distend the joint capsule by effusion and destroy the capsuloligamentous structures. All degrees of the disease are seen in the wrist. The inflammation may be acute and recurring, and may present effusion and swelling in the joint, in the tendon sheaths, or in both at the same time. At the other extreme, it may be chronic, progressive, and ultimately destructive to all wrist joint structures and neighboring tendons, with resultant deformity and tendon disintegration.

Clinically, the disease involves the wrist joint and adjacent tendons. At first, there are recurring episodes of swelling, heat, tenderness, limitation of motion, and pain in the wrist. Between these episodes, the wrist may appear normal. Involvement of the adjacent tendons (tenosynovitis) may occur at the same time, but may appear unrelated. With advancing rheumatoid disease, swelling, stiffness, and deformity become pronounced and persistent. The wrist usually becomes fixed in flexion. The distal ulna is loose and prominent dorsally. The flexor tendons digitorum superficialis and digitorum profundis may rupture, causing loss of extension at the metacarpophalangeal joint of the little, ring, and middle fingers. Less often, there are ruptures of the extensor pollicis longus or the flexor pollicis longus.

The principles of medical treatment are (1) immobilizing the wrist with a removable plaster splint and applying heat to aid in the resorption of inflammatory swelling, (2) exercising the wrist at least twice daily to prevent adhesions, (3) injecting hydrocortisone and thiotepa if swelling persists, and (4) intervening surgically. This surgical intervention may be a synovectomy, an arthrodesis, or an arthroplasty. An early synovectomy helps prevent local destruction of the wrist joint and tendon rupture. However, the proliferative synovium needs to be removed before it can seriously damage cartilage, ligaments, and tendons. After destruction of the wrist joint has occurred, only an arthrodesis or an arthroplasty may be able to restore function.

Degenerative Arthritis

Degenerative arthritis of the articular surfaces of the distal radioulnar joint usually occurs when the articular cartilage of the joint has been damaged, but the joint surfaces are held tightly opposed by intact ligaments. The damaged articular cartilage may have been produced by trauma, or, rarely, by a generalized degenerative process (Turek, 1977, pp. 980–981).

Clinically, there is pain and stiffness at rest, especially after extensive use of the wrist, which is relieved to some extent by heat. Pain is intensified by rotary motions, and by extreme supination and pronation. There is usually swelling of soft tissues about the joint, tenderness, limitation of supination and pronation, palpable crepitus with motion, and occasionally bony prominences due to spur formation.

Surgical intervention may consist of resecting the distal end of the ulna. If the carpals are affected by degenerative arthritis, radiocarpal arthrodesis may also be required.

Tuberculosis

Tuberculosis of the wrist is relatively uncommon. The synovial membrane may be the first to show signs of the disease, or it may first be demonstrated by an osseous lesion in one of the bones of the wrist joint, usually the lower end of the radius. There may be pain, swelling, local heat and tenderness, limitation of movement, and deformity. The wrist is usually held in palmar flexion. Abscesses are usually superficial and quickly break down and form sinuses. Roentgenographic examination demonstrates generalized osteoporosis or the presence of an osseous focus of infection.

Treatment begins with the generalized treatment for tuberculosis. The local treatment for tuberculosis of the wrist includes immobilization in a cast from the knuckles and the transverse crease of the palm to just below the elbow, or above the elbow when complete immobilization of the wrist is necessary. The wrist is usually held in approximately 30 degrees of dorsiflexion, and if the thumb is included in the cast it is held in opposition. Cast immobilization and chemotherapy are continued until the disease is quiescent (inactive).

Most patients require surgery because of the spread of the disease or the bony destruction present. Surgically treated lesions may heal even when other lesions in the body resist generalized treatment. Surgery for tuberculosis of the wrist is usually undertaken when the lesion is at least momentarily quiescent, and the most common procedure is an arthrodesis. After an arthrodesis, the wrist is immobilized in a cast until union is complete. Amputation is indicated in tuberculosis of the wrist when the disease is so extensive that a permanent cure appears impossible (Edmondson & Crenshaw, 1980, p. 1091).

Arthrodesis

Arthrodesis of the wrist (fusion of the radiocarpal joint) is indicated when there is gross bone and cartilage destruction or when the carpal bones are markedly subluxed. Fusion of the wrist is most often utilized for tuberculosis, for non-united or malunited fractures of the scaphoid with associated radiocarpal traumatic arthritis, and for severely comminuted fractures of the distal end of the radius. Less commonly, it is done for Volkmann's ischemic paralysis and for stabilization of the wrist in poliomyelitis and in spastic cerebral palsy of the wrist.

The wrist is fused in a position that will not be fatiguing and will allow maximum grasping strength in the hand. This position is usually neutral or 10 to 20 degrees of extension, with the long axis of the third metacarpal shaft aligned with the long axis of the radial shaft. Clinically, it is the position that the wrist normally assumes with the fist strongly clenched.

The operative procedure involves denudation of the proximal row of carpals and the distal end of the radius by removing the dorsal aspect of cortical bone (Fig. 11–12). The distal end of the ulna may or may not be removed, and Kirschner wires may or may not be used for internal fixation. Most of the many techniques used to obtain wrist fusion include the use of a bone graft from the ilium. In some, the graft extends from the radius to the proximal carpal bones, but in others it extends distally to the base of the third metacarpal. Some authorities recommend, however, that the second and third carpometacarpal joints always be included in the fusion to prevent the development of any painful motion in those joints and because the disease process of the wrist frequently extends into them. At least some carpometacarpal joints will be pre-

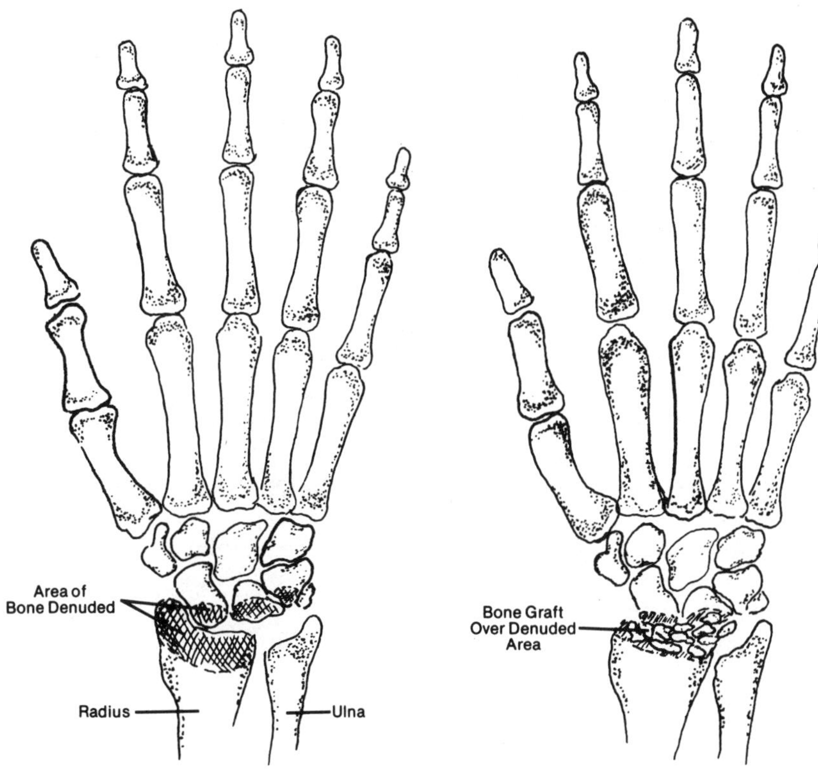

Figure 11–12. Wrist fusion. *(From Brantley, P., & Analla, M., 1980, p. 29. Courtesy of Howmedica.)*

served, and thus some motion in the wrist will be retained (Brantley & Analla, 1980, p. 29; Edmondson & Crenshaw, 1980, p. 326).

Once the arthrodesis is completed, a long arm cast is applied from the upper arm to the tips of the fingers and thumb, with the elbow at a right angle, the forearm in neutral position, the wrist at 10 to 15 degrees extension, and the fingers and thumb slightly flexed. To allow for swelling, the dorsum of the cast is windowed. Three weeks after surgery a short arm cast (from below the elbow to just proximal to the metacarpophalangeal joints) is applied. Support to the wrist is continued until firm fusion is present, ordinarily 10 weeks.

Excision of Wrist Joint. Excision of the wrist joint is indicated only when carpal destruction is so extensive that arthrodesis of the wrist is impossible. Such a situation is rare. The procedure for excising the wrist begins with a straight incision made over the dorsal surface of the wrist in line with the medial aspect of the shaft of the radius. Dissection is then done through the fascia and between the tendons of the extensor indicis proprius and the extensor pollicis longus to the radius and then through the capsule of the wrist joint to the base of the third metacarpal. The periosteum is stripped from the distal end of the radius and the bases of the metacarpals, and the carpals are excised. The articular surfaces of the radius and the ulna are resected down to bone that appears normal. The metacarpal heads and the distal portions of the ulna and the radius are placed in opposition. After closure, the arm is immobilized in a long arm plaster cast, with the wrist in extension until the immediate period of swelling has subsided. Active finger exercises are started on the fourth or fifth day. After 2 weeks, a new long arm cast is applied, and after 3 months active wrist exercises are instituted, the wrist being supported between exercise periods by a leather brace reinforced with metal bars. The support may be discarded after 6 months if wrist function is sufficient. Otherwise, a pliable wrist support is worn indefinitely. Improvements in function usually continue for at least a year (Edmondson & Crenshaw, 1980, p. 1090).

Resection of the Distal Ulna. A resection of the distal ulna is done to relieve pain and restore motion in the wrist. It may be done in instances of malunion or nonunion following Colles' fracture, pain and disability due to radioulnar arthritis, and dislocation or subluxation of the ulna. The distal ulna is resected approximately 1 inch from the end of the bone. The ulnar collateral ligament is then sutured to the periosteum to stabilize the end of the ulna. Postoperatively, no immobilization is usually required, and active exercises are allowed the following day. Complications include infection and diminished strength in the wrist (Brantley & Analla, 1980, p. 16).

SILASTIC WRIST JOINT IMPLANT (SWANSON DESIGN). A wrist implant is utilized in patients with arthritic or traumatic disabilities resulting in wrist instability due to subluxation, severe deviation of the wrist, stiffness, or fusion of the wrist in a nonfunctional position. The goals of the procedure are to provide stability and restore painless motion to the wrist.

A common procedure involves the removal of the scaphoid, the lunate, the proximal third of the capitate, and the medial portion of the triquetrum (Fig. 11–13). The distal end of the radius is removed and the intramedullary canal of the radius is reamed. The remaining portion of the capitate and the intramedullary canal of the third metacarpal are also reamed. The Silastic wrist joint implant is fitted into the radial canal and through the capitate into the third metacarpal canal. The distal portion of the ulna may or may not be excised and fitted with a Silastic ulnar head implant. The extensor tendons may be shortened or transferred as necessary for stabilization.

Following closure, a bulky hand dressing is applied. In 3 to 5 days, a short arm cast is applied with the wrist in a neutral position. The cast is worn for 2 to 4 weeks. An outrigger device may be added to the cast if the extensor tendons have been repaired. Nursing measures are focused on prevention of complications and rehabilitation of the wrist. The primary complications are infec-

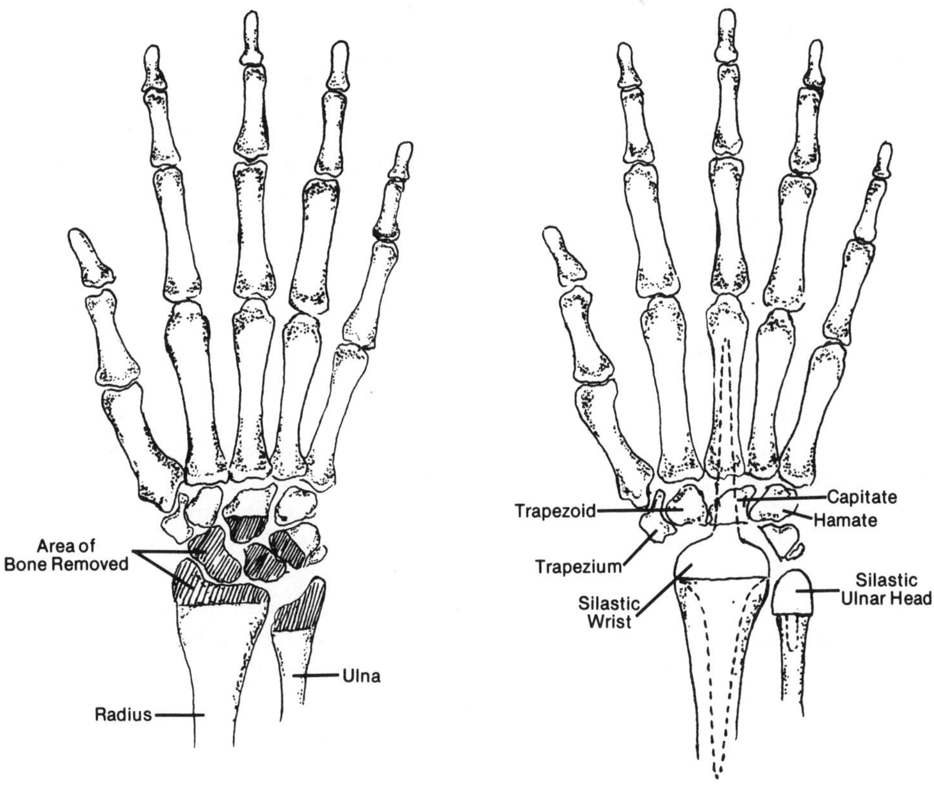

Figure 11–13. Silastic wrist joint implant, Swanson design. *(From Brantley, P., & Analla, M., 1980, p. 30. Courtesy of Howmedica.)*

tion and breakage or dislocation of the implant. Active exercises are begun after cast removal (Brantley & Analla, 1980, p. 30).

SILASTIC ULNAR HEAD IMPLANT. A Silastic ulnar head implant is indicated where there is instability, pain, or weakness of the wrist due to rheumatoid, degenerative, or traumatic arthritis of the ulnar head. The goal of the procedure is to provide painless motion and to improve stability in the wrist. The surgical procedure involves the removal of the ulnar head and the implantation of a Silastic ulnar head. After the initial incision, the ulnar head is excised at the neck and a complete synovectomy is done. The excised end of the ulna is then smoothed, and two holes are drilled into the bone. The ulnar canal is reamed to accept the stem of the ulnar head implant. Nonabsorbable retention sutures, attached to the implant, are then passed through the canal and out the drill holes. With the guidance of the retention sutures, the ulnar implant is inserted into the ulna. After skin closure, a bulky hand dressing and a palmar splint are applied. At approximately 3 to 5 days postoperatively, a short arm cast or splint is applied with the hand in slight dorsiflexion (Brantley & Analla, 1980, p. 15).

Carpal Bone Implants. Carpal bone implants have significantly improved motion and reduced pain in the wrist for patients with a number of different pathological conditions, including chronic wrist pain, instability of the joint, recurrent dislocation, avascular necrosis, traumatic arthritis, rheumatoid arthritis, degenerative arthritis, acute fractures, and pseudoarthritis following a fracture. After surgery, the arm is usually immobilized before rehabilitation with exercises is begun. The most common complications are infection, and breakage or dislocation of the implant.

CARPAL LUNATE IMPLANT. To replace the carpal lunate with an implant, the lunate is removed and a hole is drilled into the triquetrum to accept the stem of the implant. A small Kirschner wire may or may not be used for added stability. If the wire is used, it is placed through the lunate implant and either the radius or an adjacent carpal bone. Postoperative care includes immobilizing the wrist in a short arm cast for 6 weeks. Progressive exercises are begun when the cast is removed. If a Kirschner wire is used, the wire is removed through a window in the cast at 3 weeks (Brantley & Analla, 1980, p. 32).

CARPAL SCAPHOID IMPLANT. The installation of a scaphoid implant involves resecting the scaphoid and drilling a small hole in the trapezium to accept the stem of the scaphoid implant. Postoperative care includes the use of a bulky dressing and a volar splint for 3 to 5 days. A short arm cast is then applied and worn for 4 to 6 weeks (Brantley & Analla, 1980, p. 33).

CARPAL TRAPEZIUM IMPLANT. The replacement of the trapezium involves removing that bone and drilling a hole in the proximal metacarpal of the thumb to accept the stem of the trapezium implant. Adjacent tendon reconstruction or a Kirschner wire through the first and second metacarpals may be necessary to achieve stability. Postoperatively, the patient will have a bulky dressing with a splint or a thumb spica for 3 to 5 days. A short arm cast is then applied for 4 to 6 weeks. If a Kirschner wire is used, it is removed at 4 to 6 weeks (Brantley & Analla, 1980, p. 34).

SPECIAL CONDITIONS

Calcific Deposits in the Hand and the Wrist

Calcium salts deposited in the soft tissues, particularly about the wrist, may cause severe pain of sudden onset. The condition is similar to that seen more commonly in the shoulder. Clinically, the patient holds the wrist and hand protectively rigid, as any motion causes severe pain. The wrist tissues are swollen, reddened, and extremely sensitive. The roentgenogram shows an opacity in the soft tissues, particularly near tendons. The site of insertion of the flexor ulnaris is frequently involved. The pathological process is usually self-limiting, and the deposits disappear in a few weeks' time. To alleviate pain, procaine injections and immobilization in a cast are effective (Turek, 1977, p. 965).

Ganglion

A ganglion is a cystic swelling overlying a joint or a tendon sheath (Fig. 11–14). One large main cyst develops and is either uniocular or multiocular. Multiple small accessory cysts usually lie adjacent to the large cyst. The cyst walls

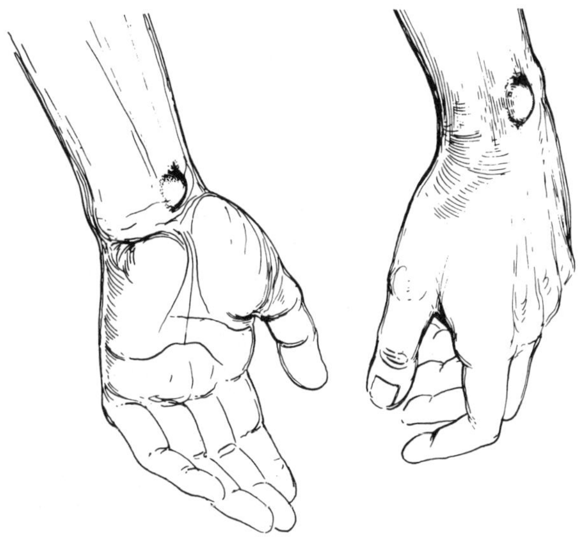

Figure 11–14. Ganglia may be found on the wrist's dorsal or volar surfaces.

are dense fibrous capsules, and the cyst fluid is thick, sticky, clear, and colorless with the consistency of soft jelly. No communication with the joint or tendon sheath is apparent, but invariably the cyst is bound to those structures by dense tissue. A ganglion occurs most frequently about the wrist, but may appear adjacent to any joint or tendon sheath. At the wrist, the cyst's usual location is the dorsum between the long extensor of the thumb and the extensor to the index finger, and it may be traced down to the articulation between the scaphoid and the lunate. Over the volar aspect of the wrist, the swelling often appears between the brachioradialis and the flexor carpi radialis tendons, and it usually is closely adherent to the latter. In the palm of the hand, the ganglion develops from the deep pulley of the finger flexors over the metacarpal heads.

There are two theories to explain why ganglions develop. One is that the dense collagenous tissue of the wrist undergoes degeneration, which leads to the formation of multiple small cysts containing mucin. Over time, several small cysts may coalesce into one large cyst. The other theory postulates a defect in the joint capsule or tendon sheath, which permits a protrusion of synovial tissue. The communicating channel between the protruding tissue and the joint becomes obliterated, and a cyst remains as a nonpatent pedicle or adhesion. If the defect in the capsule or sheath persists, additional cysts may be formed (Turek, 1977, pp. 975–976).

A ganglion of the wrist can be treated by both nonoperative and operative procedures. Nonoperative procedures include (1) aspirating the cyst fluid and injecting the remaining tissue with prednisolone (Meticortelone) or a sclerosing agent (e.g., 5 percent sodium morrhuate), (2) rupturing the cyst by means of an external force, and (3) using roentgenographic therapy (e.g., a 1.5-erythema dose, repeated in 1 month). However, nonoperative methods are frequently unsuccessful and surgical excision is required. After surgical removal, a plaster splint is used to immobilize the wrist in a relaxed position for approximately 3 weeks. Once the splint is removed, active exercises are needed because the capsular tightening done at the time of surgery produces a temporary limitation of motion.

Carpal Tunnel Syndrome

Carpal tunnel syndrome, also known as tardy median nerve palsy, results from a compression of the median nerve within the carpal tunnel. It occurs most often in patients between the ages of 30 to 60 years and is five times more frequent in women than in men. Any condition that reduces the capacity of the carpal tunnel may initiate the syndrome, for example a malaligned Colles' fracture, infection, trauma, tumor, or rheumatoid tenosynovitis. Systemic conditions such as obesity, diabetes mellitus, thyroid dysfunction, and Raynaud's disease can also produce the syndrome (Edmondson & Crenshaw, 1980, p. 361).

Paresthesia over the sensory distribution of the median nerve is the most frequent symptom. Pain frequently causes the patient to awaken during the night with a burning and numbness of the hand that is relieved by exercise.

Tinel's sign may also be demonstrated in most patients by percussing the median nerve at the wrist (Fig. 11–15A). Some atrophy of the thenar muscles, which are innervated by the median nerve, is frequently reported (Edmondson & Crenshaw, 1980, p. 361). Acute flexion of the wrist for 60 seconds (Phalen's test), or strenuous use of the hand, increases the paresthesia (Fig. 11–15B). Application of a blood pressure cuff on the upper arm sufficient to produce venous distention may also initiate the symptoms.

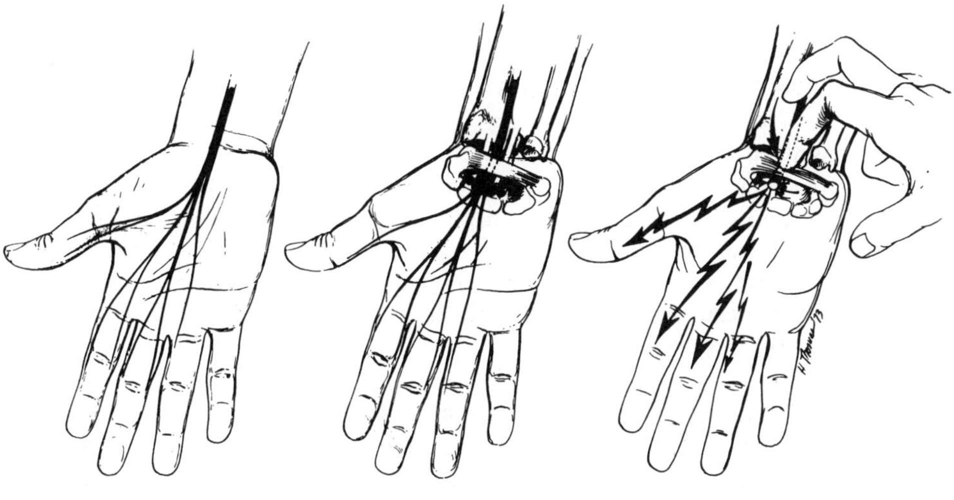

A

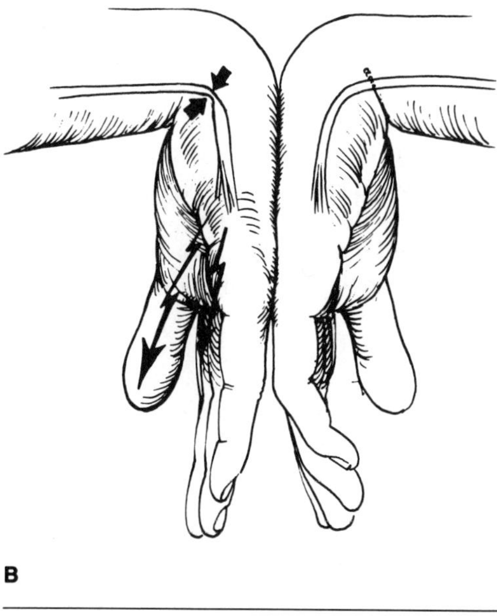

B

Figure 11–15. A. Carpal tunnel syndrome *(left and middle)*. Tinel sign *(right)*. **B.** Phalen's test to reproduce symptoms of carpal tunnel syndrome.

If mild symptoms exist and there is no thenar muscle atrophy, an injection of hydrocortisone into the carpal tunnel may give relief. When the symptoms are persistent and progressive, and there is muscle atrophy, division of the deep carpal ligament is usually indicated. After a surgical division of the ligament, a compression dressing and a volar splint are usually applied. The hand is actively used as soon as possible after surgery, but care must be taken to prevent the hand from being in a dependent position. A smaller dressing may be applied after 1 week, and normal use of the hand is then encouraged. The sutures are removed after 10 to 14 days, and the splint is maintained for 14 to 21 days (Edmondson & Crenshaw, 1980, p. 363).

□ NURSING PROCESS (Table 11–3)

Assessment

The first step in the assessment of a typical patient with a compression dressing and a volar splint following a surgical division of the carpal ligament is a neurovascular assessment of the affected arm and hand. Check that the hand is properly elevated on pillows and that the dressing is not too tight. Determine the location, duration, and severity of pain. Look for drainage on the dressing.

Nursing Diagnosis and Goal Formulation

Nursing diagnoses for a typical patient with a surgical division of the carpal ligament and a compression dressing are (1) alterations in comfort related to pain from surgery, (2) alterations in mobility related to decreased mobility in the wrist and hand from soft tissue swelling, (3) potential complications related to surgery and decreased mobility in the hand, and (4) alterations in psychological well-being related to anxiety and knowledge deficit about the surgery and the treatment methods.

Short-term goals are to have the patient experience (1) a decrease in the amount of pain through nursing measures and prescribed medications, (2) an increase in mobility through the use of controlled exercises, (3) an absence of complications from surgery and decreased arm activities, and (4) a decrease in anxiety through increased knowledge. Long-term goals are to have the patient free of pain and to have hand function.

Planning and Intervention

Alleviate Pain. Measures that help reduce pain are to elevate the affected hand above the elbow and to administer pain medications.

Increase Mobility. Soon after surgery the patient should start finger exercises. The compression dressing is usually removed a week after surgery and a small dressing and volar splint are applied. The patient is then encouraged to begin normal use of the hand. After the splint is removed,

TABLE 11–3. NURSING PROCESS FOR CARPAL TUNNEL SYNDROME TREATED BY SURGICAL DIVISION, COMPRESSION DRESSING, AND VOLAR SPLINT

Assessment	Nursing Diagnosis	Goal Formulation	Planning and Intervention	Evaluation and Reassessment
1. Assess the location, duration, and severity of pain. Assess for any swelling or neurovascular deficit. Assess tightness of dressing.	1. Alteration in comfort: pain in wrist related to soft tissue swelling.	1. Short-term goal: a relative state of comfort. Long-term goal: free of pain.	1. Alleviate Pain Elevate the hand above the elbow. Administer prescribed pain medications. Instruct on finger exercises.	1. Pain should be relieved by medication. No swelling should be noted.
2. Assess the motor and sensory function of the hand and wrist. Assess ability to do exercises.	2. Impaired physical mobility: lack of wrist function related to ligament and soft tissue trauma.	2. Short-term goal: an increase in mobility through controlled exercise. Long-term goal: return of function with no loss of function.	2. Increase Mobility Elevate the hand above the elbow. Instruct on finger, elbow, and shoulder exercises. Encourage normal hand use 14–21 days after surgery when dressing and splint removed. Avoid any pressure at the elbow.	2. The patient should be able to demonstrate the correct method of doing exercises and caring for the affected hand. The hand should be kept elevated.
3. Assess neurovascular status (especially the median nerve). Assess tightness of dressing.	3. Potential for injury: neurovascular deficit related to soft tissue swelling.	3. Short- and long-term goal: free of neurovascular deficit.	3. Prevent Complications *Neurovascular* Keep the hand elevated. Keep swelling reduced. Make sure dressing and splint are not too tight. Report any neurovascular deficit.	3. Expect no swelling and no neurovascular deficit or signs of infection. Patient should avoid putting the hand in a dependent position.
Assess for signs of infection (redness, swelling, increase in pain, drainage, and an increase in temperature.	Potential for injury: infection related to surgical incision.	Short- and long-term goal: free of any sign of infection.	*Integumentary* Keep dressing dry. Teach signs and symptoms of infection.	

(continued)

TABLE 11–3. ***(Continued)***

Assessment	Nursing Diagnosis	Goal Formulation	Planning and Intervention	Evaluation and Reassessment
4. Assess the patient's level of understanding about the rehabilitation process and home care needs.	4. Potential knowledge deficit related to the rehabilitation process.	4. Short- and long-term goal: a decrease in anxiety through increased knowledge.	4. Patient Teaching Demonstrate how to keep dressing clean and dry. Instruct on the signs and symptoms of infection. Demonstrate how to do a neurovascular assessment. Discuss restrictions such as avoiding activities that twist the wrist and not lifting objects which weigh more than 1 pound.	4. The patient should be able to demonstrate a neurovascular assessment, verbalize the important points in how to keep the dressing dry, and know the signs and symptoms of infection. The patient should be able to verbalize restrictions on activities and know potential problems and what measures should be taken to deal with them.

usually 14 to 21 days after surgery, exercises for the wrist are started. The patient should not need a sling.

Prevent Complications. Potential complications following median nerve decompression are neurovascular impairment and infection. Assess and intervene for any neurovascular impairment and implement infection control measures.

Patient Teaching. Instruct the patient how to keep the dressing clean and dry, and how to keep the hand above the elbow and avoid putting it in a dependent position. Explain the signs and symptoms of infection and how to assess the neurovascular status of the affected hand. The patient's unaffected arm can be used to help the patient learn the procedure. Following surgery, the patient should avoid activities that twist the wrist, and should not lift objects that weigh more than 1 pound.

Evaluation and Reassessment

Determine the level of pain and whether nursing measures and medications are effective in relieving pain. Note whether the patient is keeping the hand elevated and doing finger exercises. In discussions with the patient, determine the level of understanding of the rehabilitation process. Supply information and correct misconceptions. The patient should recognize the signs of potential problems and know when to notify the physician.

Ulnar Tunnel Syndrome

Ulnar tunnel syndrome results from compression of the ulnar nerve within a tight, triangular fibroosseous tunnel, about 1.5 cm long, which is located at the wrist. The tunnel is formed by the superficial and deep transverse ligaments, the pisiform bone, and the pisohamate ligaments. Symptoms follow the distribution of the ulnar nerve, and the amount of nerve compression determines whether these symptoms are motor, sensory, or both. Usually a ganglion is the cause of the compression, but other causes may be an aneurysm of the ulnar artery, thromboses of the ulnar artery, hemorrhage from a fracture of the hamate, or a lipoma. Treatment consists of surgical exploration of the ulnar nerve at the wrist and removal of the cause of compression (Edmondson & Crenshaw, 1980, p. 363).

NEOPLASM

Benign Giant-Cell Tumor

A benign giant-cell tumor is an osteolytic tumor (osteoclastoma) that occurs in young adults 15 to 35 years of age. The most common location is an asymmetric position in the epiphysis of a long bone, and the lower femur, the distal radius, and the upper tibia are the most frequent sites. There is a chronic, constant, and progressive pain in the region of the joint, which becomes worse at night and with increased activity. Limitation of joint motion is not observed until late in the disease process, as the tumor expands and distorts the end of the bone. A pathological fracture may also occur at a late stage after a large amount of cancellous and cortical bone is destroyed. Treatment consists of curretting the tumor and cauterizing the tumor wall. If necessary the cavity is filled with bone chips. When the tumor is extensive, a resection of that segment of the bone is done, and the remaining shaft is arthrodesed with the use of an intramedullary pin.

AMPUTATIONS ABOUT THE WRIST

Whenever feasible, a transcarpal amputation or a disarticulation of the wrist is preferable to an amputation through the forearm because pronation and supination are preserved as long as the distal radioulnar joint remains normal. Although only 50 percent of any pronation and supination is transmitted to a prosthesis, those motions are extremely valuable to the amputee. Furthermore, when compared to more proximal amputations, the longer lever arm left by amputation at the wrist increases the ease and power with which the prosthesis can be used. In transcarpal amputations, flexion and extension of the radiocarpal joint is preserved, and these motions can be utilized prosthetically. Prosthetic fitting for transcarpal amputation stumps is difficult but possible. Wrist disarticulation prostheses are now available, and thin prosthetic wrist units are now being used that allow the arms to be of equal length. Postoperative care focuses on the rehabilitation of the patient, regardless of whether a prosthesis is involved.

THE HAND

Trauma

Because of its multifaceted activities, the hand is often injured. Lacerating and crushing injuries to the hand may sever tendons and nerves. Joint dislocations and fractures are common. Industrial accidents may result in traumatic amputations of fingers or even the entire hand. Treatment of hand trauma frequently poses perplexing problems that require specialized knowledge from orthopaedic surgeons, plastic surgeons, and microsurgeons (Gartland, 1979, p. 295).

TENDON INJURIES

Flexor Tendon Injuries

Each finger contains two flexor tendons: the flexor sublimus, which inserts on the middle phalanx, and the flexor profundus, which inserts on the distal phalanx. The thumb has only one long flexor tendon, inserting on the distal phalanx. These tendons are contained in dense fibrous tunnels or sheaths in the area from the distal flexion crease of the palm of the hand to the distal finger joints. Many common industrial and household accidents can result in lacerating injuries to the hand and fingers that sever one or more flexor tendons.

Flexor tendon injuries require surgical intervention, but the procedures involved depend upon the time elapsed between injury and treatment, the amount of contamination in the wound, and the location and extent of the damage. In many recently inflicted wounds without extensive contamination, the wound can be cleansed and the tendon(s) immediately repaired. In older wounds, or wounds with extensive contamination, tendon repair is often delayed. In the basic repair, the tendon ends are found, trimmed, and repaired by end-to-end suturing. In some immediate repairs and in most delayed repairs, the muscles have contracted and the end-to-end repair would probably result in too much tension on the tendon. In those cases, a transfer or tendon graft is required (Brantley & Analla, 1980, p. 38). Donor tendons for grafting, in order of preference, are usually the palmaris longus, the plantaris, the long extensors of the toes, the extensor indicis proprius, and the flexor digitorum sublimis (Edmondson and Crenshaw, 1980, p. 227). After repair, a cast or splint is usually applied and worn for 4 to 6 weeks. Progressive range-of-motion exercises are begun following the removal of the immobilizing device.

Infection and adhesions may prevent the complete return of normal motion. In some areas of the hand and the fingers, a laceration may sever both the flexor sublimus and the flexor profundus tendons at the same level in the hand. If both tendons are repaired at the same level at the same time, they frequently will adhere to each other during the healing period with resulting finger stiffness. Many authorities believe that the proper treatment in such cases is to repair the profundus and excise the sublimus tendon. The profundus runs to the distal phalanx and has sufficient strength to flex the entire finger in the absence of the sublimus tendon.

If a tendon becomes adherent to its fibrous sheath by scar formation, resulting in a loss of function in a finger, treatment may include complete excision of the tendon and the insertion of a Silastic rod or a Silastic tendon prosthesis around which a new sheath can form. Months later the Silastic rod or prosthesis can be removed and a flexor tendon graft inserted through the newly formed tendon sheath (Edmondson & Crenshaw, 1980, p. 226).

Extensor Tendon Rupture (Mallet Finger)

Mallet finger (or baseball finger) is a term applied to an extensor tendon rupture deformity that results when a direct blow on the tip of an extended finger forces the distal phalanx into sudden flexion and ruptures the extensor tendon at its insertion (Fig. 11–16). The injury may be a closed or open injury, and the extensor tendon may pull away from the distal phalanx cleanly or it may avulse.

The end of a mallet finger exhibits a characteristic "droop" into flexion, and the patient loses the ability to actively extend the fingertip. Initially, the distal interphalangeal joint is swollen and painful. Later, the deformity may only be annoying because of the tendency of the drooped finger to get in the way, e.g., catch on clothing or in pockets.

If the injury is closed and treated soon after trauma, the distal phalanx may be splinted in hyperextension, with the proximal interphalangeal joint in flexion, for a period of 4 to 8 weeks. Occasionally, there may be an associated avulsion fracture or an injury severe enough to warrant surgical intervention with the use of pin fixation for 3 weeks. In either instance, the tendon usually reattaches to the bone and there is a return of function. In patients with a deformity of long duration, surgical repair is often unsatisfactory. However, fusion of the distal interphalangeal joint in the position of function gives good results.

Rupture of Extensor Pollicis Longus Tendon

The rupture of the extensor pollicis longus tendon of the thumb may follow a Colles' fracture. It may also be produced by degenerative changes in the tendon caused by the tendon rubbing against an irregular bony surface. Such ruptures are not uncommon in certain occupations, such as drummer and carpenter. Rupture causes a loss of extension of the distal thumb joint and a partial loss of extension in the proximal joint, with a consequent impairment of grasp. Direct suturing of the tendon through the ruptured area is frequently not feasible because the proximal segment retracts. By 1 month after injury, a fixed contracture of the muscle usually develops (Edmondson & Crenshaw, 1980, p. 225; Gartland, 1979, pp. 305–306).

The preferred treatment is to repair the rupture by use of a tendon graft or tendon transfer. After surgery, a splint is applied with the wrist in near full

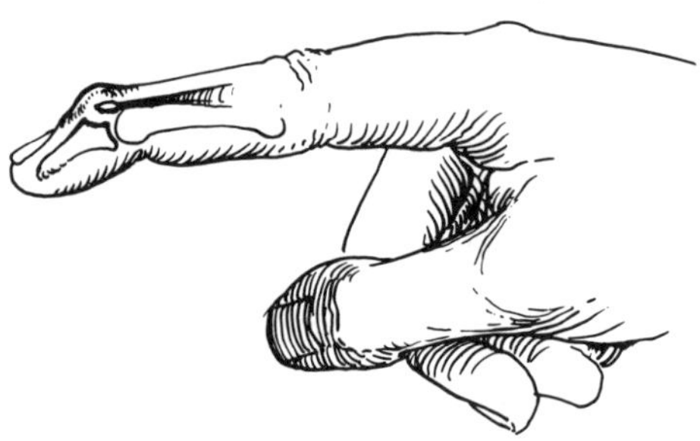

Figure 11–16. Mallet finger.

extension and the thumb extended and abducted. The splint is begun distal to the elbow and extends to the thumb tip and to the distal palmar crease. That immobilizes the thumb but allows movement in the fingers. The splint is worn for 4 weeks, after which the thumb is gradually permitted to move while the wrist is kept splinted for another week.

NERVE INJURIES

The median, ulnar, and radial nerve lie in close proximity to the flexor tendons, and are often severed in a tendon laceration. Nerve injuries usually require primary surgical intervention. In the case of grossly contaminated wounds, however, delayed repair may be necessary.

In a neurorrhaphy, the goal is to restore distal neuromuscular function. The nerve ends are found, trimmed, and the sheaths (epineurium) are sutured together using a fine, nonabsorbable suture. The hand and the arm are then immobilized in a plaster splint so that no tension is exerted on the repair for approximately 3 to 4 weeks after surgery. When the splint is removed, gradually increasing range of motion is permitted. It usually takes several months for motor or sensory function to return, and sensory or motor deficits, or both, may remain no matter how carefully the surgical repair was done. Complications include distal nerve atrophy during nerve regeneration and contractures due to joint immobilization (Brantley & Analla, 1980, p. 39; Donahoo & Spickler, 1980, p. 92).

SPRAINS

Many sprains are momentary subluxations that reduce spontaneously. In a subluxation, as in a complete dislocation, the capsule and collateral ligaments may be torn, although the damage is usually less severe. A capsular tear caused by a subluxation of the head of a metacarpal or a phalanx may be difficult to reduce and maintain in position after reduction. Effective treatment for capsular tears usually requires open reduction, surgical repair of the tear, and a period of immobilization.

DISLOCATIONS

Dislocations of finger joints can occur at the interphalangeal and metacarpophalangeal joints. They are usually caused by hyperextension injuries and, as a rule, are reduced quite readily by the application of manual traction with simultaneous slight flexion. Following reduction, the joint is immobilized in a position of slight flexion for 1 week. Occasionally, the end of a dislocating bone will "button-hole" through the capsule of the joint. When this occurs, the torn capsule may fold around the bone end, making closed manipulation reduction impossible. An open reduction and surgical capsular repair then becomes necessary.

A dislocation of the metacarpophalangeal thumb joint is the most common digit dislocation, and it frequently causes a capsular tear. The proximal phalanx usually displaces backward (dorsally) and the head of the metacarpal may protrude through the capsule, which can buttonhole the head of the metacarpal and maintain the dislocation. Occasionally a metacarpal dislocation of the thumb is accompanied by a fracture of the hook of the first metacarpal. When a dislocation of the thumb occurs without a fracture or a capsular tear and is recognized early, it can be reduced and the joint immobilized for 4 to 6 weeks to prevent recurrent dislocations. Other instances require an open reduction and surgical capsular repair.

The fifth metacarpophalangeal joint is a saddle joint and resembles the first (thumb) metacarpophalangeal joint. Open reduction is usually necessary in a dislocation of the fifth metacarpophalangeal joint, with a wire inserted to maintain the reduction. Degenerative changes usually occur following such a dislocation. These changes impair the cupping of the hand and prevent the formation of a good grip.

FRACTURES

Fractures of the phalanges and metacarpals may be spiral or transverse. Often there is no displacement of the fracture fragments and simple immobilization suffices to insure healing. Nondisplaced finger fractures are usually immobilized for approximately 10 to 14 days in a position of gentle flexion. Nondisplaced metacarpal fractures are immobilized for a 3- to 4-week period with the hand and wrist in a position of function.

Displacement of the fracture fragments leads to shortening and rotation of the involved finger. If the displacement cannot be reduced and maintained by closed methods, surgical intervention is usually necessary. Surgical treatment consists of open or closed reduction and internal fixation, usually with a Kirschner wire (Fig. 11–17). Internal fixation is indicated when (1) a displaced fracture with a fragment too small to manipulate involves a joint; (2) a fracture is displaced so severely that interposition of soft tissue prevents realignment by manipulation; (3) a fracture is so unstable that muscle contracture or joint motion will soon displace it; (4) fractures are multiple and the hand cannot be maintained in a position of function without internal fixation; (5) a fracture is open; and (6) a fracture traps a tendon between the fragments. Internal fixation usually consists of one or two oblique or intramedullary Kirschner wires or two parallel or crossed wires (Edmondson & Crenshaw, 1980, pp. 163–166).

Occasionally a patient has a severely traumatized hand with extensive skin damage, lacerated tendons and nerves, and multiple fractures. Such fractures are best treated by intramedullary pin fixation, or an external fixation device that provides a stable skeletal framework for other reconstructive procedures.

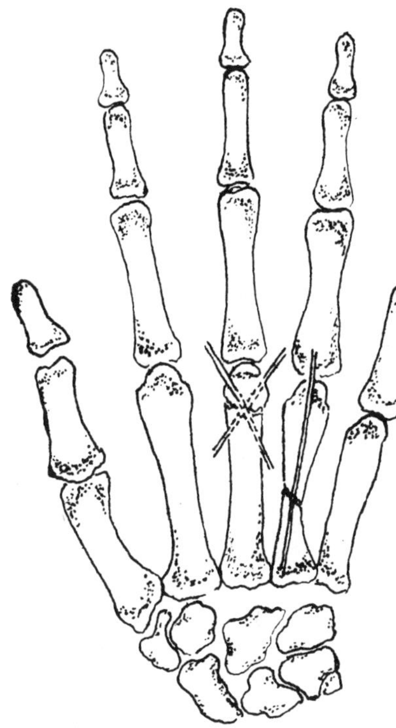

Figure 11–17. Open reduction and internal fixation, fractured metacarpal or phalanx. *(From Brantley, P., & Analla, M., 1980, p. 27. Courtesy of Howmedica.)*

Bennett's Fracture

Bennett's fracture is an intra-articular fracture through the base of the first metacarpal (Fig. 11–18A). The shaft of the metacarpal is laterally dislocated (with the hand in supination) by the unopposed pull of the abductor pollicis longus, but the medial fragment remains in place or is slightly rotated because of its capsular attachment. The fracture is usually caused by a force applied to the end of the thumb, and if not properly reduced can result in a permanent disability.

If the lateral displacement is minimal, reduction may be obtained by immobilizing the hand and the wrist in a cast with the thumb in wide abduction. Nonetheless, the use of a cast to maintain reduction by pressure on the base of the metacarpal may be unsatisfactory, because too much pressure causes skin necrosis and too little allows loss of reduction.

Fractures with fragments that are displaced and unstable usually require skeletal traction, closed percutaneous pinning, or open reduction with pin fixation. Skeletal (rubber band) traction that employs a transverse pin through the proximal phalanx is usually not dependable, as immobilization may be incomplete. Closed percutaneous pinning is accomplished by first placing a

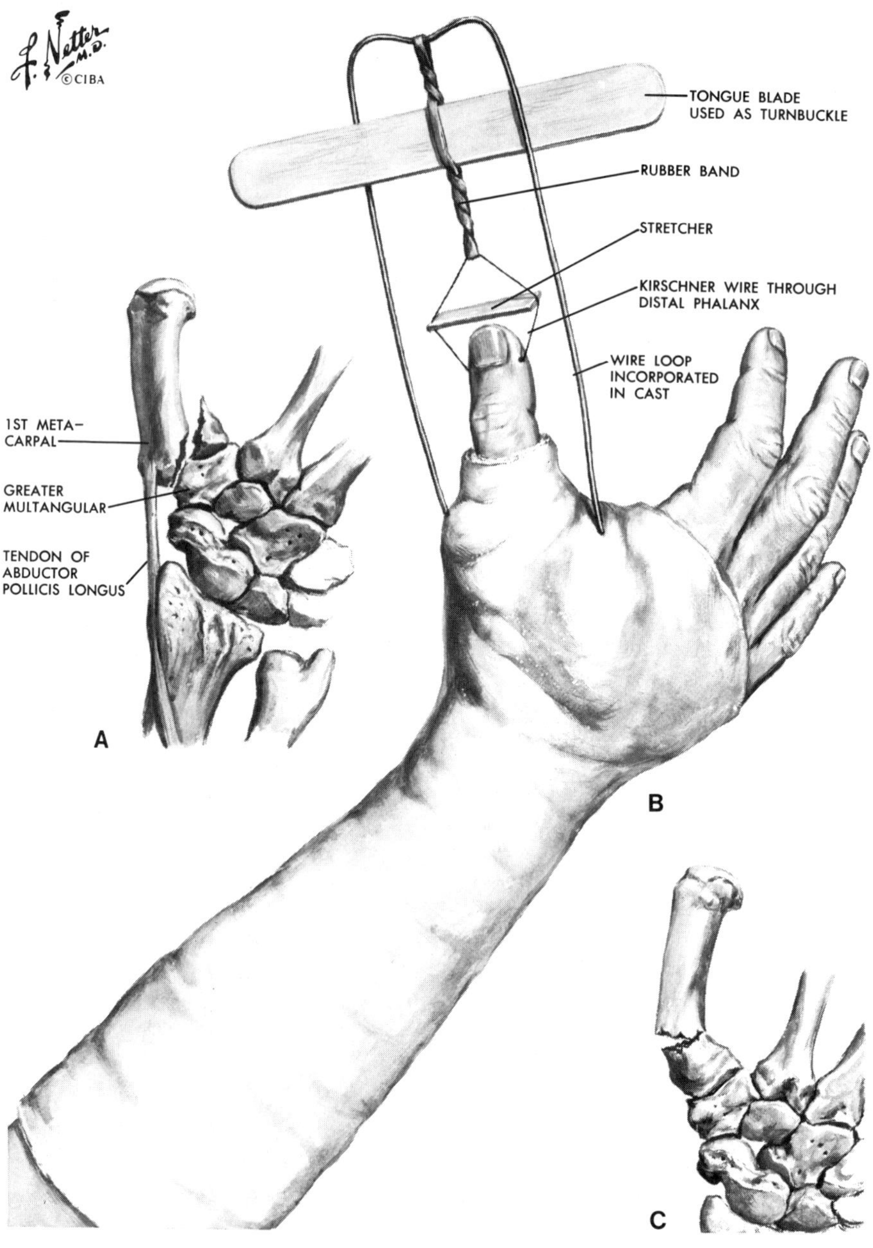

Figure 11–18. **A.** Intra-articular fracture of base of first metacarpal bone (Bennett's fracture). **B.** Immobilization with traction for Bennett's fracture. **C.** Transverse fracture of first metacarpal bone. *(Copyright © 1970, CIBA Pharmaceutical Corporation, Division of CIBA-GEIGY Corporation. Reprinted with permission from* Clinical symposia, *illustrated by Frank H. Netter, M.D. All rights reserved.)*

Kirschner wire pin into the base of the metacarpal, across the joint, and into the trapezium, then applying manual traction to reduce the fracture, and finally applying a forearm cast to effect immobilization with the wrist in extension and the thumb in abduction (Fig. 11–18B). The distal joint of the thumb is kept free of the cast. If closed percutaneous pinning is unsatisfactory, an open reduction is necessary. In an open reduction, the fracture is exposed and then reduced and maintained with the use of Kirschner wires. After surgery, a forearm cast is applied as described above. The cast is removed for wound inspection at 2 to 3 weeks and then replaced until 4 weeks after surgery. The wires are then removed and the hand immobilized for another 2 to 4 weeks.

Boxer's Fracture

The term boxer's fracture applies to a fracture of the neck of the fifth metacarpal, which can occur when an object is struck with a clenched fist. The head of the fifth metacarpal is displaced into the palm, and there is a flattening or loss of the knuckle prominence. There is also a great tendency for the pull of the extensor carpi ulnaris to proximally displace the metacarpal shaft.

It may be possible to restore the depressed metacarpal head to normal alignment by simultaneously pushing upward on the flexed proximal phalanx of the finger and downward on the metacarpal shaft. Once reduction is accomplished, it is difficult to maintain that position, and percutaneous pinning of the fracture fragments may be necessary to maintain the reduction. If manual reduction is impossible, the fracture may be reduced by mechanical traction or percutaneous pinning, followed by the application of a cast for immobilization. Boxer's fractures that are healing in a displaced position may need either correction of the malunion by osteotomy or a resection arthroplasty (Gartland, 1979, pp. 299–300).

Pathology

ARTHRITIS AND INFECTIOUS DISEASES

Rheumatoid Arthritis

Severe rheumatoid arthritis may cause grotesque and disabling deformities of the hand. Rheumatoid arthritis of the hand principally affects the synovial lining of the joints and the tendon sheaths, and the disease process also invades and destroys ligaments and tendons. The synovial covering of the flexor tendons in the hands may become inflamed and thickened and obstruct the easy sliding of tendons within the fibrous canal on the volar surface of the fingers, preventing full finger flexion. The thickening of the synovial lining may be palpable in the hands of nodular protrusions.

The development of "trigger fingers" (see pp. 686–687) may be the earliest evidence of rheumatoid disease. This condition is due to diffuse synovitis of the flexor sheath and thickening of the flexor superficialis tendon where it passes through the canal over the metacarpal heads. Distally within the finger, nodular thickening of the profundis may prevent its gliding through the bifurcation of the superficialis (sublimis).

The disease process may directly invade the tendons, which become frayed, fragile, attenuated, and ruptured. Any tendon may rupture, but rupture is more likely where bony compression and friction occur. Therefore, one of the most commonly ruptured tendons is the extensor pollicis longus (see p. 670). Other finger extensor ruptures are also seen, especially in patients with involvement of the distal radioulnar joint and dorsal dislocation of the ulna. The protruding flexor pollicis longus tendon is the most commonly ruptured tendon among the flexors, and the disruption usually takes place within the carpal tunnel.

Rheumatoid arthritis usually exists in the wrists as well as in the hands. A volar flexion deformity at the wrist increases the tension on the extensors, which pulls the metacarpophalangeal joints into hyperextension. The distal joints in the fingers are flexed secondarily, resulting in a "clawhand" deformity. An ulnar drift, i.e., a deviation of the fingers toward the ulnar side of the hand, tends to develop (see p. 689), which involves a subluxation of the metacarpophalangeal joints and a slipping of the extensor tendons off the top of the joints to the ulnar side. Ulnar deviation does not cause a great loss of function but may be unsightly.

As the disease process in the metacarpophalangeal joints invades and destroys the fascia and collateral ligaments, subluxation occurs because of the unopposed pull of the flexors. Increased tension in the extensors may lead to a buttonhole or boutonniere deformity of the finger (see pp. 687–688). Flexion and subluxation of a proximal finger joint, followed by hyperextension of the middle joint, produces a swan-neck deformity (see pp. 688–689). The distal joints of the fingers may also develop a flexion deformity due to hyperextension of the middle joint, though it is not particularly disabling. The joints of the thumb may develop subluxation, hyperextension, and flexion deformities. Most commonly, the metacarpophalangeal joint is flexed and subluxated, the interphalangeal joint is hyperextended, and the carpometacarpal joint is subluxated.

Osteoarthritis

The joints most frequently involved in osteoarthritis of the hands are the distal interphalangeal joints, the proximal interphalangeal joints, and the first carpometacarpal joint (i.e., the base of the thumb). The osteophytes that develop around the finger joints produce characteristic deformities known as Heberden's nodes (Fig. 11–19) at the distal interphalangeal joints and Bouchard's nodes at the proximal interphalangeal joints. Those conditions are more common in women, and the onset often coincides with menopause. Osteoarthritis of the hand may or may not be painful. Commonly there is pain when the

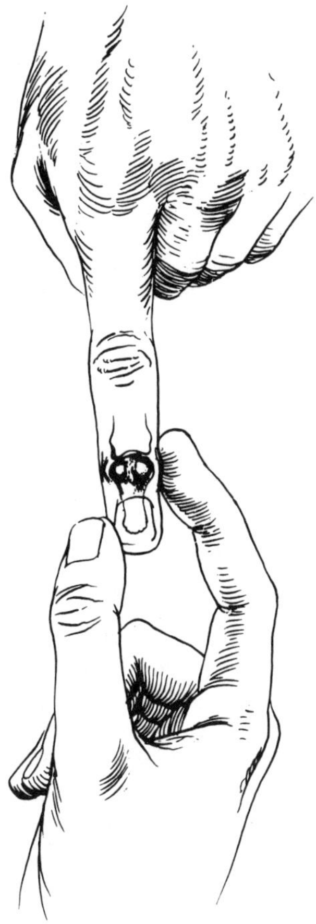

Figure 11–19. Heberden's nodes.

nodes appear, and occasionally it may be severe and associated with redness and tenderness. Eventually the pain subsides leaving a stiffer digit and a somewhat less dextrous but still functioning hand. Osteoarthritis of the first carpometacarpal joint is frequently asymptomatic, though occasionally there is temporary but severe pain (Swinson & Swinburn, 1980, pp. 14–16).

Treatment consists primarily of anti-inflammatory analgesic drugs such as aspirin or indomethacin. In cases of severe pain in the thumb, the first carpometacarpal joint may be splinted to allow the fingers to function. Occasionally, local injections of a steroid into the first carpometacarpal joint produce relief. Paraffin baths are also useful in producing temporary relief from pain in some patients. It is important to reassure patients with osteoarthritis of the hand that they do not have rheumatoid arthritis and will not develop major deformities of the hand. Surgical fusion or removal of one of the carpal bones is occasionally used in difficult cases of osteoarthritis of the first carpometacarpal joint.

Tuberculosis of the Hand

Tuberculosis of the hand is more common in children, is usually hematogenous, primarily involves the bony structures, and secondarily involves the joints. The tubercular infection is mainly in the subperiosteum of the bone. It interferes with the blood supply to the distal portion of the bone, causing necrosis. The infection also causes the bone to enlarge at the infection site, shortening it before a bony involucrum (new bony sheath) can develop. The course of the disease is chronic. Cold abscesses form within the bone and may rupture; persistent draining and secondarily infected bone sinuses result. The infected finger joints become ankylosed, and a spindle-shaped distended bone is characteristic.

Treatment consists of curettage of the bone, closure of the wound without drainage, prolonged immobilization of the finger, and the administration of antibiotics and chemotherapeutic agents specific for tuberculosis. The prognosis is good only in children. Obstinate drainage and crippling of the finger justifies amputation (Turek, 1977, pp. 956–958).

Arthrodesis

Arthrodesis of a joint of a finger or a thumb may be indicated when the joint has been so damaged by injury or disease that pain, deformity, or instability prevent useful motion. Occasionally a joint must be arthrodesed because the muscles that control the digit are not strong enough to both stabilize and move all joints. Of the three finger joints, arthrodesis is most often indicated for the proximal interphalangeal joint. The distal interphalangeal joint can frequently be stabilized by tenodesis. Arthrodesis is indicated least often for the metacarpophalangeal joint, because of the importance of motion in that joint. Thus when muscle power is sufficient, an arthroplasty is usually indicated, and when it is not, procedures to limit muscle function to the metacarpophalangeal joint are usually indicated. Of the joints of the thumb, arthrodesis is indicated most often for the metacarpophalangeal joint, because it results in little loss of function, and then for the interphalangeal joint, because fusion only results in a partial loss of the ability to pinch. Arthrodesis is indicated least often for the carpometacarpal joint because that joint is the most useful joint in the thumb. If the carpometacarpal joint of the thumb is to be arthrodesed, the function of the two distal joints should be satisfactory.

The following are the degree of flexion at which joints are usually arthrodesed: (1) in the fingers, the metacarpophalangeal joints are usually at 20 to 30 degrees of flexion, the proximal interphalangeal joints are usually at 40 to 50 degrees, and the distal interphalangeal joints at 15 to 20 degrees; (2) in the thumb, the interphalangeal joint is usually at 20 degrees, the metacarpophalangeal joint at 25 degrees, and the carpometacarpal joint at 0 degrees.

Arthrodesis of Interphalangeal Joints. In an arthrodesis of a proximal interphalangeal joint, the joint is incised and the proximal end of the middle phalanx is squared off. The distal end of the proximal phalanx is shaped by resecting its condyles until the proper angle for arthrodesis is obtained. The volar cartilaginous plate in a flexion contracture is not disturbed. (The plate stabilizes and compresses the ends of the bones anteriorly as the joint is forced into extension.) With the bones compressed, the joint is stabilized with parallel or crossed Kirschner wires. Resected bone fragments, used as bone grafts, are placed about the joint. The joint is then immobilized in a splint until roentgenograms show solid fusion. A similar procedure is used to fuse distal interphalangeal joints.

Arthrodesis of the Metacarpophalangeal Joint of the Thumb. Arthrodesis of the metacarpophalangeal joint of the thumb is usually indicated for degenerative arthritis after a malunited Bennett's fracture, for subluxation of the joint, for osteoarthritis, and for rheumatoid arthritis (Fig 11–20). The surgical procedure involves resecting the proximal phalanx and the distal end of the first metacarpal. The ends are then positioned together and held by Kirschner wires. After the surgery, the thumb is maintained in a thumb spica cast for 2 weeks. The skin sutures are then removed and the thumb spica cast reapplied and kept in place until roentgenograms demonstrate that bone fusion is obtained, usually at 12 weeks postsurgery.

Arthroplasty

The goal of an arthroplasty is to provide stability, relieve pain, and increase mobility. Of the finger joints, the metacarpophalangeals are the most likely to be treated by arthroplasty. The operation is usually indicated when degenerative changes in an otherwise useful finger joint result in less than 30 degrees of motion. The muscles that control the joint must have functional strength, or an arthroplasty will be of no value. Arthroplasty of a proximal interphalangeal joint is usually indicated only when a joint with lateral instability of 30 degrees and flexion and extension of 60 degrees or more, is preferable to a fused joint.

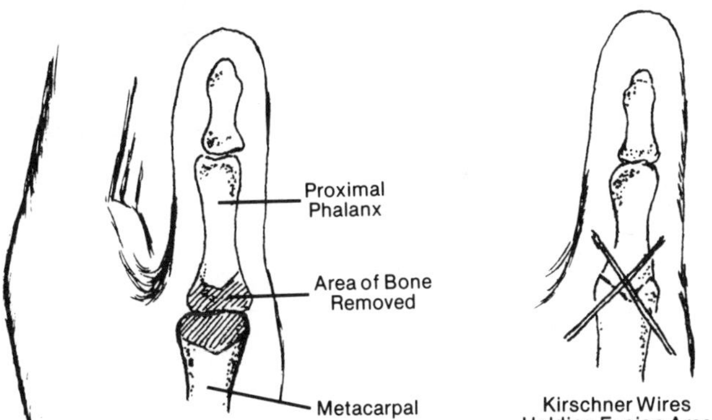

Figure 11–20. Fusion of metacarpophalangeal joint. *(From Brantley, P., & Analla, M., 1980, p. 28. Courtesy of Howmedica.)*

Again, the muscles that control the joint must have functional strength. Arthroplasty of the distal interphalangeal joint of a finger and the interphalangeal joint of the thumb is rarely indicated.

An arthroplasty (Fig. 11–21) using Silastic prosthesis for the joints of the fingers and the thumb is indicated when rheumatoid or degenerative arthritis causes pain, deformity, or disability in the metacarpophalangeal or interphalangeal joints. In the procedure, the proximal and distal portions of the involved joints are cut away and the canals reamed. The Silastic implant is then fitted into the canals. Tendon or ligament repairs are done as necessary for improved stability. With finger implants, a bulky hand dressing and volar splint are applied postoperatively. They are removed in 3 to 5 days and a dynamic brace is applied to the splint so that active finger motion can be started. After a carpometacarpal arthroplasty of the thumb, there is usually sufficient pain to require protection and immobilization for several weeks. When movement is started, the ability to pinch will be extremely weak and possibly painful for several months, until a buildup of heavy scar tissue takes place. Activities such

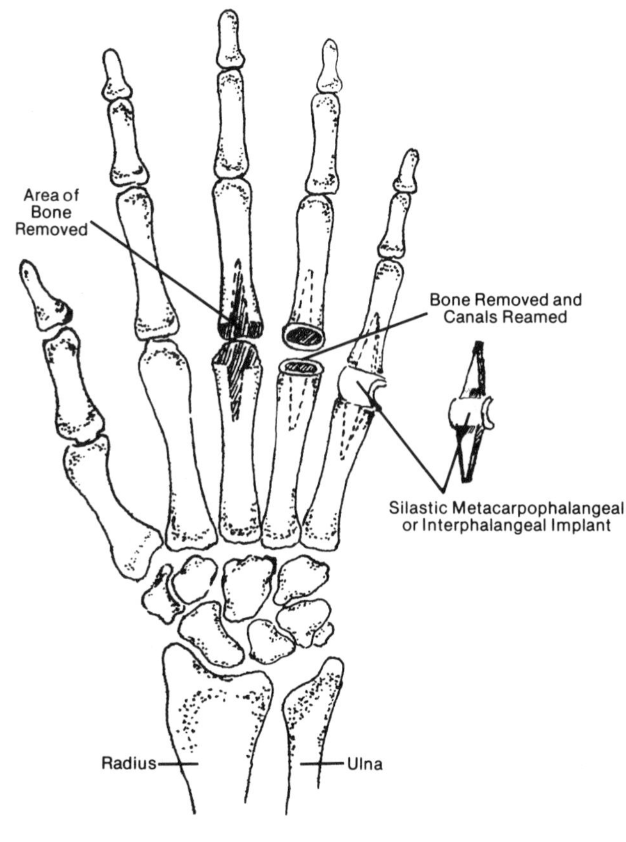

Figure 11–21. Silastic metacarpophalangeal or interphalangeal joint implant, Swanson design. *(From Brantley, P. & Analla, M., 1980, p. 31. Courtesy of Howmedica.)*

as opening car doors, cutting with scissors, putting on socks, and winding watches will eventually be possible, but will require practice and patience.

□ NURSING PROCESS (Table 11–4)

Assessment

The initial step in the assessment of a patient with a Silastic metacarpophalangeal (MP) joint implant, a bulky dressing, and a volar splint is to evaluate the neurovascular status of the hand (Chap. 2). In many instances that may be very difficult because of the dressing. Check that the hand is properly elevated. Look for any drainage on the dressing, and determine the location, duration, and severity of pain.

Nursing Diagnosis and Goal Formulation

Nursing diagnoses for a typical patient with a Silastic implant are (1) alterations in comfort related to pain from surgery, (2) alterations in mobility related to lack of joint stability, (3) potential complications related to surgery and decreased mobility in the hand, and (4) alterations in psychological well-being related to anxiety and knowledge deficit about the treatment methods.

Short-term goals are to have the patient experience (1) a decrease in the amount of pain through nursing measures and prescribed medications, (2) an increase in mobility through the use of controlled exercises, (3) an absence of complications from surgery and decreased activity in the hand, and (4) a decrease in anxiety through increased knowledge. Long-term goals are to have the patient free of pain and to have return of function in the hand.

Planning and Intervention

Alleviate Pain. Nursing measures that help reduce pain are to elevate the hand to prevent swelling and to give prescribed medications. The hand can be elevated on one or more pillows, or elevated by placing the affected hand and arm in a special sling and attaching it to an intravenous pole. Make sure the sling does not produce pressure on the patient's elbow. It is important that the patient keep the affected hand elevated at all times during the first few weeks, even during exercises, so that the swelling will decrease. The patient can also help reduce swelling in the hand by repeatedly squeezing and opening it.

Patients with metacarpophalangeal joint implants have a reduction in pain after the first few days following surgery. The pain level may increase, however, after they start their exercise program. Pain is used as a guide to the amount and vigor of the exercises. If pain lasts more than 2 hours following an activity, look at how and for how long the activity was performed, and adjust accordingly to avoid excessive strain.

TABLE 11–4. NURSING PROCESS FOR SILASTIC METACARPOPHALANGEAL (MP) JOINT IMPLANT

Assessment	Nursing Diagnosis	Goal Formulation	Planning and Intervention	Evaluation and Reassessment
1. Assess the duration, location, and severity of pain. Assess neurovascular status (may be difficult because of dressing). Check dressing for any constriction.	1. Alteration in comfort: pain in the hand and fingers related to soft tissue swelling and bone trauma.	1. Short-term goal: maintain a relative state of comfort with only minimal pain. Long-term goal: free of pain.	1. Alleviate Pain Keep the hand elevated. Make sure dressing is not tight. Instruct on relaxation techniques. Administer pain medication. Assist in repositioning hand every 2 hours. Avoid any pressure on elbow.	1. The patient should verbalize a reduction in pain after medication. Overall pain should be less following the first few days after surgery. If pain lasts more than 2 hours following exercises, reevaluate the amount and stress of the exercises.
2. Assess neurovascular status. Check that the hand is elevated. Check that exercises are done correctly.	2. Impaired physical mobility: decreased finger function related to lack of joint stability.	2. Short-term goal: an increase in mobility through controlled exercises. Long-term goal: regain optimal function in the hand.	2. Increase Mobility Elevate the hand; have patient wiggle the fingers every hour. Begin exercises 3–5 days after surgery. Keep brace with extension slings on day and night. If there is severe flexor weakness, remove extension slings 1–2 hours a day for greater active flexion of the MP joints. After 3 weeks, attach flexion cuff to brace 1–2 hours a day for passive flexion of MP joints.	2. The patient should be able to do the required exercises. If range of motion has not been obtained by second to third week it will be difficult to achieve. The patient should understand the importance of continuing the exercise program for

			Instruct on neck, shoulder, elbow, and wrist exercises. Report any excess swelling.	3 months or more to maintain movement and increase strength.
3. Assess for any signs of infection at the surgical site.	3. Potential for infection related to surgical incision.	3. Short- and long-term goal: free of any signs of infection.	3. Prevent Complications *Integumentary* Keep dressing clean and dry. Instruct on signs and symptoms of infection.	3. The patient should be able to verbalize an understanding of potential complications and activity reductions.
Assess for any signs of stress on the joints (e.g., increased pain or pain persisting 2 hours after exercises).	Potential for injury: decreased joint function related to overuse.	Short- and long-term goal: free of signs of joint stress.	*Breakage or Dislocation of Implant* Instruct the patient on the rehabilitation process. Discuss restrictions to avoid stress on the joints. *Other Complications* (See text.)	
4. Assess the patient's level of understanding about the rehabilitation process and home care needs. Assess the ability of the patient to care for self.	4. Potential knowledge deficit related to the rehabilitation process and self-care.	4. Short- and long-term goal: a decrease in anxiety through increased knowledge.	4. Patient Teaching Write down an exercise program. Go over the exercise program. Instruct on home care (e.g., hold heavy objects in the palm of the hand; use three-point pinch; avoid movements that push fingers toward the ulnar side of the hand; slide rather than carry objects; and use assistive devices in grasping).	4. The patient should be able to do exercise program without severe pain, demonstrate the motivation to do exercises without supervision, and understand the importance of not driving until that is approved by the physician.

Increase Mobility. The bulky dressing and volar splint are left on until the postoperative swelling has decreased, usually 3 to 5 days. For patients with MP joint replacements, the initial dressing is removed and a dynamic brace is then applied over a lightly padded dressing. The brace supports the patient's fingers in the desired position and allows movement in the artificial joint. If a brace is not available, guided early motion may still be obtained by applying a lightweight short arm cast fitted with outriggers and rubber band slings.

The brace, with extension slings, is usually worn day and night for the first 3 weeks, and then worn part time. If there is severe flexor weakness and good extension, the extension slings may be removed 1 to 2 hours a day during the second and third weeks to achieve greater active flexion of the MP joints. After 3 weeks, a flexion cuff may be attached to the brace and worn for 1 to 2 hours twice a day so that the MP joints may be flexed passively. Beginning with the fourth postoperative week, the extension slings are usually worn at night for another 3 weeks.

Even though the patient's fingers may be sore, it is necessary that they be bent and straightened in the brace frequently during the day. The goal of the exercise program is to obtain full extension and 70 degrees of flexion. The reconstructed joints start tightening during the second postoperative week, and will usually be quite tight after 3 weeks. If the desired range of motion has not been obtained by then, it will be difficult to achieve it. The patient needs to continue the exercise program for 3 months or more after surgery to maintain movement and increase strength. The patient should also exercise the neck, shoulder, elbow, and wrist twice a day so that they do not become stiff.

Prevent Complications. The major complications that may occur following a metacarpophalangeal joint implant are infection and breakage or dislocation of the implant. They can be prevented by infection control and educating the patient about the rehabilitation process.

Patient Teaching. Before the patient goes home, the occupational therapist should go over an outline of the patient's exercise program. The patient must return for check-ups to make sure that there are no problems, to adjust the brace or splint, and to modify the exercise program. Six weeks after surgery, most patients are able to use their hand for light activities and for personal care. It is advisable to caution the patient about doing heavy work for at least several months, and then only with the approval of the physician.

Stress that the new joint should be used but not abused. To reduce stress on the MP joints, the patient should remember (1) to hold heavy objects in the palm of the hand instead of with the thumb and fingers, i.e., to grasp instead of pinch, (2) to use three points, the thumb, the index, and the middle finger, when it is necessary to pinch, (3) to try to avoid movements that push the fingers toward the ulnar side of the hand, (4) to transfer the weight to the wrist and forearm when picking up heavy objects, (5) to slide rather than carry, and push instead of pull when moving heavy objects, (6) to use assistive devices in grasping to prevent strain on the fingers and the hand, and (7) to move fingers through their range of motion frequently and avoid prolonged resting positions.

Daily exercises are necessary to maintain range of motion. The patient needs (1) to move the wrist up and down and to each side, (2) to roll the finger tips into the palm, (3) to oppose each finger with the thumb to form a letter O, (4) to place the palm of the hand on a flat surface and then raise each finger individually, and (5) to do a finger walk with the hand, i.e., with the palm of the hand flat, adduct the index finger toward the thumb, then move the middle finger to meet the index finger, and so on.

Evaluation and Reassessment

Following an MP joint implant, the patient should have increased movement in the joint. Pain should be controlled by mild analgesics. The patient should be able to demonstrate the required exercises, have the motivation to do them without supervision, and be able to verbalize an understanding of potential complications and activity reductions.

SPECIAL CONDITIONS

Dupuytren's Contracture

Dupuytren's contracture arises from a chronic hyperplasia of the palmar fascia of the hand (Fig 11–22). Contractures that pull the fingers into a position of fixed flexion are caused by a proliferative fibroplasia of the subcutaneous palmar tissue, which occurs in the form of nodules and cords (Edmondson & Crenshaw, 1980, p. 354). Other changes include a thinning of the overlying subcutaneous fat, adhesions of the skin to the lesion, and later a pitting or dimpling of the skin. "Knuckle pads" are also common on the dorsum of the proximal interphalangeal joints.

The fingers most frequently affected are the ring finger and the little finger. The contracture is most common in men past 40 and is usually bilateral. The exact cause is unknown, but a hereditary pattern has been noted. Trauma is thought not to play a significant role, because the condition occurs frequently in those who do not do heavy manual labor. A high incidence has been observed in patients with gout and diabetes. As a rule, the condition is painless, but it does impair the function of the hand.

The only conservative treatment is finger stretching exercises. Surgery is usually the treatment of choice, and the surgical procedure is to resect the palmar fascia. Some physicians do a conservative resection, whereas others favor a more radical resection of the palmar fascia, which necessitates skin grafting. Postoperatively, a bulky hand dressing with or without a volar splint is usually applied for 5 to 7 days. Finger and hand exercises are begun after 24

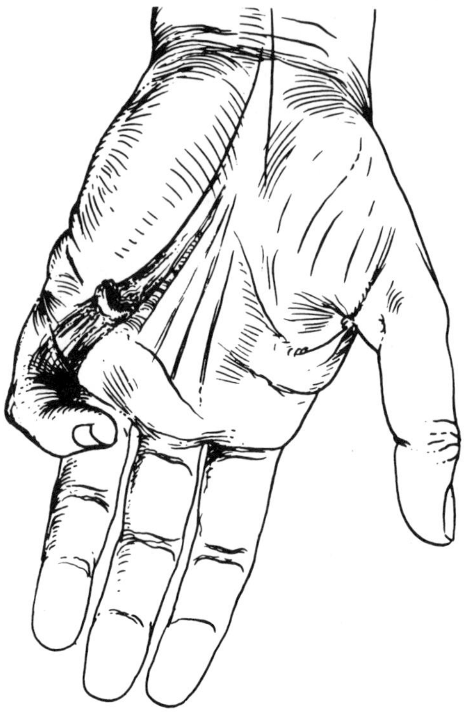

Figure 11–22. Dupuytren's contracture.

to 48 hours, but maximum rehabilitation may not be obtained for several months. Potential complications are infection, incomplete release of the contracture, scarring if motion is not instituted early, and recurrence of the contracture (Brantley & Analla, 1980, p. 45).

Trigger Finger

A trigger or snapping finger (Fig. 11–23) is one that locks in a flexed position and can be extended only with some difficulty and an associated "snap" or "pop." That condition is due to a narrowing or constricting of the flexor sheath at the level of the metacarpal neck. There is usually an accompanying nodular enlargement of the tendon that is probably secondary to the constriction. The "trigger mechanism," which is almost always located at the level of the metacarpal head, blocks free passage of the tendon, and if the tendon passes the point of obstruction, a click or snap is produced (Gartland, 1979, p. 303).

Occasionally the condition is relatively painless, but in most instances there is an aching pain as a mechanical tenosynovitis develops. Treatment often consists of hydrocortisone injected into the sheath at the level of the trigger mech-

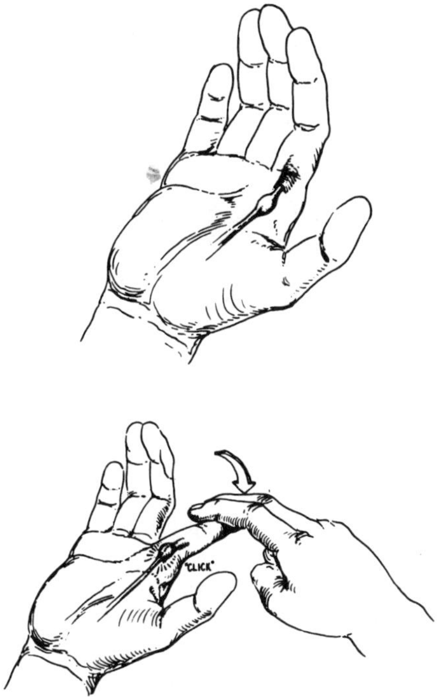

A

B

Figure 11–23. A and B. Trigger finger.

anism to reduce local edema and allow the tendon to glide freely. If that is not successful, surgical excision of the constricted portion of the sheath is necessary.

Buttonhole or Boutonniere Deformity

The so-called buttonhole or boutonniere deformity (Fig. 11–24) is commonly seen in patients with rheumatoid arthritis, although the tendon imbalance that causes the deformity is not unique to that condition. The names (*boutonniere* is French for buttonhole) arise because the extensor tendon splits around a joint which then pokes through it, and the split tendon resembles a buttonhole. The deformity is caused by a synovitis of the proximal interphalangeal joint, which causes a rupture of the central portion of the extensor and forces the lateral bands of the extensor to subluxate volarward. As the deformity progresses, the lateral bands of the extensor are forced further over the condyles of the proximal interphalangeal joint, become tightened by their new course and by pressure from the underlying swollen joint, and finally become fixed in a subluxated position volar to the transverse axis of the joint. The result is a secondary hyperextension contracture of the distal interphalangeal joint and a flexion

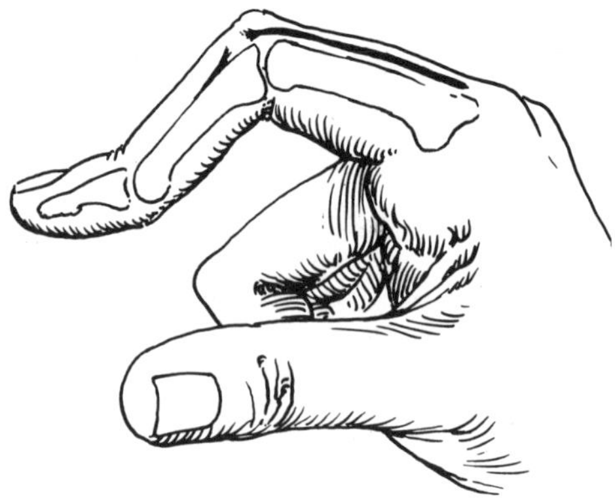

Figure 11–24. A "boutonniere" deformity.

contracture of the proximal interphalangeal joint. The MP joint is usually in a position of extension but joint motion is not lost.

The operative procedure to be used for reconstruction depends on the extent of the deformity. A mild flexion deformity (approximately 15 degrees) may be treatable by releasing the lateral tendons near their insertion in the distal phalanx. A moderate flexion contracture (approximately 40 degrees) usually requires a functional restoration of the central portion of the extensor and correction of the subluxation of the lateral bands. A severe buttonhole deformity usually requires an arthrodesis or possibly an interphalangeal joint arthroplasty.

Swan-Neck Deformity

A swan-neck deformity (Fig. 11–25) is usually caused by rheumatoid arthritis, but may also be related to cerebral palsy. Several fingers may be involved, and the condition may be quite disabling. The swan-neck deformity is characterized by flexion of the distal interphalangeal joint, hyperextension of the proximal interphalangeal joint, and flexion of the MP joint. It is caused by muscle imbalance and by secondary ligamentous and capsular relaxation at the proximal interphalangeal joint that allow that joint to hyperextend.

There are a number of surgical treatments that may improve function. One is a tenodesis of the proximal interphalangeal joint. Another is a synovectomy, possibly with the release of intrinsic muscle contractures. If there is marked proximal interphalangeal joint extension associated with joint destruction, an arthrodesis may be the procedure of choice if there is a near normal MP joint or if an MP joint arthroplasty is anticipated. An arthroplasty of the proximal interphalangeal joint may be done when there is a near normal MP joint. Most authorities would not favor an arthroplasty of both the MP joint

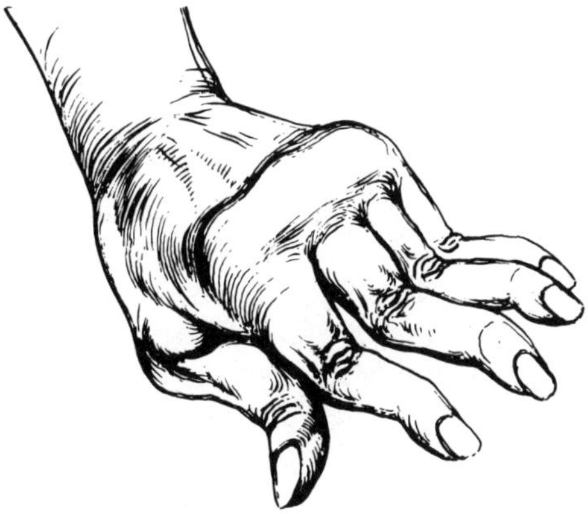

Figure 11–25. Swan-neck deformity.

and the proximal interphalangeal joint of the same finger, because of concerns about joint strength and stability.

Ulnar Deviation of the Fingers

The deformity of ulnar drift, or a marked deviation of the fingers toward the ulnar side of the hand, may be found in patients with rheumatoid arthritis and a few other conditions. Although the pathogenesis is not completely understood, ulnar deviation is thought to be caused by a combination of (1) stretching of the collateral ligaments of the MP joints by the volarly directed forces of the flexor tendons, which permits volar displacement of the proximal phalanges, (2) stretching of the accessory collateral ligaments, which permits ulnar displacement of the flexor tendons within their tunnels, (3) stretching of the flexor tunnels, which permits additional ulnar displacement of the long flexor tendons, (4) ulnar displacement of the long flexor tendons caused by surgical procedures to release their sheaths for multiple trigger fingers or for improving strength of grasp to the fingers, (5) contractures of the interosseus muscles that cause hyperextension of the proximal interphalangeal joints, flexion of the MP joints, and eventually subluxation of the MP joints, and (7) rupturing of the long extensor tendons (Edmondson & Crenshaw, 1980, pp. 320–321).

In the surgical treatment of the ulnar drift, a mild to moderate ulnar drift may be improved by extensor tendon realignment and MP joint synovectomy. Presently, there is no procedure available to realign ulnarly displaced flexor tendons (Edmondson & Crenshaw, 1980, p. 321). In severe ulnar drift with a dislocation of one or more MP joints, the function of the dislocated joints may be improved by arthroplasty (i.e., a Swanson implant). An arthroplasty of the MP joint usually relieves pain, maintains stability and alignment, and permits acceptable motion. (For surgical procedure and nursing care, see pp. 679–685.)

NEOPLASM

Osteoblastoma

A benign osteoblastoma (or osteogenic fibroma of bone, or giant osteoid osteoma) is an uncommon vascular osteoid and bone-forming tumor. It is slow growing and causes symptoms by encroaching on neighboring structures. Young men, usually younger than 20, are predisposed, and the majority of the tumors occur in the spine, in the metaphyseal or diaphyseal areas of the long bones of the lower extremities, and in the small bones of the hands and the feet. The patient usually complains of a dull, aching pain, not nocturnal and not relieved by aspirin. Symptoms generally occur from a few months to 2 years before the tumor is discovered. Complete surgical excision usually results in a cure (Turek, 1977, pp. 565–567).

Osteoid Osteoma

An osteoid osteoma is a small, rare lesion of the cartilaginous tissue of bones, composed of vascular fibrous tissue, proliferating fibroblasts, and minute formed osteoids. It occurs most frequently in young men 10 to 25 years of age. Osteoid osteoma has a predilection for the long bones, particularly the tibia and the femur, but the small bones of the hands and the feet are involved in many instances.

There is usually a solitary lesion that causes pain, mild at first but then increasingly severe and continuous, especially at night. There is a localized swelling that gradually becomes palpable as a spindle-shaped bony enlargement.

Complete excision immediately relieves the pain. Amputations are rarely warranted because surrounding sclerotic bone recedes once the center of the tumor is removed (Turek, 1977, pp. 564–565).

Chondroma

A chondroma (or endochondroma) is a benign tumor occurring in a central location in a bone that causes destruction of the surrounding bone. It is most common in young adults, and usually occurs in a phalanx or the humerus. There is usually a single lesion, with only slight soreness. Severe pain can occur suddenly as the result of a pathological fracture, or slowly from malignant transformation.

Treatment consists of the excision or curretage of the tumor and the cauterization of the tumor cavity. If a large defect develops, bone grafting is necessary. When there is a suspicion that the tumor is malignant, a radical resection is done (Turek, 1977, pp. 540–542).

AMPUTATIONS

Surgical amputation through the fingers or metacarpals is a salvage procedure, usually following trauma. The objective of the amputation is to preserve as much function as possible in the hand while shortening the time required for healing, decreasing the permanent disability, and preventing the continuation of pain. Every effort is usually made to maintain the length of the bony structures, the mobility of the joints, and the sensibility of the skin. In amputations of several digits, pinch and grasp are the chief functions to be preserved.

The only absolute indication for an amputation is an irreversible loss of blood supply. Other factors to be considered, however, are (1) the prognosis for function, (2) the soundness of other digits, (3) the extent of the involvement of the five tissue areas (i.e., the skin, tendon, nerve, bone, and joint), (4) the time since injury, and (5) the ability to salvage the thumb (Edmondson & Crenshaw, 1980, p. 235).

Amputations of the Fingertips

Amputations of the fingertips vary markedly in level depending on the amount of skin lost, the depth of the soft tissue defect, and whether the phalanx has been exposed or partially amputated. When skin alone has been lost, a free skin graft may suffice. When there is deep soft tissue defect, however, several methods are available. One is amputation of the finger proximal to the defect. This provides ample skin and other soft tissues for closure, but does shorten the finger. Another is a free skin graft, but this normally does not restore sensibility. Many different flap skin grafts and surgical techniques, including cross finger grafts, have also been used. Occasionally, a severed fingertip is recovered and replaced as a free graft. Although the graft usually survives in children, the results in adults have been poor (Edmondson & Crenshaw, 1980, pp. 235–237).

Amputation of a Single Finger

Index Finger Amputation

An amputation of the index finger at its proximal interphalangeal joint, or at a more proximal level, leaves an unsightly, useless stump that may hinder the pinch between the thumb and middle finger. Therefore, an amputation should be through the shaft of the second metacarpal.

After surgery, the hand is elevated for 48 hours. Because an amputation through the second metacarpal involves hand tissues, it may cause stiffness in the other fingers. Because a branch of the median nerve is in the first web space, the nerve may become damaged. Potential residual effects may be a sunken scar on the dorsum of the hand.

Middle or Ring Finger Amputation

The amputation of either the middle or ring finger leaves a gap in the hand through which small objects can drop when the hand is used in a scooping maneuver. The space also lets the remaining fingers deviate toward the midline. In multiple amputations, the third and fourth metacarpal heads are important because they help stabilize the metacarpal arch, but in single finger amputations that is of less importance.

In some middle finger amputations, the third metacarpal head is excised and the index ray (the index finger and second metacarpal) are transposed ulnarward. That procedure has been done with good results, because it leaves a natural symmetry and makes the presence of only three fingers less obvious. However, removing the third metacarpal head weakens the pinch. When the ring finger is amputated, transposing the little finger ray is rarely done. In most instances, the fourth metacarpal is resected at its base which permits a "folding in" of the fifth digit to close the gap (Edmondson & Crenshaw, 1980, p. 241).

Postoperatively, drains and a soft pressure dressing are usually applied. On the second day, the drains are removed, and 8 to 10 days postoperatively the dressing is usually changed and the sutures removed. A light volar plaster splint is then applied to keep the wrist in a neutral position and support the hand. The splint is worn for about 4 weeks, but must be removed daily to cleanse the hand and exercise the small joints.

Little Finger Amputation

An amputation of the little finger should save as much tissue as possible. Often the little finger survives when all of the other fingers have been destroyed, and it then becomes important in forming the pinch with the thumb. When the little finger alone is amputated, the fifth metacarpal shaft may be divided and the abductor digiti quinti transferred to the proximal phalanx of the ring finger. That procedure smooths the ulnar border of the hand.

Amputation of the Thumb

The lack of a thumb causes a severe deficiency in hand function, and is usually considered to constitute a 40-percent disability of the hand as a whole (Edmondson & Crenshaw, 1980, p. 246). If there is a traumatic amputation of the thumb, reamputation to obtain closure is not considered because the thumb should never be shortened. The wound is initially closed using a free skin graft, pedicle graft, or a local or distant flap graft. When the thumb has been severed at the MP joint or a more proximal level, reconstruction of the thumb is usually indicated.

Reconstructive surgery of the thumb should meet five requirements. They are (1) the presence of sensation in the thumb, (2) sufficient stability so that pinch pressure does not cause the thumb joints to deviate or collapse, (3) sufficient mobility to enable the hand to flatten and the thumb to oppose for pinch, (4) sufficient length to enable the opposing digital tip to touch the thumb, and (5) a satisfactory appearance.

Acceptable reconstructive procedures include (1) lengthening the thumb using a short bone graft and transferring local skin for sensibility, (2) the pollicizing of a digit (i.e., transpositioning a finger to replace an absent thumb), and (3) the direct free transfer of a toe to the hand with anastomosis of both the vessels and nerves by microsurgical techniques.

REPLANTATION

Replantation is the reattachment of a severed body part. Its success is measured by the degree of return of useful function, which may not be evident for many months because of the slow regeneration of the peripheral nerves.

Patients usually view replantation as preferable to amputation or prosthesis, even with the risk, time, and expense involved. Replantation is generally more successful for children, for multiple digit amputations, for thumb amputations proximal to the interphalangeal joint, for clean guillotine amputations, for amputations with minimal contamination, and for digits that are available for replantation 6 hours or less after amputation. Replantation is less effective in patients over 50 years of age, in single digit amputations, in severe crush or avulsion injuries, and in the presence of associated injuries.

The time interval from the accident to arrival at the replantation facility is critical, and should be reduced to a minimum. The amputated part should be wrapped in gauze and placed in a plastic bag inside an iced container. Muscle tissue begins to deteriorate after only 4 to 6 hours at room temperature. That time may be increased to 12 hours or more by cooling the part as described above, with care taken to avoid freezing the amputated part. (Freezing will eliminate any possibility of later replantation.) There should be no attempt to wash, irrigate, or perfuse the amputated part prior to transportation. Although necessary primary care must be given to the patient, any crushing of exposed blood vessels by the use of clamps should be avoided if at all possible, because excision of the crushed ends further shorten the vessels. When the bleeding vessels are so large that direct pressure and elevation of the part with the patient lying supine are inadequate, a pneumatic tourniquet should be used (Edmondson & Crenshaw, 1980, p. 268).

Authorities do not agree on many preoperative, intraoperative, and postoperative aspects of replantation surgery, but do agree on certain basic principles. First, the history and general physical assessment of the patient should indicate that the patient can tolerate surgery that may last 10 or more hours. Second, the patient and the family need to understand the possibility of complications, including the loss of the amputated part and the probable need for multiple surgeries.

When a patient returns from surgery after a replantation, there will be a bulky dressing and dorsal and volar plaster splints on the affected hand. Most physicians apply a layer of petroleum gauze directly over the skin wound, followed by layers of gauze dressing over the dorsal and volar surfaces. Cotton soaked in a physiological solution is then applied to keep the dressing moist. The dorsal and volar plaster splints are applied over the cotton dressing to hold the wrist and fingers in functional position, and are held in place by a circular bandage. During the first week, the splints are removed and the dressing is soaked with a physiological solution every 8 hours to prevent drying of blood or crust formation that may constrict the vascular flow.

The replanted part is held at heart level for approximately a week after surgery, while the patient is kept on bedrest. Frequent evaluations of the circulation of the replanted part are carried out on the fingertips and small areas of the skin that were left exposed. Should a vascular occlusion occur, the patient may have to return to surgery.

The environment of the patient should be kept reasonably warm to avoid vasoconstriction of the replanted part, and smoking must be prohibited to prevent vasoconstriction from nicotine. Sedation of the patient relieves anxiety and assists peripheral vasodilation. Systemic heparin, low-molecular-weight dextran, aspirin, and stellate ganglion blocks have been advocated postoperatively, but some authorities routinely use only aspirin and low-molecular-weight dextran. Dressings are changed infrequently to avoid manipulation of the replanted part. The first dressing change is best delayed for 7 to 10 days, and active motion should not be started for at least 3 weeks after surgery.

REFERENCES

Brantley, P., & Analla, M. *The nurse and orthopedic surgery.* Rutherford, N.J.: The Orthopedic Nurses' Association Inc., in cooperation with Howmedica, Inc., 1980.

Cailliet, R. *Hand pain and impairment* (2nd ed.). Philadelphia: F. A. Davis, 1981.

Donahoo, C. S., & Spickler, L. (Eds.). *Curriculum of orthopedic nursing.* Atlanta, Ga.: The Orthopedic Nurses' Association, Inc., 1980.

Edmondson, A. S., & Crenshaw, A. H. (Eds.). *Campbell's operative orthopaedics* (6th ed.), St. Louis: C. V. Mosby, 1980.

Gartland, J. J. *Fundamentals of orthopaedics* (3rd ed.). Philadelphia: W. B. Saunders, 1979.

Iversen, L. D., & Clawson, D. K. *Manual of acute orthopaedic therapeutics.* Boston: Little, Brown, 1977.

Swinson, D. R., & Swinburn, W. R. *Rheumatology.* New York: Wiley, 1980.

Turek, S. L. *Orthopaedics, principles and their applications* (3rd ed.). Philadelphia: Lippincott, 1977.

BIBLIOGRAPHY

Albright, J. A., & Brand, R. A. (Eds.). *The scientific basis of orthopaedics.* New York: Appleton-Century-Crofts, 1979.

Anderson, M., & Willis, S. Fingertip injuries and the orthopedic nurse. *Orthopedic Nurses' Association Journal,* 1978, *5* (7), 14–19.

Arthritis Health Profession Section of the Arthritis Foundation. *Self-help manual for patients with arthritis.* Atlanta, Ga.: Arthritis Foundation, 1980.

Beasley, R. W. Surgery of hand and finger amputations. *Orthopedic Clinics of North America,* 1981, *12* (4), 763-804.

Berger, M. R. Dupuytren's contracture. *American Journal of Nursing,* 1978, *2,* 244–245.

Berger, M. R. Painful tendon problems of the hand: Trigger thumb, trigger finger and de Quervain's syndrome. *Orthopaedic Nursing,* 1982, *1* (5), 20–23.

Berger, M. R. Fingertip dressings. *Orthopaedic Nursing,* 1983, *2* (5), 45–49.

Berger, M. R., & Froimson, A. I. Hands that hurt: Carpal tunnel syndrome. *American Journal of Nursing,* 1979, *2,* 264–266.

Bowers, W. H., & Fajgenbaum, D. M. Closed rupture of the volar plant of the distal interphalangeal joint. *Journal of Bone and Joint Surgery,* 1979, *61A* (1), 146.

Broudy, A. S., & Smith, R. J. Advances in surgery of the rheumatoid hand. *Current Practice in Orthopaedic Surgery,* 1977, *7,* 1–36.

Cailliet, R. *Soft tissue pain and disability* (5th ed.). Philadelphia: F. A. Davis, 1981.

Cochran, G. Van B. *A primer of orthopaedic biomechanics.* New York: Churchill Livingstone, 1982.

Cho, K. O. Entrapment occlusion of the ulnar artery in the hand. *Journal of Bone and Joint Surgery,* 1978, *60A* (6), 841–843,

Compere, E. L. *Orthopaedic surgery: A handbook of operative surgery.* Chicago: Year Book Med. Pub., 1974.

Cooney, W. P. Complications of Colles' fractures. *Journal of Bone and Joint Surgery,* 1980, *62A* (4), 613–619.

Cooney, W. P., Linscheid, R. L., & Dabyns, J. H. External pin fixation for unstable Colles' fractures. *Journal of Bone and Joint Surgery,* 1979, *61A* (6), 840–845.

DeGowin, E. L., & DeGowin, R. L. *Bedside diagnostic examination* (3rd ed.). New York: Macmillan, 1976.

Doi, K., Tominaga, S., Hono, H., et al. Reconstruction of an amputated thumb in one stage. *Journal of Bone and Joint Surgery,* 1979, *61A* (8), 1254–1255.

Fambrough, R. A., & Green, D. P. Tendon rupture as a complication of screw fixation in fractures in the hand. *Journal of Bone and Joint Surgery,* 1979, *61A* (5), 781–782.

Fries, J. F. *Arthritis, A comprehensive guide.* Menlo Park, Calif.: Addison-Wesley, 1982.

Gelberman, R. N., Amiel, D., Rudolph, R. M., & Vance, R. M. Dupuytren's contracture. *Journal of Bone and Joint Surgery,* 1980, *62A* (3), 425–432.

Ghista, D. N., & Roaf, R. *Orthopaedic mechanics: Procedures and devices.* San Francisco: Academic Press, 1978.

Hoppenfeld, S. *Physical examination of the spine and extremities.* New York: Appleton-Century-Crofts, 1976.

Hubbard, L. F., & Herndon, J. H. Microsurgery in orthopedics. *Surgical Clinics of North America,* 1983, *63* (3), 737–748.

Kessler, I. A simplified technique to correct hypertension deformity of the metacarpophalangeal joint of the thumb. *Journal of Bone and Joint Surgery,* 1979, *61A* (6), 903–905.

Kleinert, H. E., Smith, D. J. Jr., Juhala, C. A., et al. Replantation utilizing microsurgery. *Current Practice in Orthopaedic Surgery,* 1977, *7,* 78–89.

Kramer, S. Partial hand amputation. *Orthopedics,* 1978, *1* (4), 314.

Lucas, G. L. Internal fixation in the hand: A review of indications and methods. *Orthopedics,* 1980, *3,* 1083–1089.

McKenna, M. P. Torn lateral collateral ligament of the right fifth finger. *Orthopedic Nurses' Association Journal,* 1978, *5* (11), 20–21.

McMahan, R. H. The carpal navicular bone. *Orthopedic Nurses' Association Journal,* 1979, *6* (1), 13–14.

Meyer, V. E., Zhong-Wei, C., & Beasley, R. W. Basic technical considerations in reattachment surgery. *Orthopedic Clinics of North America,* 1981, *12* (4), 871–895.

Miller, B. K. Hands that hurt less. *American Journal of Nursing,* 1979, *2* (2), 266–267.

Miller, B. K. How to spot and treat carpal tunnel syndrome—early. *Nursing 80,* 1980, *10* (3), 50–53.

North, E. R., & Eaton, R. G. Volar dislocation of the fifth metacarpal. *Journal of Bone and Joint Surgery,* 1980, *62A* (4), 657–659.

Pillet, J. The aesthetic hand prosthesis. *Orthopedic Clinics of North America,* 1981, *12* (4), 961–969.

Powell, M. *Orthopedic nursing.* New York: Churchill Livingston, 1976.

Roaf, R., & Hodkinson, L. J. *Textbook of orthopaedic nursing* (2nd ed.). Oxford: Blackwell Scientific, 1975.

Ross, D. G. Musculoskeletal assessment: Range of motion of the fingers and hand. *Orthopedic Nursing,* 1982, *1* (5), 11–19.

Zhong-wei, C. Reconstruction by autogenous toe transplantations for total hand amputation. *Orthopedic Clinics of North America,* 1981, *12* (14), 835–842.

12

OVERVIEW: ORTHOPAEDICS AS AN EXPANDING FIELD

RECENT ADVANCES IN ORTHOPAEDIC CARE

The management of orthopaedic problems has changed greatly in recent years with the development of new diagnostic procedures such as arthroscopy, amipaque myelograms, bone scanning, computerized axial tomographic (CAT) scans, and the introduction of nuclear magnetic resonance (NMR) spectroscopy. There have also been noteworthy advances in fracture management, reconstructive surgery, and microsurgery (*Surgical Clinics of North America,* 1983).

Fracture Management

New techniques have occurred in fracture management, involving the use of external fixators, the technique of closed intramedullary nailing, and the employing of electrical bone stimulators. In the late 1970s, an old technique for the management of complex, open fractures, external fixation, reappeared in the United States. The acceptance of the new external fixation devices has been attributed to many factors, including new concepts of open wound treatment developed during the Viet Nam war, improved antibiotics, and perhaps most importantly, vastly improved external frames.

Intramedullary nailing, particularly of fractures of the middle third of the femur, has been a standard method of treatment since the late 1950s. Over the last few years, however, Enders and others have developed techniques for closed intramedullary nailing that reduce the risk of infection and blood loss. Although closed nailing still requires a surgical incision, the new methods make the incision more remote from the fracture site, have a smaller chance of hematoma development, and cause less damage to soft tissue. The major drawback of those techniques is that they require a specialized fracture table and biplane roentgenographic image intensification.

The treatment of nonunions has been improved by the development of electrical stimulation devices that promote bone growth. The process of stimulation usually requires several weeks or months to demonstrate calcification.

The treatment can usually be accomplished while the patient is sleeping and requires no hospitalization.

Reconstructive Surgery

Reconstructive orthopaedic surgery has advanced enormously in the last 10 years, especially with the introduction of total joint replacements, both in the upper and lower extremities. The majority of total joint arthroplasties now involve an implant made of one of several metal alloys that articulates with a high-density polyethylene polymer component. The two components are fixed to the bone with methyl methacrylate cement, which is polymerized in surgery at the time of implantation. Total joint replacement procedures are being developed for additional joints, and rapid development continues in the design of prostheses. New materials are rapidly changing the implants on the market, and there are new joint arthroplasty components that require no cement for implantation. Improving the effectiveness of noncemented prostheses is one of the major challenges in orthopaedics today.

Over the last few years, a continuous passive motion machine was developed to assist patients following surgery for knee reconstruction or knee trauma. The machine takes the involved joint through continuous passive motion without the active involvement of the patient, and even allows the patient to sleep with the machine in motion. Because of the success of that approach for the knee, similar machines are now available for the shoulder and the elbow.

Microsurgery

The expansion of microsurgery from its origins in otolaryngology and neurosurgery has made replantation of part of an extremity or of a whole extremity possible. In 1963, the Chinese reported a series of replantations of severed digits, and Malt reported on his experience with severed arms in 1964. Based on that early experience, and with laboratory data generated by Buncke, Kleinert, and others, replantation has become a procedure commonly performed in many major institutions, and has undergone considerable evolution. A high degree of survival of replanted digits, up to 90 percent, has been achieved.

In orthopaedics, the advent of microsurgical procedures has encouraged innovation. Replantation was soon followed by the development of other procedures, such as free tissue transfers. As microsurgical techniques become more refined, there will undoubtedly be many more applications.

Treatment of Back Problems

Back problems have long been prevalent because of the anatomical arrangement of the lower spine and the consequent difficulties in maintaining good posture while standing and walking. In recent years, several new diagnostic and treatment methods have appeared. In 1982, the U.S. Food and Drug Admin-

TABLE 12–1. THE GROWTH OF ORTHOPAEDIC MEDICINE IN THE UNITED STATES

Active Physicians (M.D.s)	Year		% Increase
	1965	1979	
All specialties	277,575	389,157	40.2
Orthopaedic surgeons	7,507	13,419	78.8
Orthopaedic surgeons as a percentage of all M.D.s	2.70	3.45	—

(From the U.S. Department of Health, Education and Welfare, Health Resources Statistics, *1965, p. 103, and the U.S. Department of Health and Human Services,* Health: United States, *1981, p. 179.)*

istration approved the use of chymopapain for intradisc injections in the treatment of herniated nucleus pulposus. That treatment is less invasive than a laminectomy, and reduces some of the complications associated with laminectomies, such as infection. Although a period of rehabilitation is still required, the hospital stay is much reduced and in some instances the treatment may be done on an outpatient basis. The surgical treatment of adult scoliosis has been advanced by the introduction of Dwyer and Luque instrumentation and the Dunn device for vertebral fractures.

THE GROWTH OF ORTHOPAEDICS

The field of orthopaedics has experienced substantial growth in recent decades. Although figures on the number of orthopaedic nurses are not available, Table 12–1 shows that between 1965 and 1979, the number of orthopaedic surgeons grew nearly twice as fast as the total number of physicians.

Orthopaedic nurses now practice in many different settings. A large number of orthopaedic nurses work in acute care hospitals or in doctor's offices and clinics, but many are now working in education, as nurse practitioners, and in home health care organizations, and a few have developed joint practices with physicians.

The professional organization of orthopaedic nursing, the National Association of Orthopaedic Nurses (NAON), focuses on the professional development and continuing education of orthopaedic nurses. *Orthopaedic Nursing,* a bimonthly journal, is the official publication of the organization. NAON also sponsors district workshops and an annual Congress, and is presently developing a core curriculum for orthopaedics and developing criteria and guidelines for the certification of orthopaedic nurses.

APPENDIX A
TRACTION

The skeleton is the bony framework of the body. Movements of its joints are kept under control by the balanced action of opposing groups of muscles, and that balancing principle is the basis of all traction and suspension devices. Traction is the application of a pulling force to a part of the body, such as the spine, the pelvis, and the long bones of the upper and lower extremities, and is an important form of orthopaedic immobilization. It can be applied as an alternative to surgery, is used to ensure proper positioning of an affected extremity, and can be used in the correction of deformities.

A. The Mechanics of Traction
   1. Purpose of Traction
      a. To reduce a fracture and realign bone fragments by overcoming muscle spasms
      b. To reduce and treat dislocations
      c. To maintain skeletal length and alignment until calcification occurs
      d. To immobilize to prevent further soft tissue damage
      e. To prevent the development of contractures
      f. To relieve muscle spasms, such as with low back pain
      g. To lessen deformities, such as with scoliosis or arthritis
      h. To rest a diseased joint
   2. Classifications of Traction
      a. Manual. Manual traction is traction that is accomplished by a person's hands exerting a pulling force. It is utilized to reduce fractures and to apply a steady pull while mechanical traction is released for readjustment or while a cast is being applied. Manual traction must be done with a smooth firm grip, as sudden jerky motions of the extremity can cause severe pain. Never use manual traction without specific orders to do so.
      b. Mechanical. Mechanical traction is traction that utilizes mechanical devices. It is applied by a variety of methods.

i. Type of Attachment to Patients
   (a) Skin. Skin traction immobilizes a body part intermittently over an extended period through direct application of a pulling force to the patient's skin and soft tissues. The force may be applied using adhesive or nonadhesive traction tape or other skin traction devices such as a cast, boot, belt, or halter.
   (b) Skeletal. Skeletal traction immobilizes a body part for prolonged periods by exerting a pulling force directly on the patient's bones by means of pins, screws, wires, or tongs. Skeletal traction allows greater traction time and heavier weights than does skin traction.
   (c) Plaster. Plaster traction is skeletal traction applied by incorporating the ends of Steinmann pins or Kirschner wires in a cast that maintains continuous traction.
   (d) Brace. Brace traction employs a brace to exert a pull on a portion of the body, as in the case of hyperextension braces or long leg braces for correction of leg alignment deformities.

ii. Nature of the Pull
   (a) Continuous or Intermittent
      (1) Continuous. Continuous traction means that the traction must be maintained at all times (e.g., traction on an unrepaired fracture).
      (2) Intermittent. Intermittent traction refers to traction that is either applied for short periods of time (e.g., intermittent cervical traction) or traction that can be released for a short period of time (e.g., pelvic traction to relieve muscle spasms).
   (b) Running or Suspension
      (1) Running (or Straight). Running traction is traction that is applied to a body part with a pull in one direction. The countertraction is the patient's body, and any movement made by the body changes the pull of the traction.
      (2) Balanced Suspension. Balanced suspension traction provides countertraction so that the pull of the traction remains unchanged when the patient moves. The affected extremity is supported by means of a hammock or splint that is held in place by balanced weights attached to an overhead bar.

3. Applications of Mechanical Traction
   a. Traction to the Upper Extremity
      i. Purpose
         (a) To reduce and immobilize fractures of the humerus or elbow
         (b) To reduce and immobilize fractures or injuries involving the shoulder
         (c) To reduce and immobilize fractures of the wrist and thumb
         (d) To hold the arm in either extension or flexion

ii. Types

(a) Sidearm Skin. Sidearm skin traction is applied with adhesive straps and ace bandage wrap. There are two separate skin applications, one on the upper arm and one on the forearm.

(b) Sidearm Skeletal. Sidearm skeletal traction is applied by the use of a pin through the olecranon and adhesive straps and an ace bandage wrapped around the forearm.

(c) Overhead 90-90. Overhead 90-90 traction is applied with the affected arm suspended over the patient's chest and the upper part of the arm perpendicular to the body with the elbow flexed 90 degrees. In most cases, 90-90 traction is applied with a pin through the olecranon and the forearm suspended in a sling.

(d) Dunlop's. Dunlop's traction is a temporary skin traction most often used for children. Dunlop's traction stretches the bicep muscle by applying lateral traction to the elbow with the shoulder abducted 90 degrees and the elbow in a 45-degree extended position. A second, downward force is applied by a sling hanging from the distal portion of the upper arm.

(e) Hanging Arm Cast. A hanging arm cast is a long arm cast with a loop on the radial surface between the wrist and the elbow, usually close to the wrist. A strap is placed around the patient's neck and attached to the cast through the loop. The hanging arm cast is heavier than a normal cast because its purpose is to exert a pull on the upper arm to reduce and immobilize an upper arm fracture.

(f) Plaster. Plaster traction is utilized in the upper extremity (wrist or thumb) by first inserting a Steinmann pin or Kirschner wire through the bone(s) and then incorporating the ends of the pin in a cast to maintain the position of the extremity, provide a fixed traction, and allow the patient to move about.

iii. Complications

(a) Potential circulatory or nerve impairment due to pressure

(b) Skin breakdown from pressure of straps, cast, or bedrest

(c) Infection due to skin breakdown or wounds at the pin sites

(d) Physical and psychological complications of enforced recumbency

b. Traction to the Lower Extremity

i. Buck's Extension. Buck's extension traction is a form of running skin traction

(a) Purpose

(1) To immobilize a fractured hip or femur preoperatively

(2) To reduce muscle spasms after hip surgery

(3) To prevent hip flexion contractures

(4) To reduce low back muscle spasms (used bilaterally)

(5) To reduce and immobilize injuries of the pelvis
(6) To reduce a dislocated hip
(b) Complications
(1) Potential neurovascular impairment
(2) Foot drop from pressure on the Achilles tendon
(3) Skin breakdown
(4) Lack of immobilization of the fracture site causing trauma and pain
(5) Physical and psychological complications of enforced recumbency

ii. Russell. Russell's traction is a form of suspension skin traction to the leg consisting of a straight Buck's extension traction with a second, upward pull from a sling under the patient's leg just above the knee.
(a) Purpose
(1) To reduce and immobilize hip fractures
(2) To reduce and immobilize fractures of the femur
(b) Complications
(1) Potential neurovascular impairment
(2) Foot drop from pressure on the Achilles tendon
(3) Skin breakdown
(4) Lack of immobilization of the fracture site causing trauma and pain
(5) Physical and psychological complications of enforced recumbency

iii. Balanced Suspension. Balanced suspension skeletal traction is usually accomplished by a Steinmann pin or Kirschner threaded or unthreaded wire of stainless steel. Skeletal traction to the lower extremity is generally applied through the proximal or distal end of the tibia, the heel, or the distal end of the femur.
(a) Purpose and Types
(1) To treat the following fractures by means of a pin generally applied through the distal femur or proximal tibia, with the leg supported by a Thomas or Hodgen splint and a Pearson attachment
a. Fractures of the femur
b. Fractures of the pelvis
c. Unstable fractures of the acetabulum
d. Fractures of the acetabular rim with dislocations of the hip
(2) To treat the following fractures by means of a pin usually applied through the calcaneus, with the leg supported by a Boehler-Braun frame
a. Compound fractures of the tibia with severe soft tissue damage
b. Markedly unstable fractures of the tibia

(b) Complications
  (1) Potential neurovascular impairment
  (2) Potential pressure areas in the groin, or the adductor muscles, the ischial area, heel, and popliteal space
  (3) Potential infection at the pin site or from skin breakdown
  (4) Lack of immobilization of the fracture causing trauma and pain
  (5) Physical and psychological complications of enforced immobility

c. Traction to the Spinal Column and Pelvis

i. Cervical Skin. Cervical skin traction is accomplished by utilizing a head halter or two straps in a horizontal or vertical position to apply traction to the cervical spine. Continuous traction relieves muscle spasms with minimal weight, whereas intermittent traction stimulates blood flow and relieves muscle spasms with relatively heavy weights for a short period of time.

(a) Purpose
  (1) To relieve pain of cervical arthritis with radiculitis
  (2) To counteract muscle spasms associated with cervical disc syndrome
  (3) To relieve static postural neck strain
  (4) To relieve symptoms of cervical sprain

(b) Complications
  (1) Painful chin from the continued pressure
  (2) Marked discomfort to men from the growth of their beard
  (3) Circulatory and nerve impairment due to pressure
  (4) Pain in the temporomandibular joints
  (5) Physical and psychological complications of enforced recumbency

ii. Cervical Skeletal. Cervical skeletal traction is always horizontal and continuous and is accomplished by the use of skull tongs (Vinke, Crutchfield, Barton, Gardner-Wells) with the patient positioned on a turning frame (such as a Stryker frame. Foster bed, or circolectric bed).

(a) Purpose
  (1) To reduce fractures and dislocations of the cervical spine
  (2) To immobilize cervical fractures
  (3) To reduce subluxations of the cervical spine

(b) Complications
  (1) Circulatory and nerve impairment
  (2) Infection at the tong sites
  (3) Skin breakdown
  (4) Physical and psychological complications of enforced recumbency
  (5) Lack of immobilization of the fracture site causing trauma and pain

iii. Pelvic. Pelvic traction is a form of running skin traction accomplished by a pelvic belt around the pelvis. Traction can be continuous or intermittent.
(a) Purpose
(1) To relieve muscle spasms of the lower back
(2) To reduce pressure on spinal nerve roots
(b) Complications
(1) Skin breakdown at bony prominences of the pelvic girdle
(2) Footdrop
(3) Physical and psychological complications of enforced recumbency
(4) Constipation
iv. Bilateral Buck's Traction (see b.i. above)
v. Pelvic Sling. A pelvic sling, a form of continuous skin traction, is a large canvas sling that fits under the patient's buttocks to support the entire pelvis. Crossbars are inserted into the sling on each side and attached to weights that provide an upward pull.
(a) Purpose
(1) To stabilize and immobilize fractures of the pelvis
(2) To suspend patients with pelvic fractures
(3) For suspension and compression of the pelvic girdle
(4) To treat separations of the anterior pelvic ring
(b) Complications
(1) Lack of immobilization of the fracture site from too much lifting and turning causing trauma and pain
(2) Skin breakdown (back, sacral, and buttock)
(3) Difficulty in voiding (especially for women)
(4) Perineal irritation because of difficulty in cleansing (especially in women)
(5) Footdrop
(6) Physical and psychological complications of enforced recumbency

4. Care of Traction Equipment
a. Check for weakness in the traction cord; never reuse a cord.
b. Tie proper type of knots and then secure knots with adhesive tape.
c. Check for correct poundage, apply weights in a slow manner, avoid any bumping or jerking of weights, and make sure weights hang free of any obstruction.
d. Make sure all parts of the traction equipment are working correctly.
i. Never oil any pulley without notifying the patient's physician first
ii. Apply manual traction if any piece of the equipment needs to be readjusted or replaced
e. Check countertraction and insure that the patient does not slide into the headboard, footboard, or side of the bed.
f. Check for obstructions that may interfere with the pull of the traction, such as
i. Knots pressing against pulleys

   ii. Traction pieces such as spreader bars, footplates or splints coming in contact with the bedframe
   iii. Bed linen on top of traction straps and ropes
g. Check the line of pull and be certain that the fracture fragments are in correct alignment.
h. In continuous traction, make sure the pull is maintained 24 hours a day.
i. Check the position of the patient for
   i. Correct body alignment
   ii. Comfort
   iii. Support for all body parts
   iv. No undue stress or pull

B. Observing the Patient in Traction

Learn to make routine observations each time nursing care is given until such observations become so habitual that they are no longer conscious. Learn to ask yourself questions.

1. Is the circulation and nerve status of the extremity adequate?
2. Is the condition of the skin around the tape and straps satisfactory?
   a. Look for irritation, reddened areas, and maceration
   b. Look for pimples, abrasions, and purulent discharge
3. Learn to use your nose as well as your eyes to detect signs of trouble; the odors of macerating soft tissue and infection are distinctive.
4. Are the tapes slipping or the wrapping coming loose?
5. Is there any pressure on the popliteal region?
6. Is the heel free of pressure?
7. Is there any pressure over the outer aspect of the head of the fibula (the lateral upper calf)?
8. Is there sufficient countertraction?
9. Is the angle of elevation of the heel enough or too much?
10. In balanced skeletal traction, check that hip flexion does not exceed 20 degrees (between the bed and the thigh).
11. In arm traction, check for pressure on the dorsum of the hand, at the elbow, at the wrist, and on the axilla.
12. Is there any deformity at the fracture site?
13. Is the patient comfortable and warm?
14. Is the patient having an undue amount of pain?
15. Is the patient's body positioned correctly?
16. Assess for complications of prolonged bedrest and reduced activity.

C. Patient Teaching

Inform the patient about

1. The nature of the traction equipment
2. The purpose of the traction
3. Exercises and positioning to prevent effects of immobility and increase muscle strength
4. Maintaining activities of daily living while in traction
5. Possible diversional activities
6. The rehabilitation process

APPENDIX B
CASTS

A cast is an immobilizing device, made of layers of plaster bandages, fiberglass, or a thermolabile plastic material.

A. The Mechanics of Casts
   1. Purpose
      a. To hold bone fragments in reduction
      b. To apply uniform compression on soft tissues
      c. To permit early mobilization
      d. To improve function by stabilizing a joint
      e. To correct and prevent deformities
   2. Major Types
      a. Upper Extremity
         i. Thumb Spica or Gauntlet Cast. The cast extends from below the elbow to the proximal palmar crease, with a spiral bandaging between the thumb and the hand. Used in the treatment of fractures of the carpal navicular and the thumb metacarpal and phalanges, and in the treatment of ligamentous thumb joint injuries.
         ii. Short Arm Cast (SAC). The cast extends from below the elbow to the proximal palmar crease. Used in the treatment of stable fractures of the finger metacarpals, carpals, and the distal radius, and in the treatment of severe wrist sprains.
         iii. Long Arm Cast (LAC). The cast extends from the upper level of the axillary fold to the proximal palmar crease with the elbow at a right angle. Used in the treatment of stable injuries of the elbow joint, stable fractures of the distal humerus, fractures of one or both bones of the forearm, unstable ligamentous injuries of the wrist joint, and unstable fractures of the carpal bones.
         iv. Hanging Arm Cast. The cast is a long arm cast with a loop on the radial surface between the wrist and the elbow, usually close to the wrist. A strap is placed around the patient's neck and attached to the cast through the loop. The hanging arm cast is heavier than

a normal cast because its purpose is to exert a pull on the upper arm to reduce and immobilize a fracture site. Used to treat some shoulder injuries, displaced fractures of the surgical neck of the humerus, and spiral or comminuted fractures of the humeral shaft.

v. Shoulder Spica Cast. The cast is a combination of a body jacket and a long arm cast with a spiral bandage between the trunk and the affected arm. The shoulder is in abduction and the elbow is in a flexed position. Used to treat unstable fractures of the shoulder girdle and humerus, unstable elbow joint injuries, and dislocations of the shoulder girdle.

b. Lower Extremity

i. Short Leg Cast (SLC). The cast extends from below the knee to the base of the toes. Used to treat fractures of the ankle and stable fractures of the distal tibia and fibula.

ii. Long Leg Cast (LLC). The cast extends from the mid-upper thigh to the base of the toes, with the ankle at a right angle and the foot in a neutral position. Used to treat stable injuries of the knee joint and distal femur and unstable fractures of the tibia, the fibula, and the ankle joint.

iii. Walking Cast. A short or long leg cast with a walking device implanted on the bottom of the cast.

iv. Patellar Tendon Weight-Bearing Cast. The cast is a special type of short leg weight-bearing cast that extends higher on the leg than the typical short leg cast. Resembles a patellar tendon-bearing prosthesis. Used in the treatment of unstable fractures of the tibia and fibula.

v. Long Leg Cylinder Cast (LLCC). A cast similar to a long leg cast except that the foot and the ankle are not casted and the cast may not extend as high on the upper leg. Used in the treatment of stable injuries of the distal femur, proximal tibia, and knee joint.

vi. Brace Cast. The cast brace is a combination of cast and brace made up of three components. First, there is a patellar weight-bearing cast on the lower leg, either as a short leg cast or a cylinder cast. Second, there is an ischial weight-bearing cast on the thigh, molded well around Scapra's triangle, the ischial seat and the greater trochanter. The thigh component is applied snugly to increase the hydrodynamic compressive effect of the thigh muscles, and to immobilize the fracture fragments. Third, there are external polycentric knee hinges that connect the below-the-knee portion to the thigh portion and that allow 90 degrees of knee flexion. The cast brace allows for mobility of both hip and knee joints while permitting a fairly normal gait when ambulating. Used in the treatment of midshaft or distal-shaft fractures of the femur.

vii. Hip Spica Cast. A cast that extends from midtrunk (just below the nipple line) down the entire length of an affected leg, with a spiral bandage from the trunk to the affected leg. It may be a single, a one and one-half, or a double hip spica cast, depending on how the other leg is casted. Used in the treatment of a dislocated hip and to immobilize a hip following reconstructive surgeries or injuries to the pelvis, the hip joint, and the femur.

c. Body Cast. Body casts are used to immobilize the spine to relieve degenerative disorders, and to promote healing of surgical fusions and unstable spinal injuries.
   i. Minerva Jacket. The cast covers the frontal and occipital regions of the skull and extends over the neck, chest, back, abdomen, and iliac crest. The face, ears, buttocks, pubic area, and extremities are exposed.
   ii. Body Jacket. The cast extends from the upper chest over the trunk to the pubis. The iliac crests are enclosed but the buttocks and perineal areas are exposed. Some body jackets may include the thighs and pelvis or the cervical spine.
   iii. Hyperextension Body Cast. This body jacket is applied with the patient in a position of hyperextension. It extends from the symphysis pubis to the suprasternal notch in front, and from the tip of the coccyx to the scapulae behind, so as to prevent the smallest degree of forward flexion of the spine. Used to treat compression fractures of the spine.
   iv. Halo Cast. The body jacket portion of the halo brace is made of a casting material. Used to immobilize fractures of the cervical spine.

d. Splint or Mold. A cast that supports an extremity without completely enclosing it.
   i. Anterior or posterior splints or molds are applied with an elastic bandage and are used postoperatively after knee surgery, following an arm fracture, and after the removal of a cast.
   ii. Sugar-Tong Splints. Splints used to immobilize the arm and the wrist in fractures of the wrist and the forearm. They are often anterior and posterior and are applied with an elastic bandage.
   iii. Elephant-Ear Cast. A splint that extends from the wrist along the posterior aspect of the arm and up over the shoulder to immobilize and support the humerus.

3. Cast Materials
   a. Plaster of Paris. An open weave cotton roll or strip saturated with anhydrous calcium sulfate (a chalky white powder made from gypsum crystals).
      i. Application
         (a) The patient should be prepared physically and psychologically.

(b) For closed reductions, the correct size of stockinette should be used (too tight a stockinette constricts, and too loose allows wrinkles and resultant pressure areas).
(c) Sheet wadding or webril for padding should be placed over the entire area to be casted.
(d) Felt padding should be placed around bony prominences if needed (especially for body or spica casts).
(e) Rolls of plaster should then be applied in a circular motion. The plaster should be immersed in tepid water until the bubbles stop, and then the water should be squeezed out until the plaster roll has the desired consistency.
(f) The plaster should then be smoothed out with a damp hand to make the cast smooth.
(g) The number of rolls in a cast depends on the extremity and the desired strength of the cast.
(h) Plaster splints may be incorporated in the cast for reinforcement.

ii. Drying Methods
(a) A chemical reaction makes the cast warm to hot in the beginning, but it soon becomes cold and damp.
(b) The cast should be exposed to the air so it can "breathe" and dry.
(c) The cast should not be covered as that would interfere with the drying process.
(d) The patient should be turned every 2 to 3 hours so the cast will dry evenly. The casted portion of the body should be moved with flat hands so fingers and thumbs do not cause indentations or pressure areas in the cast.
(e) If approved by the institution, the following methods may be utilized for cast drying.
(1) A commercial dryer with the heat set at a very low temperature
(2) A heat cradle with a 25-watt bulb
(3) A hair dryer set on low
(4) An electric fan to circulate the air (but not to blow directly on the cast)

iii. Drying Time
(a) Up to 24 hours for a regular arm or leg cast
(b) 24 to 48 hours for weight-bearing casts
(c) 36 to 72 hours for large body casts
(d) The cast is dry when
(1) The plaster is white, shiny, and odorless.
(2) The cast is hard, firm, and resonant when tapped.

b. Fiberglass. An open weave fiberglass tape saturated with polyurethane resin.

i. Application
(a) The patient should be prepared physically and psychologically.
(b) The application procedures described above can be followed, except
(1) A rayon stockinette and padding should be used.
(2) Each roll of casting should only be opened immediately before using (a lubricant such as K-Y jelly should be used on hands to prevent resin from sticking).

ii. Drying Method and Time
(a) Open air
(b) 10 to 15 minutes
(c) No weight-bearing for 30 minutes after application

c. Synthetic. A polyester and cotton weave fabric impregnated with water-activated polyurethane.

i. Application
(a) The patient should be prepared physically and psychologically.
(b) The application procedures described above can be followed except
(1) A cotton stockinette and padding should be used.
(2) Each roll should be opened just before using, and should be immersed in water at 70 to 80°F (21.1 to 26.6°C).
(3) Water should *not* be squeezed from the roll before applying (if the water is removed, its cooling effect will be lost).

ii. Drying Method and Time
(a) Open air
(b) Approximately 7 minutes
(c) Weight bearing possible 20 minutes after application

4. Care of the Cast

a. Petaled Edge. "Petaling the cast" is a method of making the edge of the cast smooth. Only casts without stockinettes will usually need to be petaled. Inspect the skin for pressure areas and signs of irritation from rough edges on the cast. Trim the cast edges and smooth out the padding. To prevent irritation or abrasion, petal-shaped strips of adhesive tape or moleskin adhesive may be applied to the exterior surface and rough edges of the cast, and anchored smoothly to the interior surface of the cast. To prepare the "petal," use a roll of adhesive tape, unroll a small portion of the tape, and fold the two non-adhesive sides together. For each petal, cut the tape at a 45-degree angle. When each segment of the tape is unfolded, it will have a sharp point like the point of a petal. The point of the tape goes into the interior surface, and reduces the likelihood of a wrinkle developing in the tape that could irritate the skin under the cast.

b. Window. A window results from cutting out a portion of the cast, usually over a suture line (to change a dressing or check on drainage) or over a pressure area. If the window is removed and a dressing changed, the same amount of dressing must be replaced before the window is taped back into place. That is necessary to prevent unnecessary swelling and possible skin necrosis.

c. Split. A split is a cut in the cast to help relieve possible neurovascular impingement. When splitting a cast, try not to cut directly over a bony area where there is very little flesh (such as directly over the tibia).
d. Bivalve. Bivalving is when the cast is cut lengthwise into two equal parts. Bivalving a cast is usually done to facilitate care or when a rigid cast is not needed at all times but is used for support or turning.
e. Wedge. Wedging enables the physician to turn and realign the foot portion of a leg cast. A cut is made on one side of the cast, and a slender wedge of the cast is removed from the other side. After the foot is repositioned, the cast is turned so the cut side opens and the wedge is then inserted into that cut. After the wedge is inserted, new casting material is applied to seal the cuts.
f. Cleansing Plaster of Paris Casts
    i. Discuss ways to prevent soiling the cast with the patient.
    ii. The cast may be cleansed with a damp cloth and cleanser, but it should not become wet.
    iii. Small stains that cannot be removed may be covered with white shoe polish if the patient does not have an incision or open lesion.
    iv. Old bleeding through the cast can be covered by applying new casting material.

5. Removal of Casts
    a. Explain the procedure to the patient.
    b. A cast cutter sounds and looks dangerous, even though it is quite safe because it cuts using vibrations. The patient should only feel heat and some pressure. Demonstrate the safety of the cutter by touching it to the palmar surface of your thumb.
    c. Bivalve the cast with the cutter, cutting with even pressure. Release the pressure once you feel the cutter cut through the cast.
    d. Separate the cast with a cast spreader.
    e. Cut through the padding with scissors.
    f. Gently remove the anterior portion of the cast.
    g. Expect old, loose, or semi-attached skin; the hair on the extremity to appear longer; and skin discoloration if there has been bleeding into the tissues.
    h. Gently remove the posterior portion of the cast while supporting the joints of the extremity.
    i. The casted extremity may appear slightly smaller than the other one, especially if the cast was worn for a long period of time and no muscle setting or other exercises were done.
    j. If another cast is not to be applied, carefully cleanse the skin. Do not try to remove all of the dead skin. Apply a little oil, and in a couple of days it can easily be washed away.

k. After cast removal, some patients may need an elastic bandage to support the joint for a few days until their muscle strength returns.

B. Complications of Casts
1. Impaired circulation
2. Nerve damage
3. Pressure areas
4. Infection, tissue necrosis, and irritation
5. Cast syndrome (especially with body casts)
6. Lack of immobilization of fracture site causing trauma and pain
7. Cast claustrophobia

C. Nursing Care of Patients in Casts
1. Assessing neurovascular status
   a. Neurovascular compression
   b. Compartmental syndrome
2. Assessing for and intervening to relieve pain and pressure
3. Assessing the amount of drainage into the cast
4. Turning the patient every 2 hours during the day and every 4 hours at night
5. Keeping the extremity elevated on pillows to prevent swelling
6. Utilizing ice as needed to prevent or reduce swelling
7. Providing skin care to prevent irritation and dryness
8. Encouraging the patient to do as many activities of daily living as possible
9. Setting up an exercise program to prevent the effects of immobility
10. Setting up an exercise program for the affected part

D. Patient Teaching
1. Discuss the nature and purpose of the cast.
2. Explain exercises and positioning.
3. Discuss ways to maintain activities of daily living while in a cast.
4. Demonstrate the application and utilization of a sling for the upper extremity.
5. Demonstrate ambulation techniques.
   a. Weight-bearing casts with a walking heel
   b. Three-point gait crutch walking for nonweight-bearing casts
6. Discuss how to do cast care and activities of daily living at home.

APPENDIX C
CRUTCH WALKING AND CANE USE

In the treatment of various forms of arthritis, of most fractures of the lower extremity, after operations on the leg, and immediately following an amputation, crutches provide a convenient method for getting from one place to another. Crutch walking must be taught, and the learning process should begin early. One of the first prerequisites for crutch walking is for the patient to develop power in the shoulder girdle and upper extremities to bear the weight while crutch walking. Of equal importance is the patient's motivation, and the patient's age, interests, future intentions, and prognosis should be considered in helping him or her adjust to crutches.

UPPER EXTREMITY EXERCISES

Performing arm exercises (flexion and extension of the arms) strengthens the muscles in the shoulder girdle and upper extremities so that the patient can use an assistive device (crutch or cane) for walking. The use of the trapeze, which strengthens the biceps of the arm, helps, but the major muscle in the arm that needs strengthening is the triceps. This can be accomplished by the following two exercises. The patient, in a sitting position, takes a weight in each hand, flexes both arms, and then extends the hands above the head directly toward the ceiling. Another exercise uses sawed-off crutches or books placed on the bed on each side of the patient. The patient pushes down on the books or crutches and lifts the buttocks off the bed.

Good posture and balance are essential to crutch walking. Before the patient tries to use crutches, he or she should learn balance by standing next to a chair on the unaffected leg.

MEASUREMENT FOR CRUTCHES

Adjustable crutches are practical because the disease may cause changes in the muscles and joints, or the patient may improve and progress to a different crutch base and gait. There are four ways to make approximate measurements of crutches. If the patient has to be measured for crutches while lying flat in bed, measure from the anterior fold of the axilla to the sole of the foot, and then add 5 cm (2 inches). Another method is to determine the height of the patient and subtract 40 cm (16 inches). If the patient is able to sit up in bed without a back support, have the patient sit up straight and abduct both arms straight out from the body. Ask the patient to flex one arm at the elbow, and then measure across the patient's back from the fingertip to the elbow. The back must not be bowed or hyperflexed. That method can also be utilized if the patient can stand. Another method for a standing patient is to measure from 3.75 to 5.0 cm (1 1/2 to 2 inches) below the axillary fold to a point on the floor 10 cm (4 inches) in front of the patient and 15 cm (6 inches) laterally from the small toe.

For final measurements, have the patient assume the tripod position, that is stand with the crutches under the arms with the tips of the crutches 10 cm (4 inches) in front and 15 cm (6 inches) to each side. Next, check that there is a two-finger width space between each axillary fold and the armpiece of each crutch. With the patient standing erect, the handpiece of each crutch should allow for 30 degrees of flexion at the elbow, with the wrist extended and the hand dorsiflexed. The patient should be wearing shoes that fit well and have a firm sole. The crutches should be fitted with large rubber suction tips before measuring.

CRUTCH STANCE

The tripod position is the basic crutch stance and gives the strongest and most balanced support. Because a greater height requires a broader base, however, a taller patient needs a wider stance and a shorter patient a narrower stance.

The patient should be taught to support the weight on the handpieces. If the weight is borne on the axilla, pressure from the crutch can damage the brachial plexus nerves and produce "crutch paralysis." A foam rubber pad on the underarm piece eases pressure on the upper arm and thoracic cage.

CRUTCH GAITS

The selection of the crutch gait depends on the type and the severity of the disability, the patient's physical condition, arm and trunk strength, and the patient's body balance. The nurse must know how much (if any) weight can be placed on the affected side and whether the crutches are being used for balance or for support. Teach the patient two gaits (if possible) so he or she may change from one to the other. For example, a faster gait can be alternated with a slower one. Shifting crutch gaits relieves fatigue because each gait requires the use of a different combination of muscles. If a muscle is forced to contract steadily without relaxing, the circulation of blood to that muscle is reduced.

All gaits begin in the tripod position. The more common gaits are:

The Four-Point Gait

The four-point gait can be used when supported weight bearing is permitted for both legs. It is safe and gives maximal balance because there are always three points of contact with the floor. It is slow because it requires constant shifting of weight. The sequence is to advance the (1) right crutch, (2) left foot, (3) left crutch, and (4) right foot.

The Two-Point Gait

The two-point gait is faster, because there are only two points of contact at one time. The sequence is (1) right crutch and left foot, and (2) left crutch and right foot.

The Three-Point Gait

The three-point gait is a fast gait that requires the most strength and balance. The patient must be able to support the entire body weight on the arms. The sequence is to advance (1) the weaker leg and both crutches simultaneously, and then (2) the stronger leg. The three point gait is utilized when no weight bearing is allowed on one leg.

The Swing-To and Swing-Through Gaits

The swing-to and swing-through gaits are usually employed when the patient's lower extremities are weak or paralyzed. The patient may or may not be wearing long leg braces. The starting position for both gaits is to have the crutches comfortably at the patient's side with the patient standing in a normal stance with feet together. The swing-to is used by patients who not only have weakened leg muscles but also have very poor abdominal and back muscles. which make it more difficult to regain and maintain balance once they have moved forward. In that gait, the patient moves both crutches forward, lifts the body by transfering the weight to the crutches, and swings up to the crutches. The patient then straightens and stabilizes the body before once more placing the crutches forward. The swing-through gait is utilized by patients who are better able to stabilize themselves. The patient places the crutches forward, swings the body (with both feet together) past the crutches, and then straightens and balances the body before moving the crutches forward again.

MANEUVERING TECHNIQUES

Going Down and Up Stairs

To go downstairs, the patient should begin by going to the forward edge of the top step. The patient should then advance the crutches and the weaker or affected leg to the next lower step by tilting the pelvis and bending the unaffected leg at the knee and hip. Once the crutches are safely placed on the lower step, the stronger or unaffected leg is advanced. In that way, the stronger or unaffected leg and the arms share the work of lowering the body's weight.

To go upstairs, the patient should walk forward to about a half-step width away from the lowest step. The patient should then place the weight on the hands and lift the stronger or unaffected leg up to the next step. Once that foot is safely on the next step, the affected or weaker leg and crutches are advanced. The arms need to be strong to support the patient's body weight during the move.

There are a number of memory devices that can be used to help the patient remember which foot goes first. Two of them are "strong leg goes up first and comes down last," and "up with the good and down with the bad."

Getting In and Out of a Chair

Patients using crutches need to know how to get into and out of a chair, on and off the toilet, and in and out of a car. The technique used is essentially the same. The patient using crutches should walk up to the chair, turn using the crutches, and back up until the back of the unaffected leg touches the seat. The patient should then grip both crutches in one hand by the hand pieces, using the hand on the unaffected side, bend at the waist, place the affected side's hand on the seat, move the affected leg forward, and lower onto the seat gradually. It is safer to place the crutches on the unaffected side because there is less chance that a casted, braced, or weakened leg will knock the crutches away while the patient is trying to sit. Holding the crutches on the unaffected side also assures the patient of ample room to sit, as contact is made with the seat with both the unaffected leg and the hand on the affected side.

To rise from the seat, the patient should reverse the procedure, pushing off against the seat with the hand on the affected side, and pulling upward with the other hand, which is holding both crutches. It is also acceptable for the patient to push off while grasping the hand piece of a crutch in each hand.

AMBULATION WITH A CANE

A cane is used to help the patient walk with greater balance and support and to relieve pressure on weight-bearing joints. To fit the patient for a cane, flex the patient's elbow at a 25- to 30-degree angle and adjust the cane so that the handle is approximately level with the greater trochanter. An adjustable aluminum cane fitted with a rubber suction tip for traction gives optimum stability and helps the patient walk with greater speed and less fatigue.

Cane–Foot Sequence

1. Hold the cane fairly close to the body on the unaffected side.
2. Advance the cane with the affected leg.

The patient can use two canes with the four-point and two-point gaits discussed under crutch gaits.

To Go Up and Down Stairs

1. Step up with the unaffected leg.
2. Then advance the cane and the affected leg.
3. Reverse this procedure for descending steps ("up with the good and down with the bad").

INDEX

Letters after page numbers represent figures (*f*) and tables (*t*).